ALLERGY

Commissioning Editor: Sue Hodgson
Development Editor: Sharon Nash
Project Manager: Sukanthi Sukumar
Designer: Kirsteen Wright
Illustration Manager: Merlyn Harvey
Illustrators: Robert Britton (4e), Martin Woodward (3e)
Marketing Manager(s) (UK/USA): Gaynor Jones/Helena Mutak

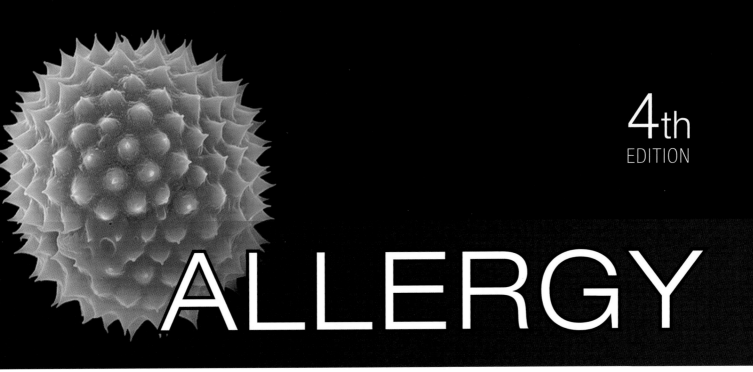

4th EDITION

ALLERGY

Stephen T Holgate CBE BSc MB BS
MD DSc CSci FRCP FRCP(Edin) FRCPath
FSB FIBMS FMedSci

MRC Clinical Professor of
Immunopharmacology
School of Medicine
Infection, Inflammation and Immunity Division
University of Southampton
Southampton General Hospital
Southampton, UK

Martin K Church MPharm PhD DSc
FAAAAI

Professor of Immunopharmacology
Department of Dermatology and Allergy
Allergy Centre Charitè
Charitè Universitätsmedizin
Berlin, Germany
Emeritus Professor of Immunopharmacology
University of Southampton
Southampton, UK

David H Broide MB ChB
Professor of Medicine
University of California, San Diego
La Jolla, CA, USA

Fernando D Martinez MD
Regents' Professor
Director, BIO5 Institute
Director, Arizona Respiratory Center
Swift-McNear Professor of Pediatrics
The University of Arizona
Tucson, AZ, USA

ELSEVIER
SAUNDERS   Edinburgh   London   New York   Oxford   Philadelphia   St Louis   Sydney   Toronto   2012

ELSEVIER
SAUNDERS

SAUNDERS an imprint of Elsevier Limited
© 2012, Elsevier Limited. All rights reserved.

First edition 1993
Second edition 2001
Third edition 2006

The right of Stephen T. Holgate, Martin K. Church, David H. Broide, and Fernando D. Martinez to be identified as authors of this work has been asserted by them in accordance with the Copyright, Designs and Patents Act 1988.

Notices
Knowledge and best practice in this field are constantly changing. As new research and experience broaden our understanding, changes in research methods, professional practices, or medical treatment may become necessary.
Practitioners and researchers must always rely on their own experience and knowledge in evaluating and using any information, methods, compounds, or experiments described herein. In using such information or methods they should be mindful of their own safety and the safety of others, including parties for whom they have a professional responsibility.
With respect to any drug or pharmaceutical products identified, readers are advised to check the most current information provided (i) on procedures featured or (ii) by the manufacturer of each product to be administered, to verify the recommended dose or formula, the method and duration of administration, and contraindications. It is the responsibility of practitioners, relying on their own experience and knowledge of their patients, to make diagnoses, to determine dosages and the best treatment for each individual patient, and to take all appropriate safety precautions.
To the fullest extent of the law, neither the Publisher nor the authors, contributors, or editors, assume any liability for any injury and/or damage to persons or property as a matter of products liability, negligence or otherwise, or from any use or operation of any methods, products, instructions, or ideas contained in the material herein.

British Library Cataloguing in Publication Data

Allergy. – 4th ed.
  1. Allergy.
  I. Holgate, S. T.
  616.9'7–dc22

ISBN-13: 9780723436584

Printed in China
Last digit is the print number: 9   8   7   6   5   4   3   2   1

preface

In 1992, we published the first edition of an entirely new text on allergic diseases and their mechanisms based on specifically designed, clear and informative diagrams. This allowed us to produce a text that found a unique niche between the more heavily referenced books and the more superficial guides. In this edition, the reader was introduced to the individual cells and mediators that participate in the allergic response and this information was then built on to describe the histopathological features, diagnoses and treatment of allergic responses occurring in all major organs.

When preparing the second edition, we took note of the feedback of many clinicians who asked us if we could put primary emphasis on the clinical manifestations of allergy and augment this with a solid scientific background. We kept this format for the third edition. This format has appeared to be very successful with our readers, so much so that it was awarded 'Book of the Year' prize by the British Medical Association.

Now, 19 years after the original *Allergy* we are at the fourth edition with two new editors. Dr Lawrence Lichtenstein has retired and we welcome Dr David Broide and Dr Fernando Martinez to the editorial team. We have also updated the format slightly by emphasising the clinical aspects while reducing the cellular science to a single chapter introducing mechanisms of allergic disease. Furthermore, two new chapters have been added, one on eosinophilia, including eosinophilic oesophagitis and the other on systemic mastocytosis.

One thing that has not changed is our policy of inviting international authorities, often two or more authors from different countries, to work together to produce their sections. Although this approach is not without its logistical problems, we believe it has produced a more authoritative text and we thank all the authors for their forbearance. Indeed, we owe a great debt of gratitude to the many experts who have contributed such informative chapters.

As readers, we hope that you will appreciate the fourth edition of *Allergy* and that you find its content enjoyable and educative to read. As we requested in the first three editions, please give us your feedback on the book so that we can refine it even further in the future.

STH, MKC, DHB, FDM 2012

list of contributors

Mitsuru Adachi MD PhD
Professor of Medicine
Division of Allergology and Respiratory
Medicine
School of Medicine
Showa University
Tokyo, Japan

Sarah Austin MS
Scientific Operations Manager
Laboratory of Allergic Diseases
National Institute of Allergy and Infectious
Diseases
National Institutes of Health
Bethesda, MD
USA

Leonard Bielory MD
Director
STARx Allergy and Asthma Research
Center
Springfield, NJ
Rutgers University
Center for Environmental Prediction
New Brunswick, NJ
Professor
Medicine, Pediatrics, Ophthalmology and
Visual Sciences
New Jersey Medical School
Newark, NJ
USA

Stephan C Bischoff MD
Professor of Medicine
Department of Clinical Nutrition and
Prevention
University of Hohenheim
Stuttgart, Germany

Attilio L Boner MD
Professor of Pediatrics
Pediatric Department
University of Verona
Verona, Italy

Larry Borish MD
Professor of Medicine
Asthma and Allergic Disease Center
University of Virginia
Charlottesville, VA
USA

Piera Boschetto MD PhD
Associate Professor of Occupational
Medicine
Department of Clinical and Experimental
Medicine
University of Ferrara
Ferrara, Italy

David H Broide MB ChB
Professor of Medicine
University of California, San Diego
La Jolla, CA
USA

William W Busse MD
Professor of Medicine
Allergy, Pulmonary and Critical Care
Medicine
Department of Medicine
University of Wisconsin School of
Medicine and Public Health
Madison, WI
USA

Virginia L Calder PhD
Senior Lecturer in Immunology
Department of Genetics
UCL Institute of Ophthalmology
London, UK

Thomas B Casale MD
Professor of Medicine
Chief, Division of Allergy/Immunology
Creighton University
Omaha, NE
USA

**Martin K Church MPharm PhD DSc
FAAAAI**
Professor of Immunopharmacology
Department of Dermatology and Allergy
Allergy Centre Charitè
Charitè Universitätsmedizin
Berlin, Germany
Emeritus Professor of
Immunopharmacology
University of Southampton
Southampton, UK

Jonathan Corren MD
Associate Clinical Professor of Medicine
Division of Pulmonary and Critical Care
Medicine
Section of Clinical Immunology and Allergy
University of California
Los Angeles, CA
USA

Peter S Creticos MD
Associate Professor of Medicine
Medical Director
Asthma and Allergic Diseases
Division of Allergy and Clinical Immunology
Johns Hopkins University
Baltimore, MD
USA

Adnan Custovic DM MD PhD FRCP
Professor of Allergy
Head, Respiratory Research Group
University of Manchester
Education and Research Centre
University Hospital of South Manchester
Manchester, UK

Charles W DeBrosse MD MS
Allergy and Immunology Fellow
Cincinnati Children's Hospital Medical
Center
Cincinnati, OH
USA

Pascal Demoly MD PhD
Professor and Head
Allergy Department
Maladies Respiratoires – Hôpital Arnaud
de Villeneuve
University Hospital of Montpellier
Montpellier, France

Stephen R Durham MA MD FRCP
Professor of Allergy and Respiratory
Medicine
Head, Allergy and Clinical Immunology
National Heart and Lung Institute
Imperial College and Royal Brompton
Hospital
London, UK

Mark S Dykewicz MD
Professor of Internal Medicine
Director, Allergy and Immunology
Section on Pulmonary, Critical Care,
Allergy and Immunologic Diseases
Allergy and Immunology Fellowship
Program Director
Wake Forest University School of Medicine
Center for Human Genomics and
Personalized Medicine Research
Winston-Salem, NC
USA

Pamela W Ewan CBE FRCP FRCPath
Consultant Allergist and Associate Lecturer
Head, Allergy Department
Cambridge University Hospitals
National Health Service Foundation Trust
Cambridge, UK

Clive EH Grattan MA MD FRCP
Consultant Dermatologist
Dermatology Centre
Norfolk and Norwich University Hospital
Norwich, UK

Rebecca S Gruchalla MD PhD
Professor of Internal Medicine and
Pediatrics
Section Chief, Division of Allergy and
Immunology
UT Southwestern Medical Center
Dallas, TX
USA

**Melanie Hingorani MA MBBS
FRCOphth MD**
Consultant Ophthalmologist
Ophthalmology Department
Hinchingbrooke Hospital
Huntingdon, Cambridgeshire
Richard Desmond Children's Eye Centre
Moorfields Eye Hospital
London, UK

**Stephen T Holgate CBE BSc MB BS
MD DSc CSci FRCP FRCP(Edin)
FRCPath FSB FIBMS FMedSci**
MRC Clinical Professor of
Immunopharmacology
School of Medicine
Infection, Inflammation and Immunity
Division
University of Southampton
Southampton General Hospital
Southampton, UK

John W Holloway PhD
Professor of Allergy and Respiratory
Genetics, Human Development & Health
Faculty of Medicine
University of Southampton
Southampton, UK

Patrick G Holt DSc FRCPath FAA
Head, Division of Cell Biology
Telethon Institute for Child Health
Research and Centre for Child Health
Research
University of Western Australia
Perth, WA, Australia

Alexander Kapp MD PhD
Professor of Dermatology and Allergy
Chairman and Director
Department of Dermatology and Allergy
Hannover Medical School
Hannover, Germany

Phil Lieberman MD
Clinical Professor of Medicine and
Pediatrics
University of Tennessee College of
Medicine
Memphis, TN
USA

**Susan Lightman PhD FRCP
FRCOphth FMedSci**
Professor of Clinical Ophthalmology
UCL/Institute of Ophthalmology
Moorfields Eye Hospital
London, UK

Martha Ludwig PhD
Associate Professor
School of Biomedical, Biomolecular and
Chemical Sciences
The University of Western Australia
Perth, WA, Australia

Piero Maestrelli MD
Professor of Occupational Medicine
Department of Environmental Medicine
and Public Health
University of Padova
Padova, Italy

Hans-Jorgen Malling MD DMSci
Associate Professor
Allergy Clinic
Gentofte University Hospital
Copenhagen, Denmark

Fernando D Martinez MD
Regents' Professor
Director, BIO5 Institute
Director, Arizona Respiratory Center
Swift-McNear Professor of Pediatrics
The University of Arizona
Tucson, AZ
USA

Marcus Maurer MD
Professor of Dermatology and Allergy
Director of Research
Department of Dermatology and Allergy
Allergie-Centrum-Charité/ECARF
Charité – Universitätsmedizin Berlin
Berlin, Germany

Dean D Metcalfe MD
Chief, Laboratory of Allergic Diseases
National Institute of Allergy and Infectious
Diseases
National Institutes of Health
Bethesda, MD
USA

Dean J Naisbitt PhD
Senior Lecturer
MRC Centre for Drug Safety Science
Department of Pharmacology
University of Liverpool
Liverpool, UK

Hans Oettgen MD PhD
Associate Chief
Division of Immunology
Children's Hospital
Associate Professor of Pediatrics
Harvard Medical School
Boston, MA
USA

B Kevin Park PhD
Professor, Translational Medicine
MRC Centre for Drug Safety Science
Department of Pharmacology
University of Liverpool
Liverpool, UK

David B Peden MD MS
Professor of Pediatrics, Medicine and
Microbiology/Immunology
Chief, Division of Pediatric Allergy,
Immunology, Rheumatology and Infectious
Diseases
Director, Center for Environmental
Medicine, Asthma and Lung Biology
Deputy Director for Child Health,
NC Translational & Clinical Sciences
Institute (CTSA) School of Medicine
The University of North Carolina at Chapel
Hill
Chapel Hill, NC
USA

R Stokes Peebles MD
Professor of Medicine
Division of Allergy, Pulmonary, and Critical
Care Medicine
Vanderbilt University School of Medicine
Nashville, TN
USA

Thomas AE Platts-Mills MD PhD FRS
Department of Medicine
Division of Allergy and Immunology
University of Virginia
Charlottesville, VA
USA

**Susan Prescott BMedSci(Hons)
MBBS PhD FRACP**
Winthrop Professor
School of Paediatrics and Child Health
University of Western Australia
Paediatric Allergist and Immunologist
Princess Margaret Hospital for Children
Perth, WA, Australia

Marc E Rothenberg MD PhD
Professor of Pediatrics
Director, Division of Allergy and
Immunology
Director, Cincinnati Center for Eosinophilic
Disorders
Cincinnati Children's Hospital Medical
Center
University of Cincinnati College of
Medicine
Cincinnati, OH
USA

Hugh A Sampson MD
Dean for Translational Biomedical
Sciences
Kurt Hirschhorn Professor of Pediatrics
Department of Pediatrics and Immunology
The Mount Sinai School of Medicine
The Jaffe Food Allergy Institute
New York, NY
USA

Glenis K Scadding MA MD FRCP
Hon. Consultant Allergist and Rhinologist
Royal National Throat, Nose and Ear
Hospital
London, UK

Peter D Sly MBBS MD DSc FRACP
Senior Clinical Research Fellow
Queensland Children's Medical Research
Institute
University of Queensland
Brisbane, Australia

Geoffrey A Stewart PhD
Winthrop Professor
School of Biomedical, Biomolecular and
Chemical Sciences
The University of Western Australia
Perth, WA, Australia

**Philip J Thompson MBBS FRACP
MRACMA FCCP**
Director, Lung Institute of Western
Australia Inc
Winthrop Professor of Respiratory
Medicine
Director, Centre for Asthma, Allergy and
Respiratory Research
University of Western Australia
Clinical Professor
Curtin University
Consultant Respiratory Physician
Sir Charles Gairdner Hospital
Western Australia
Perth, WA, Australia

Peter Valent MD
Associate Professor of Internal Medicine
Division of Hematology and
Hemostaseology
Department of Internal Medicine I and
Ludwig Boltzmann Cluster Oncology
Medical University of Vienna
Vienna, Austria

Erika von Mutius MD MSc
Professor of Pediatrics
Dr. von Haunersche Children's Hospital
Ludwig Maximilian University
Munich, Germany

**John O Warner MD FRCP FRCPCH
FMedSci**
Professor of Paediatrics and
Head of Department
Imperial College
Honorary Consultant Paediatrician
Imperial College Healthcare NHS Trust
London, UK

Thomas Werfel MD
Professor of Medicine
Department of Dermatology and
Allergology
Hannover Medical School
Hannover, Germany

Bruce L Zuraw MD
Professor of Medicine
University of California, San Diego and
San Diego VA Healthcare System
La Jolla, CA
USA

1

Introduction to mechanisms of allergic disease

Hans Oettgen and David H Broide

DEFINITION

An improved understanding of the mechanisms mediating allergic inflammation provides a rationale for the development of targeted therapies to prevent and treat allergic disorders.

Introduction to the immune response

The immune system has evolved to play a pivotal role in host defence against infection as without a functioning immune system individuals would be predisposed to develop a variety of infections from viruses, bacteria, fungi, protozoa, and multicellular parasites. The key components of a well-functioning immune system include the ability to generate both innate and adaptive immune responses (Fig. 1.1). The innate immune system comprises cellular elements that are both resident in tissues (i.e. epithelium, macrophages, mast cells) for a rapid response and circulating leukocytes that are recruited from the blood stream (neutrophils, eosinophils, basophils, mononuclear cells, natural killer (NK) cells, and NK T cells). In addition to the cellular response the innate immune system has humoral elements (complement, antimicrobial peptides, mannose-binding lectin), which provides a mechanism for an immediate response to infection that is not antigen specific and does not have immunological memory. In contrast, the adaptive immune response generated by its component T and B cells is slower to respond to infections (taking days) but has the advantage of exhibiting antigen specificity and immunological memory. A malfunctioning immune system may lead not only to immunodeficiency with recurrent infections, but also to autoimmunity and allergic diseases. In this chapter, we focus on the cellular and molecular mechanisms through which an aberrant immune response to low levels of otherwise innocuous and ubiquitous environmental exposures such as airborne grass pollens or ingested foods may trigger a range of allergic responses from chronic symptoms affecting quality of life to acute severe allergic reactions that are life threatening.

Overview of the allergic immune response

Allergic diseases such as allergic rhinitis, asthma, and food allergy are characterized by the ability to make an IgE antibody response to an environmental allergen. There is both a strong genetic (see Ch. 2) as well as environmental contribution to the development of allergic disease (see Chs 3 and 4). Immunoglobulin E (IgE)-mediated allergic responses most frequently occur on mucosal (nose, conjunctiva, airway, gastrointestinal tract) or skin surfaces as these anatomical sites contain high levels of mast cells to which IgE is affixed.

© 2012 Elsevier Ltd
DOI: 10.1016/B978-0-7234-3658-4.00005-6

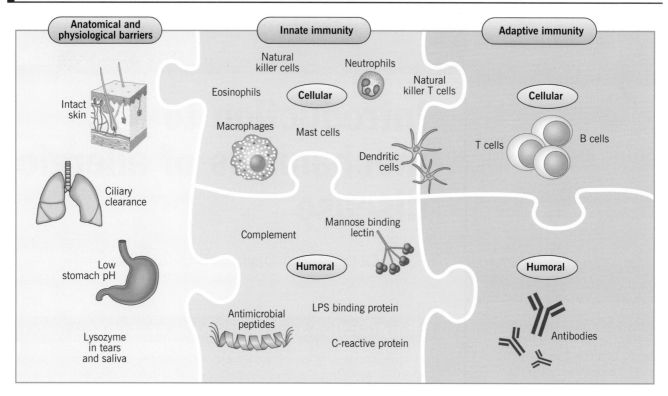

Fig. 1.1 Innate and adaptive immune response. The human microbial defence system can be simplistically viewed as consisting of three levels: (1) anatomical and physiological barriers; (2) innate immunity; and (3) adaptive immunity. In common with many classification systems, some elements are difficult to categorize. For example, NK T cells and dendritic cells could be classified as being on the cusp of innate and adaptive immunity rather than being firmly in one camp. (Adapted from: Figure 2 in Turvey SE, Broide DH. J Allergy Clin Immunol. 2010; 125:S24–32.)

Initial exposure of a genetically predisposed individual to low levels of allergens such as grass pollens results in uptake of the pollen allergen by antigen-presenting cells (APCs), intracellular digestion of the allergen into peptide fragments, and display of the allergen peptide fragments in an human leukocyte antigen (HLA) groove on the APC surface (Fig. 1.2). When circulating T cells (expressing an antigen cell surface receptor specific for the allergen peptide) interact with the APC, the interaction activates the T cell to express cytokines characterized by a helper T cell type 2 (Th2) cytokine profile (Fig. 1.3). Th2 cytokines (Table 1.1) play an important role in inducing B cells to switch class and express IgE (e.g. interleukin-4, IL-4), induce eosinophil proliferation in the bone marrow (i.e. induced by IL-5), and up-regulate adhesion molecules on blood vessels to promote tissue infiltration of circulating inflammatory cells associated with allergic inflammation such as eosinophils and basophils. The allergen specific IgE (induced by initial exposure to allergen) binds to high-affinity IgE receptors on mast cells and basophils. These IgE sensitized mast cells upon re-exposure to specific allergen are activated to release histamine and many other proinflammatory mediators that contribute to the allergic inflammatory response (Fig. 1.4). Although this induction of a Th2 response is characteristic of allergic inflammation, it is increasingly evident that additional immune and inflammatory responses contribute to allergic inflammation. In this chapter we explore these mechanisms in greater detail to gain insight into the cellular and molecular events that contribute to the development of the allergic inflammatory response. Such important insights provide the rationale for the development of novel therapies for the targeted treatment of allergic disease, as well as the potential development of biomarkers to assess allergic disease severity, progression, or response to therapy.

Central role of IgE and mast cells

Atopy, the tendency to produce IgE antibodies specific for environmental allergens, affects 30–40% of the population of developed nations. The production of IgE results in a range of hypersensitivity disorders including, anaphylaxis, allergic rhinitis, atopic dermatitis and asthma. IgE antibodies, IgE receptors, and several lineages of effector cells activated by IgE have persisted through vertebrate evolution implicating this antibody isotype in important physiological immune functions. IgE probably serves to eliminate helminthic parasites during primary infection and in parasite endemic regions to protect previously

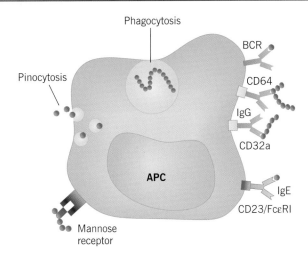

Fig. 1.2 Antigen uptake. Antigens may be taken up by antigen-presenting cells through several different mechanisms including: (i) phagocytosis – performed by phagocytes such as monocytes and macrophages, (ii) B-cell receptor (BCR) – very efficient performed by antigen-specific B cells only, (iii) FcγR1 receptors (CD64) expressed by monocytes and macrophages; FcγR2a receptors (CD32a) expressed by many different antigen-presenting cells (APCs), (iv) FcεRI receptors expressed by dendritic cells, and monocytes, and FcεRII (CD23) expressed by dendritic cells, macrophages, and B cells; especially important in allergy; CD23 can be induced on dendritic cells and monocytes by IL-4, (v) mannose receptors – very efficient and allow APCs (mostly dendritic cells) to bind sugar (mannose) residues of glycosylated proteins, (vi) pinocytosis – not efficient as large quantities of antigen are needed; theoretically performed by all types of APC.

Table 1.1 Signature cytokine production patterns of Th1 vs Th2 cells

Th1	Th2
IFN-γ	IL-4
	IL-5
Th1 and Th2	IL-9
IL-2	IL-13
IL-3	IL-25
GM-CSF	IL-31
	IL-33

exposed individuals against re-infection. In current practice however, the clinically relevant function of IgE is to trigger mast cells and basophils following allergen encounter leading to the release of preformed and newly synthesized mediators of immediate hypersensitivity and expression of acute allergic symptoms. In addition, the production of immune-modulating and proinflammatory cytokines by these activated effector cells sets into motion an array of processes leading ultimately to the persistent allergic tissue inflammation experienced by individuals with chronic allergies. In recent years, IgE blockade using the monoclonal antibody omalizumab has been introduced as an important new therapeutic option. As IgE plays a central role in allergic inflammation, it is important to understand the structural properties of IgE antibodies, the organization of the immunoglobulin heavy chain locus and the cellular and molecular events regulating IgE production by B cells.

IgE structure

Hardly a day passes when a practising allergist does not employ skin testing or in vitro diagnostic techniques to detect IgE antibodies. Establishing the presence of IgE specific for environmental aeroallergens, food antigens, and insect venom components is the cornerstone of allergic diagnosis. In this light it may seem surprising from a historical perspective that the IgE antibody isotype was the last one identified, discovered only in the 1960s, decades after IgM, IgD, IgG, and IgA. Biochemical characterization of the *reaginic* fraction of serum, the activity capable of passively transferring cutaneous sensitivity from an allergic donor to the skin of a non-allergic recipient (Prausnitz–Küstner reaction), along with the serological classification of some unusual myeloma antibodies established the existence of a novel isotype that was heat labile, failed to fix complement, did not cross the placenta and did not give antibody : antigen precipitates (precipitin lines) in immunodiffusion assays. This apparently novel isotype resided in the γ-globulin fraction of serum and was identified as IgE by investigators in Japan, Sweden, and England.

IgE remained elusive for so long primarily because of its very low plasma concentrations and short half-life compared with other immunoglobulin isotypes. Whereas IgG antibodies are typically present at levels >500 mg/dL, IgE normally circulates at logs lower concentration even in atopic individuals with a normal range of <0.2 mg/dL. Although its presence in the circulation is transient, with a half-life of only about 2 days, considerably shorter than that of IgG (3 weeks), IgE is quite stable when bound to tissue mast cells where it may persist for months. This has important clinical implications. Transplantation of solid organs harboring IgE-coated mast cells from donors with allergy to food or drugs can confer sensitivity for systemic anaphylaxis to previously allergen-tolerant recipients.

IgE shares its basic structural features with other immunoglobulin isotypes. It consists of two heavy chains (the ε-chains) and two light chains (κ or λ) assembled into a tetrameric structure (Fig. 1.5). The heavy chains are composed of five immunoglobulin domains, a shared structural motif of many proteins with immunological

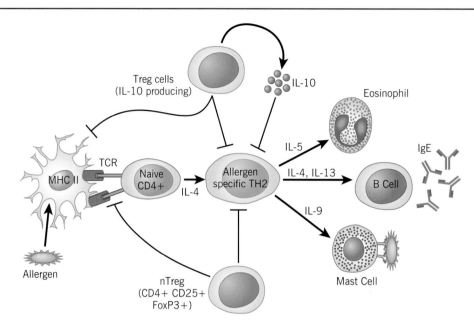

Fig. 1.3 Allergen-induced immune and inflammatory responses. Allergen challenge induces activation of Th2 cells that express cytokines including IL-4, which induces class switching to IgE, and IL-5, which induces eosinophil proliferation. IL-9 induces mucus and mast cell proliferation, while IL-13 induces class switching to IgE and airway hyperreactivity. Treg cells (natural and adaptive) have the ability to inhibit Th2 responses. Theoretically, a deficiency of Treg function in allergic inflammation could promote continued Th2-mediated inflammation. TCR, T-cell receptor; nTreg, natural T-regulatory cell. (Adapted from: Figure 2 in Broide DH. J Allergy Clin Immunol 2008; 121:560–572.)

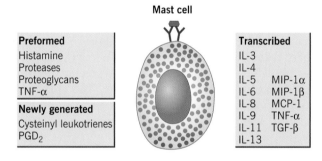

Fig. 1.4 Mast cell. Upon cross-linking of IgE affixed to FcεRI by allergen, mast cells immediately release preformed mediators from storage in secretory granules via exocytosis. In addition, leukotrienes and PGD_2 are generated from arachidonic acid, and cytokine and chemokine transcription is induced.

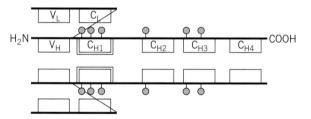

Fig. 1.5 Structure of IgE. Immunoglobulin E (IgE) consists of two heavy chains, each with a total of five immunoglobulin domains, and two light chains, containing two immunoglobulin domains each. Each immunoglobulin domain contains an intrachain disulphide bond. Intrachain disulphide bonds covalently attach the heavy and light chains to form a tetrameric structure. Sites of glycosylation are indicated with circles. Antigen specificity is conferred by the variable (V_H and V_L) domains. The biological functions of IgE are mediated by interaction with its receptors (FcεRI and CD23) via amino acids in the C_{H2} and C_{H3} domains.

function characterized by a stretch of approximately 100 amino acids with a series of antiparallel β-strands assembled into a sandwich of β-sheets which forms an immunoglobulin fold. Disulphide bonds between conserved cysteine residues at each end of the domain stabilize the structure. Four of the ε-chain domains are constant-region domains, encoded by the Cε exons ($C_{ε1-4}$) in the IgH locus. Thus IgE heavy chains have one more constant domain than do IgG γ-chains, which have only three. The N-terminal variable domain of the ε-heavy chain contains complementarity-determining sequences encoded by the VDJ cassette at the 5′ end of the IgH

locus and is responsible for specific antigen binding. In addition to the secreted form of IgE, whose heavy chains are composed of one variable and four constant domains, IgE-committed B cells also express a transmembrane form of the antibody, generated by alternative mRNA splicing and containing an additional C-terminal M-domain responsible for anchoring the antibody in the plasma membrane. ε-heavy chains are encoded by a gene (Fig. 1.6) assembled by somatic genomic recombination only in B cells that have differentiated to produce IgE.

B-cell development and differentiation: generation of antibody diversity

IgE antibodies are produced by B cells and their specialized antibody-producing progeny, plasma cells. The generation of B cells producing allergen-specific IgE has two major phases: an antigen-independent phase of B-cell development occurring in the bone marrow, which provides a systemic pool of B cells with a wide range of antigen specificities, followed by an antigen- and T-cell-dependent process in the periphery, during which allergen-responsive B-cell clones expand and differentiate to produce antibodies of the IgE isotype.

During B-cell development in the bone marrow, common lymphoid progenitors undergo a complex process of regulated gene expression and somatic gene rearrangements that ultimately give rise to mature B cells of fixed antigenic specificity (Fig. 1.7). Commitment to the B-cell lineage is first evidenced by the expression of B-cell surface markers, including CD19, on pro-B cells. These do not yet produce any immunoglobulin chains. An ordered series of DNA rearrangements is set into motion in these precursors in which V, D, and J elements at the 5′ end of the IgH locus (Fig. 1.8) are assembled into a VDJ cassette that constitutes a complete V_H exon encoding the variable region domain of the Ig heavy chain (Fig. 1.9). This is a stochastic process in which one of many V, D, and J elements separately encoded in the germline IgH locus is randomly selected for insertion into the evolving VDJ cassette, leading to combinatorial diversity of V_H domains. Additional diversity is provided by imprecise joining of the V–D–J borders (junctional diversity) and by the insertion of extra nucleotides at these joints. Assembling the V_H exon in this manner gives rise to an enormous spectrum of possible structures and resultant array of antigenic specificities, a range of diversity that could not be achieved by separately encoding each potential sequence in the germline. Completion of

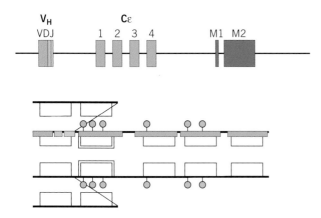

Fig. 1.6 IgE gene structure. The ε-heavy chain of IgE is located in the IgH (Ig heavy chain) locus. A VDJ cassette encodes the V_H domain, while exons Cε 1–4 encode the constant region domains. Additional M exons encode transmembrane sequences in alternatively spliced transcripts for the membrane-associated form of IgE.

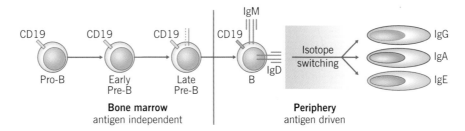

Fig. 1.7 B-cell development. B cells arise in the bone marrow from pluripotent progenitors in an antigen-independent process marked by sequential expression of B-cell lineage markers (including CD19), μ-heavy chain and, finally intact cell surface IgM. Expression of membrane IgM defines a B cell. Antigen-driven processes outside the bone marrow can drive expansion of antigen-specific B-cell clones and, in the setting of T-cell help, lead to switching of immunoglobulin isotypes to confer antibody effector functions appropriate for the immune challenge.

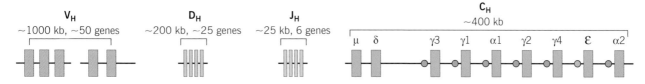

Fig. 1.8 Immunoglobulin heavy chain (IgH) locus. The genetic elements encoding variable and constant sequences in immunoglobulins are encoded in a very large locus (>1000 kb) on chromosome 14. A major portion of IgH contains the V_H genes, which, together with D_H and J_H sequences, encode the variable domains of immunoglobulin heavy chains. Heavy chain constant region domains are encoded in clusters of C_H exons corresponding to each isotype. The exons encoding each isotype are preceded by switch regions (indicated as circles), which mediate isotype switch recombination.

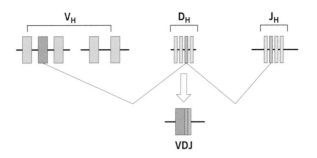

Fig. 1.9 V–D–J recombination. Assembly of a highly diverse repertoire of heavy chain variable regions is mediated by a process of somatic DNA rearrangement occuring during B-cell development in the bone marrow. V_H, D_H, and J_H segments are randomly selected and annealed. Combinatorial diversity is provided by the random assortment of V, D, and J elements while additional variability is introduced by imprecision in joining (junctional diversity) and by the introduction of extra junctional nucleotides. This random and plastic process of somatic DNA rearrangment leads to a far greater variety of V_H sequences than could ever be separately encoded in the germline genome.

recombination results in the assembly of an intact V_H exon just upstream of the Cμ exons. This constitutes a complete transcriptional unit that gives rise to mRNA encoding μ heavy chains (early pre-B cell). Although isolated μ heavy chains cannot be expressed at the surface in the absence of immunoglobulin light chains, they can be detected in the cytosol and can be assembled with so-called surrogate light chains (λ5 and V-pre-B) for surface expression, marking the late pre-B-cell stage. Assembly of this pre-B-cell B-cell receptor (BCR) triggers both a second round of VDJ rearrangements, this time at the light chain loci (κ or λ) and, at the same time, the cessation of further rearrangements at the IgH locus on the chromosome (allelic exclusion), assuring that a B cell can make antibodies only of a single specificity. Completion of the light chain rearrangement process renders a cell competent to produce full IgM (and IgD), completing the process of B-cell development.

Immunoglobulin isotype switching: regulation of the B-cell switch to IgE

The ongoing process of B-cell development is antigen independent and generates a large pool of cells producing antibodies with a highly diverse repertoire of specificities. Upon exiting the bone marrow, each of these B-cell clones is initially committed to the production of IgM and IgD antibodies of defined antibody specificity. In order to generate antibodies of other immunoglobulin isotypes (IgG, IgE, and IgA), B cells must execute a process known as 'immunoglobulin isotype switching'. This is an antigen-driven and T-cell-dependent process

that occurs outside the bone marrow in secondary lymphoid organs and mucosal sites. Isotype switching greatly enhances the range of effector functions of the antibody response by producing antibodies in which the immunoglobulin heavy chains express the same V region (hence retaining the originally committed antibody specificity of the B-cell clone) but now in association with a new set of C_H domains, resulting in production of a new isotype. At the molecular genetic level, immunoglobulin isotype switching is mediated by deletional class switch recombination, a process that, like the VDJ recombination involved in B-cell development, involves irreversible somatic gene rearrangements.

Isotype switching in B cells is tightly regulated by both cytokine signals and the interaction of accessory cell surface molecules. In the case of IgE, the combined effects of signals provided by IL-4 and/or IL-13 secreted by activated T cells and by CD40 ligand (CD154) expressed on the surface of those same helper T cells sets this process in motion. Both the cytokine and accessory signals are necessary to efficiently drive switching. Exposure to these stimuli triggers an ordered cascade of events in the nucleus of the responding B cell in which targeted activation of transcription at specific regions in the IgH locus leads to DNA breaks, followed by repair resulting ultimately in the juxtaposition of the VDJ cassette with the appropriate CH exons.

The immunoglobulin heavy chain (IgH) locus spans over 1000 kb of genome on chromosome 14q32.33, beginning with the V, D, and J exons, followed by the Cμ and Cδ exon clusters and then by groups of CH exons encoding each of the other Ig heavy chain isotypes (see Fig. 1.8). The earliest detectable event in a cytokine-stimulated B cell initiating the process IgE isotype switching is the generation of germline mRNA transcripts. IL-4 and IL-13 trigger STAT-6-driven germline transcription at the Cε locus (Fig. 1.10). In its germline configuration, the Cε locus contains not only the four Cε exons encoding the ε-heavy-chain constant region domains but also an IL-4 responsive promoter (harbouring response elements for STAT-6), an Iε exon, a switch recombination region (Sε), and, downstream of Cε1-4, M sequences encoding the transmembrane form of IgE. Although the transcripts that arise in this process do not encode functional protein (the Iε codon present at the 5′ end of these mRNAs actually contains stop codons), the process of transcription is nevertheless critical for the initiation of switch recombination.

Transcription initiated at the ε-promoter results in recruitment of the enzyme activation-induced cytidine deaminase (AID), which is induced by CD40L signalling, to the ε–locus. AID functions to deaminate deoxycytidine residues in the C-rich Sε region to deoxyuracils. These, in turn, are substrates for another enzyme, uracil DNA-glycosylase (UNG), which acts to introduce single-stranded DNA nicks within Sε. High-density introduction of such nicks can lead to endonuclease-induced double-stranded breaks (DSB) in the DNA. Both UNG and AID are critical for switching. Individuals with mutations in either gene suffer from the autosomal recessive form of immunodeficiency with hyper-IgM, a syndrome in which patients are capable of producing high levels of IgM antibodies but are completely unable to switch to other isotypes resulting in antibody deficiency and susceptibility to recurrent and severe bacterial sinopulmonary infections.

In parallel with the events driven by transcription at the ε-locus, a similar process takes place many kilobases upstream at the Sμ locus, resulting in DSB introduction there. Finally, via the action of components of the DNA repair mechanism (Artemis, DNA ligase IV, ATM), the DSB of these distant sites are annealed leading to both juxtaposition of the VDJ cassette from the 5′ end of the IgH locus with the downstream Cε exons and the simultaneous formation of a switch excision circle (Fig. 1.11). Both ε-germline transcripts and ε-switch excision circles are detectable in the respiratory mucosa of aeroallergen-exposed subjects indicating that this is a locally active process in the airway. B cells that have undergone this process have now irreversibly lost their capacity to

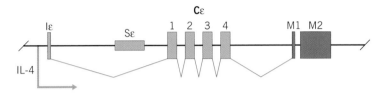

Fig. 1.10 Germline structure of the Cε locus. Prior to class switch recombination, the genetic elements encoding IgE constant region domains reside in the Cε locus near the 3′ end of the IgH locus (see Figure 1.8). The locus has the genetic structure of a fully autonomous gene, including an IL-4 responsive promoter (containing STAT-6-binding elements), Cε 1–4 exons, encoding the heavy chain constant region domains of IgE and M exons, encoding the hydrophobic sequences present in the transmembrane form of IgE in switched B cells. Exposure of B cells to IL-4 or IL-13 leads to activation of transcription and gives rise to ε-germline transcripts (εGLT). These do not encode any functional product. Rather, transcription serves to recruit important elements of the class switch recombination apparatus to the Cε locus. Sε is a C-rich region at which double-stranded DNA breaks are introduced during the process of class switching.

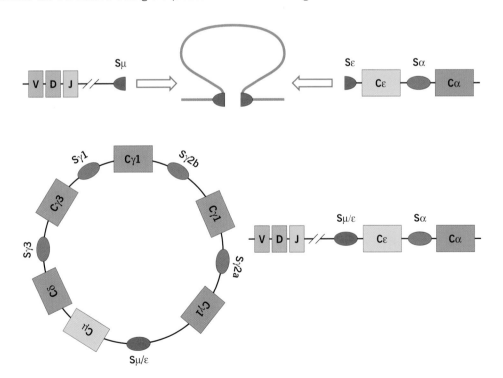

Fig. 1.11 Deletional class switch recombination. In IL-4- and CD40L-stimulated B cells, transcription at the Cε locus targets enzymes that introduce double-stranded breaks (DSB) into the Sε region of the Cε locus in the germline configuration of genomic DNA. DSB are concurrently generated far upstream at the Sμ locus. Annealing of the distant DSB is mediated by cellular DNA repair mechanisms resulting in the generation of two products: a complete ε-heavy-chain gene, with VDJ sequences juxtaposed to Cε exons, and a circular episomal piece of DNA (switch excision circle) which is gradually diluted during subsequent cell divisions of the switched B cell.

produce IgM and the IgG isotypes encoded 5′ of the ε-locus and are committed to the production of IgE antibodies.

T-cell help in IgE class switching

IgE switching, while occurring in B cells, is completely dependent on help provided by CD4+ Th cells. Help is provided both in the form of secreted cytokines and by the interaction of cell surface molecules during direct cell–cell contact (Fig. 1.12). Antigenic peptides displayed on the B-cell surface, bound to major histocompatibility complex (MHC) class II molecules, engage the T-cell receptor of Th cells of the same antigenic specificity (a *cognate* interaction) leading both to cytokine transcription (including IL-4) and to expression of CD40L (CD154), an activation molecule not present on resting Th cells. CD40L in turn engages CD40 back on the B-cell surface, where CD40 is constitutively expressed, providing a stimulus that, in concert with IL-4, induces ε-germline transcription and AID expression, setting into motion the molecular machinery of immunoglobulin class switch recombination to IgE. CD40–CD40L engagement also drives the expression of B7-family accessory molecules on the B-cell surface that bind to receptors on the T-cell surface to amplify the cytokine signal further. This tightly choreographed sequence ensures the delivery of antigen-specific help for class switching.

Targeting transcription and consequent immunoglobulin switching to the ε-locus require that the cytokine signal be in the form of IL-4, which is provided by the Th2 subset of Th cells (Fig. 1.13). Th2 cells, which produce the allergy-associated cytokines, IL-4, IL-5, IL-10, and granulocyte–macrophage colony-stimulating factor (GM-CSF), arise from antigen-stimulated Th0 precursors. Their differentiation is supported by the presence of IL-4 and by the activation of the transcription factor STAT-6 upon IL-4 receptor signalling. STAT-6-induced transcription results in the production of both Th2 cytokines and transcription factors (including GATA-3, Maf, and NIP45), which stabilize the Th2 gene expression profile. As Th2 clones expand through further cell divisions, the early induction of a specific gene expression pattern by STAT-6 signalling and lineage-specific transcription factor expression as well as the silencing of non-Th2 cytokine genes is permanently stabilized by epigenetic mechanisms including DNA demethylation and chromatin remodelling. In addition to their cytokine profile, Th2 cells are characterized by surface expression of CRTH2 (a receptor for prostaglandin D$_2$ (PGD$_2$), a product of activated mast cells) and ST2 (a receptor for the IL-1 family member IL-33, a cytokine that enhances Th2 cytokine responses).

A central paradox in the Th-differentiation paradigm is that Th2 cells require IL-4, which they themselves produce, for their own induction. Similarly, Th1 cells require their own product interferon-γ (IFN-γ) to differentiate. An important and not fully understood question in allergy is 'what is/are the earliest priming sources of IL-4 in tissues during an evolving allergic response?' Several candidates, all effector cells of innate immune functions, have been considered and probably play

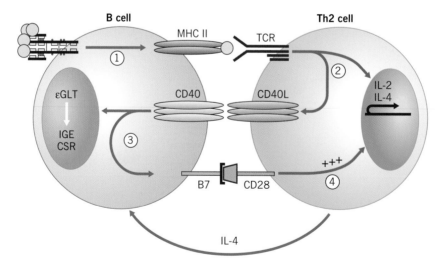

Fig. 1.12 T-cell help in IgE switching. An ordered sequence of T–B cell interactions involving both cell–cell contact and secreted cytokines drives class switching. B cells take up their specific antigen in a process enhanced by the presence of antigen-specific cell surface Ig. Following processing, antigenic peptides are presented by B-cell surface MHC II molecules to the T-cell receptor (TCR) of responding T-cell clones. This interaction drives expression of both CD40L (CD154) on the T-cell surface and cytokines, including IL-4. CD40L binding to CD40 (back on the presenting B cell), along with IL-4, drives germline transcription and activates the expression of components of the pathway of deletional class switching. CD40 activation also drives expression of B7 family costimulatory molecules, which engage receptors on the Th cell and amplify cytokine responses and proliferation. εGLT, ε-germline transcripts; CSR, class switch recombination.

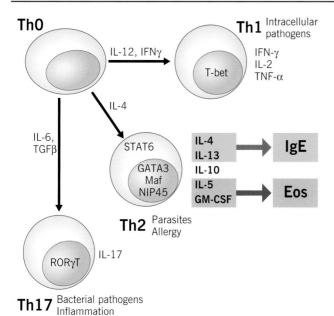

Th0

IL-12, IFNγ

Th1 Intracellular pathogens

T-bet

IFN-γ
IL-2
TNF-α

IL-4

IL-6, TGFβ

STAT6
GATA3
Maf
NIP45

IL-4
IL-13
IL-10
IL-5
GM-CSF

IgE

Eos

Th2 Parasites Allergy

RORγT

IL-17

Th17 Bacterial pathogens Inflammation

Fig. 1.13 T-helper cell subsets. Induction of IgE switching in B cells is dependent on a subset of Th cells (Th2 cells) that produce IL-4. During antigen-driven activation and expansion, uncommitted Th0 antigen-specific T cells can take on one of several T-helper phenotypes. The presence of IL-4 in the environment of responding T cells favours their differentiation into Th2 T cells producing IL-4 and IL-13 (which can drive IgE production as well as other aspects of the allergic response), as well as IL-10, IL-5, and GM-CSF, which are important in eosinophilopoiesis (Eos). Th0 cells exposed to IL-12 and interferon-γ (IFN-γ) differentiate into Th1 cells, which produce IFN-γ, IL-2 and TNF-α and are important in the elimination of intracellular pathogens. The presence of IL-6 and TGF-β drives Th17 induction. IL-17 family cytokines derived from this cell type are important in responses to extracellular bacterial pathogens and in some inflammatory diseases. Each of the Th lineages is characterized by expression of a specific set of transcription factors: T-bet for Th1, GATA-3, Maf and NIP45 for Th2 and RORγT for Th17.

overlapping roles. It is known that activated mast cells produce IL-4. As these cells reside in the skin and mucosal tissues, sites of initial allergen encounters, and since they can be activated by non-specific stimuli, it is possible that mast-cell-derived IL-4 could start the cascade towards Th2 expansion. Recently basophils, which like mast cells express surface FcεRI and are important sources of mediators of immediate hypersensitivity but, unlike mast cells, do not express the surface receptor c-kit, have been identified as Th2 inducers. Basophils constitutively produce large amounts of IL-4 and their depletion in animal models of allergic disease has been shown to result in attenuation of Th2 responses. NK T cells, which express cell surface markers of both NK and T cells, have an invariant Vα14 T-cell receptor specific for glyco- and phospho-lipid antigens presented in the context of MHC class I-like CD1 molecules, also express abundant IL-4 and have been implicated in allergic responses in humans and animal model systems.

IgE receptors

IgE mediates its biological functions via two separate receptors: FcεεRI (the high-affinity receptor) and CD23 (also known as FcεRII or the low-affinity IgE receptor). FcεRI can be expressed in one of two forms: an $\alpha\beta\gamma_2$ tetramer, which is found on mast cells and basophils, and a trimeric form, $\alpha\gamma_2$, lacking the β-chain, present on a number of other cell lineages (Fig. 1.14). The α-chain, which contains two extracellular immunoglobulin domains, is responsible for binding IgE and interacts specifically with sequences in the $C\varepsilon_{2-3}$ region of the ε-heavy chain. This is a very high-affinity interaction with a Kd of 10^{-8} M and, in contrast to Fcγ receptors, FcεRI is constitutively occupied by ligand (IgE) at physiological IgE levels. The β-chain of the receptor, present only in the tetrameric form found on mast cells and basophils, belongs to a tetraspanner family of proteins that cross the cytoplasm four times with both N- and C-termini residing in the cytosol. This β-chain has been shown to have an important amplification function in FcεRI signalling. However the most important chain with respect to signal transduction by the receptor is probably the γ-chain, present as a disulphide-linked dimer. Both γ- and β-chains contain intracellular sequences known as immunoreceptor tyrosine-based activation motifs (ITAMs) that are targets for phosphorylation by receptor-associated tyrosine kinases.

The src-family tyrosine kinase, lyn, is associated with FcεRI and aggregation of FcεRI in the membrane by extracellular receptor-bound IgE with polyvalent allergens favours lyn-mediated phosphorylation of the cytosolic ITAMs. These, in turn, serve as docking sites for the SH2-domain containing tyrosine kinase, syk, which is recruited and, via phosphorylation of linker molecules including LAT, Gads, and SLP-76, leads to the assembly of a signalling complex. Among the signalling molecules recruited to this complex is phospholipase-Cγ (PLCγ), which hydrolyses membrane phosphatidylinositol 4,5-bisphosphate (PtdIns(4,5)P2) to generate inositol 1,4,5-trisphosphate (PIP$_2$) and diacylglycerol (DAG). PIP$_2$ induces the release of Ca^{2+} from endoplasmic reticulum stores, resulting in increased intracellular Ca^{2+}. This rise in Ca^{2+} is a critical trigger for mast cell degranulation. Activation of protein kinase C (PKC) by both DAG and increased Ca^{2+} leads to signalling events driving mast cell gene activation. In addition to the PLCγ pathway, several parallel cascades of signalling events including the stress-activated protein kinase (SAPK) and cytoskeletal (WASP) pathways are set into motion by FcεRI aggregation, all converging to regulate mast cell degranulation and gene expression. Cell surface levels of FcεRI are regulated by

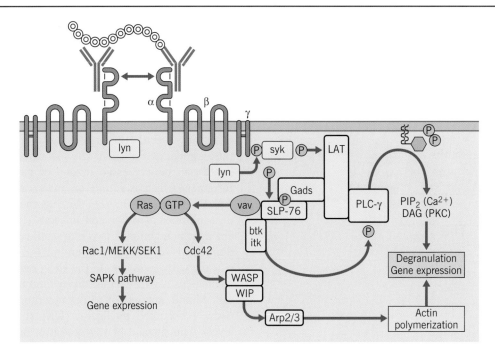

Fig. 1.14 FcεRI structure and signalling. The high-affinity IgE receptor (FcεRI) on mast cells and basophils is a tetrameric structure (αβγ₂). A trimeric form lacking the tetra-membrane spanning β-chain exists on other cell types. The α-chain of the receptor, which contains two extracellular immunoglobulin domains, binds to IgE via residues in the Cε_{2-3} domains. Interaction of FcεRI-bound IgE with polyvalent antigen leads to receptor clustering. In the cytosol, the protein tyrosine kinase, lyn, which is associated with FcεRI, phosphorylates tyrosine residues in immunoreceptor tyrosine-based activation motifs (ITAMs) contained in the β- and γ-chains. These phosphotyrosines serve as docking sites for the SH2-family tyrosine kinase, syk, which the phosphorylates a number of cellular targets leading to the assembly of a signalling complex around the linker proteins, LAT, SLP-76, Gads and others. Recruitment of phospholipase Cγ to this complex and its subsequent activation via phosphorylation, leads to hydrolysis of membrane phosphatidylinositol 4,5-bisphosphate (PtdIns(4,5)P2) to generate inositol 1,4,5-trisphosphate (PIP₂) and diacylglycerol (DAG). PIP₂ triggers increased cytosolic calcium concentrations (via Ca²⁺ release from endoplasmic reticulum stores). Activation of protein kinase C (PKC) by DAG and Ca²⁺ lead to signalling events driving gene expression. Simultaneous activation of Ras-GTP exhange factors by vav lead to activation of the SAPK pathway and cytolskeletal (WASP/WIP) pathways, both of which also drive downstream gene expression.

ambient IgE levels in a positive-feedback loop. As a result, one of the consequences of anti-IgE therapy is a down-regulation of FcεRI levels with a resultant increase in the antigen stimulation threshold required for mast cell activation.

CD23, the so-called low-affinity IgE receptor, has an entirely different structure and exerts biological functions distinct from those of FcεRI. It is a C-type lectin family member and type II membrane protein (N-terminus intracellular) expressed in two alternatively spliced isoforms, CD23a and CD23b, with CD23a present predominantly on B cells and CD23b present on a wide range of cell types including Langerhans cells, follicular dendritic cells, T cells, eosinophils, and gastrointestinal epithelium. CD23 is assembled as a trimeric structure with a long extracellular coiled-coil stalk that is abundantly N glycosylated terminating in three globular head domains that bind to IgE (Fig. 1.15). CD23 is susceptible to cleavage from the cell surface by a variety of proteases including those present in some allergens (like Der p 1 of dust mites) and the metalloprotease ADAM 10. Like

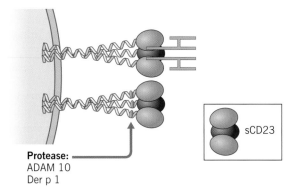

Fig. 1.15 CD23 structure. CD23 is expressed as a type II (amino terminus intracellular) transmembrane protein with globular IgE-binding heads sitting on top of long coiled-coil stalks. The receptor contains a protease-sensitive site that can be targeted by endogenous (ADAM 10) or allergen (including Der p 1) proteases to shed a soluble form of the receptor, sCD23. Occupancy of the receptor by IgE inhibits this process, stabilizing cell surface CD23.

FcεRI, CD23 expression is regulated by ambient IgE levels. Occupancy of the receptor by IgE protects it from protease-mediated shedding.

A variety of functions have been attributed to membrane-bound and soluble CD23. It has been shown that, in the presence of allergen-specific IgE, CD23 can mediate B-cell uptake of allergen/IgE complexes in a process described as IgE-facilitated antigen presentation. CD23 is expression on the luminal surface of gut epithelial cells and, in a similar fashion, may mediate transcytosis of food allergens in individuals with preformed allergen-specific IgE. Engagement of the membrane form of CD23 on B cells appears to suppress IgE production. In contrast, it has been reported that soluble CD23 fragments enhance IgE production – perhaps by preventing the interaction of IgE with transmembrane CD23. Alternatively, CD23 is known to bind the B-cell surface antigen CD21 (the receptor for Epstein–Barr virus, EBV), and the interaction of soluble CD23 with CD21 might exert its IgE-inducing effect.

The immune response in allergy

Dendritic cells

Dendritic cells in the skin and mucous membranes perform a unique sentinel role in that they recognize antigens through their expression of pattern recognition receptors [e.g. Toll-like receptors (TLR), NOD-like receptors, C-type lectin receptors] that recognize motifs on virtually any pathogenic organism, allergen, or antigen. Dendritic cells (DC) can also sense tissue damage through receptors for inflammatory mediators (e.g. damage-associated molecular patterns like uric acid, high-mobility group box 1) allowing them to serve as a bridge between innate and adaptive immune responses. DCs arising from a CD34+ precursor in the bone marrow further differentiate under the influence of various cytokines into subsets including myeloid DC (e.g. Langerhans cell, inflammatory dendritic epidermal cell) and plasmacytoid DC, which express specific markers. A unique feature of DCs is their typical morphology with long dendrite-like extensions that express high levels of MHC to present antigen (Fig. 1.16).

Allergens are taken up by DCs and this plays a very important role in the subsequent immune response. Allergens can also activate DCs through indirect mechanisms involving cells such as epithelium. For example, house dust mite allergen can activate epithelial cells through several epithelial-expressed receptors (TLR, C-type lectin, protease-activated receptor 2), which leads to the release from epithelial cells of innate cytokines [thymic stromal lymphopoietin (TSLP), IL-25, IL-33] that programme dendritic cells to become Th2 inducers.

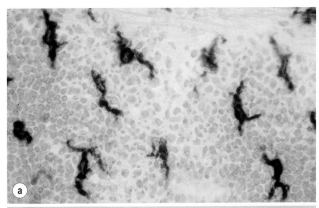

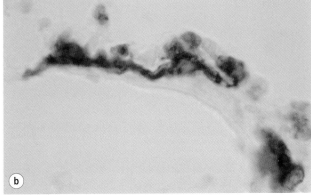

Fig. 1.16 Dendritic cell networks in the respiratory tract. (a) Airway dendritic cells (rat) stained for major histocompatibility complex (MHC) II (normal healthy airway epithelium, tangential section; (b) MHC II+ dendritic cells in rat alveolar septal wall.

Of particular importance to allergic inflammation, dendritic cells express the high-affinity IgE receptor that can mediate allergen presentation to T cells. The FcεRI complex in dendritic cells differs from that described in mast cells and basophils in that it expresses only two (α, γ) of the three (α, β, γ) chains known to be expressed by mast cells and basophils (Fig. 1.17). The presence of allergen-specific IgE bound to the high-affinity IgE receptor on dendritic cells can lead to a 100-fold lowering of the threshold dose for allergen recognition by Th2 cells. Once activated, dendritic cells migrate to regional lymph nodes where they present the processed antigen to T cells. Following allergen challenge, dendritic cells are a prominent source of the Th2-cell-attracting chemokines TARC (CCL17) and MDC (CCL22). Thus, dendritic cells not only present allergen to activate T cells but also play an important role in Th2-cell recruitment to sites of allergic inflammation.

Effector T-cell subsets

Naïve CD4+ cells can differentiate into Th1, Th2, Th9, or Th17 effector cells based on microenvironmental stimuli to which they are exposed in the presence of

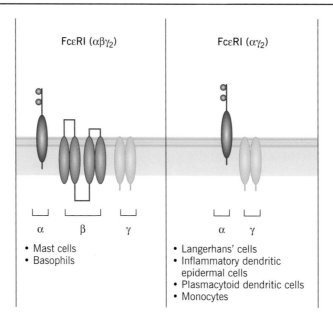

Fig. 1.17 Comparison of high-affinity IgE receptor structure on mast cells and dendritic cells. Mast cells express a four-chain $\alpha\beta\gamma_2$ FcεRI receptor whereas dendritic cells express a three-chain $\alpha\gamma_2$ FcεRI receptor lacking the β chain.

antigen. Each of these T-cell subsets can promote different types of inflammatory response based on the profile of cytokines they express. In particular Th2 cells have a prominent association with allergic inflammation.

Th1 vs Th2 cells

CD4+ T cells were initially identified and classified in the mouse into functionally distinct Th1 or Th2 subsets on the basis of distinct cytokine profiles expressed by each subset (see Table 1.1). Whereas Th1/Th2 polarization is clear-cut in murine models, the situation is not as clear-cut for human T-cell subsets, which can secrete a mixed pattern of cytokines. Thus, Th1 and Th2 cells are not two distinct CD4+ T-cell subsets, but rather represent polarized forms of the highly heterogenous CD4+ Th-cell-mediated immune response. Additional T-cell populations including Th17 and Th9 cells have been identified underscoring the limitation of a pure Th1 vs Th2 paradigm of immune responses (Fig. 1.18). With these caveats in mind, Th1 cells nevertheless play a prominent role in cellular immunity by expressing cytokines that promote the development of cytotoxic T cells and macrophages [e.g. IFN-γ, IL-2, and tumor necrosis factor-α (TNF-α)], while Th2 cells regulate IgE synthesis (IL-4), eosinophil proliferation (IL-5), mast cell proliferation (IL-9), and airway hyperreactivity (IL-13). A Th2 pattern of cytokine expression is noted in allergic inflammation and in parasitic infections, conditions both associated with IgE production and eosinophilia. The cytokine environment encountered by a naïve T cell plays a prominent role in determining whether that naïve T cell develops into a Th1 or Th2 cell. Thus, the same naïve Th cell can give

rise to either Th1 or Th2 cells under the influence of both environmental (e.g. cytokine) and genetic factors acting at the level of antigen presentation. In particular cytokines such as IL-4 play a prominent role in deviating naïve T cells to develop into Th2 cells, whereas IFN-γ and IL-12 are important in the development of Th1 cells. In addition to the local cytokine environment, the level of antigen-induced activation of the T-cell receptor (high- versus low-dose antigen), the delivery of co-stimulatory signals from the APC, and the number of postactivation cell divisions influence the development of Th1 versus Th2 cells. A large number of studies have supported the hypothesis that Th2-type responses are involved in the pathogenesis of several allergic diseases including atopic asthma, allergic rhinitis, and atopic dermatitis. However, there are still aspects of this paradigm that require further investigation.

Transcription factors and expression of Th2 cytokine responses

There is increasing interest in the role of transcription factors in the regulation of cytokine gene expression in asthma and allergy, as therapeutically targeting transcription factors may provide a novel approach to inhibiting the function of several cytokines important to the genesis of allergic inflammation. Transcription factors are intracellular signalling proteins that bind to regulatory sequences of target genes, resulting in the promotion (transactivation) or suppression (transrepression) of gene transcription, with resultant effects on subsequent cytokine mRNA and protein production. Transcriptional control of genes involved in the allergic inflammatory response is mediated by several classes of signal-dependent

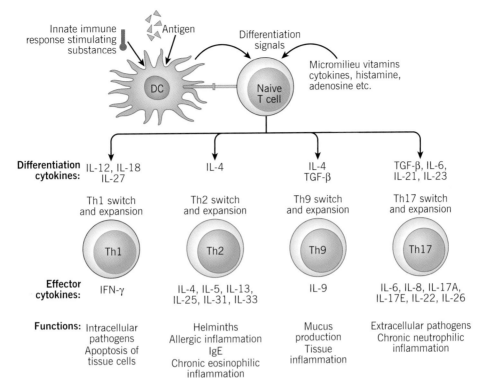

Fig. 1.18 Effector T-cell subsets. After antigen presentation by DCs, naïve T cells differentiate into Th1, Th2, Th9, and Th17 effector subsets. Their differentiation requires cytokines and other cofactors that are released from DCs and also expressed in the microenvironment. T-cell activation in the presence of IL-4 enhances differentiation and clonal expansion of Th2 cells, perpetuating the allergic response. IL-12, IL-18, and IL-27 induce Th1-cell differentiation; IL-4 and TGF-β induce Th9 differentiation; and IL-6, IL-21, IL-23, and TGF-β induce the differentiation of Th17 cells. (Adapted from: Figure 1 in Akdis CA, Akdis M. J Allergy Clin Immunol. 2009; 123:735–746.)

transcription factors that can be categorized according to their structure. Examples of transcription factors important in mediating Th2 immune responses include GATA-3, STAT-6, c-MAF, and NF-ATc. In contrast, STAT-4 and T-bet are transcription factors that are important in mediating Th1 immune responses.

STAT-6
The transcription factor STAT-6 is involved in the upregulation of IL-4-dependent genes, such as the genes encoding the IL-4 receptor, IgE, and chemokine receptors (CCR4, CCR8), which play key roles in allergic responses. STAT-6 expression in bronchial epithelium has correlated with the severity of asthma. STAT-6 is also activated by other Th2 cytokines such as IL-5 and IL-13, contributing to the local amplification of the Th2 response.

GATA-3
The transcription factor GATA-3 is selectively expressed in Th2 cells and plays a critical role in Th2 differentiation in a STAT-6-independent manner. GATA-3 regulates the transcription of IL-4 and IL-5, and like STAT-6, has been suggested to act as a chromatin-remodelling factor, favouring the transcription of Th2 cytokines IL-4 and IL-13.

c-MAF
The transcription factor c-MAF is a Th2-specific transcription factor that is induced in the early events of Th2 differentiation and transactivates the IL-4 promoter. Asthmatic patients display an increased expression of c-MAF.

NF-AT
The NF-AT transcription factors comprise four different members, which are expressed in T and B lymphocytes, mast cells, and NK cells. One of the NF-AT transcription factors NF-ATc (also known as NF-AT2) plays an important role in the development of Th2 responses.

T-bet
Deficiency in T-bet (a transcription factor that regulates expression of Th1 rather than Th2 cytokines) is associated with increased airway responsiveness in mouse models of asthma. Reduced levels of T-bet have also been noted in the airway of human asthmatics.

Th9 cells

IL-9 has been considered a Th2-cell-derived cytokine that contributes to mucus expression and mast-cell hyperplasia (see Fig. 1.3). More recently, a novel Th9 cell population that differs from Th2 cells has been described that does not express any well-defined transcription factors such as GATA-3, T-bet, RORγt or Foxp3, emphasizing that Th9 cells are different from Th2, Th1, Th17, and Treg populations (see Fig. 1.18). It is currently unknown whether, during the allergic response in vivo, IL-9-secreting T cells are distinct from Th2 cells or whether Th2 cells can be reprogrammed into Th9 cells.

Th17 cells

Th17 cells are associated with neutrophil-mediated inflammation and have therefore been studied in diseases associated with neutrophils including bacterial infection, chronic obstructive pulmonary disease (COPD), and cystic fibrosis. Since the discovery of IL-17, several other homologous proteins have been identified, resulting in a six-member IL-17 cytokine family in which the members are designated as IL-17A through IL-17F. The IL-17 family members IL-17A and IL-17F share the greatest homology and are perhaps the best-characterized cytokines in the family. In contrast, IL-17E, also referred

to as IL-25, is the most divergent member. In asthma, elevated IL-17A levels correlate with increased neutrophilic inflammation, a characteristic of severe asthma and corticosteroid-resistant asthma. Increased IL-17A has also been correlated with increased airway responsiveness in asthmatics. Th17-cell-released cytokines include IL-17A, IL-17F, and IL-22 (see Fig. 1.18), which induce multiple chemokines and growth factors to promote neutrophil and macrophage accumulation. Induction of Th17 cells requires signalling through STAT-3 and activation of transcription factors RORγT and RORα.

Treg cells

The term regulatory T cell (Treg) refers to cells that actively control or suppress the function of other cells, generally in an inhibitory fashion. Thus, in allergic inflammation Treg cells that suppress the function of Th2 cells may have an important role in limiting allergic responses (Fig. 1.19). For example, allergen immunotherapy induces Treg cells, which express inhibitory cytokines [transforming growth factor-β (TGF-β), IL-10] that can

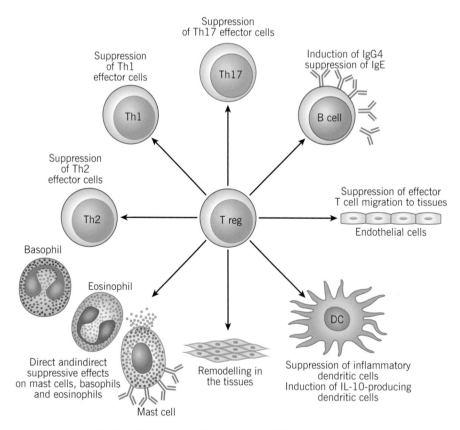

Fig. 1.19 Treg and suppression of allergic inflammation. Foxp3+ CD4+ CD25+ and T_R1 cells contribute to the control of allergen-specific immune responses in several major ways. Suppression of DCs that support the generation of effector T cells; suppression of Th1, Th2, and Th17 cells; suppression of allergen-specific IgE and induction of IgG4, IgA, or both; suppression of mast cells, basophils, and eosinophils; interaction with resident tissue cells and remodelling; and suppression of effector T-cell migration to tissues. (Adapted from: Figure 2 in Akdis CA, Akdis M. J Allergy Clin Immunol. 2009; 123:735–746.)

down-regulate the allergic inflammatory response. Thus, one potential mechanism through which allergen immunotherapy is hypothesized to be effective in allergic rhinitis is through induction of Treg cells. Several different Treg cell populations have been described (CD4+CD25+, Th3, TR1, TR, and NK T cells) of which the CD4+CD25+ Treg cells express the transcription factor Foxp3 have been most studied in allergic inflammation. They are naturally occurring regulatory cells that prevent autoimmune disease, and also inhibit Th2 responses.

The inflammatory response in allergy

Allergens

Allergens initiate the immune and subsequent inflammatory response by being processed by APCs to activate T cells. In addition certain allergens such as house dust mite also have protease activity that can increase epithelial cell permeability to enhance allergen penetration of the mucosa, as well as activate protease receptors on epithelial cells to release cytokines that promote Th2 cytokine responses. Although allergens are mostly large glycoproteins, there does not appear to be a common amino acid structure that confers the ability of a protein to initiate allergic disease. Occupational allergens also share no common structural features and are represented by a wide variety of low- and high-molecular weight compounds, including metal anhydrides, amines, wood dusts, metals, organic chemicals, animal and plant proteins, and biological enzymes. Platinum salts and low-molecular-weight acid anhydrides can interact with mast cells by acting as haptens and are recognized by IgE only after conjugation with a protein.

Mast cells

Mast cells play a pivotal role in the initiation of the IgE-mediated allergic response to allergen exposure on mucosal surfaces. Cross-linking of high-affinity IgE receptors induces release of preformed mediators stored in cytoplasmic granules (e.g. histamine, tryptase, TNF-α), the generation of lipid mediators (e.g. PGD_2 and LTC_4), as well as the transcription of cytokine genes. The important role of the mast cell is further discussed below in the section on early phase response to allergen challenge, as well as above in the section on IgE.

Early response cytokines: TNF-α and IL-1β

IL-1β and TNF-α up-regulate a broad range of proinflammatory activity in these cells and have been termed the early response proinflammatory cytokines. Macrophages are the major source of IL-1β and TNF-α. However, TNF-α is also released by mast cells, lymphocytes, eosinophils, fibroblasts, and epithelial cells. TNF-α and IL-1β initiate further synthesis and release of cytokines and mediators, up-regulate the expression of adhesion molecules on endothelial cells, and promote production of extracellular matrix by fibroblasts.

Epithelium

The integrity and barrier function of epithelial cells minimizes the underlying tissue exposure to potential antigens. The proteolytic function of some allergens (e.g. Der p 1) confers additional properties that facilitate their penetration through the cleavage of intercellular adhesion molecule. Epithelial cells are activated by the early response cytokines including IL-1β and TNF-α. In response to these stimuli, epithelial cells generate chemokines, cytokines, and autacoid mediators, which promote the allergic response (Fig. 1.20). In particular, epithelial products have powerful chemoattractant activity for eosinophils, lymphocytes, macrophages, and neutrophils. The epithelium is a major source of eosinophil chemoattractants (including eotaxin-1, RANTES, and monocyte chemotactic peptide-4), as well as CD4+ T memory lymphocyte chemoattractants (RANTES, MCP-1, and IL-16).

TSLP, IL-25, IL-33

The cytokines thymic stromal lymphopoietin (TSLP), IL-25, and IL-33 have been recognized to play an important role in initiating, amplifying, and maintaining Th2 responses important to allergic inflammation (see Fig. 1.20).

TSLP
Increased levels of TSLP have been noted in skin biopsies from subjects with atopic dermatitis as well as in the airways of subjects with asthma. The increased levels of TSLP in the airway in asthma correlate with disease severity. TSLP is derived from epithelial cell and non-epithelial cell sources and acts on dendritic cells to up-regulate the co-stimulatory molecule OX40 ligand and hence favours Th2 responses.

IL-25
IL-25 (also known as IL-17E) is a member of the IL-17 cytokine family. Increased levels of IL-25 have been detected in asthma and atopic dermatitis. Studies in mouse models of asthma suggest that IL-25 may play an important role in promoting or sustaining an ongoing Th2 immune response. IL-25 is produced by multiple cell types including epithelial cells, mast cells, eosinophils, and basophils.

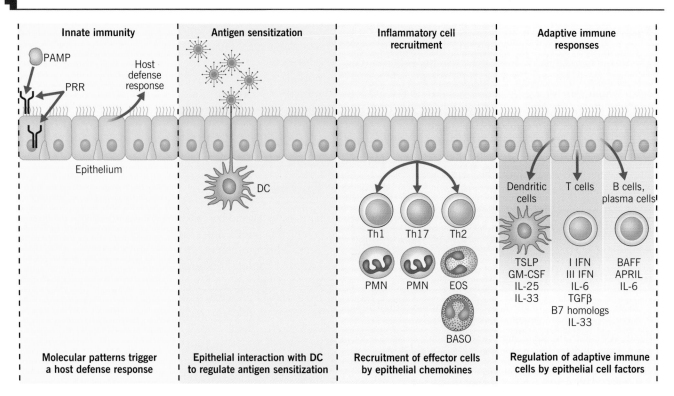

Fig. 1.20 Epithelial cell influence on innate and adaptive immune responses. Epithelial cells express pattern-recognition receptors and release antimicrobial products into the airways. They also interact with interepithelial DCs and subepithelial DCs to alter the ability of DCs to skew T cells. During inflammatory and immune responses, epithelial cells release specific chemokines that recruit subsets of granulocytes and T cells that are appropriate to the particular immune response. Finally, epithelial cells regulate the adaptive immune response by expression of soluble and cell-surface molecules that alter the function of DCs, T cells, and B cells in the airways. PAMP, pathogen-associated molecular pattern; PRR, pathogen-recognition receptor; PMN, polymorphonuclear leukocyte; EOS, eosinophil; BASO, basophil; APRIL, a B-cell proliferation-inducing ligand; TSLP, thymic stromal lymphopoietin; BAFF, B-lymphocyte-activating factor of the TNF family. (Adapted from: Figure 1 in Schleimer RP, Kato A, Kern R, et al. J Allergy Clin Immunol. 2007; 120:1279–1284.)

IL-33

IL-33 (a member of the IL-1 cytokine family) increases cytokine production from polarized Th2 cells. Cellular sources of IL-33 include epithelial cells, macrophages, and dendritic cells. Increased levels of IL-33 have been detected in the airway of subjects with severe asthma.

Epithelial cells and Th2 responses

As TSLP, IL-25, and IL-33 are all produced by epithelial cells, the potential for these three cytokines to enhance Th2-mediated allergic inflammation at mucosal surfaces is evident. In addition, both IL-25 and IL-33 induce TSLP production from epithelial cells suggesting a potential mechanism by which these three cytokines interact and potentiate their function at mucosal surfaces.

Eosinophils

The allergic inflammatory response is characterized by the presence of increased numbers of eosinophils in the bone marrow, blood, and tissues. IL-5, a Th2-cell-derived cytokine, is an important lineage-specific eosinophil growth factor that plays an important role in the generation of eosinophils in the bone marrow. Eosinophils travel from the bone marrow through the blood stream and bind to adhesion molecules expressed by endothelium at sites of allergic inflammation. Eosinophils chemotax into tissues in response to CC chemokines in particular eotaxin-1 and RANTES. Once in the extracellular matrix, eosinophil survival is enhanced by IL-5 and GM-CSF and by adhesion of eosinophils to fibronectin components of the extracellular matrix. Normal eosinophil life span in tissue is about 2–5 days but, under the influence of these factors, survival may be extended to 14 days or more by rescue from apoptosis. This prolongation of the eosinophil life span probably contributes to the increased eosinophil numbers observed at sites of allergic inflammation. Mature eosinophils have cytoplasmic granules that contain several proteins toxic to parasites and in allergic inflammation to a variety of host cells including epithelium. In established allergic disease, activated eosinophils are a major source of cysteinyl leukotrienes, which cause smooth muscle contraction, mucus hypersecretion, microvascular leakage, and airway hyperresponsiveness. The precise mechanism responsible for eosinophil activation in vivo is not known, although in vitro cross-linking of IgA receptors on eosinophils, or eosinophil adhesion to the CS-1 region of fibronectin, are capable of stimulating mediator release.

Eosinophils are considered to be proinflammatory cells that mediate many of the features of asthma and related allergic diseases. They have a characteristic bilobed nucleus and the cytoplasm of each cell contains about 20 membrane-bound, core-containing, specific granules that contain basic proteins such as major basic protein (MBP) (Fig. 1.21). In addition, eosinophils contain a number of primary granules, which lack a core and are of variable size. These granules contain Charcot–Leyden crystal protein (CLC protein), a characteristic feature of asthmatic sputum. Normal eosinophils contain about five non-membrane-bound lipid bodies, which are the principal store of arachidonic acid and also contain the enzymes cyclooxygenase and 5-lipoxygenase, which are required to synthesize prostaglandins and leukotrienes. Generally, the amount of cytokines produced by eosinophils is low compared with that produced by other cell types, though the increased number of eosinophils at sites of allergic inflammation may partially compensate.

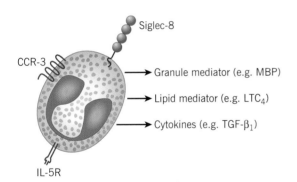

Fig. 1.21 Eosinophils. Eosinophils express receptors that, when engaged by ligand, induce their proliferation (IL-5 receptor, IL-5R), chemoattraction into tissues (CCR-3), and apoptosis (Siglec-8). Eosinophils can contribute to inflammation through release of preformed cytoplasmic granule mediators (e.g. major basic protein, MBP), newly generated lipid mediators (e.g. LTC$_4$) and transcribed cytokines (e.g. TGF-β$_1$). (Adapted from: Figure 3 in Broide DH. J Allergy Clin Immunol. 2008; 121:560–570.)

Studies with anti-IL-5 have demonstrated that it significantly reduces eosinophil levels in the blood by >90%. In the idiopathic hypereosinophilic syndrome, administration of anti-IL-5 reduces eosinophil levels as well as the amount of corticosteroid therapy needed to control the disease. In asthma, anti-IL-5 reduces exacerbations in asthmatics who have elevated levels of eosinophils in sputum but does not influence symptoms or airway hyperreactivity in asthmatics who are not recruited for clinical studies based on sputum eosinophil levels. In addition anti-IL-5 reduces levels of extracellular matrix remodelling in mild asthmatics. This reduction in remodelling is associated with reduced numbers of eosinophils and reduced expression of the pro fibrotic growth factor TGF-β1 by eosinophils in the airway.

Neutrophils

Tissue neutrophilia is the hallmark of inflammation induced by bacterial infection. Allergen challenge induces a more prominent influx of eosinophils than neutrophils. Increased numbers of neutrophils can be detected in asthma exacerbations and in subjects with severe asthma as well as in subjects who die suddenly of asthma. The increased numbers of neutrophils in these more severe asthma populations may be related to infections, the use of corticosteroids that inhibit neutrophil apoptosis, or the active recruitment of neutrophils in severe asthma. Increased levels of the neutrophil chemoattractant IL-8 and Th17 cells have also been detected in severe asthma. Neutrophils have the ability to generate a variety of proinflammatory mediators including enzymes, oxygen radicals as well as lipid mediators and cytokines that attract and activate more neutrophils (Fig. 1.22). At present it is not known whether the neutrophil contributes to airway responsivenes in asthma. The development of selective inhibitors of neutrophils (i.e. targeting IL-8 or the IL-8 receptor) will allow further study of the effect of selectively depleting neutrophils on the development of subsequent asthma or allergic inflammatory responses.

Macrophages

Macrophages are an important component of the innate immune system and clear organisms through their

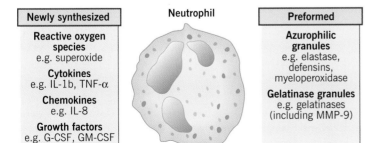

Fig. 1.22 Neutrophil mediators. The neutrophil is a source of range of preformed and newly synthesized mediators. MMP-9, matrix metalloprotease 9; G-CSF, granulocyte colony-stimulating factor; GM-CSF, granulocyte–macrophage colony-stimulating factor.

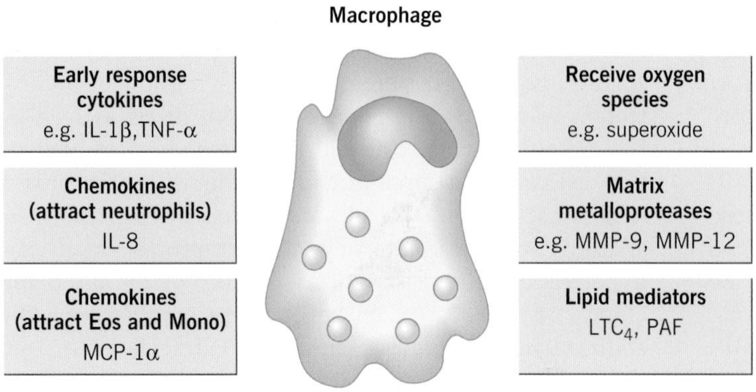

Macrophage

| Early response cytokines
e.g. IL-1β, TNF-α |
| Chemokines
(attract neutrophils)
IL-8 |
| Chemokines
(attract Eos and Mono)
MCP-1α |

| Receive oxygen species
e.g. superoxide |
| Matrix metalloproteases
e.g. MMP-9, MMP-12 |
| Lipid mediators
LTC₄, PAF |

Fig. 1.23 Macrophage mediators. The macrophage is a source of a range of preformed and newly synthesized mediators. MCP, macrophage chemoattractant protein.

phagocytic function (Fig. 1.23). Toll-like receptors expressed by macrophages play an important role in their activation. Macrophages at tissue sites of allergic inflammation originate from mononuclear cell in the bone marrow. In addition to their phagocytic and antigen presenting role, macrophages have the potential to be proinflammatory or antiinflammatory based on the spectrum of mediators they are able to release. For example, macrophages release proinflammatory cytokines (e.g. IL-1β, TNF-α) and chemokines (e.g. IL-8), which have all been detected at sites of allergic inflammation. In addition macrophages release biologically active lipids, reactive oxygen and nitrogen metabolites. Macrophages may be activated by allergen via the low-affinity IgE receptor (FcεRII) as well as by Th2 cytokines (IL-4 and IL-13) and LTD₄. Thus, there are several mechanisms through which macrophages could be acivated to express proinflammatory cytokines at sites of allergic inflammation. Macrophages are also able to express antiinflammatory cytokines including the IL-1 receptor antagonist, IL-10 and IL-12, which provides a potential for macrophages to down-regulate allergic inflammatory responses. There is some evidence that the antiinflammatory cytokine IL-10 is reduced in both blood monocytes and alveolar macrophages from allergic patients with asthma.

Macrophage subsets: M1 vs M2 macrophages

There is emerging evidence of distinct macrophage subsets (M1 and M2) with the M2 macrophage playing a greater role in Th2-mediated inflammation. The ability of the Th2 cytokine IL-4 to induce the differentiation of M2-like macrophages suggests that M2 macrophages may be important at sites of allergic inflammation. In contrast, Th1 cytokines such as IFN-γ or bacterial products such as LPS promote M1 macrophages, which induce strong IL-12-mediated Th1 responses. There is also emerging evidence of distinct monocyte subsets (Gr1⁻/Ly-6C^{low} and Gr1⁺/Ly-6C^{high}) with distinct functions and fates, such as the differentiation into cells with features of M1 or M2 macrophages respectively.

Primary functions of macrophages in allergy

Alveolar macrophages in health may subserve a suppressive role in inflammation, but are phenotypically altered in asthma towards a more stimulatory role. In addition, antigen presentation through the high-affinity receptor for IgE, which is increased on the surface of human monocytes of atopic patients, results in an approximately 100-fold or greater increased efficiency in activating antigen-specific T cells. Thus, in allergic inflammation, changes occur in the alveolar macrophage population, which results in an enhanced capacity to present antigen and a loss of their immunosuppressive phenotype. This is attributed to changes in the local environment with evidence for an important role of GM-CSF. In addition, an increase in newly recruited monocytes that demonstrate increased antigen-presenting function is likely to contribute to enhanced antigen presentation in the asthmatic lung.

Bone marrow

The bone marrow is likely to play an important effector role in allergic inflammation through production of leukocyte effector cells and leukocyte progenitors. Most of the leukocyte effector cells associated with allergic inflammation, namely basophils, eosinophils, neutrophils, and monocytes, are produced in the bone marrow and travel to sites of allergic inflammation. In addition, allergen challenge induces trafficking of bone marrow progenitors such as eosinophil progenitors to sites of allergic inflammation in the tissues where under local microenvironmental stimuli they can differentiate into mature eosinophils. Thus, the bone marrow may be a source not only of mature leukocytes but also of precursor leukocyte populations that travel to sites of allergic inflammation.

Nerves

Neural mechanisms may play a role in allergic inflammation through interactions with inflammatory cells or through direct effects on target organs such as smooth muscle, mucous glands, and blood vessels. Studies have investigated the role of cholinergic nerves, adrenergic nerves, non-adrenergic non-cholinergic nerves, and neuropeptides such as substance P, calcitonin gene-related peptide (CGRP), vasoactive intestinal polypeptide (VIP) and nerve growth factor (NGF) in contributing to allergic inflammation. One of the best-studied neural pathways is the sensory nerve reflex. Activation of local tissue sensory nerves at sites of allergic inflammation may activate cholinergic reflexes. Stimulated cholinergic nerves can rapidly induce smooth muscle contraction, mucus hypersecretion, and vasodilation. The vasodilation may contribute to nasal congestion at sites of allergic inflammation. Sensory nerves at sites of allergic inflammation can be triggered by non-specific chemical and physical irritants, bradykinin, histamine, leukotrienes, and prostaglandins particularly after the loss of overlying epithelium. In addition, inflammatory mediators may act on various prejunctional nerve receptors to modulate the release of neurotransmitters. For example, mast cell products (especially histamine and PGD_2) and eosinophil mediators can up-regulate the activity of the cholinergic ganglia.

Modulation of allergic responses by cytokines, chemokines, and adhesion molecules

What are cytokines?

Cytokines are extracellular signalling molecules that bind to specific cell surface cytokine receptors to regulate both the immune and the inflammatory response. Currently over 70 cytokines have been identified (e.g. interleukins 1 to 35, growth factors, etc.) of which a subset is known to be expressed during episodes of allergic inflammation (Table 1.2). Cytokines predominantly act on closely adjacent cells (the paracrine effect), but can also act on the cells of their origin (the autocrine effect), and rarely on distant cells in another organ (the systemic effect). Cytokines are involved in orchestrating the initiation, maintenance, and resolution of the allergic inflammatory response. In allergic inflammation, cytokines are both active in the bone marrow where they regulate the development and differentiation of inflammatory cells (e.g. IL-5 induces eosinophilopoesis), and are also expressed at tissue sites of allergic inflammation (e.g. lower airway in asthma) where they regulate the immune and inflammatory response. Cytokines function through complex cytokine networks to promote or inhibit inflammation. During an inflammatory response the profile of cytokines expressed, as well as the profile of cytokine receptors expressed on responding cell types and the timing of their expression, will determine whether the response is predominantly pro- or anti-inflammatory. Activation of high-affinity cytokine receptors on target cells induces a cascade of intracellular signalling pathways that regulate the transcription of specific genes and the ultimate cellular inflammatory response. Considerable progress has been made in characterizing the cellular sources and actions of the numerous cytokines involved in allergic inflammation (see Table 1.2). Overall, these studies suggest that cytokines exhibit redundancy (i.e. several cytokines can often subserve the same function), and that several cell types can generate or respond to the same cytokine. Thus, therapeutic strategies in allergic inflammation aimed at neutralizing a single cytokine may not

Table 1.2 Cytokines in allergic inflammation

Cytokine	Cell source	Actions
IL-1β	Predominately monocytes, macrophages; also smooth muscle, endothelium, epithelium	Activation of T cells and endothelium
IL-2	Predominantly T cells; also NK cells	Promotes T-cell proliferation and clonal expansion
IL-3	T cells, mast cells, eosinophils	Stimulates development of mast cells and basophils; promotes eosinophil survival
IL-4	Predominantly Th2 cells; also basophils, NK T cells, mast cells, eosinophils	Promotes T-cell differentiation to Th2 phenotype, class switching to IgE, up-regulation of VCAM-1 on endothelial cells
IL-5	T cells, mast cells, eosinophils	Promotes eosinophil growth, differentiation and survival
IL-6	Predominantly monocytes, macrophages; also eosinophils, mast cells, fibroblasts	Differentiation of T cells into Th17 cells and B cells into plasma cells

Table 1.2 Continued

Cytokine	Cell source	Actions
IL-8	Predominantly macrophages; also T cells, mast cells, endothelial cells, fibroblasts, neutrophils	Neutrophil activation and differentiation; chemotactic factor for neutrophils
IL-9	T cells, T9 cells	Enhances mast-cell growth; increases mucus expression
IL-10	T cells, B cells, macrophages, monocytes	Inhibits T-cell proliferation and down-regulates proinflammatory cytokine production by Th1 and Th2 cells
IL-12	Predominantly dendritic cells, monocytes, macrophages	Promotes Th1 phenotype and IFN-γ production; inhibits Th2 development and cytokine expression; suppresses IgE production
IL-13	Predominantly Th2 cells; also mast cells, basophils, eosinophils	Promotes class switching to IgE, increased expression of VCAM-1 on endothelial cells, increased airway hyperactivity
IL-16	Predominantly CD8+ T cells; also mast cells, airway epithelium	Recruitment of CD4+ T cells and eosinophils
IL-17	Th17 cells, CD4+ T cells, neutophils, basophils	Induces neutrophil recruitment and activation
IL-18	Predominantly macrophages; also airway epithelial cells	Member of IL-1 family; activates B cells. Induces IFN-γ, promoting Th1 phenotype
IL-21	Predominantly T cells	Activates NK cells and promotes proliferation of B and T cells
IL-22	Predominantly Th17, Th1 as well as NK and mast cells	Activates innate immune response
IL-23	Predominantly dendritic cells	Induces IFN-γ; influences Th17 differentiation
IL-25	Predominantly Th2 lymphocytes; IL-25 is also known as IL-17E	Stimulates IL-4, IL-5 and IL-13 release from non-lymphoid accessory cell; increases eotaxin-1 and RANTES expression
IL-26	Predominantly monocytes and T memory cells	Induces IL-8, IL-10, and ICAM-1
IL-27	Predominantly macrophages and dendritic cells	Synergizes with IL-12 to induce IFN-γ
IL-31	Predominantly expressed by T cells	Induces chemokines that mediate neutrophil, monocyte, and T-cell recruitment
IL-33	Predominantly epithelium, fibroblasts, smooth muscle, DC	Member of IL-1 family; increases Th2 cytokines, IgE, and eosinophils
GM-CSF	Macrophages, eosinophils, neutrophils, T cells, mast cells, airway epithelial cells	Priming of neutrophils and eosinophils; prolongs survival of eosinophils
TNFα	Mast cells, macrophages, monocytes, epithelial cells	Up-regulates endothelial adhesion molecule expression; chemoattractant for neutrophils and monocytes
TSLP	Epithelium	Activates DC to promote Th2 cytokine response
TGFβ_1	Macrophagse, eosinophils, epithelium, Treg cells	Profibrotic effects involved in airway remodeling; chemotactic for monocytes, fibroblasts and mast cells; promotes tolerance
IFN-γ	T cells, NK cells	Suppression of Th2 cells; inhibits B-cell switching to IgE; increases ICAM-1 expression on endothelial and epithelial cells

IL, interleukin; GM-CSF, granulocyte–macrophage colony-stimulating factor; ICAM-1, intercellular adhesion molecule-1; IFN-γ, interferon-γ; NK cells, natural killer cells; TGF-β_1, transforming growth factor-β_1; TNF-α, tumor necrosis factor-α; VCAM-1, vascular cell adhesion molecule-1; TSLP, thymic stromal lymphopoietin.

always be successful if an alternate cytokine can subserve the same function. However, in rheumatoid arthritis, a disease associated with expression of multiple cytokines, neutralizing a single cytokine (e.g. TNF) has resulted in a significant therapeutic benefit. Thus, in allergic inflammation an improved understanding of the mechanism through which cytokines promote allergic inflammation may identify key cytokine targets for therapeutic intervention.

Cytokine regulation of IgE synthesis

Cytokines such as IL-4 play a very important role in class switching of B cells to generate IgE an essential component of allergic responses (see Section on IgE).

Cytokine regulation of blood vessel adhesion molecule expression

Leukocyte adhesion molecules

Adhesion molecules are glycoproteins expressed on the surface of leukocytes that mediate leukocyte to endothelium, as well as leukocyte to extracellular matrix adhesion and communication. The role of adhesion molecules expressed by circulating leukocytes and adhesion counterreceptors expressed by endothelial cells has been extensively investigated to determine pathways for general tissue recruitment of leukocytes, as well as to identify mechanisms that mediate selective tissue recruitment of leukocyte subpopulations (e.g. eosinophils at sites of allergic inflammation). In order to accumulate in the airway in diseases such as asthma, circulating leukocytes derived from the bone marrow must adhere to the endothelium lining the blood vessels of the bronchial microcirculation, penetrate the vessel wall, and migrate to the airway lumen. Cell adhesion molecules are involved in all stages of this process.

Cell adhesion molecules and leukocyte adhesion to endothelium

Adhesion molecules involved in leukocyte trafficking are grouped into three families based on structural features: the selectins, the integrins, and the immunoglobulin (Ig) gene superfamily (Table 1.3). Studies of leukocyte adhesion to endothelium in vitro, as well as in vivo, and observation of the living microcirculation using intravital microscopy (Fig. 1.24), have delineated the coordinated sequence of events responsible for the tissue accumulation of circulating leukocytes. In the absence of inflammation, circulating leukocytes rarely adhere to the blood vessel wall that does not constitutively express adhesion molecules. However, allergic individuals when exposed to an allergen on a mucosal surface (e.g. nasal mucosa) release cytokines (e.g. IL-1, IL-4, IL-13, and TNF-α) and

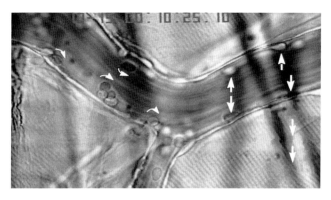

Fig. 1.24 Postcapillary leukocyte recruitment. The photograph shows the stages of leukocyte recruitment in a postcapillary venule of a mouse cremaster muscle. The picture was taken 10 minutes after initiating surgery. (Courtesy of Dr Keith Norman, University of Sheffield.)

mediators (e.g. histamine) derived from cell types including mast cells and macrophages. These released cytokines and mediators bind to their respective receptors on endothelial cells and up-regulate local endothelial cell adhesion molecule expression. The local up-regulation of adhesion molecule expression by endothelium at the site of allergen challenge localizes circulating leukocytes to that site. Circulating leukocytes are tethered to adhesion molecules expressed by endothelium via a transient adhesive interaction that results in leukocytes rolling along the endothelium of postcapillary venules (Fig. 1.25). The selectin family of adhesion molecules expressed by endothelium and their glycoprotein ligands expressed by leukocytes largely mediate this process, although the very late antigen-4 (VLA-4) integrin is also able to subserve this tethering function in eosinophils and lymphocytes. Subsequent activation of leukocyte integrins by chemoattractants (e.g. chemokines, anaphylatoxins, formylated peptides, and lipid mediators) causes the rolling leukocyte to arrest, firmly adhere, and flatten (reducing exposure to shear forces generated by blood flow and increasing surface area in contact with endothelium) (see Fig. 1.25). Integrins and immunoglobulin superfamily member adhesion molecules mediate these steps of leukocyte firm adhesion to endothelium. Finally, the leukocytes migrate between endothelial cells (diapedesis) into the interstitium and move towards the source of the stimulus (chemotaxis). The importance of leukocyte adhesion molecules to leukocyte tissue recruitment is suggested from genetic disorders that result in defective leukocyte integrin adhesion molecules [leukocyte adhesion deficiency I (LAD I)], or defective leukocyte sialyl Lewis X (sLex) expression (LAD II). Patients with either of these leukocyte adhesion deficiencies have neutrophil adhesion defects, tissues that lack neutrophils, associated blood neutrophilia, and recurrent infections as neutrophils cannot bind to endothelial cells and emigrate into infected tissues to mediate host defence against infection.

Table 1.3 Adhesion molecules in leukocyte–endothelial cell adhesion

Adhesion proteins mediating leukocyte cell adhesion interactions						
Adhesion family	Adhesion molecule	Alternative designation	Gene	Location	Ligand	Function
Selectin	L-selectin	CD62L	1q21-24	All leukocytes	CD34, MAdCAM	Rolling
	P-selectin	CD62P	1q21-24	Endothelial cells, platelets	PSGL-1	Rolling
	E-selectin	CD62E	1q21-24	Endothelial cells	PSGL-1, ESL-1	Rolling
Integrin	$\alpha_L\beta_2$	CD11a/CD18, LFA-1	$16(\alpha_1)\ 21(\beta_2)$	All leukocytes	ICAM-1, ICAM-2, ICAM-3	Adhesion
	$\alpha_M\beta_2$	CD11b/CD18, Mac-1	$16(\alpha_M)\ 21(\beta_2)$	Granulocytes, monocytes	ICAM-1, C3bi, fibrinogen	Adhesion
	$\alpha_x\beta_2$	CD11c/CD18, P150.95	$16(\alpha_x)\ 21(\beta_2)$	Granulocytes, monocytes	C3bi, fibronectin	Adhesion
	$\alpha_4\beta_1$	CD49d/CD29, VLA-4	$2(\alpha_4)\ 10(\beta_1)$	Lymphocytes, monocytes, eosinophils, basophils	VCAM-1, CS-1 Domain of fibronectin	Adhesion or rolling
	$\alpha_4\beta_7$	CD49d/β_7	$2(\alpha_4)\ 12(\beta_7)$	Lymphocytes, eosinophils	MAdCAM-1, VCAM-1, fibronectin CS-1 domain	Adhesion
Immungolobulin	ICAM-1	CD54	19p13.2	Endothelium, monocytes	LFA-1, Mac-1	Adhesion
	ICAM-2	CD102	17q23-25	Endothelium	LFA-1	Adhesion
	VCAM-1	CD106	1p31-32	Endothelium	VLA-4	Adhesion or rolling
	PECAM-1	CD31	17q23	Endothelium, leukocytes, platelets	PECAM-1 (homophilic) $\alpha_v\beta_3$ (heterophilic)	Emigration
	MAdCAM-1	–	19p13.3	Endothelium	$\alpha_4\beta_7$ L-selectin	Adhesion or rolling

ESL, E-selectin ligand; ICAM, intercellular adhesion molecule; LFA, lymphocyte-function-associated antigen; MAdCAM, mucosal vascular addressin cell adhesion molecule; PECAM, platelet/endothelial cell adhesion molecule; PSGL, P-selectin glycoprotein ligand; VCAM, vascular cell adhesion molecule; VLA, very late antigen.

Selectins and leukocyte adhesion to endothelium

All three members of the selectin family (E-, L-, P-selectin) (Fig. 1.26) may contribute to recruitment of circulating leukocytes to sites of allergic inflammation as E- and P-selectin are induced to be expressed on endothelium and L-selectin is expressed constituitively on circulating leukocytes. L-selectin is expressed constitutively on the surface microvilli of all leukocyte classes including eosinophils and basophils. P-selectin is synthesized and stored in Weibel–Palade bodies in endothelial cells. Stimulation of endothelial cells with inflammatory mediators such as histamine rapidly induces preformed P-selectin to be expressed at the endothelial cell surface. P-selectin

is also up-regulated transcriptionally by several inflammatory cytokines expressed during episodes of allergic inflammation including TNF-α and the Th2 cytokine IL-4. In animal models of allergic inflammation inhibiting any of the three selectins reduces eosinophil tethering to endothelium and tissue recruitment of eosinophils. As the selectin pathway is used for recruitment of all circulating leukocytes, targeting this pathway would not selectively reduce tissue recruitment of a particular leukocyte subset.

Selectin ligands

All three selectins can recognize glycoproteins and/or glycolipids containing the tetrasaccharide sialyl-Lewis[x]. P-selectin glycoprotein ligand 1 (PSGL-1) is the best

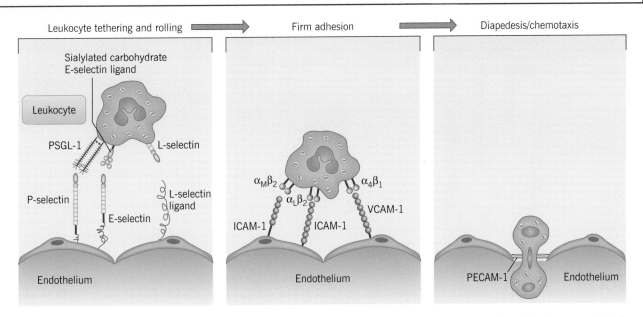

Fig. 1.25 The leukocyte endothelial cell adhesion cascade. Circulating leukocytes initially tether via selectins to endothelium, firmly adhere to endothelium via β1 and β2 integrins, and subsequently diapedese between endothelial cells. ICAM-1, intercellular adhesion molecule-1; PECAM-1, platelet endothelial cell adhesion molecule-1; PSGL-1, P-selecting glycoprotein ligand-1; VCAM-1, vascular cell adhesion molecule-1.

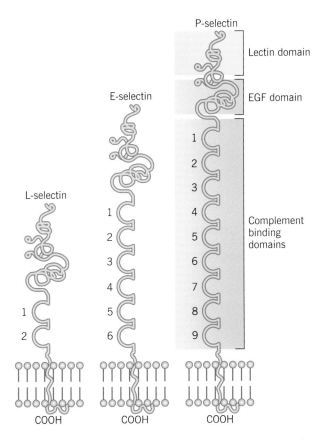

Fig. 1.26 Molecular structure of the Selectin family. Each selectin contains a lectin ligand binding domain, an epidermal growth factor (EGF)-like domain, and different numbers of complement binding domains or consensus repeats (numbered 1–9).

characterized selectin ligand, whose counter-receptor is P-selectin. PSGL-1 is localized to microvilli on all leukocytes and is therefore in a prime position to adhere to P-selectin when it is induced to be expressed by endothelium at sites of allergic inflammation. Limited human studies of pan selectin antagonists have demonstrated only a minor inhibitory effect on allergen-induced sputum eosinophilia in asthmatics.

Leukocyte integrins (β1, β2, and β7) and adhesion to endothelium

Integrins are heterodimeric proteins consisting of non-covalently linked α and β chains that mediate leukocyte adhesion to endothelial cells and matrix proteins (Fig. 1.27). Integrin-mediated adhesion is an energy-requiring process that also depends on extracellular divalent cations. There are 18 α and 8 β known integrin chains. Although leukocytes express 13 different integrins, the most important for mediating leukocyte adhesion to endothelial cells are the β1, β2, and β7 integrins (Fig. 1.28).

β1 integrins

The β1 integrin VLA-4 (α4β1) is expressed on circulating leukocytes important to allergic inflammation (including eosinophils, T cells, basophils, mononuclear cells), but is not significantly expressed on neutrophils. VLA-4 binds to counter-receptors expressed by endothelial cells [i.e. vascular cell adhesion molecule-1 (VCAM-1)], as well as to receptors in the extracellular matrix (the CS-1 region of fibronectin). The α4 integrins support firm adhesion of leukocytes to VCAM-1, and can also support leukocyte rolling on endothelium in vivo.

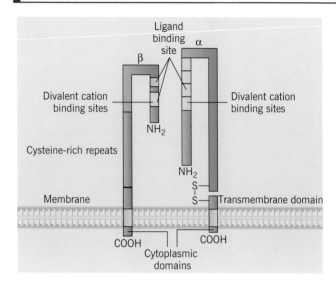

Fig. 1.27 The structure of an integrin heterodimer with its α and β subunits. Examples of integrin heterodimers include: β1 integrins (α4β1 or VLA-4), β2 integrins (αLβ2 or LFA-1), and β7 integrins (α4β7).

β2 integrins

The β2 integrin subfamily is highly expressed on all circulating leukocytes and consists of a common β2 subunit (CD18) linked to one of four α subunits: CD11a, CD11b, CD11c, or CD11d. The leukocyte β2 integrins mediate firm adhesion of leukocytes to intercellular adhesion molecule-1 (ICAM-1) expressed by endothelial cells. Thus, firm adhesion of leukocytes to endothelium can either be mediated by leukocyte β1 integrin binding to endothelial-expressed VCAM-1, or by leukocyte β2 integrin binding to endothelial expressed ICAM-1. β2 integrins expressed by lymphocytes are primarily CD11a/CD18 (LFA-1) while neutrophils, eosinophils, and monocytes express all four β2 integrins. On neutrophils, surface expression of the β2 integrin CD11b (Mac-1) is rapidly increased after exposure to chemoattractants due to mobilization from intracellular granule stores. In contrast, CD11a (LFA-1) is constitutively expressed and a change in the conformation of this integrin regulates its affinity for its counter-receptor ICAM-1.

β7 integrins

β7 integrins such as α4β7 are expressed on eosinophils and a subset of gut-homing lymphocytes. On eosinophils, α4β7 mediates binding to two different ligands on endothelial cells (VCAM-1, and MAdCAM-1). As MAdCAM is not significantly expressed in the lung compared with the GI tract, MAdCAM plays a more important role in homing of cells expressing α4β7 to the gut, but less of a role in mediating eosinophil recruitment to the lung via α4β7 integrins.

The immunoglobulin superfamily of endothelial cell expressed adhesion molecules

Endothelial cells express several immunoglobulin superfamily adhesion molecules (ICAM-1, VCAM-1, MAdCAM-1, and PECAM-1), which bind to integrin counter-receptors expressed by circulating leukocytes (see Table 1.3).

ICAM-1

Cytokines such as TNF-α induce endothelial cell ICAM-1 expression, which binds to β2 integrins on leukocytes (see Table 1.3). ICAM-1 deficient mice show substantially impaired lymphocyte and eosinophil trafficking into airways following antigen challenge.

VCAM-1

VCAM-1 is another member of the Ig superfamily that is expressed on endothelial cells and binds to the β1 integrin VLA-4. Basal expression of VCAM-1 on endothelial cells is very low, and is up-regulated by cytokines including IL-4, IL-13, and TNF-α.

MAdCAM-1

MAdCAM-1 (mucosal address in cell adhesion molecule-1) is expressed by endothelial cells and is a major ligand for the β7 integrin α4β7 expressed by leukocytes such as eosinophils.

PECAM-1

PECAM-1 (platelet endothelial cell adhesion molecule-1) is expressed constitutively on endothelial cells and leukocytes. Cytokines such as TNF-α induce a redistribution of PECAM-1 to the endothelial cell periphery without affecting the total amount expressed by each cell. This redistribution of PECAM-1 facilitates leukocyte migration between adjacent endothelial cells particularly for neutrophils and mononuclear cells.

What are chemokines?

Chemokines are a group of structurally related cytokine proteins of low molecular weight (8–10 kDa) expressed by a wide variety of cell types that induce activation and the directed migration of specific leukocyte subsets to sites of inflammation.

Chemokine families

The chemokines are a large family of chemotactic cytokines that have been divided into four groups, designated CXC, CC, C, and CXXXC (or CX3C), depending on the spacing of conserved cysteines in their amino acid sequence (C is cysteine; X is any amino acid). Over 50 different chemokines are now recognized and many of these are involved in the recruitment of inflammatory cells from the circulation during episodes of allergic

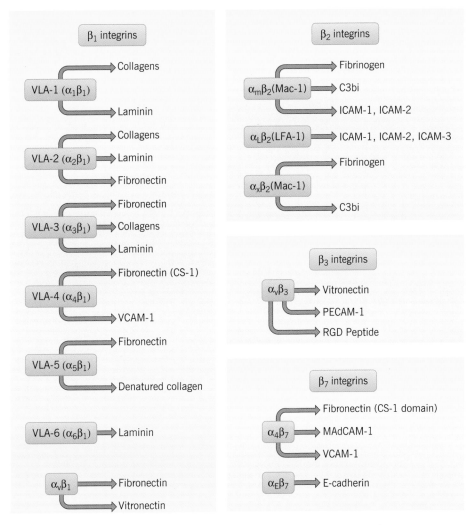

Fig. 1.28 Leukocyte integrins and their ligands. Leukocytes bind through β1, β2, β3, and β7 integrins to counter-receptors expressed on endothelial cells (VCAM-1, ICAM-1), as well as to extracellular matrix components (e.g. laminin, collagen, fibronectin). ICAM-1, intercellular adhesion molecule-1; MAdCAM-1, mucosal address in cell adhesion molecule-1; PECAM-1, platelet/endothelial cell adhesion molecule-1; VCAM-1, vascular cell adhesion molecule-1.

inflammation. The CC chemokines (Table 1.4) target a variety of cell types important to allergic inflammation including eosinophils, basophils, lymphocytes, macrophages, and dendritic cells, whereas the CXC chemokines mainly target neutrophils and mononuclear cells.

Stimuli that induce chemokine expression

Many of the stimuli for secretion of chemokines are the early signals elicited during innate immune responses including proinflammatory cytokines (such as IL-1β and TNF-α), which are released at sites of allergic inflammation. Chemokines are induced rapidly (i.e. within 1 hour) by these triggers and provide an important link between early innate immune responses and adaptive immunity (by recruiting and activating T cells). Chemokines are produced by a variety of cells at mucosal surfaces especially structural cells such as epithelium, as well as recruited inflammatory cells (monocytes, lymphocytes).

Chemokine function

The chemokine gradient from the epithelium (high concentration of chemokine) to the blood vessel (lower concentration of chemokine) assists in directing the migration of extravascular leukocytes to the epithelium (Fig. 1.29). Chemokines also play a role in activation-dependent adhesion of circulating leukocytes to endothelium. In the vascular lumen, chemokines presented by endothelial cells bind to chemokine receptors on circulating leukocytes when the leukocytes are tethering to the endothelium. This binding of chemokines to chemokine receptors on the tethering leukocyte induces a rapid change in affinity of integrin adhesion receptors on the circulating

Table 1.4 CC chemokines and CC receptors to which they bind

CC Chemokine (CCL 1–28)	Corresponding Chemokine Receptors (CCR 1–10)	CC Chemokine (CCL 1–28)	Corresponding Chemokine Receptors (CCR 1–10)
CCL1 (I-309)	CCR 8	CCL15 (HCC-2)	CCR 1, 3
CCL2 (MCP-1)	CCR 2	CCL16 (HCC-4)	CCR 1
CCL3 (MIP-1 α)	CCR 1, 5	CCL17 (TARC)	CCR 4
CCL4 (MIP-1 β)	CCR 5	CCL18 (PARC)	Unknown
CCL5 (RANTES)	CCR 1,3,5	CCL19 (ELC)	CCR 7
CCL6 (C-10)	CCR 1	CCL20 (LARC)	CCR 6
CCL7 (MCP-3)	CCR 2,3	CCL21 (SLC)	CCR 7
CCL8 (MCP-2)	CCR 1,2,3,5	CCL22 (MDC)	CCR 4
CCL9 (MIP-1α)	CCR 1	CCL23 (MPIF 1)	CCR 1
CCL10 (Unknown)	Unknown	CCL24 (eotaxin-2)	CCR 3
CCL11 (Eotaxin-1)	CCR 3	CCL25 (TECK)	CCR 9
CCL12 (Unknown)	CCR 2	CCL26 (eotaxin-3)	CCR 3
CCL13 (MCP-4)	CCR 2, 3, 5	CCL27 (CTAK)	CCR 10
CCL14 (HCC-1)	CCR 1	CCL28 (MEC)	CCR 10

CCL, CC chemokine ligand; CCR, CC chemokine receptor; MCP, monocyte chemotactic protein; MIP, macrophage inflammatory protein; HCC, hemofiltrate derived CC chemokine; RANTES, regulated on activation normal T cell expressed and secreted.

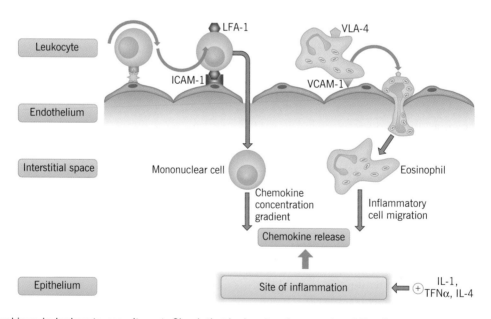

Fig. 1.29 Chemokines in leukocyte recruitment. Circulating leukocytes (e.g. eosinophil) adhere to endothelial adhesion molecules, diapedese between endothelial cells, and migrate along the chemokine gradient towards the site of inflammation. Chemokines up-regulate the affinity of integrins on leukocytes [e.g. VLA-4, or lymphocyte-function-associated antigen (LFA-1)] promoting tight adhesion of leukocytes to corresponding counter-receptor molecules expressed by vascular endothelium [e.g. vascular cell adhesion molecule-1 (VCAM-1) or intercellular adhesion molecule-1 (ICAM-1)]. In addition, chemokines play a primary role in promoting chemotaxis of leukocytes into inflamed tissues.

leukocyte. This change in leukocyte integrin affinity from a low-affinity to a high-affinity integrin binding state leads to tight adherence of the leukocyte to endothelium and subsequent leukocyte extravasation. Once the leukocyte extravasates between endothelial cells into the extracellular space, the chemokine concentration gradient promotes directed cell migration to the site of inflammation.

CC chemokines and allergic inflammation

As CC chemokines are expressed at increased levels at sites of allergic inflammation and attract cells important to the perpetuation of the allergic inflammatory response (e.g. eosinophils, basophils, monocytes, and lymphocytes), they have received attention as a target to modulate the allergic inflammatory response. Studies in asthmatics have established that CC chemokines are expressed by airway epithelial cells, and that allergen challenge can up-regulate expression of chemokines in the airway. The levels of chemokines expressed during allergen-induced late phase responses demonstrate correlations between individual chemokines and subsets of leukocytes which respond to these chemokines. During inflammatory responses epithelial cells, macrophages and, to a lesser extent, eosinophils and lymphocytes localized to the sub-epithelial layer are significant sources of chemokines. CC chemokines important to allergic inflammation include TARC (CCL17) and MDC (CCL22), which attract Th2 cells, and eotaxins-1,-2-3 (CCL11, CCL24, CCL26), which attract eosinophils, while MCP-1 (CCL2) is a potent mononuclear cell attractant (see Table 1.4).

Chemokine receptors

Chemokine receptors belong to the seven transmembrane receptor superfamily of G-protein-coupled receptors and include ten human CC chemokine receptor genes (they are known as CCR1 through CCR10), and seven CXCR receptors have been identified (they are referred to as CXCR1 through CXCR7).

CCR chemokine receptor family
The CCR chemokine receptors are expressed on cells important to allergic inflammation including eosinophils, basophils, lymphocytes, macrophages, and dendritic cells, whereas the CXCR are expressed mainly on neutrophils and lymphocytes. Activation of chemokine cell surface receptors by specific chemokines results in activation of a cascade of intracellular signalling pathways, including guanosine triphosphate-binding proteins of the Ras and Rho families, leading ultimately to the formation of cell surface protrusions termed uropods and lamellipods, which are required for cellular locomotion. Some chemokine receptors are expressed only on certain cell types, whereas other chemokine receptors are more widely expressed. In addition, some chemokine receptors are

expressed constitutively whereas others are expressed only after cell activation. A given leukocyte often expresses multiple chemokine receptors, and more than one chemokine typically binds to the same receptor. Examples of chemokine receptor expression by circulating cells important to allergic inflammation include: eosinophils and basophils, which express the CC chemokine receptor CCR3, T cells, which express CCR4 and CCR8, and dendritic cells, which express CCR6.

CXCR chemokine receptor family
Neutrophils express CXCR1 and CXCR2 receptors, which bind IL-8 and this mediates neutrophil tissue recruitment. In addition to the predominant expression of CC chemokine receptors, eosinophils, basophils, and mononuclear cells express the CXC chemokine receptor CXCR4, which is also expressed on neutrophils. The ligand for CXCR4 is the CXC chemokine SDF-1 (stromal cell derived factor-1).

T-cell subsets and chemokine receptors
Although certain chemokine receptors have been associated with specific T-cell subsets, chemokine receptor expression in vivo is complex and overlapping. Examples of chemokine receptors expressed on T-cell subsets include CCR4 and CCR8 on Th2 cells, and CCR5, CXCR3, and CXCR6 on Th1 cells (Fig. 1.30).

CCR3 antagonists and allergic inflammation
The CC chemokine receptor CCR3 is expressed on multiple leukocytes important to the allergic inflammatory response including eosinophils, basophils, and activated Th2-type lymphocytes. As several CC chemokines (eotaxin-1, eotaxin-2, eotaxin-3, RANTES, MIP-1, macrophage chemoattractant protein-2, -3, -4 or MCP-2, -3, -4) activate a common CCR-3 receptor, there has been particular interest in the therapeutic potential of using chemokine-receptor antagonists targeting one receptor (i.e. CCR3) to inhibit the actions of multiple CC chemokines on eosinophils and other inflammatory cells. Several small molecule inhibitors of CCR3 are effective in inhibiting eosinophil recruitment in animal models of

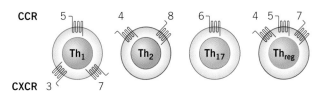

Fig. 1.30 Chemokine receptors and T-cell subsets. The pattern of chemokine receptor expression allows for recruitment of a variety of T cells under inflammatory. However, the pattern of CCR and CXCR chemokine receptors expressed by a given T-cell subset indicated in the figure does not define that subset nor is it necessarily specific for that subset. Th, T-helper cell.

allergic inflammation and are currently undergoing clinical trials.

Lipid chemoattractants

In addition to chemokines, lipid chemoattractants also play an important role in recruiting leukocytes to sites of allergic inflammation. For example leukotriene B4 attracts neutrophils, platelet-activating factor (PAF) attracts multiple leukocyte cell types, and PGD_2 recruits T cells expressing CRTH2 receptors.

Resolution of allergic inflammation and remodelling

The vast majority of episodes of allergic inflammation resolve with no significant structural changes to the tissues involved. However, in a minority of subjects remodelling of tissues occur and this has been best studied in the lung in asthma.

Apoptosis as a mechanism for resolution of inflammation

Apoptosis and necrosis are two mechanisms by which cell death occurs. Apoptosis, or programmed cell death, is a mechanism for resolution of allergic or other forms of inflammation. Apoptotic cells are removed by neighboring phagocytic cells without loss of their potentially harmful cell contents. In contrast to apoptosis, necrosis is a pathological form of cell death resulting from acute cellular injury. Necrosis is always associated with loss of intracellular mediators and enzymes into the extracellular environment and the consequential potential induction of an inflammatory response. Biochemically, apoptosis is characterized by a controlled autodigestion of the cell. Intracellular proteases called caspases are essential mediators of the apoptotic death machinery. Caspases are processed by cleavage at specific aspartate residues to form active heterodimeric enzymes. It appears that caspases work in a hierarchical system similar to other proteolytic cascades such as complement activation or blood coagulation. Caspase-mediated proteolysis results in cytoskeletal disruption, cell shrinkage, membrane blebbing, and nucleus condensation. More recently a third form of cell death autophagy has been described in which starving cells, or cells deprived of growth factors, generate energy and metabolites by digesting their own organelles and macromolecules.

Eosinophils provide an example of a cell type that has receptors that if activated can increase eosinophil survival [e.g. IL-5, GM-CSF, or IL-3 receptor] as well as receptors that when triggered induce eosinophil apoptosis (Siglec-8, Fas). Thus, depending upon the profile of ligands for these receptors expressed at sites of allergic inflammation, eosinophils may undergo apoptosis. Interestingly, incubating eosinophils with the survival cytokine IL-5 does not prevent their apoptosis being induced by activation of Siglec-8 receptors.

Remodelling as a consequence of chronic allergic inflammation

In contrast to the complete resolution of allergic inflammation without significant structural changes in the vast majority of individuals, a subset of subjects best studied in asthma may be predisposed to develop structural tissue changes termed 'airway remodelling'. These structural changes include subepithelial fibrosis, smooth muscle hypertrophy/hyperplasia, angiogenesis, mucus metaplasia, and deposition of increased amounts of extracellular matrix. Allergen challenge in asthmatics can also induce expression of TGF-β1, a proremodelling cytokine, and increased expression of extracellular matrix genes. Anti-IL-5, which reduces levels of eosinophils expressing TGF-β1 in the airway, can reduce levels of deposition of extracellular matrix proteins in the airway. However, other factors in addition to allergic inflammation, such as viral infections, tobacco smoke, pollutants, as well as genetic factors are likely to contribute to the development of significant remodelling in a subset of allergic asthmatics.

Fibroblasts

Fibroblasts proliferate in response to several cytokines and mediators generated during an allergic inflammatory response. Recognized fibroblast mitogens include histamine, heparin, and tryptase derived from mast cells, and major basic protein (MBP) and eosinophil cationic protein (ECP) from eosinophils. The cytokines TGF-β as well as platelet-derived growth factor (PDGF), b-fibroblast growth factor (b-FGF), insulin-like growth factor 1 (IGF-1), IL-1, and endothelin released during chronic allergic inflammation promote fibroblast proliferation, differentiation, and activation.

TGF-β enhances production of a range of extracellular matrix components, and decreases the synthesis of matrix-degrading enzymes while increasing the synthesis of protease inhibitors. Thus, TGF-β promotes the deposition of extracellular matrix while inhibiting its degradation, and contributes to the widespread subepithelial extracellular matrix deposition that may be associated with chronic allergic inflammation.

Chronic allergic inflammation may lead to the deposition of types III and V 'repair' collagens in the lamina reticularis beneath the types IV and VII 'reticular' collagens, which largely make up the basement membrane. The altered sub-basement membrane region also contains increased deposition of extracellular matrix components including fibronectin, tenascin, and lamin. Myofibroblasts present below the basement membrane are increased in number in asthma and are the source of many of the extracellular matrix products that are expressed after allergen challenge.

Extracellular matrix

Extracellular matrix proteins

The extracellular matrix produced by fibroblasts consists of a variety of proteins and complex carbohydrates. Approximately one-third of the dry mass of lung tissue is collagen, largely types 1, 3, and 5, whereas collagen types 4 and 7 are the main components of basement membrane. Elastin makes up another one-third of the dry mass of lung tissue, and the remainder is composed of glycoproteins – fibronectin, tenascin, laminin, the proteoglycan heparan sulphate, hyaluronan, and other minor matrix components. The composition of matrix elements may be altered by several products of the allergic inflammatory response especially matrix-degrading proteases (i.e. matrix metalloproteases or MMPs). Thus, the allergic inflammatory process may alter the dynamic balance between matrix breakdown and synthesis.

Extracellular matrix metalloproteases

MMPs play a role in remodelling of the extracellular matrix and thus may play a role in the development of airway remodelling and airway hyperresponsiveness. MMPs are zinc-dependent endopeptidases present in many leukocytes that have specific and selective activity against many components of the extracellular matrix which they degrade into fragments. MMP-9, MMP-2 and ADAM-33 are examples of proteases that have been most extensively studied in allergic inflammation because of their increased levels of expression in allergic inflammation or in the case of ADAM-33 genetic linkage to asthma. All MMPs are inhibited by related compounds called tissue inhibitors of metalloproteases (TIMPs). For example, TIMP-1 binds to both pro-MMP-9 and active MMP-9, inhibiting MMP-9 function.

In vivo studies of the allergic inflammatory response

Early phase response (EPR) and late phase response (LPR)

In allergic subjects the immune and inflammatory response to an allergen challenge can be investigated in the nose, lung, or skin. In allergic subjects the response to allergen challenge is characterized by an immediate or early phase response (EPR), which is followed in approximately 50% of adults and 70% of children by a late phase response (LPR) (see Fig. 1.32). The EPR is initiated by the release of mast cell mediators following allergen challenge of a sensitized individual. Although the spectrum of mediators is essentially the same in all tissues, the symptoms provoked are different due to differences in the anatomy of their target tissues (e.g. bronchoconstriction in the lower airways, rhinorrhoea and congestion in the nose, and a wheal and flare response in the skin). The EPR generally develops within approximately 10 minutes of allergen exposure, reaching a maximum at 30 minutes, and resolving within 1–2 hours. In the absence of further allergen inhalation, a LPR may also occur, reaching a maximum at 6–12 hours and resolving by 24 hours. The EPR results from IgE-dependent activation of mast cells which release preformed mediators including histamine, as well as newly generated lipid mediators including leukotrienes (LTC_4, LTD_4, and LTE_4), prostanoids [prostaglandins D_2, $F2\alpha$ (PGD_2, $PGF_{2\alpha}$), and thromboxane A_2 (TXA_2)].

A characteristic feature of the LPR is the recruitment of inflammatory cells particularly eosinophils, as well as CD4+ Th2 cells, mononuclear cells, and basophils. These inflammatory cells recruited from the circulation release cytokines and proinflammatory mediators. The profile of cytokines released during the LPR is characterized by the expression of Th2 cytokines (IL-4, IL-5, IL-9, IL-13) rather than Th1 cytokines [interferon-γ (IFN-γ, IL-12)]. Corticosteroids have an inhibitory effect on the LPR and also reduce the number of cells expressing IL-4 mRNA and IL-5 mRNA, and the number of eosinophils.

EPR and LPR in the lung

Inhalation of allergen by sensitized individuals results in an early phase response with airway narrowing which develops within 10–15 minutes, reaches a maximum within 30 minutes, and generally resolves within 1–3 hours response. The main clinical manifestation of the early phase response is dyspnea, chest tightness, wheezing, and cough. In some of these subjects, a late phase response occurs after 3–4 hours and reaches a maximum at 6–12 hours (Fig. 1.31). The mechanism of bronchoconstriction is complex and results from a combination of bronchial smooth muscle contraction, increased vascular permeability leading to oedema, and increased airway mucus production. Histamine, PGD_2, and CysLTs all have the ability to contract human bronchial smooth muscle. In addition to causing bronchoconstriction, histamine and the CysLTs can increase vascular permeability and stimulate mucus production. The LPR in the lung is associated with significant recruitment of eosinophils. Anti-IgE inhibits both the EPR as well as the LPR response in the lung. Interestingly, anti-IL-5 does not significantly inhibit the LPR response to allergen challenge.

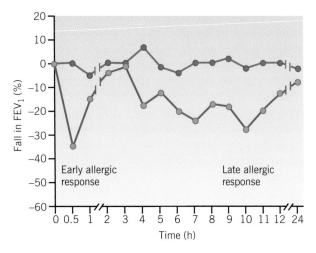

Fig. 1.31 Early and late phase responses in asthma. The asthmatic response to allergen inhalation challenge with house dust mite allergen (green line) and diluent control (red line), demonstrating both an early and a late phase allergic response. FEV_1, forced expiratory volume in 1 second.

EPR and LPR in the nose

In the nose, topical allergen challenge of sensitized individuals causes immediate nasal reactions involving itching, sneezing, congestion, and watery discharges. The early response usually abates within 1–3 hours. In contrast to the dual allergic response in the lower airways, distinct late phase responses are not common in the nose although low-grade nasal inflammation and symptoms may continue well beyond the first 3 hours after challenge with large amounts of allergen. Furthermore, nasal allergen challenge has a 'priming' effect, with the nasal mucosa exhibiting an increased responsiveness to histamine or to a second allergen challenge on the day after the initial challenge. Rhinorrhoea, caused by a combination of local vasodilatation and mucous gland stimulation, is largely histamine mediated, thus explaining the effectiveness of antihistamines in treating these symptoms. As most of the early phase obstruction to airflow in the upper airways is reversed by α-adrenergic receptor vasoconstrictor drugs, this suggests that acute filling of venous sinuses rather than tissue oedema is responsible for nasal blockage. Nasal congestion is poorly inhibited by antihistamines, suggesting that mediators other than histamine are playing a more prominent role.

EPR and LPR in the skin

Intradermal injection of allergen induces a characteristic 'triple response' characterized by an almost immediate reddening of the skin (histamine-mediated arteriolar vasodilatation) at the site of allergen injection, which is followed within 5–10 minutes by the development of an

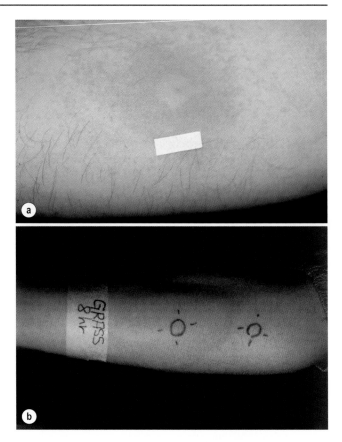

Fig. 1.32 The cutaneous response to allergen. (a) A wheal-and-flare response 10 minutes after the intradermal injection of allergen into a sensitized individual; (b) a late cutaneous response 8 hours after the intradermal injection of allergen into a sensitized individual.

area of oedema, or wheal (histamine-mediated increased permeability) (Fig. 1.32). The third component of the triple response is an area of erythema, or flare, around the wheal. This is initiated by the stimulation of histamine receptors on afferent non-myelinated nerves, which results in the release of neuropeptides with consequent vasodilatation and skin erythema. Histamine-induced nerve stimulation also results in itch. The size of the flare is again dose dependent and may measure several centimetres across. The wheal-and-flare generally resolves within about 30 minutes. However, in up to 50% of subjects challenged intradermally with a high dose of allergen the immediate reaction evolves into a late phase reaction characterized by an indurated erythematous inflammatory reaction. The latter reaches a peak at about 6–8 hours and often persists for 24 hours. The reduction in the size of the LPR to intradermal allergen challenge correlates well with the clinical response to subcutaneous allergen immunotherapy in patients with allergic rhinitis.

Mast cell dependence of EPR

The detection of extracellularly released mast-cell-derived mediators (i.e. histamine, PGD_2, tryptase) at sites of early phase responses, as well as the ability of mast-cell-directed therapies such as anti-IgE and cromolyn to block the early phase response provide evidence for the important role of the mast cell in the early phase response. At therapeutic doses antihistamines can inhibit approximately 75% of the skin wheal-and-flare response induced by intradermal allergen, suggesting an important role for histamine in this mast-cell-mediated event.

Leukotrienes and EPR and LPR

Pretreatment of patients with specific $CysLT_1$-receptor antagonists and LT-biosynthesis inhibitors significantly attenuate allergen-induced early asthmatic responses, as well as partially attenuate late asthmatic responses, providing evidence for a role of CysLTs in the development of allergen-induced responses. No studies with antileukotrienes have demonstrated complete protection against EPR.

Prostaglandins

Several prostaglandins are generated during episodes of allergic inflammation. These include stimulatory prostaglandins, such as PGD_2 and $PGF2\alpha$, which are potent bronchoconstrictors, and inhibitory prostaglandins, such as PGE_2, which can reduce allergen-induced bronchoconstrictor responses and attenuate the release of acetylcholine from airway nerves. PGD_2 is a cyclooxygenase product generated by mast-cell activation. PGD_2 binds to two different receptors: DP1 (the classic PGD_2 receptor) and DP2 or CRTH2 (a chemokine receptor expressed by Th2 cells). Based on this dual PGD_2 action, there has been renewed interest in determining whether blocking both these PGD_2 receptors will influence the clinical outcome in allergic disease.

Methods for studying the early and late phase reactions

Atopic subjects with mild asymptomatic allergic rhinitis or asthma can be challenged with an allergen to which the individual is sensitized in the nose or lower airway to understand the molecular and cellular pathways that are up-regulated by allergen challenge. In addition, pretreatment with a therapeutic intervention prior to allergen challenge can assist in determining whether the intervention reduces the EPR and/or LPR as well as effects on inflammation (cells, mediators measured in nasal lavage, sputum, or bronchoalveolar lavage), symptoms, and physiological end-points (rhinomanometry, FEV_1, methacholine airway responsiveness).

Conclusion

IgE and mast cells play a central role in the expression of allergic inflammation. In addition, Th2 cytokine responses and eosinophilic inflammation are a characteristic feature of chronic allergic inflammation. Cytokines, chemokines, and adhesion molecules play a key role in regulating the immune and inflammatory response in allergic inflammation. An improved understanding of the complex molecular mechanisms of allergic diseases will help to identify potential novel targets for therapeutic intervention. Anti-IgE, leukotriene antagonists, and anti-IL-5 are examples of therapies that have targeted specific pathways associated with allergic inflammation and provided important insight into the contribution of these pathways to the pathogenesis of individual diseases associated with allergic inflammation. Clinical trials with cytokine antagonists, chemokine inhibitors, adhesion molecule antagonists, or compounds that interfere with intracellulalar signalling pathways or the transcription of genes important to allergic inflammation will improve our understanding of the function of these individual molecules in allergic inflammation. The use of any of these antagonists in clinical practice will be dependent on their relative potency in inhibiting allergic inflammation (e.g. therapeutic efficacy), as well as evidence that they do not significantly impair host defence to infection or immune surveillance (e.g. side-effect profile).

Summary of important messages

- The key components of a well-functioning immune system include the ability to generate both innate and adaptive immune responses
- Th2 cells expressing IL-4, a switch factor for IgE synthesis, and IL-5, an eosinophil growth factor, are associated with allergic inflammation
- IgE antibodies affixed to high-affinity IgE receptors on mast cells and basophils play a central role in mediating allergic responses
- Eosinophils are bone-marrow-derived leukocytes that travel to tissue sites of allergic inflammation (i.e. nose, lung, skin)
- Cytokines, chemokines, and adhesion molecules play a key role in regulating the immune and inflammatory responses during episodes of allergic inflammation
- Anti-IgE, leukotriene antagonists, and anti-IL-5 are examples of therapies that have targeted specific pathways associated with allergic inflammation

Acknowledgement

The authors acknowledge the contributions of Natalija Novak, Thomas Bieber and Patrick G Holt (Ch. 19; 3rd edition), Catherine M Hawrylowicz, Donald W

MacGlashan, Hirohisa Saito, Hans-Uwe Simon, Andrew J Wardlaw (Ch. 21; 3rd edition), Burton Zweiman, Paul M O'Byrne, Carl GA Persson, Martin K Church (Ch. 22; 3rd edition) to elements of the contents of this chapter covered in the 3rd edition. The chapter has been substantially revised for this 4th edition.

Further reading

Bochner BS, Gleich GJ. What targeting eosinophils has taught us about their role in diseases. J Allergy Clin Immunol 2010; 126:16–25.

Finkelman FD, Hogan SP, Hershey GKK, et al. Importance of cytokines in murine allergic airway disease and human asthma. J Immunol 2010; 184:1663–1674.

Geissmann F, Manz MG, Jung S, et al. Development of monocytes, macrophages, and dendritic cells. Science 2010: 327:656–661.

Gould HJ, Sutton BJ. IgE in allergy and asthma today. Nat Rev Immunol 2008; 8:205–217.

Hotchkiss RS, Strasser A, McDunn JE, et al. Mechanisms of disease: cell death. N Engl J Med 2009; 361:1570–1583.

Jolly CJ, Cook AJ, Manis JP. Fixing DNA breaks during class switch recombination. J Exp Med 2008; 205:509–513.

Kelly M, Hwang JM, Kubes P. Modulating leukocyte recruitment in inflammation. J Allergy Clin Immunol 2007; 120:3–10.

Lambrecht BN, Hammad H. Biology of lung dendritic cells at the origin of asthma. Immunity 2009; 31:412–424.

Lloyd CM, Hawrylowicz CM. Regulatory T cells in asthma. Immunity 2009; 31:438–449.

Medoff BD, Thomase SY, Luster AD. T cell trafficking in allergic asthma: the ins and outs. Annu Rev Immunol 2008; 26:205–232.

Ochs HD, Oukka M, Torgerson TR. T_H17 cells and regulatory T cells in primary immunodeficiency diseases. J Allergy Clin Immunol 2009; 123:977–983.

Paul WE, Zhu J. How are T_H2-type immune responses initiated and amplified? Nat Rev Immunol 2010; 10:225–235.

Saenz SA, Taylor BC, Artis D. Welcome to the neighborhood: epithelial cell-derived cytokines license innate and adaptive immune responses at mucosal sites. Immunol Rev 2008; 226:172–190.

Stone KD, Prussin C, Metcalfe DD. IgE, mast cells, basophils, and eosinophils. J Allergy Clin Immunol 2010; 125:S73-S80.

Turvey SE, Broide DH. Innate immunity. J Allergy Clin Immunol 2010; 125: S24-S32.

The genetic basis of allergy and asthma

John W Holloway and Stephen T Holgate

DEFINITION

Allergic diseases cluster in families indicating an important role for susceptibility genes. Multiple genes interact with environmental factors to generate the different allergic phenotypes.

Introduction

In the twentieth century, a major theme in biomedical science was the 'nature vs nurture debate'. For most phenotypes and disease it is now recognized that both factors play an important role and it is the interaction between these factors that determines an individual's susceptibility to disease. The dawn of the new century has seen a revolution in our understanding of the genetic basis of common diseases such as obesity, diabetes, heart disease, cancer, and neuropsychiatric conditions. These diseases are termed 'complex genetic diseases' as they result from the effect of multiple genetic and interacting environmental factors (see Appendix 2.1, p. 50 for common genetic terms).

Like these other common conditions, the role of a heritable component to susceptibility to allergic disease has long been recognized, with atopy and the clinical manifestation of allergy such as asthma and atopic dermatitis resulting from the interaction between an individual's genetic make-up and their environmental exposures. Recent years have seen considerable progress in unravelling the contribution of specific genetic factors to an individual's susceptibility, subsequent development, and severity of allergic disease. This has resulted in increasing insight into novel areas of allergic disease pathophysiology. Furthermore, studies of gene–environment interaction have lead to greater insight into the importance of environmental triggers for the initiation, exacerbation, and persistence of allergic diseases. Studies of the timing of action of genetic variants in determining disease susceptibility have highlighted the importance of in utero development and early life in determining susceptibility to allergic disease. In the future, genetic discoveries in allergic disease will potentially lead to better endophenotyping, prognostication, prediction of treatment response, and insights into molecular pathways in order to develop more targeted therapy for these conditions.

Heritability of allergic disease

Heritability is the proportion of observed variation in a particular trait that can be attributed to inherited genetic factors in contrast to environmental ones. The fact that a disease has been observed to 'run in families' is insufficient evidence to begin molecular genetic studies because this can occur for a number of reasons, including common environmental exposure and biased ascertainment, as well as having a true genetic disposition. There are a number of approaches that can be taken to determine whether genetics contributes to a disease or disease phenotype of interest – including family studies, segregation analysis, twin and adoption studies, heritability studies, and population-based relative risk to relatives of probands.

In twin studies, heritability is estimated by comparing the concordance rates of monozygotic twins for particular traits with those of dizygotic twins for the same traits, with monozygotic twins being genetically identical (for nuclear DNA) and dizygotic twins (on average) sharing 50% of their segregating DNA variation in common. Therefore, a disease that has a genetic component is expected to show a higher rate of concordance in monozygotic than in dizygotic twins. In adoption studies, if the disease has a genetic basis the frequency of the disease should be higher in biologic relatives of probands than in members of their adopted family.

Family studies involve the estimation of the frequency of the disease in relatives of affected compared with unaffected individuals. The strength of the genetic effect can be measured as λ_R, where λ_R is the ratio of risk to relatives of type R (e.g. sibs, parents, offspring, etc.) compared with the population risk. The stronger the genetic effect, the higher is the value of λ. For example, for a recessive single gene mendelian disorder such as cystic fibrosis the value of λ is about 500; for a dominant disorder such as Huntington's disease it is about 5000. For complex disorders the values of λ are much lower e.g. 20–30 for multiple sclerosis, 15 for insulin-dependent diabetes mellitus (IDDM), and 4 to 5 for Alzheimer's disease. It is important to note though that λ is a function of both the strength of the genetic effect and the frequency of the disease in the population. Therefore a disease with a λ of 3 to 4 does not mean that genes are less important in that trait than in a trait with a λ of 30 to 40. A strong effect in a very common disease will have a smaller λ than the same strength of effect in a rare disease.

In 1860, Henry Hyde Salter in his magnus opus, *On asthma its pathology and treatment*, wrote 'Is asthma hereditary? I think there can be no doubt that it is.' Subsequent to this, many studies have now conclusively shown that susceptibility to asthma and other allergic diseases has a heritable component.

The results of many studies have now established that both atopy and atopic disease such as asthma, rhinitis, and eczema have strong genetic components. Family studies have shown an increased prevalence of atopy, and phenotypes associated with atopy, among the relatives of atopic compared with non-atopic subjects. Studies of specific genetic diseases have shown that there is a striking association between asthma in the parent and asthma in the child, between hay fever in the parent and hay fever in the child, and between eczema in the parent and eczema in the child, suggesting that 'end-organ sensitivity' or the type of allergic disease that an allergic individual will develop is controlled by specific genetic factors, differing from those that determine susceptibility to atopy *per se*.

Many twin studies have shown a significant increase in concordance for atopy among monozygotic twins as compared with dizygotic twins, providing evidence for a genetic component to that condition. Atopic asthma has also been widely studied, and both twin and family studies have shown a strong heritable component to this phenotype, although estimates of the contribution of genetics to atopy and allergic disease susceptibility vary widely from 40 to >80% and it is apparent that the genetic contribution to risk of allergic disease such as asthma (λ_{Sib} ~2–3) is weaker than that of other common conditions such as rheumatoid arthritis (λ_{Sib} 8), type 1 diabetes (λ_{Sib} 14) and Crohn disease (λ_{Sib} 30) . The heritability of many allergic disease related phenotypes has also been studied and has shown that genetic factors influence not just disease susceptibility per se but all aspects of disease. For example, for asthma, heritability studies have shown there is genetic influence in many aspects, from susceptibility to atopy and regulation of total and specific IgE levels, to blood eosinophil levels, susceptibility to asthma per se, degree of bronchial hyperresponsiveness, severity of asthma symptoms, and even risk of mortality from asthma. Genetic factors also play a major role in determining asthma remission, with a family history of both atopy and asthma being associated with lower rates of remission.

Once familial aggregation with a probable genetic aetiology for a disease has been established, the mode of inheritance can be determined by observing the pattern of inheritance of a disease or trait by observing how it is distributed within families. For example, is there evidence of a single major gene, and is it dominantly or recessively inherited? Segregation analysis of allergic disease phenotype failed to find evidence of any consistent clear inheritance pattern for a number of allergic phenotypes and diseases. This confirms that, in contrast to rare monogenic diseases such as Netherton syndrome, *ichthyosis vulgaris*, and hyper-IgE syndrome, whose phenotypes include aspects of allergic disease such as high serum IgE levels and atopic dermatitis, common forms of these conditions are determined by the actions, and the interactions, of multiple genetic factors (Fig. 2.1).

Finding genes for allergic disease

Variation in DNA sequences occurs once in approximately every 200–500 base pairs in the human genome.

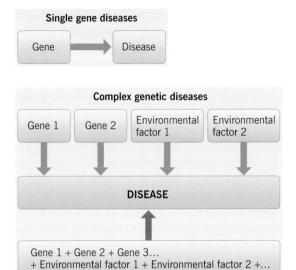

Fig. 2.1 Monogenetic versus complex genetic disease. Single gene diseases such as cystic fibrosis result from mutations in a single gene. Complex, or polygenic, diseases arise from the additive effect of multiple risk variants in multiple genes together with environmental effects.

This means that in every human population most genes can be expected to show variation. Sequence variations (mutations) occurring in over 1% of the population are termed 'polymorphisms' and those that occur in less than 1% are termed 'rare alleles'. Polymorphism in DNA sequence between individuals can take many forms including differences at a single base pair involving substitution, insertion, or deletion of a single nucleotide (commonly termed 'single nucleotide polymorphisms' or SNPs) and repetition, insertion, or deletion of longer stretches of DNA ranging from a few base pairs to many thousands of base pairs, often termed 'copy number variations' or CNVs. The different versions of the nucleotide sequence present at any one location in the genome (locus) are termed 'alleles'. Polymorphisms form the basis of human diversity, including our responses to environmental stimuli. Genetic epidemiology has provided statistical methods for measuring the effects of gene polymorphisms on a clinical phenotype.

There have been a number of approaches utilized to identify genetic factors that contribute to allergic disease susceptibility. The approach utilized will depend on a number of variables including the phenotype to be analysed, the population available for analysis (case-control cohorts, or family cohorts) and the genetic approach to be utilized.

In general there are two broad approaches to genetic analysis: linkage and association analysis. Linkage analysis involves proposing a model to explain the inheritance pattern of phenotypes and genotypes observed in a pedigree. When two genes are close together they are said to be linked. Therefore, alleles at such loci have a tendency to pass together into each gamete. Thus any disturbance of independent assortment, as defined by Mendel's second law, provides an important clue that two genes are linked. If the chromosomal location of one of the genes is known, then the other can be mapped to the same region. If the genetic variant predisposing to the disease of interest and the genetic marker loci are on separate chromosomes, independent assortment will occur and the disease and markers should be found as often together as apart in the offspring. If the disease and marker loci lie close together on the same chromosome, independent assortment will not occur and the disease and marker will occur together in each child unless they are separated by crossover at meiosis. As the distance between the disease locus and a marker locus increases so the chance of recombination in the interval between them increases and the proportion of recombinant increases. If the disease and marker loci are separated by a considerable distance on the same chromosome, then crossover between the loci is highly likely and the disease and marker traits will occur separately in each recombinant but together in non-recombinants.

The evidence for linkage of a genomic region to a phenotype of interest is usually expressed in terms of the ratio of their odds of the two hypotheses (linkage or non-linkage), the likelihood ratio (LR), or more equivalently by the lod score (Z), where $Z = \log_{10}(LR)$. Both parametric (involving prior specification of a genetic model) and, more commonly in complex disease, non-parametric linkage approaches such as allele sharing can be taken. Allele-sharing methods test whether the inheritance pattern of a particular chromosomal region is inconsistent with random mendelian segregation by showing that pairs of affected relatives inherit identical copies of the region more often than would be expected by chance. Affected sib-pair analysis is the simplest form of allele-sharing analysis. Two sibs can show identical-by-descent (IBD) sharing for no, one, or two copies of any locus (with a 1:2:1 distribution expected under random segregation). Excess allele sharing can be measured with a simple χ^2 test.

Association studies do not examine inheritance patterns of alleles; rather, they are case-control studies based on a comparison of allele frequencies between groups of affected and unaffected individuals from a population. A particular allele is said to be associated with the trait if it occurs at a significantly higher frequency among affected individuals than in the control group. The odds ratio of the trait in individuals is then assessed as the ratio of the frequency of the allele in the affected population compared with the unaffected population.

It is important to remember with association studies that there are a number of reasons leading to an association between a phenotype and a particular allele (Box 2.1).

Box 2.1 Key concepts

Explanations for association (or lack of association) between polymorphism and allergic disease phenotype

A: Positive association

Causal link

- The polymorphism tested directly affects gene(s) expression or protein function, resulting in increased susceptibility

Linkage disequilibrium

- The polymorphism tested is not directly casual but is in linkage disequilibrium with an adjacent polymorphism that is. Linkage disequilibrium refers to the non-random association of alleles at two (or more) loci; the allele of one polymorphism in an LD block (haplotype) can predict the allele of adjacent (not genotyped) polymorphism. The size of the LD blocks depends on the recombination rate in that region and the time since the first disease-contributing variant arose in an ancestral individual in that population.

Population stratification

- Population stratification is the presence of a systematic difference in allele frequencies between subpopulations in a population due to different ancestry. Allele frequencies often differ between populations of different ancestry, hence if case and control populations are not adequately matched for ancestry, this can lead to false positive associations. This can be controlled for by the assessment of ancestry using polymorphisms known to differ in allele frequency between populations (ancestry informative markers, AIMs) or through the use of family-based association.

Type I error

- A positive association may represent a false positive observation. Especially in studies of multiple SNPs

and/or phenotypes it is important to consider the strength of p-values observed in the context of the number of statistical tests undertaken.

B: No observed association

Variants assessed do not contribute to phenotype

- The variants assessed do not contribute to the heritability of the phenotype assessed. It is important to recognize that this does not exclude the encoded protein from playing an important role in the pathogenesis of the disease; rather it only indicates that genetic variation in the gene does not contribute to it.

Type II error

- No association observed owing to lack of power. The effect size for common variants on susceptibility to complex disease is typically small (OR < 1.5). The majority of studies are not adequately powered to detect an effect of this size.

Failure to replicate previous report of positive association

- There are a number of reasons why a study may fail to replicate a previous report of positive association between a polymorphism and a phenotype. Apart from the consideration of whether either of the studies represents a false negative or positive association, it is important to determine whether the studies truly replicate one another. For example, were they carried out in populations of similar genetic ancestry, or with similar environmental exposures? Were exactly the same polymorphisms studies in the gene and was the phenotype tested the same?

Source: Holloway JW, Yang IA, Holgate ST. Genetics of allergic disease. J Allergy Clin Immunol 2010; 125(2 suppl 2):S81–94.

- A positive association between the phenotype and the allele will occur if the allele is the cause of, or contributes to, the phenotype. This association would be expected to be replicated in other populations with the same phenotype, unless there are several different alleles at the same locus contributing to the same phenotype, in which case association would be difficult to detect, or if the trait was predominantly the result of different genes in the other population (genetic heterogeneity), or depended on interaction with an environmental exposure not present in the replication population.

- Positive associations may also occur between an allele and a phenotype if that particular allele is in linkage disequilibrium with the phenotype-causing allele. Linkage disequilibrium is the correlation between nearby variants such that the alleles at neighbouring polymorphisms (observed on the same

chromosome) are associated within a population more often than if they were unlinked. Thus, an allele may show positive association with disease if the allele tends to occur on the same parental chromosome that also carries the trait-causing mutation more often than would be expected by chance.

- Positive association between an allele and a trait can also be artefactual as a result of recent population admixture. In a population of mixed ancestry, any trait present in a higher frequency in a subgroup of the population (e.g. a particular ethnic group) will show positive association with an allele that also happens to be more common in that population subgroup. To avoid spurious association arising through admixture, studies should be performed in large, relatively homogeneous populations.

Other considerations in assessing the significance of association studies include whether the size of the study was adequately powered if negative results are reported, whether the cases and controls were appropriately matched, which phenotypes were measured (and which have not) and how they were measured and whether reported statistical evidence levels have been adjusted to take account of multiple testing.

Candidate gene versus genome-wide analysis

There are two main approaches to the study of the genetics of disease: the candidate gene approach and the genome-wide or hypothesis-independent approach (Fig. 2.2). In the candidate gene approach, genetic variation in individual genes is directly assessed for association with the disease phenotype of interest. In general, candidate genes are selected for analysis because of a known or postulated role for the encoded product of the gene in the disease process or an expression pattern associated with the disease. Polymorphisms within the gene that are believed to be functional (i.e. affecting gene expression or encoded protein function), or that are selected for maximal information on the basis of linkage disequilibrium patterns surrounding the gene (often termed 'tagging SNPs'), are then tested for association with the disease or phenotype in question. A hybrid approach is the selection of candidate genes based not only on their function but also on their position within a genetic region previously linked to the disease (positional candidate). However, by definition, the candidate gene approach is not capable of identifying all the major genetic factors predisposing towards a disease or identifying role for novel gene products in disease pathogenesis.

If, as in most complex disorders, the exact biochemical or physiological basis of the disease is unknown, it is often desirable to undertake a hypothesis-independent approach to the identification disease genes that considers the entire genome. One such method is to test genetic markers (most commonly microsatellites – short repetitive stretches of DNA that often vary between individuals) randomly spaced throughout the entire genome for linkage with the disease phenotype. If linkage is found between a particular marker and the phenotype, then further typing of genetic markers including SNPs and association analysis will enable the critical region to be further narrowed; the genes positioned in this region can be examined for possible involvement in the disease process and the presence of disease-causing genetic variants in affected individuals. This approach is often termed 'positional cloning', or 'genome scanning' if the whole genome is examined in this manner. Although this approach requires no assumptions to be made about the particular gene involved in genetic susceptibility to the

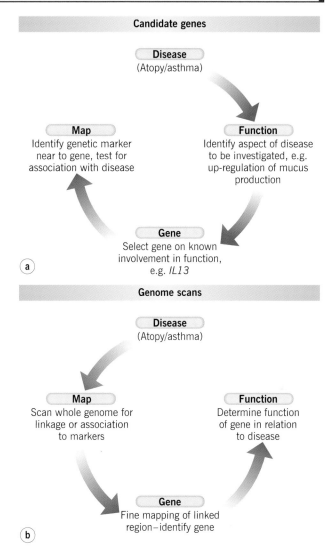

Fig. 2.2 Candidate gene versus genome-wide analysis. (a) In candidate gene analysis genetic variation in a gene selected on the basis of a known (or suspected) role in disease pathogenesis is tested for association with disease. (b) In genome-wide approaches (whether by linkage analysis in families or by genome-wide association studies), genetic variation across the genome is genotyped to identify a genetic region that underlies disease susceptibility. The genes in the region can then be identified and how their encoded products contribute to disease pathogenesis established.

disease in question, it does require considerable molecular genetic analysis to be undertaken in large family cohorts, involving considerable time, resources, and expense.

More recently, positional cloning by linkage analysis in family cohorts has been superseded by the population-based genome-wide association study (GWAS) approach. This approach tests for association between SNPs evenly spaced throughout the genome and the disease or phenotype in question and, like linkage, is also an assumption-free approach. However, unlike positional cloning by linkage, GWAS does not require the recruitment and phenotyping of large family-based samples; rather, by the utilization of case-control cohorts it achieves much greater statistical power for the same number of individuals. The advent of the GWAS approach has been made possible by several technological developments in recent years including the characterization and mapping of millions of SNP variants in the human genome and technological advances in array-based SNP genotyping technologies that have made possible the simultaneous determination of the genotype of hundreds of thousands of SNPs throughout the genome of an individual. Genome-wide association studies have now revolutionized the study of genetic factors in complex common disease. For hundreds of phenotypes – from common diseases such as Crohn's disease and myocardial infarction to physiological measurements such as birth weight, height, and body mass index (BMI) and biological measurements such as circulating lipid levels and blood eosinophil levels – GWAS have provided compelling statistical associations for hundreds of different loci in the human genome.

Whether by linkage or GWAS, the identification of an associated disease is only the beginning of the work required to understand its role in the disease pathogenesis. Further molecular genetic studies will be required to identify the precise genetic polymorphism that is exerting functional consequences for the gene's expression or function, as opposed to those that are merely in linkage disequilibrium with the causal SNP. It is unlikely that the SNP showing the strongest association in the initial study will be the causal locus, as SNPs are chosen to provide maximal coverage of other variation in that region of the genome and not on biological function. Therefore, often fine mapping and haplotype (combinations of alleles at adjacent polymorphisms) analysis of the region will be undertaken with the aim of identifying the causal locus. Gene expression analysis, both comparisons of a selection of cases with controls and inter-individual comparisons of different genotypes, can provide further evidence for a gene's involvement in disease. If linkage disequilibrium prevents the identification of a specific gene in a region of high linkage disequilibrium spanning multiple genes, then the analysis of different racial and ethnic populations may aid localization.

Often the gene identified may be completely novel and cell and molecular biology studies will be needed to understand the gene product's role in the disease and to define genotype:phenotype correlations. Furthermore, by using cohorts with information available on environmental exposures, it may be possible to define how the gene product may interact with the environment to cause disease. Ultimately, knowledge of the gene's role in disease pathogenesis may lead to the development of novel therapeutics.

How do genetic studies increase understanding of allergic disease?

In the two decades since the first report of linkage between polymorphic markers on chromosome 11 with atopy, there have now been over 1000 published studies whose aim is to identify genetic factors that are associated with allergic disease or related phenotypes. This explosion of activity can be attributed, in part, to the insights that genetic studies can bring to our understanding of disease pathogenesis (Box 2.2).

Insight into disease pathogenesis

One of the keys provided by identification of genetic susceptibility factors by disease is an increased insight into disease pathogenesis. The fact that genetic variation within the population that alters either a gene's expression or the function of an encoded protein is associated with increased risk of disease suggests that the gene's product, whether that be a functional non-coding RNA

Box 2.2 Key concepts

What insights can genetics studies of allergic disease provide?

Greater understanding of disease pathogenesis
- Identification of novel genes and pathways leading to new pharmacological targets for developing therapeutics

Identification of environmental factors that interact with an individual's genetic make-up to initiate disease, and confirmation of causality of environmental factors through mendelian randomization
- Targeted prevention of disease by environmental modification, possibly targeted to genetically at risk individuals

Identification of susceptible Individuals
- Early-in-life screening and targeting of preventative therapies to at-risk individuals to prevent disease

Targeting of therapies
- Subclassification of disease on the basis of genetics and targeting of specific therapies based on this classification
- Identification of individuals at risk of severe disease and targeting of preventative treatments
- Determination of the likelihood of an individual responding to, or suffering adverse reactions to, a particular therapy (pharmacogenetics) and individualized treatment plans

Adapted from Holloway JW, Yang IA, Holgate ST. Genetics of allergic disease. J Allergy Clin Immunol 2010; 125(2 suppl 2):S81–94.

or a protein, must play an important role in the disease pathogenesis. Thus genetic studies, especially hypothesis-independent genome-wide approaches, have the potential to identify novel biological mechanisms underlying disease, potentially leading to new pharmacologic targets for therapeutics. For example, the first novel asthma susceptibility locus to be identified by a GWAS approach contains the *ORMDL3* and *GSDMB* genes on chromosome 17q12-21. The observation of association between polymorphisms at this locus has been extensively replicated in subsequent studies and the polymorphisms are associated with altered expression of both genes. Although the cellular function of either of the proteins encoded by these genes is unknown, the genetic observations suggest that they must play an important role in asthma pathogenesis. Furthermore, the observation that this genetic locus has been associated with a number of chronic immune-mediated disorders such as ulcerative colitis, type 1 diabetes, primary biliary cirrhosis, and Crohn's disease suggests a common mechanism may operate in these conditions. The recent observation that Orm family proteins mediate sphingolipid homeostasis and regulate endoplasmic reticulum-mediated Ca^{2+} signalling suggests a new avenue to explore pathogenic mechanisms in asthma.

Gene–environment interaction

It is clear that allergic diseases, as is the case for all complex genetic disorders, arise from the interaction between individuals' genetic susceptibility and their cumulative environmental exposures during the life course (Fig. 2.3). A range of inhaled and ingested environmental factors have been hypothesized to contribute to the development of allergic disease, including allergens, diet, respiratory viruses, air pollutants, environmental tobacco smoke, endotoxin, and occupational exposures.

Studies that focus on the interaction between genetic factors and environmental exposure increase understanding of disease in several ways.

Firstly, by adding environmental exposure as a cofactor into the analysis of the effect of genetic polymorphisms on disease outcomes, it is possible for researchers to explain a proportion of the variability in observed differences in association between populations who may differ in environmental exposure. Furthermore, an observed synergistic interaction between gene and environmental exposure provides insight into how both the environmental effect and genetic effect cause disease. For example, recent studies have shown the association between SNPs in the susceptibility locus on chromosome 17q21 encompassing the *ORMDL3/GSDMB* genes has been shown to be confined to early onset asthma, and in particular those who were exposed to environmental tobacco smoke in early life. The association of these 17q21 variants is also enhanced in those children who experience respiratory infections before the age of 2 years, with the strongest association in those children exposed to both tobacco smoke and respiratory infections.

Secondly, the use of genetic epidemiology is likely to present real opportunities for solving problems of casual inference in observational epidemiology. Epidemiological studies of environmental exposures may identify spurious causes of disease due to confounding by behavioural, physiological, and socioeconomic factors related both to exposures and to disease end points. For example, the epidemiological findings that hormone replacement therapy protects against coronary heart disease, and vitamin E and vitamin C reduce risk of cardiovascular disease, have all been refuted by randomized controlled trials (RCTs) and have raised concerns about the value of epidemiological studies. One solution to this is the use of mendelian randomization. This approach is based on Mendel's second law that inheritance of one trait is

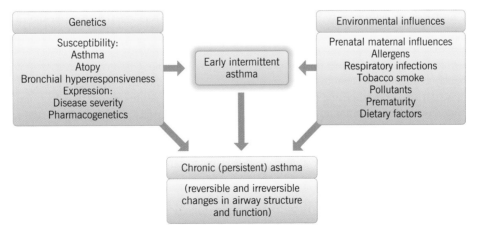

Fig. 2.3 Gene–environment interactions in the pathogenesis of asthma. In a complex disease such as asthma, disease is a result of complex interactions between inherited susceptibility genes and environmental exposures throughout the life course that determine not only disease initiation, but also disease progression, severity, and response to treatment.

independent of inheritance of other traits. It uses common genetic polymorphisms that are known to influence exposure patterns (such as availability of dietary nutrients such as vitamin E or D) or have effects equivalent to those produced by modifiable exposures (such as raised blood cholesterol concentration). Associations between genetic variants and outcome are not generally confounded by behavioural or environmental exposures. Thus if a genetic factor that modulates exposure to the environment [e.g. apolipoprotein E (apo E) for cholesterol or vitamin D receptor polymorphisms] modulates the effect of the exposure on outcome, it strengthens casual inference for the exposure of interest. The utilization of a mendelian randomization approach is likely to be of value in the future for increasing evidence for causality for a range of environmental exposures shown to be associated with increased risk of allergic disease, from farm exposure and diet to aeroallergen and air pollution exposure.

For example, pattern recognition receptors such as CD14 and Toll-like receptor 4 (TLR4) are involved in the recognition and clearance of bacterial endotoxin (LPS), by activating a cascade of host innate immune responses. Single nucleotide polymorphisms alter the biology of these receptors and could influence the early life origins of asthma, when the immune system is developing. Polymorphisms in CD14, TLR4, and other Toll-like receptor genes have been shown to modify the associations with risk of developing atopy and asthma, particularly in the presence of country living and farm milk consumption or household LPS exposure. Such studies indicate that the protective effect of rural lifestyle may be, in part, determined by the effect of early LPS exposure on the developing immune system.

Studies assessing the effects of air pollution on asthma susceptibility have found variable results. However gene–environment studies of polymorphisms in genes encoding metabolizing enzymes such as the glutathione-S-transferase genes (*GST*) have shown that these also influence the effects of ambient air pollution on asthma risk during childhood, particularly when controlled for levels of ozone and diesel exhaust particles.

Supporting evidence for a direct effect of prenatal acetaminophen exposure during pregnancy on subsequent risk of childhood asthma and wheezing has recently been provided by the observation that the effects of the exposure are modified by maternal (thus excluding confounding of postnatal exposure) polymorphisms affecting oxidant responses (a plausible biological response to acetaminophen).

Thus future identification of the factors that influence variability to environmental exposure would help to identify at-risk groups who would benefit most from preventive strategies. This identification of at-risk groups, the degree of their sensitivity to exposure, and their frequency in the population will aid in the cost–benefit

analysis of 'safe' exposure levels in the public health setting.

What is known about the genetics of allergic disease

Atopy

Although most genetic studies of allergic disease have focussed on clinical manifestations of atopy such as asthma or atopic dermatitis, there have been many hundreds of candidate gene association studies undertaken that examined association with phenotypes of atopy, specific IgE responses, and total serum IgE levels. A number of genes have shown consistent association with atopy phenotype, for instance genes related to theTh2 immune response such as IL-4, IL-13, IL-4 receptor-α (*IL4RA*), and *STAT6*.

More recently, the use of the genome-wide association approach has provided significant insights into the genetic basis of an atopic predisposition per se. For example, a GWAS analysis of 1530 individuals to identify loci associated with serum IgE levels and allergic sensitization showed strong association between functional variants in the gene encoding the alpha chain of the high-affinity receptor for IgE (*FCER1A*) on chromosome 1q23 and both of these phenotypes. In addition this study also confirmed previous candidate gene studies that implicated variants in both *STAT6* and the genetic region on chromosome 5q31 that contains the genes encoding the typical Th2 cytokines IL-4 and IL-13. The exact causal polymorphism at the locus is unclear as there have been multiple polymorphisms identified in the promoters of both genes that regulate their transcriptional levels. In addition, both of these genes together with the nearby cytokine gene *IL5* appear to be coordinately regulated, through the actions of regulatory locus control elements extending into the adjacent *RAD50* gene.

Another atopy-related phenotype to be examined using a GWAS approach is blood eosinophil counts. In an Icelandic population, polymorphism in proinflammatory cytokine genes, including *IL1RL1* and the gene encoding the Th2-promoting cytokine IL-33, alongside those that encode molecules regulating haematopoietic progenitor cell differentiation and proliferation such as *MYB*, were shown to be associated with base-line blood eosinophil counts.

As might be expected, loci identified in both these studies are also associated with disease phenotypes involving Th2-mediated immunity or a role for eosinophils. For example, in the Icelandic population several of the loci associated with blood eosinophil levels were also associated with asthma and myocardial infarction. Variation within the *IL4-IL13* locus has long been recognized as being associated with a wide range of atopy and atopic disease phenotypes. This overlap between genetic variation identified as predisposing to atopy and that underlying asthma is not surprising given current understanding of the role played by IgE and Th2-mediated immune responses in the pathogenesis of allergic disease, and studies of heritability that have suggested that genes that predispose to atopy overlap with those that predispose to asthma.

Asthma

There are many hundreds of studies published that examine polymorphism in several hundred genes for association with asthma and related phenotypes such as airway hyperresponsiveness, bronchodilator response, and lung function. An increasing number of genes have been also identified as asthma susceptibility genes using hypothesis-independent genome-wide linkage, and more recently GWAS approaches.

Positional cloning by linkage

To date, several genes have been identified as the result of positional cloning using a genome-wide scan for allergic disease phenotypes including for example *ADAM33*, *DPP10*, *PHF11*, *HLAG*, *OPN*, *NSPR1 (GPRA)*, *UPAR*, and *IRAKM* for asthma, and *PCDH1* for bronchial hyperresponsiveness. The identification of these genes, most of which had not been implicated in allergic disease previously, has revealed the importance of utilizing hypothesis-independent approaches to identify susceptibility genes. Furthermore, unlike many candidate gene studies, the susceptibility genes identified through positional cloning have, in general, been more likely to be replicated in subsequent studies of additional cohorts. Despite the success of such positional-cloning studies, in general linkage analysis for allergic disease phenotypes has proved to be slow and expensive and the majority of studies, despite recruiting several hundred families, have proved to be underpowered to identify susceptibility genes for complex disease.

Genome-wide association studies

There have now been several genome-wide association studies performed with great success in asthma. The first novel asthma susceptibility locus to be identified by a GWAS approach was on chromosome 17q12-21.1 (Fig. 2.4). In this study, 317000 SNPs were genotyped in 994 subjects with childhood onset asthma and 1243 non-asthmatic controls. After adjustments for quality control, 7 SNPs remained above the 1% false discovery rate (FDR) threshold and all mapped to a region spanning 100000 base pairs on chromosome 17. Replication of the findings was achieved by genotyping nine of the associated in 2320 subjects (200 asthmatic cases and 2120 controls) with 5 of the SNPs being significantly associated

with disease. In order to prioritize which of the several genes at this locus as candidates for further functional studies, the association of the diseases associated SNPs with gene expression has been examined and this has implicated both the *ORMDL3* and *GSDMB* genes. Importantly, many subsequent studies in multiple ethnically diverse populations have now replicated the association between variation in the 17q21 genomic region and childhood asthma. Other asthma susceptibility genes identified using GWAS have included the phosphodiesterase 4D (*PDE4D*) gene, involved in airway smooth muscle contraction, the gene *TLE4* on chromosome encoding a transcription factor implicated in cell fate decision and boundary formation, and *DENND1B*, a gene that is expressed by natural killer cells and dendritic cells and encodes a protein that interacts with the tumour necrosis factor alpha (TNF-α) receptor. Most recently, the GABRIEL study, which undertook genome-wide association analysis of 10365 cases and 16110 controls, not only confirmed a role for the chromosome 17q21 locus but also highlighted a number of genes involved in inflammatory responses such as *IL1RL1* and *IL18R1*, members of the interleukin 1 (IL-1) receptor family on chromosome 2, and the genes encoding the Th2-promoting cytokine IL-33 (*IL33*) and the SMAD3 intracellular signalling protein. In occupational asthma, researchers using GWAS to identify the determinants of asthma in workers exposed to toluene-diisocyante identified multiple polymorphisms of the alpha-T-catenin gene (*CTNNA3*) as strongly associated with disease. These polymorphisms were associated with increased bronchial hyperresponsiveness (BHR), increased specific IgG to CK19, which may be an intermediate phenotype of TDI-asthma and lower CTNNA3 mRNA expression.

These studies show the power of the GWAS approach for identifying complex disease susceptibility variants and the number is likely to rapidly increase in near future. However, as for other complex diseases such as Crohn's disease and diabetes mellitus (which have been extensively studied using GWAS approaches), the results from studies performed to date do not fully explain the heritability of common complex disease. It is thought that this inability to find all the genetic factors underlying disease susceptibility may be explained by limitations of GWAS, such as the presence of other variants in the genome not captured by the current generation of genome-wide genotyping platforms, analyses not adjusted for gene–environment and gene–gene (epistasis) interactions, or epigenetic changes in gene expression.

Genetic studies of asthma increase understanding of disease pathogenesis

The study of the genetic basis of asthma has revealed astonishing insights into the pathogenesis of this complex condition. Initially, most candidate gene studies of asthma

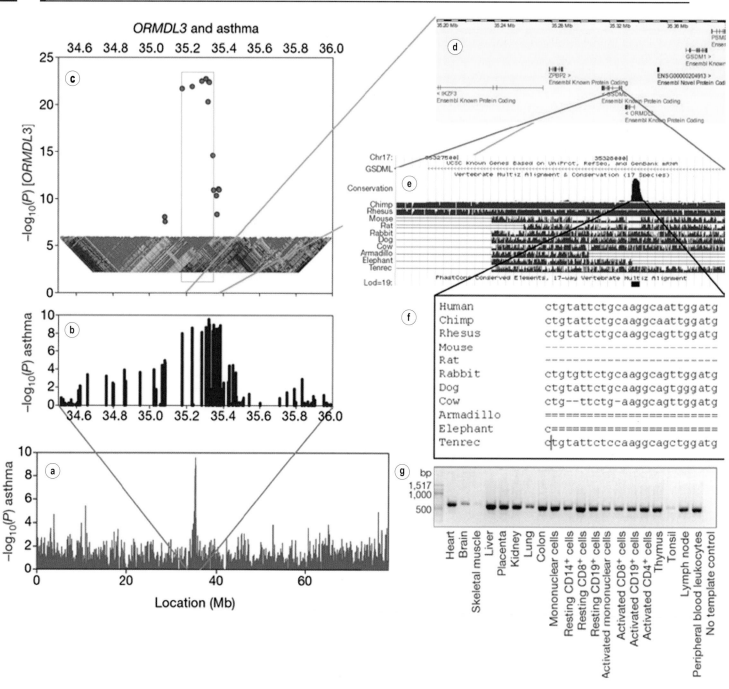

Fig. 2.4 Identification of ORMDL3 on chromosome 17q21 as an asthma susceptibility gene. This figure shows how a susceptibility gene is identified using a genome-wide association approach. Following typing of 317 000 SNPs across the genome (not shown), Moffatt et al identified a number of polymorphisms on chromosome 17 to be strongly associated with asthma. Panel (a) shows the level of significance of association with asthma for SNPs in a 80 million base pair region of chromosome 17 and this is shown in more detail in panel (b). (c) To aid identification of the causal gene at this locus, the authors then examined the association between the same SNPs and *ORMDL3* transcript abundance in EBV-transformed B-cell lines. Panel (d) shows a plot of linkage disequilibrium between markers, with red indicating high linkage disequilibrium and blue denoting low. The central island of linkage disequilibrium, which contains maximum association to *ORMDL3* and asthma, is contained within the grey rectangle. (e) Genes contained within the associated interval. Panel (f) shows a plot of sequence homology between the human genome and a number of other species from the region of maximum association, with increased homology suggesting conservation of sequence motifs throughout evolution, implying functionality. SNPs showing maximum association to *ORMDL3* levels lie within the first intron of the neighbouring *GSDML* gene. This non-coding sequence shows significant homology between species (f), and contains an element with high homology to the proinflammatory transcription factor C/EBPb sequence homology from intron I of *GSDML*. Another way to prioritize genes in a region of maximal association is to test for expression in disease-relevant tissues; panel (g) shows RT-PCR analysis of *ORMDL3* expression in a range of tissues. (Reprinted with permission of Macmillan Publishers Ltd: Nature from Moffatt MF, Kabesch M, Liang L, et al. Genetic variants regulating ORMDL3 expression contribute to the risk of childhood asthma. Nature 2007; 448:470–473, copyright 2007.)

were focused on association of functional polymorphisms in components of Th2-mediated immune responses. For example, the gene encoding the Th2 effector cytokine IL-13 is one of the genes most consistently associated with asthma and related phenotypes. Given the importance of Th2-mediated inflammation in allergic disease, and the biological roles of IL-13, including switching B cells to produce IgE, wide-ranging effects on epithelial cells, fibroblasts, and smooth muscle promoting airway remodelling, and mucus production, *IL13* is a strong biological candidate gene. Furthermore, it is also a strong positional candidate. The gene encoding IL-13 and early linkage studies also strongly implicated the genetic region containing the Th2 cytokine gene cluster on chromosome 5q31 as containing an asthma susceptibility gene. Several functional polymorphisms of *IL13* have been characterized. These include promoter polymorphisms such as the -1112 C/T variant that appears to alter transcription factor binding, and an amino acid polymorphism involving a single base pair change that results in the substitution of glycine for arginine at amino acid 131 (110 in the mature protein). This has been shown to alter the affinity of IL-13 for the decoy receptor IL13Rα2, increase functional activity through IL13Rα1, and enhance stability of the molecule in plasma.

Polymorphism of a number of other genes encoding either proteins regulating Th2 T-cell production such GATA-binding protein 3 (GATA-3), T-bet, the transcription factor necessary for Th1 cell development (encoded by the gene *TBX21*), and the cytokine IL-4, its receptor IL-4Rα, and downstream signal transducer STAT-6 have also all been repeatedly associated with increased susceptibility to asthma and related phenotypes, and there is evidence that there may be a synergistic effect on disease risk in inheriting more than one of these variants.

Although studies of these biological candidate genes have increased understanding of the genetic basis of asthma susceptibility, they have not given new insight into the biological mechanisms important in asthma, as a role of the proteins encoded by these genes is well established in asthma in the absence of genetic studies. However, the startling observation from genetic studies of asthma, especially genes identified through hypothesis-independent genome-wide approaches, is that genes encoding proteins involved in Th2-mediated immune responses are not the only, or even the most important, factors underlying asthma susceptibility. It is clear from heritability studies of allergic disease that the propensity to develop atopy is influenced by factors different than those that influence disease clinical manifestations of allergic disease such as asthma. However, these disease factors require interaction with atopy (or something else) to trigger disease. For example, in asthma bronchoconstriction is triggered mostly by an allergic response to inhaled allergen accompanied by an eosinophilic

inflammation in the lungs, but, in some people who may have 'asthma susceptibility genes' but not atopy, asthma is triggered by other exposures such as toluene diisocyanate. It is possible to group the genes identified as contributing to asthma into four broad groups (Fig. 2.5).

Firstly, there is a group of genes that are involved in directly modulating response to environmental exposures. These include genes encoding components of the innate immune system that interact with levels of microbial exposure to alter risk of developing allergic immune responses such as the genes encoding components of the LPS response pathway such as *CD14* and *TLR4*, highlighting the importance of innate immunity in asthma. Interactions between genes and environment will be discussed further below. Other environment response genes include detoxifying enzymes such as the glutathione-S-transferase genes that modulate the effect of exposures involving oxidant stress, such as tobacco smoke and air pollution.

The second major group is a group of genes involved in maintaining the integrity of the epithelial barrier at the mucosal surface and signalling of the epithelium to the immune system following environmental exposure. Like the role of filaggrin in the epidermal barrier (see below) genes encoding chitinases such as AMCase and YKL-40 appear to play an important role in modulating allergic inflammation and are produced in increased levels by the epithelium and alternatively activated macrophages in patients with asthma. The gene *PCDH1*, encoding protocadherin-1, a member of a family of cell adhesion molecules and expressed in the bronchial epithelium, has also been identified as a susceptibility gene for BHR. IL-33, identified by both candidate gene and genome-wide approaches, is produced by the airway epithelial in response to damage and drives production of Th2-associated cytokines such as IL-4, IL-5, and IL-13.

The third group of genes is those that regulate the immune response, including those regulating Th1/Th2 differentiation and effector function as discussed above, but also others such as *DENND1B*, *IL1RL1/IL18R*, *IRAKM*, and *PHF11*, which may regulate the level of inflammation that occurs at the end organ for allergic disease (i.e. the airway, skin, nose, etc.).

Finally, a number of genes appear to be involved in determining the tissue response to chronic inflammation such as airway remodelling. They include genes such as *ADAM33*, which is expressed in fibroblasts and smooth muscle, *PDE4D* in smooth muscle (and inflammatory cells) and *SMAD3*, regulating an intracellular signalling protein that is activated by the profibrotic cytokine TGF-β.

Thus, genetic studies have shown that variation in genes regulating atopic immune responses arise not the only, nor even the major, factor in determining susceptibility to asthma. This has provided strong additional

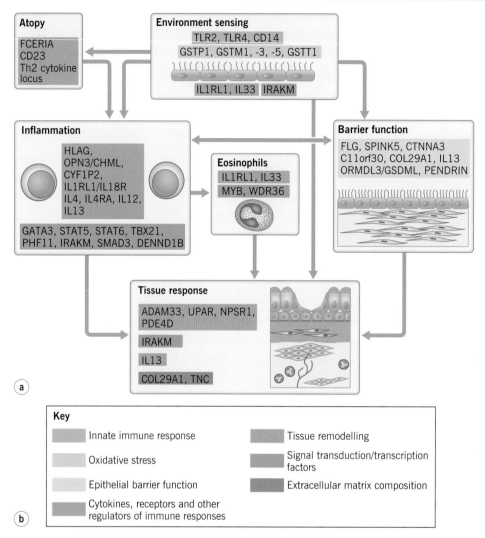

Fig. 2.5 Susceptibility genes for allergic disease. (a, b) Group 1: sensing the environment. The group of genes encodes molecules that directly modulate the effect of environmental risk factors for allergic disease. For example, genes such as *TLR2*, *TLR4*, and *CD14*, encoding components of the innate immune system, interact with levels of microbial exposure to alter the risk of allergic immune responses. Polymorphisms of glutathione-S-transferase genes (*GSTM1*, *GSTM2*, *GSTM3*, *GSTM5*, *GSTT1*, and *GSTP1*) have been shown to modulate the effect of exposures involving oxidant stress, such as tobacco smoke and air pollution on asthma susceptibility. Group 2: barrier function. A high proportion of the novel genes identified for susceptibility to allergic disease through genome-wide linkage and association approaches has been shown to be expressed in the epithelium. This includes genes such as *FLG*, which directly affects dermal barrier function and is associated not only with increased risk of atopic dermatitis but also with increased atopic sensitization. Other susceptibility genes, such as *ORMDL3/GSDML*, *PCDH1*, and *C11orf30* are also expressed in the epithelium and might have a role in possibly regulating epithelial barrier function. Group 3: susceptibility to atopy. It is clear from genome-wide studies that the genes that predispose to atopy and serum IgE responses are mostly distinct from those that predispose to atopic disease. Genes identified for atopy include *FCER1A* and polymorphisms in the *IL4*, *IL13*, *IL5 Th2* cytokine locus on chromosome 5q31.1. Group 4: regulation of (atopic) inflammation. This group includes genes that regulate Th1/Th2 differentiation and effector function [e.g. *IL13*, *IL4RA*, and *STAT6*; *TBX21* (encoding T-box transcription factor); and *GATA3*], as well as genes such as *IL33*, *IL1RL1*, *DENND1B*, *IRAKM*, *PHF11*, and *UPAR* that potentially regulate both atopic sensitization and the level inflammation that occurs at the end-organ location for allergic disease. This also includes the genes shown to regulate the level of blood eosinophilia (*IL1RL1*, *IL33*, *MYB*, and *WDR36*). Group 5: tissue response genes. This group includes genes that modulate the consequences of chronic inflammation (e.g. airway remodelling), such as *ADAM33* and *PDE4D*, which are expressed in fibroblasts and smooth muscle, and *COL29A1*, encoding a novel collagen expressed in the skin linked to atopic dermatitis. Some genes can affect more than one disease component. For example, *IL13* regulates atopic sensitization through IgE isotype switching but also has direct effects on the airway epithelium and mesenchyme, promoting goblet-cell metaplasia and fibroblast proliferation. IL-33 is an epithelial derived cytokine that promotes Th2 responses and has been associated with both susceptibility to asthma and blood eosinophil levels. (Adapted with permission from Holloway JW, Yang IA, Holgate ST. Genetics of allergic disease. J Allergy Clin Immunol 2010; 125(2 suppl 2):S81–94.)

evidence as to the importance of local tissue response factors and epithelial susceptibility factors in the pathogenesis of both asthma and other allergic diseases. This conclusion has only been reinforced by GWAS studies such as the GABRIEL study described above, in which the majority of asthma susceptibility loci identified were not associated with serum IgE levels.

Development in early life and asthma

Another area in which genetic studies of asthma have reinforced observations from traditional epidemiology is in the importance of early life events in determining asthma susceptibility. A number of genetic studies have now provided evidence to support a role for early life developmental effects in allergic disease. For example, *ADAM33* was identified as an asthma susceptibility gene using genome-wide positional cloning. The observed positive association between polymorphisms in this gene and asthma susceptibility and BHR, but not with atopy or serum IgE levels, coupled with the selective expression of *ADAM33* in airway smooth muscle cells and fibroblasts, strongly suggests that alterations in its activity may underlie abnormalities in the function of these cells critical for both BHR and airway remodelling. As in adult airways, multiple ADAM33 protein isoforms exist in human embryonic lung when assessed at 8–12 weeks of development, and polymorphism in *ADAM33* is associated with early life measures of lung function (sRaw age 3). Whilst replication studies are awaited, this finding suggests that variability in this gene is acting *in utero* or in early life to determine lung development. A recent replication study of the association between SNPs on chromosome and asthma showing that the association was observed only in individuals who developed early onset asthma (≤4 years of age), has also provided further support for a critical early life period for the development of asthma.

Atopic dermatitis

As with asthma, a genetic basis for atopic dermatitis (AD, eczema) has long been known as a complex trait with disease susceptibility involving the interactions between multiple genes and environmental factors. Heritability studies support a role for both genetic factors related to atopy in general and also for disease-specific AD genes, the risk of AD in a child being much greater if one or both parents have AD, compared with one or both parents having asthma or allergic rhinitis.

Again, as for asthma there have been a large number of studies of the genetic basis of AD using both candidate gene and hypothesis-independent positional cloning and genome-wide association approaches. A recent (mid 2009) comprehensive review of genetic studies of AD found more than 100 published reports on genetic association studies investigating 81 genes, in 46 of which at least 1 positive association with AD was demonstrated.

Although the majority of studies have examined polymorphisms in genes related to atopic immune responses, more recently a number of studies have investigated genes encoding proteins involved in the epidermal barrier. This has been prompted by the identification of the gene encoding filaggrin (*FLG*), which has a key role in epidermal barrier function, as being one of the strongest genetic risk factors for AD. Filaggrin (filament-aggregating protein) is a major component of the protein–lipid cornified envelope of the epidermis, which is important for water permeability and blocking the entry of microbes and allergens. The filaggrin gene *FLG* is located on chromosome 1q21 in the epidermal differentiation complex. In 2006, it was recognized that loss-of-function mutations in this gene caused *ichthyosis vulgaris*, a skin disorder characterized by dry flaky skin and a predisposition to atopic dermatitis and associated asthma. The mutations in FLG appear to act in a semidominant fashion, with carriers of homozygous or compound heterozygous mutations (R501X & 2282del4) having severe *ichthyosis vulgaris* whereas heterozygotes had milder disease. The combined carrier frequency of null filaggrin mutations is approximately 9% in Caucasian populations.

Subsequently, it was recognized that individuals heterozygous (carrying one copy) for these null alleles had a significantly increased risk of atopic dermatitis, and also atopic sensitization and asthma, but only in the presence of atopic dermatitis. It has been estimated that, although *FLG* null alleles are relatively rare in the Caucasian population, they nevertheless account for up to 15% of the population-attributable risk of atopic dermatitis, with penetrance estimated to be between 40 and 80%; meaning that between 40 and 80% subjects carrying one or more *FLG* null mutations will develop AD. The increased risk of atopic sensitization and atopic asthma in the presence of AD suggests that, by conferring a deficit in epidermal barrier function, *FLG* mutation could initiate systemic allergy by allergen exposure through the skin and start the 'atopic march' in susceptible individuals. This has been confirmed by the analysis of the spontaneous recessive mouse mutant flaky-tail (*flt*), whose phenotype has been shown to result from a frame-shift mutation in the murine filaggrin gene. Topical application of allergen in mice homozygous for this mutation resulted in enhanced cutaneous allergen priming and resultant allergen-specific IgE and IgG antibody responses.

As well as candidate gene studies, both positional cloning by linkage and GWAS have been used to identify genes for AD in a hypothesis-independent manner. Although a number of family based genome-wide linkage scans have been undertaken for AD, the only gene identified by this approach has been that encoding the novel collagen, COL29A1, which provides further support for the notion of a genetically determined deficit in epidermal barrier function underlying AD. More recently, a study using a GWAS approach a SNP adjacent to a gene of unknown function (*C11orf30* encoding a nuclear protein EMSY) on chromosome 11q13 was identified as being strongly associated with susceptibility to atopic dermatitis. This locus has previously been identified as a susceptibility locus for Crohn's disease, another disease involving epithelial inflammation and defective barrier function, and increases in copy number of the *C11orf30* locus have been reported in epithelium-derived cancer of the breast and ovary. Together this suggests that the 11q13 locus represents another gene for an allergic disease that acts at the mucosal surface rather than by modulating the level or type of immune response.

Atopic rhinitis

At the present time, little is known about the genetics of atopic rhinitis. Whereas familial aggregation has been observed in genetic epidemiology studies, genetic studies have been limited. Several genome-wide linkage studies have identified potential disease susceptibility loci but no genes underlying rhinitis have been positionally cloned to date. A number of candidate gene studies for rhinitis have shown association between polymorphisms in inflammatory genes such as *IL13* but the majority of these studies have been limited in size. It remains to be seen whether genetic susceptibility to rhinitis involves specific genetic factors that are distinct from those underlying susceptibility to atopy and asthma.

Food allergy and anaphylaxis

Although it is clear from heritability studies that propensity to allergic reactions to food has a heritable component, the precise genetic factors underlying this have been comparatively underresearched compared with other allergic diseases. Candidate gene studies have shown evidence for polymorphisms of *CD14*, signal transducer and activator of transcription 6 (*STAT6*), serine peptidase inhibitor kazal type 5 (*SPINK5*)1, and *IL1011* being associated with susceptibility to food allergy. Recently, a study of Japanese patients with food allergy and anaphylaxis showed that functional SNPs in the NOD-like receptor (NLR) family, pyrin domain containing 3 (*NLRP3*) gene, which encodes a protein that controls the activity of inflammatory caspase-1 by forming inflammasomes, were strongly associated with susceptibility to food-induced anaphylaxis and aspirin-intolerant asthma. Although these observations await replication in other cohorts, they do show that it may be possible to predict those atopics at risk of developing severe reactions to allergens in the future, allowing targeting of preventative treatments such as allergen immunotherapy.

The clinical utility of greater understanding of allergic disease genetics

The revolution in molecular genetics in the past two decades has seen the dawn of an era that has been dubbed 'genomic medicine', where increased understanding of the interactions between the entire genome and non-genomic factors that result in health and disease results in new diagnostic and therapeutic approaches to common multifactorial conditions. Apart from increased understanding of disease pathogenesis, there are a number of other ways in which greater understanding of the genetic basis of allergic disease will improve diagnosis and treatment in the future.

Predicting disease

The major hope for studies of the genetic basis of common disease is that discovery of the genetic risk factors for disease would lead to accurate risk prediction for individual patients, leading to targeting of preventative therapies. It is already routine for a surrogate measure of heritable risk to be used to aid diagnosis in clinical practice, namely family history, and this has been shown to have some validity. However, attempts to develop scores to predict common disease based on genetic risk factors have shown that these currently show relatively poor discrimination and add little to clinical risk scores that incorporate family history, even in diseases where a greater degree of information is available from GWAS than is currently the case for allergic disease. This simply reflects the complex interactions between different genetic and environmental factors underlying common diseases, resulting in the predictive value of variation in any one gene being low, with a typical genotype relative risk of 1.1–1.5. In the future, identification of further risk factors that explain a larger proportion of the heritability of the disease, and the development of better methods for incorporating genetic factors into risk models, are likely to substantially increase the value of genotypic risk factors. The final clinical utility of any genetic test will depend on its sensitivity, positive and negative predictive values, and whether there are any possible interventions, their cost and potential benefits to the patient. Other considerations that will need to be addressed include patients' understanding of the benefits and risks of, and attitudes towards, the use of genetic testing, adequacy of consent, data confidentiality, and the reporting of results to patients.

Subclassifying disease using genetics

Allergic diseases such as asthma are defined on the basis of clinical symptoms and it is often assumed that the same underlying pathology is presented in all patients with similar symptoms, and thus all will respond to the same therapeutic strategies. This is a simplistic view and readily contradicted by observations such as steroid-resistant asthma and the limited efficacy of biologics targeting individual T-cell surface receptors and cytokines in asthma (e.g. CD25, IL-5, IL-13 or TNF-α). Although individual patients may benefit from such therapies, they form only a small subgroup of the whole disease spectrum. Thus the concept is emerging of subphenotypes of asthma driven by differing gene–environmental interactions. In the future, understanding of individual genetic susceptibility may allow better targeting of therapeutics to those patients most likely to respond.

Equally, understanding of the genetic factors that drive asthma severity may allow identification of those who are most likely to develop severe persistent disease and hence targeting of preventative treatments. The identification of 'severity genes' in allergic diseases such as asthma is difficult owing to the complex interactions between susceptibility, environment, and treatment. However, a number of studies have identified genetic variations that are associated with measures of asthma severity such as the SNPs in the gene encoding the cytokine TNF-α. Identification of a panel of markers of severe disease may in the future allow targeting of healthcare resources to those individuals who are likely to exhibit the greatest morbidity and mortality.

Pharmacogenetics

Pharmacogenetics is the study of genetic influences on interindividual variability in both therapeutic and adverse response to therapies. The study of pharmacogenetics holds out the possibility that clinicians will be able to select prospectively the most appropriate therapeutic strategy for an individual patient based not just on their symptoms, but on their propensity to respond or suffer adverse effects as ascertained by their individual genetic make-up. It is clear from both anecdotal clinical experience and large clinical trials that, in asthma, patient response to drugs such as bronchodilators, corticosteroids, and antileukotrienes is heterogeneous. A number of studies have investigated whether polymorphism in candidate genes may account for some of this interpatient variability.

Naturally occurring polymorphisms in the β_2-adrenoceptor gene (*ADRB2*) may alter the function and expression of the β_2-adrenoceptor, and therefore affect response to short- and long-acting bronchodilators. A number of non-synonymous single nucleotide polymorphisms have been shown to be functional in vitro, including at amino acids 16, 27, and 164 and in the promoter region. Clinical studies have shown that β_2-adrenoceptor polymorphisms influence the response to bronchodilator treatment. Asthmatic patients carrying the *Gly16* polymorphism have been shown to be more prone to developing bronchodilator desensitization, whereas children who are homozygous or heterozygous for *Arg16* are more likely to show positive acute responses to bronchodilators. However, other common polymorphisms in the *ADRB2* gene also appear to show effects on bronchodilator response, and some studies have shown that acute responses to bronchodilator treatment are genotype independent.

More recently, the study of *ADRB2* pharmacogenetics has been applied to longer-term clinical studies of long-acting bronchodilators. Although some studies have shown that *Arg/Arg16* subjects have reduced peak expiratory flow rate compared with *Gly/Gly16* subjects in response to salmeterol (with or without concomitant inhaled corticosteroid treatment), subsequent studies have failed to confirm these findings. Variation in study design (e.g. sample size, use of combination inhalers) may explain some of the difference in results between these clinical studies.

Given the discordant results, further work is required to evaluate fully the exact role of *ADRB2* polymorphisms in the response to bronchodilators in asthmatics. Furthermore, there are likely to be other genetic determinants of response to bronchodilator treatment; for example, one study assessing the effect of 844 SNPs in 111 candidate genes recently identified the *ARG1* gene encoding arginase 1 as a predictor of acute response to salbutamol (albuterol).

Clinical responses to inhaled corticosteroids also vary between individuals and polymorphisms in steroid signalling pathways may also be clinically important in asthma management. Polymorphisms in a numbers of genes such as the corticotropin-releasing hormone receptor 1 (*CRHR1*) gene involved in cortisol synthesis, *TBX21* encoding a transcription factor regulating Th1-cell induction, and the low-affinity IgE receptor gene *FCER2* have been associated with a range of phenotypes such as improved lung function (FEV$_1$) response to inhaled steroids, improvement in airways hyperresponiveness, and protection from exacerbations after inhaled corticosteroid treatment.

An obvious candidate for corticosteroid response is the glucocorticoid receptor gene *NR3C1*. Although common polymorphisms of *NR3C1* do not appear to be important in determining interindividual corticosteroid resistance and response, in another component of the large heterocomplex of proteins that cooperatively functions to activate the glucocorticoid receptor, STIP1, has been associated with the magnitude of FEV_1 improvement in response to inhaled corticosteroid treatment.

A number of SNPs in genes involved in the leukotriene biosynthetic pathway and leukotriene receptors have been associated with response to leukotriene modifiers. Promoter polymorphisms affecting the transcription of the 5-lipoxygenase (*ALOX5*) gene, and polymorphisms of the leukotriene C_4 synthase (*LTC4S*) and LTA_4 hydrolase (*LTA4H*) genes appear to be associated with improvements in lung function and exacerbation rates following montelukast treatment. Similar observations have been made in regards to responses to zileuton.

Although such studies show that pharmacogenetic effects have the potential to influence the efficacy of asthma therapies, it is clear that the effects at the individual SNP or gene level are small. Together with variability between studies and populations, this has limited the applicability of these observations in clinical practice. In the future, genome-wide studies together with the use of clinical scoring systems incorporating multiple genetic and non-genetic predictors of response may enable the translation of pharmacogenetics to the clinic.

Environmental effects on genes: epigenetics and allergic disease

The role of epigenetics is being increasingly recognized as playing an important role as a mechanism by which the environment can alter disease risk in an individual. The term 'epigenetics' refers to biological processes that regulate gene activity but do not alter the DNA sequence itself. Epigenetic factors include modification of histones (the structural protein complexes around which DNA is coiled) by acteylation, methylation, and phosphorylation, and DNA methylation. Modification of histones regulates transcription, altering levels of protein expression. DNA methylation involves adding a methyl group to specific cytosine (C) bases in islands of CpG in the DNA to suppress gene expression. Importantly, both changes to histones and DNA methylation can be induced in response to environmental exposures such as tobacco smoke and alterations in early life environment (e.g. maternal nutrition). Furthermore, DNA methylation patterns are heritable, providing a mechanism for transgenerational effects of environmental exposures on disease risk.

There is increasing evidence as to the importance of epigenetic factors in allergic disease. For example, a number of studies have linked altered birth weight and/or head circumference at birth (proxy markers for maternal nutrition) with an increase in adult IgE levels and risk of allergic disease. A recent study has also shown that increased environmental particulate exposure, from

traffic pollution, results in a dose-dependent increase in peripheral blood DNA methylation.

The effect of epigenetics has been observed over more than just a single generation. For example, in humans, transgenerational effects have been observed where the initial environmental exposure occurred in the F_0 generation and was still present in the F_2 one (the grandchildren). Studies of grandparental exposure, such as poor nutrition or smoking during the slow growth period of the F_0 generation, revealed effects on life expectancy and growth through the male line and female line in the F_2 generation, although there had been no further exposure. Observations such as grandmaternal smoking increasing the risk of childhood asthma in their grandchildren support the concept that transgenerational epigenetic effects may be operating in allergic disease. Other support comes from the study of animal models such as pregnant mice given dietary supplementation with methyl donors

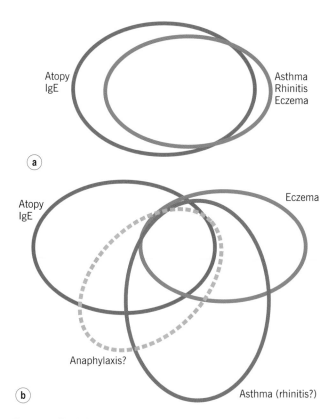

Fig. 2.6 Evolving insights into relationship between atopy and atopic disease susceptibility. (a) When molecular genetic studies were first undertaken in allergic disease, it was expected that the genes underlying both susceptibility to atopy and susceptibility to atopic disease would substantially overlap. (b) With increased insight provided by hypothesis-independent approaches such as genome-wide association and linkage studies, together with evolving understanding of disease pathogenesis, it is now recognized that genes predisposing to atopy per se make up a small fraction of atopic disease susceptibility genes.

whose offspring exhibit enhanced airway inflammation following allergen challenge.

It is likely, in the near future, that the study of large prospective birth cohorts with information on maternal environmental exposures during pregnancy is likely to provide important insights into the role of epigenetic factors in the heritability of allergic disease.

Conclusion

New techniques for scanning the human genome promise great advances in tracking the origins of disorders caused by multiple genes such as asthma and atopic dermatitis. Genetic studies have highlighted the importance of a number of new areas of biology in the pathogenesis of allergic disease, such as the importance of the end disease organ such as airway epithelial barrier in asthma and epidermal barrier in atopic dermatitis, and the importance of the tissue response in determining the consequences of inflammation in organs such as the airway (Fig. 2.6). However, it is clear from the studies presented in this overview that, even with the advent of genome-wide association studies, we are far from understanding the complete genetic basis of allergic disease and how genetic factors interact with the environment. As a result, the derivation of direct benefits from understanding the genetic basis of these conditions, or the incorporation of genetic testing into routine clinical practice for the management of allergic disease, although holding great promise, still lies in the future.

Summary of important messages

- Both allergy and allergic diseases such as asthma have a heritable component
- Allergic diseases are complex genetic conditions resulting from the interaction between multiple genetic and environmental factors
- Genetic variation influences not only disease susceptibility, but also disease severity and response to treatment
- Genetic studies of allergic disease have provided much insight into the mechanisms of allergic disease, but have not, to date, improved assessment of disease risk for individual patients

Further reading

Barnes KC. An update on the genetics of atopic dermatitis: scratching the surface in 2009. J Allergy Clin Immunol 2010; 125(1):16–29, e1-11.

Baye TM, Martin LJ, Khurana Hershey GK. Application of genetic/genomic approaches to allergic disorders. J Allergy Clin Immunol 2010; 126(3):425–436.

Feero WG, Guttmacher AE, Collins FS. Genomic medicine: genomic medicine – an updated primer. N Engl J Med 2010; 362:2001–2011.

Holloway JW, Arshad SH, Holgate ST. Using genetics to predict the natural history of asthma? J Allergy Clin Immunol 2010; 126(2):200–209.

Holloway JW, Yang IA, Holgate ST. Genetics of allergic disease. J Allergy Clin Immunol 2010; 125(2 suppl 2):S81–94.

Kazani S, Wechsler ME, Israel E. The role of pharmacogenomics in improving the management of asthma. J Allergy Clin Immunol 2010; 125(2):295–302.

Kazani S, Wechsler ME, Israel E. The role of pharmacogenomics in improving the management of asthma. J Allergy Clin Immunol 2010; 125(2):295–302.

Moffatt MF, Gut IG, Demenais F, et al for the GABRIEL consortium. A large-scale, consortium-based genomewide association study of asthma. N Engl J Med 2010; 363:1211–1221.

Moffatt MF, Kabesch M, Liang L, et al. Genetic variants regulating ORMDL3 expression contribute to the risk of childhood asthma. Nature 2007; 448:470–473.

Vercelli D. Discovering susceptibility genes for asthma and allergy. Nat Rev Immunol 2008; 8(3):169–182.

Appendix 2.1 Definitions of common terms in genetics

Gene: A defined DNA sequence that is transcribed to form an RNA product. This is then either translated to from a protein or may, as in the case of microRNAs, have a biological function. Transcription of the RNA is driven by a specific DNA sequence, a promoter, in front of the gene that contains recognition sequences for transcription factors to bind to the DNA.

Allele: Any one of a series of two or more different DNA sequence variations that occupy the same position (locus) on a chromosome.

Haplotype: A set of closely linked genetic polymorphisms present on one chromosome.

Polymorphism: One of two or more alternate forms (alleles) of a chromosomal locus that differ in nucleotide sequence. Generally the term is reserved for variants that are present at >1% frequency in the general population.

Single nucleotide polymorphism: DNA sequence variation that occurs when a single nucleotide in the genome sequence is changed, by substitution, insertion or deletion of a single base pair.

Functional polymorphism: Genetic variation that has been shown to have a biological effect, either by altering the genetic code resulting in production of an altered protein or by altering expression levels of a gene product by mechanisms such as altering transcription factor binding affinity to gene promoters.

Copy number variants: Defined regions of the genome (from several base pairs to many 1000s of base pairs) that are present in variable copy number compared with a reference genome as a result of deletion, or duplication of genetic material.

Linkage disequilibrium: The occurrence of combinations of genetic variants at different loci at a frequency that varies from what would be accounted for by chance. For example, if alleles A and B occur at one locus and X and Y occur at another, and each time X is detected A is also detected, then alleles X and A are in linkage disequilibrium.

Types of studies used in genetics

Family-based studies are studies of the inheritance of genetic variants between an affected subject and his or her parents or siblings in an attempt to identify the aberrant gene by either linkage or association.

Candidate gene studies are studies of genetic variation in genes chosen because their encoded product is part of a biological pathway that is plausibly related to the disease or the expression of which is altered in the disease sate.

Genome-wide association studies are an approach to gene mapping that involves scanning markers across the entire genome to find associations between a particular phenotype and allelic variation in a population. This methodology relies on the fact that the markers will be in linkage disequilibrium with polymorphisms truly associated with the phenotype.

3

Early life origins of allergy and asthma

Patrick G Holt, Peter D Sly and Susan Prescott

DEFINITION

A term used for the hypothesis that asthma and allergy arise from influences present during fetal life and early childhood.

Introduction

Allergic sensitization, and the ensuing manifestations of allergic diseases exemplified by atopic asthma, can arise de novo at any stage of life. However, as demonstrated in a broad range of prospective birth cohort studies, some of which have now tracked populations for over 20 years, it is much more common for these diseases to appear initially in a mild form during childhood. Indeed, particularly in the case of allergy, the transient appearance of IgE against ubiquitous environmental allergens in early childhood is so frequent within the overall population that it can be classed as 'normal' and it is only in a small subset of children that these responses fail to resolve spontaneously and instead persist and consolidate, leading to clinically significant symptoms. It is also becoming increasingly evident that this period in early life represents a unique potential 'window of opportunity' for modulation of these responses before they become persistent. There is accordingly widespread interest in definition of the underlying regulatory mechanisms at play within the immature immune system at this time, as these constitute potential therapeutic targets. Moreover, it is also evident that, although atopic sensitization is an important risk factor for diseases such as asthma, only a small proportion of atopic individuals develop persistent asthma, which infers that other important cofactors are involved that operate against the background of atopy to create atopic disease. These and related issues are discussed in the review below.

Aetiology of respiratory allergy: development of sensitization versus tolerance to environmental allergens

Animal model studies

Sensitization to aeroallergens has traditionally been ascribed to a failure in immune exclusion barriers operative at mucosal surfaces, in particular secretory IgA. However, more recent animal model studies have demonstrated that, analogous to the situation in the gastrointestinal tract (GIT), active immunological recognition of inhaled non-pathogenic proteins is the rule

© 2012 Elsevier Ltd
DOI: 10.1016/B978-0-7234-3658-4.00005-6

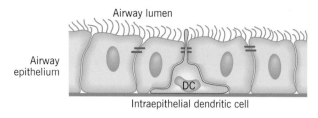

Fig. 3.1 Airway intraepithelial dendritic cell (DC). DC within the airway mucosa between adjacent epithelial cells. Airway epithelial cells maintain apical tight junctions (pink bars), through which DC extend dendrites to sample the luminal surface ('snorkelling').

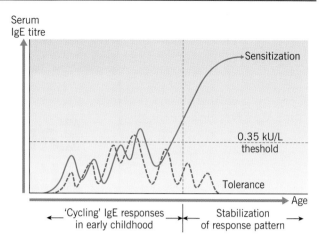

Fig. 3.2 Early immunity to aeroallergens in atopic vs non-atopic children. During early childhood, IgE antibody levels in non-atopics typically fluctuate over time ('cycling') below the sensitization threshold, prior to the eventual onset of stable tolerance. In contrast, in atopics, typically from age 2 onwards, this cycling is replaced by a pattern of upwardly trending IgE production coinciding with the development of stable allergen-specific T-cell and B-cell memory.

as opposed to the exception, and the normal outcome is the development of a form of immunological tolerance ('inhalation tolerance'). This process is mediated by populations of T-regulatory (Treg) cells, previously designated as suppressor T cells, and the sampling process by which such proteins gain access to the submucosal immune system involves the activity of intraepithelial dendritic cells that 'snorkel' through epithelial tight junctions via extrusion of dendrites which are armed with an array of receptors to facilitate antigen binding/uptake (Fig. 3.1).

A hallmark feature of the tolerance process is the transient production of specific IgE during the induction phase, which, depending on the IgE-responder phenotype of the animal strains employed, can attain moderate-to-high titres prior to the final onset of tolerance. Moreover, genetic factors related to IgE-responder phenotype are important determinants of susceptibility to normal tolerance induction via either the GIT or the lung, with high-responder strains (homologues of human atopics) requiring higher-level and more sustained exposure to elicit stable tolerance. Intriguingly, respiratory viral infections appeared capable of interfering with this tolerance process, in particular de novo exposure to aerosolized allergen during the acute phase of infection results in sensitization rather than tolerance.

Primary sensitization in humans: prospective and cross-sectional cohort studies

Antibody studies

The first indications that allergic sensitization was typically initiated during early postnatal life came from cross-sectional studies showing that inhalant-allergen-specific IgE titres in atopic children increased progressively after infancy. Prospective cohort study designs have proven more instructive, and have demonstrated that both aeroallergen-specific and food-allergen-specific IgE titres commonly fluctuate in a 'saw tooth' fashion during the first 2–3 years of life in children who are not sensitized

by age 5 years (Fig. 3.2). It is interesting to note that the definition of 'clinically relevant sensitization' based on IgE titre is of limited value in this age range if the international standard cut-off of 0.35 kU/L IgE is employed, as titres below this are significantly associated with disease risk. Moreover it has been observed that an apparent threshold exists in relation to time-dependent fluctuations in IgE titres and risk for persistent sensitization, notably ≥83% of children whose anti-house dust mite (HDM) IgE titres exceeded 0.20 kU/L by their second birthday progressed to clinical sensitization by age 5 years.

Th-cell studies

IgE antibody production by plasma cells is dependent on provision of IL-4/IL-13 signals from type 2 (Th2) memory cells, and it is the priming of these cells that represents the initiating step in the allergic sensitization process. In multiple studies dating back to the 1980s the presence of Th cells putatively responding to in vitro allergen exposure via proliferation and/or cytokine production has been reported in cord blood. This has led to widespread suggestions that initial Th-cell priming may occur in utero via transplacental leakage of allergen from the maternal circulation. In apparent support of this proposition a recent study employing a high-sensitivity IgE assay has detected what is claimed to be fetal-derived specific IgE at low level in cord blood, implying in utero initiation of the priming/sensitization process. However, additional evidence from prospective follow-up studies demonstrating persistence of these antibodies will be required to substantiate this possibility.

Contrary evidence is also available from prospective studies on aeroallergen-specific Th-cell priming. In particular, although several studies have demonstrated the presence of aeroallergen-specific Th2 activity in cord blood and accompanying age-dependent increases in this activity between birth and the end of infancy, more long-term studies have cast doubt on the relevance of the cord blood data. Notably, although progressively stronger correlations are found between cytokine responses from 6 months onwards and corresponding reactivity at 5 years, cord blood responses display no such correlations. The answer to this apparently enigmatic finding may lie in the results of studies on 'recent thymic emigrants (RTE)', which comprise the bulk of CD4 T cells in cord blood. These cells have functionally immature antigen receptors that interact at low affinity with a broad range of peptides (in contrast to the fine specificity of mature T cells), enabling RTE to respond in a 'pseudo-memory T-cell' fashion to antigens/allergens they have not previously encountered, leading to a burst of proliferation and cytokine production, terminated by apoptotic death. The function of these RTE in neonates is the subject of much debate, but in particular the question of whether these early responses bear any relationship to the subsequent development of genuine stable Th-cell memory remains unresolved.

Factors influencing intrauterine development of immune function

A substantial body of work suggests a link between epigenetic gene regulation, immunity, and physiological development. Notably, perinatal differences in immune function precede the development of allergic disease, including relative T-cell immaturity as well as differences in Treg and innate cell function that are already evident at birth. These differences in gene expression at birth reflect both inherited genetic programmes and how these have been modified by in utero events and exposures. The emerging field of epigenetics provides a new frontier for understanding mechanisms underlying these gene–environment interactions. As discussed further below, there is now evidence that many of the environmental factors implicated in the rise of allergic disease (including diet, microbial infections, tobacco smoke, and other pollutants) can epigenetically modify expression of immune-related genes with associated effects on immune programming.

Prenatal immune development

Complex immunological mechanisms have evolved to allow the fetal and maternal immune systems to coexist during pregnancy. The maternal cellular immune system adapts subtly towards a more 'Th2-state' in order to down-regulate Th1-cell-mediated alloimmune responses to fetal antigens. This profile is reflected in the fetal immune responses, which also show Th2 dominance and silencing of Th1–IFN-γ gene expression in CD4+ T cells. There is also an emerging role of CD4+CD25+ Treg in mediating tolerance at the materno-fetal interface.

T-cell differentiation is under epigenetic control through changes in DNA/histone methylation and/or histone acetylation. Specifically, these epigenetic mechanisms are known to regulate Th1, Th2, Th17, and Treg differentiation. These observations have led to speculation that factors modulating gene methylation/acetylation may modify the risk of allergic disease by altering the developmental patterns of gene expression in these pathways. There are now several examples where this is seen to occur (see below).

Emerging differences associated with atopic risk

Allergy-prone individuals have recognized differences in many aspects of immune function at birth, including effector T cells, regulatory T cells (Tregs), haemopoetic progenitor populations and innate cells. These altered patterns of gene expression reflect inherited genetic programmes and how these have been modified by in utero events and exposures. Significant differences in magnitude and relative maturity of effector T-cell responsiveness by the end of gestation have been associated with the later development of allergic disease, in particular a relative deficiency in type 1 Th-cell interferon gamma (IFN-γ) production compared with non-allergic children, and there is growing evidence that in high-risk infants (of allergic mothers) this is accompanied by differences in Treg activity. These subjects display reduced placental expression of the key regulatory gene *FOXP3*, as well as reduced Treg numbers and function in cord blood, fuelling growing speculation that impaired Treg function is implicated in the development of allergic disease. Intriguingly, the allergy-protective effect of microbial burden in pregnancy (see below) has been shown to be associated with increased Treg activity and this was mediated through demethylation of the *FOXP3* promoter. This further supports conjecture that environmental changes begin their influence on immune development during pregnancy.

Influence of the maternal environment: emerging epigenetic paradigms

There is now firm evidence that environmental exposures during critical stages in pregnancy can alter gene expression and disease predisposition through epigenetic mechanisms. The placenta and the fetus are both vulnerable to exogenous and endogenous maternal influences during this period. Specific maternal exposures such as microbial contact and diet, as well as cigarette smoke and other airborne pollutants, are known to modify fetal immune function and contribute to an increased risk of subsequent allergic disease. Notably, most of these factors are now known to exert their effects on immune programming by epigenetically activating or silencing immune-related genes. Recent environmental change and associated epigenetic dysregulation are likely to explain a significant component of the inappropriate expression of pathways that promote allergic disease.

The endogenous maternal environment

Maternal allergy is a stronger determinant of allergic risk and immune neonatal function than paternal allergy, suggesting effects of direct materno-fetal interactions in utero. Pregnancy has been shown to modify maternal cytokine production to both environmental antigens and fetal alloantigens, and allergic mothers have lower Th1 IFN-γ responses to HLA-DR mismatched fetal antigens compared with non-allergic women. These factors may affect the cytokine milieu at the materno-fetal interface and could be implicated in the attenuated Th1 responses observed commonly in infants of atopic mothers (above). Foreseeably, the rise in maternal allergy may also be amplifying the effect of other environmental changes.

Microbial exposure

Although the initial focus of the 'hygiene hypothesis' was in the postnatal period, there is now good evidence that in utero microbial exposure can also have allergy-protective effects. In several studies, maternal environments rich in microbial compounds (such as traditional European farming environments) appear to protect against the development of childhood allergic disease independently of postnatal exposure. Animal models also confirm that exposure to both pathogenic and non-pathogenic microbial strains prevent allergic airway inflammation in the offspring, through epigenetic effects. This is echoed by human studies that now also show that the protective effects of maternal microbial exposure are associated with enhanced neonatal Treg function, *FOXP3* expression, and associated epigenetic effects (demethylation) on the *FOXP3* gene. Thus, although postnatal exposure remains the largest source of direct microbial exposure, the effects of this important environmental influence clearly begin in utero.

Maternal diet in pregnancy

Dietary changes are at the centre of the emerging epigenetic paradigms that underpin the rise in many modern diseases, and are among the many complex environmental changes implicated in the allergy epidemic. Specific nutrients, including antioxidants, oligosaccharides, polyunsaturated fatty acids, folate, and other vitamins, have documented effects on immune function and have been implicated in epidemiological studies of allergic disease. Significantly, it has been shown that maternal (fish oil) supplementation in pregnancy can favourably modify the expression of T-cell maturation markers (PKCζ) towards an allergy-protective profile. In one of the first epigenetic models of allergic disease, maternal folic acid (a dietary methyl donor) has been shown to modify fetal gene expression epigenetically and promote experimental asthma in animals. This is consistent with preliminary reports linking folic acid supplementation in human pregnancy with increased risk of asthma and respiratory disease in the infants and highlights the urgent need for further studies, especially given the move towards mandatory dietary folate supplementation in some parts of the world. In summary, complex modern dietary changes appear to be contributing to the more proinflammatory conditions of the modern lifestyle. These effects also begin in uterine life and may offer important opportunities for non-invasive prevention strategies.

Other environmental exposures in pregnancy

Maternal medications including antibiotics, paracetamol, and acid reflux medications have been implicated in an increased risk of asthma and allergic disease. Pollutants including cigarette smoke, traffic exhaust, and indoor pollutants also have document effects on lung development, immune function, and asthma risk, with recognized epigenetic effects. Other modern pollutants including organic products of industry and agriculture have also been recently associated with epigenetic effects, including effects on global DNA methylation patterns at the low-dose exposure found in the ambient environment. Some of these products [including polychlorinated biphenyl compounds (PCBs), organochlorine pesticides, dioxins, and phthalates] have been readily measured in breast milk, cord blood and placental tissue, highlighting the potential to influence early development. These modern exposures should remain an important consideration in the rise of modern diseases.

In summary, there is overwhelming evidence that antenatal events play a pivotal role in setting the scene for postnatal disease development (Fig. 3.3). Many environmental exposures have the capacity to influence multiple aspects of immune development and predispose to subsequent allergic disease, supporting the growing momentum behind notions of 'developmental origins of disease'. Emerging epigenetic paradigms provide a new framework for understanding how these early gene–environment interactions drive vulnerability, and may also provide opportunities for disease prevention.

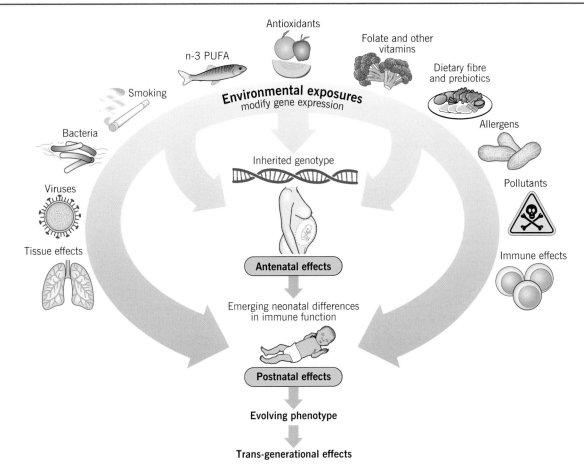

Fig. 3.3 Gene-by-environment interactions in the pathogenesis of allergic disease. A wide range of environmental factors, acting antenatally and/or postnatally, are known to influence the maturation of immunological competence, and hence modulate risk for development of allergic diseases (see text).

Variations in the efficiency of postnatal maturation of immune competence and risk for development of allergic diseases

Maturation of adaptive immunity

A number of observations in the earlier clinical literature suggested links between 'immunological immaturity' and risk for development of allergic diseases during early life, but mechanistic understanding of the nature of this linkage is still incomplete. It is now evident that the functional capacity of the adaptive arm of the immune system is heavily constrained in utero, probably to protect tissues at the feto-maternal interface from potentially toxic Th1 cytokines, which can damage placental function. As a consequence Th-cell activation capacity per se is restricted, and the ability of these cells to secrete both Th1 and Th2 cytokines is reduced. In order to resist pathogens in the extrauterine environment it is necessary for the infant adaptive immune system to up-regulate these effector functions after birth, and accumulating evidence suggests that this maturation process proceeds more slowly in children who subsequently develop atopy. In particular T-cell cloning efficiency in atopic infants is reduced relative to their non-atopic counterparts and this is accompanied by reduced capacity to secrete all classes of cytokines, but particularly Th1 cytokines, resulting in a state of relative 'Th2 bias' in their overall adaptive immune function.

Reduced capacity to secrete Th1 cytokines in children at high risk (HR) of allergic diseases has also been implicated in attenuated responsiveness to vaccine antigens and increased susceptibility to respiratory infections, which as discussed below is an important aetiological factor in conjunction with atopic sensitization in asthma pathogenesis. It is additionally of note that the typical pattern of postnatal maturation of Th1 function in HR children is biphasic (Fig. 3.4), with initial hyporesponsiveness in infancy being progressively replaced by a state of hyperresponsiveness by the end of the preschool years. Moreover, several independent studies suggest that in these children elevated Th1 responses to aeroallergens contribute to the pathogenesis of diseases such as atopic

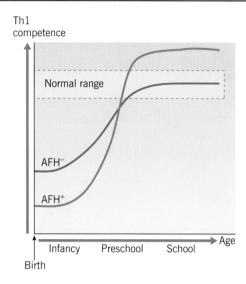

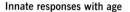

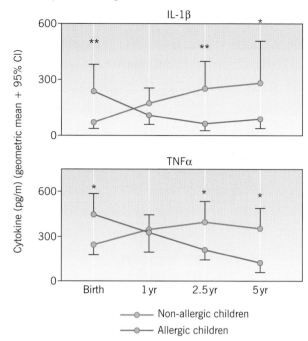

Fig. 3.4 Postnatal maturation of Th1 competence in atopic family history positive (AFH⁺) vs atopic family history negative (AFH⁻) children. AFH⁺ children at birth display diminished Th1 competence relative to their AFH⁻ counterparts, but eventually they typically 'overshoot' the normal range and become hyperresponsive with respect to both Th1 and Th2 cytokine phenotypes.

Fig. 3.5 Innate immune response profiles with age. Production of proinflammatory cytokines exemplified by IL-1β and TNF-α in response to innate stimuli is elevated at birth in atopic children, but eventually lags behind that of non-atopics.

asthma in which the major underlying driver is Th2 immunity.

Development of innate immune function

Although innate immune cells are functional at birth, the production of innate cytokines (including TNF-α, IL-1β, and IL-6) and key Th1-trophic cytokines (such as IL-12) is significantly reduced in the neonatal period, and may not achieve adult levels until late childhood. This has been attributed, at least in part, to deficiencies in the number and/or function of DC. Recent longitudinal studies show progressive postnatal maturation of microbial recognition pathways (signalling through Toll-like receptors [TLR]2, TLR3, TLR4, TLR5, TLR2/6, TLR7/8, and TLR9) in healthy non-allergic children, which correspond directly to the age-related maturation in adaptive Th1 responses noted in our original studies. This further suggests that T-cell development, and in particular inhibition of Th2 differentiation, may be driven through the innate immune system as it undergoes microbial-driven maturation.

Notably, allergic children show striking differences in the developmental trajectory of both innate and adaptive immunity, as well as apparent 'dissociation' between these functional cellular compartments of the immune system. Specifically, allergic children show exaggerated inflammatory responses (TNF-α, IL-1β and IL-6) to virtually all TLR ligands at birth compared with non-allergic

children (Fig. 3.5). The increased neonatal production of these inflammatory cytokines correlates with their subsequent propensity for Th2 adaptive responses. In the postnatal period, allergic children show a relative decline in microbial responses, so that by 5 years of age their TLR responses are significantly attenuated compared with non-allergic children. Although innate immune responses are important for host defence, excessive inflammatory responses are maladaptive and can lead to unwanted tissue damage. It is possible that the early propensity for innate inflammatory responses is a driver for Th2 cytokine production, potentially 'tipping the balance' during this critical period of T-cell development. What role these cytokines then have in the declining innate responses of allergic children is as yet unknown.

Developmental differences in TLR function have functional implications for the many subsets of cells expressing these receptors including DC and regulatory T cells that play critical roles in programming and controlling effector T-cell responses. Unless DC receive obligatory Th1-trophic signals from the local tissue environment during antigen processing, they are likely to induce Th2 differentiation as a default response. These signals are likely to occur with microbial exposure, which is known to evoke protective type 1 effector T-cell responses in mature individuals.

The role of other innate cells, such as polymorphonuclear cells, in the pathogenesis of allergic disease is less clear. Eosinophils and basophils are the downsteam targets of the Th2 response, but there is preliminary evidence of presymptomatic differences in levels of their progenitor populations in cord blood of children at risk of allergic disease. More recent studies suggest an altered TLR expression and functional responsiveness of these neonatal CD34+ haemopoietic progenitors in cord blood of infants at high atopic risk. Again this suggests a role of maternal allergic status and other environmental exposures in utero, and that engagement of TLR pathways in early life though microbial exposure could modulate eosinophil–basophil progenitors.

Development of Treg function

With their recently recognized role in immune regulation and the suppression of maladaptive responses, Treg are now high among the candidate immunological pathways that underpin the hygiene hypothesis, as well as being prime therapeutic targets. Although these cells do appear to play a role in the suppression of established allergic responses via strategies such as immunotherapy, their role in the primary pathogenesis of disease is not clear. This is in part because these are among the most challenging cells to study. The lack of relevant lineage-specific surface markers has made them difficult to identify and isolate, and developmental studies are further hampered by difficulties in isolating sufficient cells from the small volumes of blood available from children. As such, the developmental studies of Treg in childhood are largely confined to thymus tissue, which show that the proportion of putative CD4+CD25+CD127lo/-FOXP3+ Treg increases with age during early childhood. Cord blood studies also show preliminary evidence of impaired neonatal Treg function in infants at high risk of allergy and those who go on to develop early allergic disease. Notably, the previously recognized allergy-protective effects of microbial exposure in pregnancy have recently been associated with enhanced neonatal Treg function, which appears to be mediated by epigenetic effects with demethylation of the *FOXP3* gene and increased gene expression (as discussed above). At this stage there are no longitudinal studies of postnatal Treg maturation.

Role of environmental factors in postnatal development

After birth the infant remains vulnerable to the more direct effects of many immunomodulatory environmental exposures. Notably, as summarized in Figure 3.3, many of the most critical postnatal environmental influences interact with the developing immune system in the gastrointestinal tract, which provides the largest lymphoid network in the body and the most significant interface between the newborn and its new environment. The rise in food allergy and other disorders of oral tolerance are clear evidence that modern environments are not providing optimal tolerogenic conditions during allergen encounter. Beyond the gastrointestinal tract, exposures at other mucosal surfaces play a role in local events that contribute to disease pathogenesis. In the respiratory tract, viral infection and inhaled pollutants are important postnatal exposures that may contribute to the development of tissue-specific inflammation.

Gut microflora

Although still incompletely understood, colonization is essential for normal immune development, underscoring the symbiotic relationship that has evolved over millennia. Changes in colonization patterns with progressive industrialization have probably been a strong element of the hygiene hypothesis, with evidence of altered colonization patterns and reduced diversity in children who go on to develop allergic disease. The specific immunoprotective effects of microflora appear to be mediated through multiple pathways within and beyond the gut-associated lymphoid tissue (GALT). This includes effects on local IgA production and induction of tolerogenic dendritic cells and regulatory T-cell populations. These collectively promote production of immunomodulatory cytokines such IL-10 and TGF-β, which inhibit local inflammation, improve gut integrity, and thereby reduce the risk of inappropriate systemic immune responses. A better understanding of these myriad effects of the gut microbiota may provide avenues for the development of improved preventive and therapeutic strategies.

Infant diet

Breast milk is the first and most important early nutritional source in the postnatal period, containing a large range of nutrients, growth factors, and immunomodulators such as immunoglobulins, lactoferrin, lyzozymes, oligosaccharides, long-chain fatty acids, cytokines, nucleotides, hormones, antioxidants, and maternal immune cells. In animal studies the tolerogenic properties of maternal milk are mediated by CD4+ regulatory T cells and are dependent on TGF-β present in maternal milk. Although the mechanisms need further investigation, breast milk appears to assist the infant in initiating the fine balance between immunoprotection and oral tolerance, and may reveal insights into the optimal development of a tolerogenic environment in the gut.

The weaning diet also contains many immunomodulatory factors (as with maternal diet, above) that can influence both systemic immune responses and local events in the gut. One of the most topical new areas at present is the emerging role of soluble dietary fibre and oligosaccharides. In addition to their previously recognized role promoting favourable colonization, their fermentation products (short-chain fatty acids) have newly discovered antiinflammatory properties. Earlier epidemiological studies suggested a protective link between dietary fibre and allergic conditions and preliminary allergy prevention studies suggest an allergy-protective effect of neonatal supplementation with 'prebiotic' oligosaccharides. This provides a strong basis for further exploring the role of dietary fibre and oligosaccharides in the promotion of oral tolerance.

Infant foods also contain a range of potential allergens, which in a growing number of children are associated with manifestations of food allergy. Although these food antigens are first encountered in small concentrations in breast milk and possibly in utero, the largest exposure occurs during complimentary feeding. Under optimal conditions, immune tolerance is the default response to these harmless oral exposures. The rise in food allergy is more likely to reflect less tolerogenic conditions during allergen encounter (such as altered colonization) rather than specific changes within the allergens themselves. Early attempts to prevent allergic disease by 'allergen avoidance' have been unsuccessful. There has been a major recent shift in this regard for food antigens, which are seen now as potential 'tolerogens' that may be utilized in prevention and treatment of allergic disease. Based on these concepts, avoidance of food allergens in pregnancy, lactation or infancy is no longer recommended, and a series of new studies are now examining their role in tolerance induction.

In summary, these and the many other dietary factors continue to play an important role in shaping development of the immune system in the postnatal period, and may provide opportunities for promoting more tolerogenic conditions.

Viral infection

Despite the declining burden of bacterial and parasitic infections, viral infection remains the most common cause of acute illness in childhood. Viral respiratory infection, particularly with respiratory syncytial virus (RSV), is one of the strongest postnatal associations with allergic airways disease, although the complexity of this relationship has been difficult to dissect. Wheezing lower respiratory infection in the first year of life is a powerful risk factor for asthma at 6 years of age in both non-atopic and atopic children, and this issue is dealt with separately below.

Pollutants in the postnatal period

Cigarette smoke exposure remains of the most common noxious, yet avoidable, exposures in early childhood. Beyond the established intrauterine effects (see above and below), postnatal exposure at mucosal surfaces also has well-documented irritant effects with local epithelial damage and inflammatory changes. This contributes to the recognized increase in respiratory symptoms and pathology in smoke-exposed infants. The role of other indoor pollutants is less well understood. In some populations the use of home gas appliances has been associated with an increase risk of HDM sensitisation and subsequent respiratory symptoms, but this finding requires further investigation. At present, avoidance of cigarette smoke remains the only unequivocally recommended avoidance strategy for reducing the burden of respiratory disease.

Development of respiratory function in early life

There is an increasing recognition that persistent asthma results from insults occurring in early childhood. An important risk factor for persistent asthma is low lung function, with most longitudinal cohort studies showing a deficit in lung function in asthmatics when it is first measured. Lung function grows along percentiles during the rapid growth period in childhood and, as such, the lung function an individual is born with is a major determinant of lung function throughout life. The respiratory system is immature at birth and has a prolonged period of postnatal maturation. Thus environmental exposures that limit lung growth, especially during the rapid growth period in early childhood, may reduce an individual's peak lung function and increase the risk of persistent asthma.

Prenatal lung development

Lung development begins at approximately 3 weeks of gestation when the laryngotracheal grooves develops from the foregut. The primitive trachea is formed and lobar and segmental bronchi develop by the fifth week. By the end of week 14, approximately 70% of the airways tree has developed with the conducting airways fully formed down to the level of the terminal bronchioles. Major blood vessels develop in parallel with the airways. Fetal breathing movements become established during this period. By the end of the 16th week of gestation, the basic branching pattern of the airways is complete and airways are lined with columnar epithelial cells proximally and cuboidal cells distally. Respiratory bronchioles develop during the canalicular phase of development (weeks 17–27) and by the end of this period the respiratory acini including respiratory bronchioles, alveolar ducts, and primitive alveoli are present. Types I and II pneumocytes also develop during this period and lamellar bodies, the precursors to surfactant production, begin to appear in type II pneumocytes by about 24 weeks' gestation. True alveoli appear only at about 36 weeks and approximately 30–50% of the eventual adult complement of alveoli is present at birth, if this occurs at full term.

Prenatal exposures that affect lung growth and development

For an exposure to impact adversely on growth of the airway tree, it needs to occur while the airways are developing (i.e. before 17 weeks' gestation). Exposures occurring later in gestation may impact on epithelial cell differentiation, development of gas exchange capacity, surfactant production, and alveolar development. A growing number of maternal exposures (e.g. Table 3.1) have been shown to decrease fetal lung growth including: personal and environmental tobacco smoke, air pollution, household chemicals and cleaning agents, respiratory infections, and poor maternal nutrition.

Maternal smoking during pregnancy and, to a lesser extent, exposure to environmental tobacco smoke limit fetal lung growth. Although direct data on mechanisms in humans are limited, maternal smoking inhibits fetal breathing movements. Animal data also demonstrate inhibition of fetal breathing movements, decreased alveolar attachments around airways, and increased collagen deposition around large and small airways. Infants born to mothers who smoked during pregnancy have reduced lung function. Ambient air pollution may decrease fetal somatic growth and lung function in infancy. The mechanism(s) by which environmental toxicants alter lung growth are not known; however, induction of oxidative stress in the mother is likely to be involved.

Postnatal lung growth and development

Knowledge of lung growth in the early postnatal period is largely inferred from measurements of lung function in later childhood and from anatomical studies performed on a small number of supposedly healthy lungs. Lung volume is thought to roughly double from birth to 18

months of age, double again by 5 years of age and double again by adulthood. This growth in volume is accomplished by continued alveolar growth initially and by lung expansion in parallel with somatic growth. Postnatal alveolar growth is thought to proceed rapidly during the first 18 months to 2 years of postnatal life and then to continue more slowly. Airways increase in length and diameter in conjunction with somatic growth, but there is no alteration to the airway branching pattern after birth.

Growth in lung function tracks along growth trajectories, at least from mid-childhood (Fig. 3.6). Data from early childhood are lacking. A recent international collaborative effort has compiled cross-sectional data on lung function measured by spirometry from 4 to 80+ years of age. However, these data need to be treated with caution, especially in young children, where the physiological meaning of the forced expiratory volume in 1 second (FEV_1) differs substantially from that in older children and adults. Similar data from birth through the period of rapid lung growth are lacking.

Postnatal factors influencing lung growth and development

As the postnatal increase in lung function largely parallels somatic growth, factors impacting on somatic growth

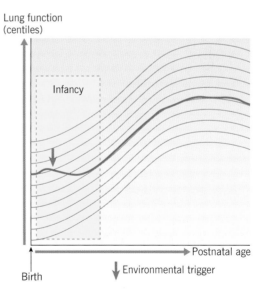

Fig. 3.6 Age-dependent tracking of respiratory function during childhood. Lung function during childhood typically tracks stably on the same centile, which defines their relative capacity at birth. However, exposure to environmental insult(s) such as environmental tobacco smoke (ETS) or severe viral infection can trigger rapid movement to a lower centile, and this may be essentially irreversible, with reduced lung function being the long-term result.

Table 3.1 Environmental exposures known to adversely affect lung growth in relation to timing of exposure

Exposure	Antenatal	Postnatal
Maternal smoking	Yes	Yes
ETS	Probable	Yes
Ambient air pollution	Yes	Yes
Indoor air pollution	Probable	Yes
Poor nutrition	Yes (maternal)	Probable
Viral LRT1	NA	Possible

have the potential to adversely affect growth in lung function. Although a full review of this area is beyond the scope of this chapter, the importance of adequate nutrition for lung growth, especially in low-income developing countries, needs to be recognized. Recent reviews have highlighted the fact that asthmatics, as a group, have lower lung function than non-asthmatics. The extent to which this low lung function is a contributor to the development of asthma or a consequence of other early life factors that predispose to the development of asthma is uncertain.

Early life exposures that are recognized as risk factors for asthma and have been implicated in lower growth in lung function include: postnatal exposure to tobacco smoke, ambient air pollution, and, to a lesser extent, indoor air pollution; several of these factors can also affect lung growth in utero (see Table 3.1). The evidence of a role for early life respiratory viral respiratory infections in limiting lung growth and/or increasing the risk of asthma is increasing. The argument as to whether early life infections damage the lungs (viral-induced effect) or whether such infections unmask vulnerable individuals (susceptible host) has not been settled. Severe viral infections requiring hospitalization, especially with adenoviruses and the respiratory syncytial virus, can damage the developing lung and lead to recurrent respiratory problems, including recurrent wheeze in childhood. As shown in Figure 3.6, if the maturation of lung function is retarded by a significant respiratory infection that drops an individual to a lower growth trajectory, particularly if this occurs against a background of inhalant allergy (see below), lifelong consequences may occur. Recent findings from longitudinal birth cohort studies have shown that early life human rhinovirus infection is particularly potent in this regard, and is both a risk factor for subsequent asthma and associated with lower lung function at the age of 6 years.

Multifactorial nature of allergic disease pathogenesis in early life: interactions between atopic and antimicrobial immunity in asthmatics as a paradigm

Infections and allergy in the inductive phase of asthma

Evidence from prospective birth cohort studies suggests that early infections play a critical role in development of persistent asthma in children. Moreover, the chronology of infection is a key factor; in particular it has been demonstrated that the bulk of the asthmatogenic effects of infections occurring before 2 years of age manifest in

the children who display sensitization within the time frame of these early infections. This suggests that underlying interactions between the host response to pathogens and that to allergens may create a strong inflammatory milieu in the growing lung and airway that has a maximally negative impact on the subsequent development of respiratory function. This general conclusion is consistent with the recent report demonstrating that, although the overall frequency of lower respiratory tract infections is comparable in atopic and non-atopic children, the frequency of highly symptomatic infections is considerably higher amongst the atopic individuals.

An additional finding from these cohort studies is the quantitative nature of the relationship between early sensitization and early infections, in relation to risk for subsequent asthma development. Notably, risk for asthma development by age 5 years increases with the frequency of severe lower respiratory viral infections during the first 2 years, and for each infection frequency the asthma risk increases in a linear fashion with the concomitant titre of aeroallergen-specific IgE (Fig. 3.7). The quantitative nature of the contribution of 'intensity of allergic sensitization' to risk for current asthma continues into the teen years, underscoring the limitations of using binary

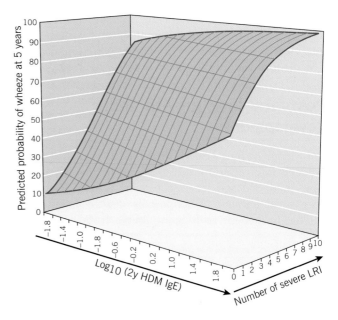

Fig. 3.7 Interaction(s) between severe lower respiratory tract viral infection and aeroallergen-specific IgE in pathogenesis of persistent asthma. These data are from a birth cohort study (J Allergy Clin Immunol 2010; 125:645–51), in which information on the number of severe (wheezing and/or febrile) LRI before age 2 years plus titre of HDM-specific IgE at 2 years and wheezing status at age 5 years, was integrated by logistic regression. The highest probability for current wheeze at age 5 was in children with multiple early infections/early aeroallergen sensitization.

measures of atopy [e.g. skin prick test (SPT) reactivity] in asthma risk assessment.

Respiratory infections as triggers of acute severe asthma: emergency room admissions as a paradigm

The most overt manifestation of the interactions between atopy-associated and infectious disease-associated inflammatory pathways in asthma pathogenesis is that of paediatric ER admissions for acute viral-induced severe exacerbations. The vast majority of these cases occur during the winter viral season, and the affected children are almost invariably atopic. A recent study on such children employing genomics-based techniques to profile circulating inflammatory cell populations within peripheral blood mononuclear cells (PBMC) and detected prominent gene signatures downstream of type 1 IFNs and the Th2 cytokines IL-4 and IL-13, predominantly in monocytes and dendritic cells (DC). This implies the translocation of molecular signals generated at the site of infection to the precursors of migratory leukocyte populations in bone marrow, and their subsequent 'programming' before release into the blood – a process that has been known for many years to operate during episodes of lung inflammation. Prominent amongst this expression signature is the chemokine receptor CCR2, which plays a key role in recruitment of inflammatory cells to inflamed lung, IL-13R, FcεR1γ, and multiple genes indicative of the 'alternatively activated macrophage' (AAM) pathway, and these expression patterns can be reproduced in vitro by culture of PBMC with IFN-α and/or IL-4/IL-13. Moreover, flow cytometric analyses have identified strong up-regulation of expression of FcεR1 on monocytes and both plasmacytoid and myeloid DC in blood during acute exacerbations.

It is noteworthy that recent studies in mouse models of respiratory viral infection have described type 1 IFN-dependent up-regulation of the high-affinity IgE receptor on DC in lungs, and also the accumulation in postinfected lung of IL-13R-bearing AAM, which can become a source of chronic IL-13 production.

An additional finding was the dualistic role of type 1 IFN in this process. Notably, IFN-α has been shown to up-regulate expression of the gamma chain of FcεR1 directly – a process known to be rate limiting in relation to expression of the overall FcεR1 complex on the surface of DC. However, IFN-α also inhibits IL-4/IL-13-mediated up-regulation of FcεR1α gene activation, effectively terminating surface expression of the receptor complex. Thus, initial viral infection initiates a cascade via stimulation of a burst of type 1 IFN production in infected airway tissue, resulting in local up-regulation of the FcεR1 complex on the surface of adjacent airway DC (Fig. 3.8). In the presence of a ready supply of specific IgE and specific aeroallergen (e.g. in atopic children sensitized to

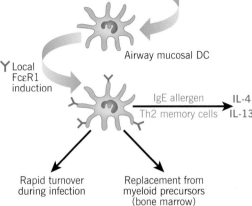

Local effects following viral infection in lungs

Fig. 3.8 Local short-term effects of respiratory viral infection. Viral infection triggers local production of type 1 IFN, which directly up-regulates FcεR1 on airway DC, facilitating their role in allergen presentation to local allergen-specific Th2 memory cells, triggering an initial burst of Th2 cytokines. The DC turn over rapidly in the infected mucosa, and draw on bone marrow for replacements from the myeloid precursor pool.

perennial indoor allergen), this results in markedly enhanced allergen uptake/processing/presentation to, and resultant activation of, Th2 memory cells (see Fig. 3.8). The ensuing burst of IL-4/IL-13 production in the infected airway is sensed by myeloid precursors in bone marrow, which are needed to replenish the airway DC population that turns over very rapidly at the infection site. Under the influence of this IL-4/IL-13 signal, up-regulation of the FcεR1 complex occurs on the surface of the immature DC generated from these precursors, before their release into the circulation and subsequent trafficking to lung and airways – that is, they no longer require local type 1 IFN exposure in the airway to maintain FcεR1 expression (Fig. 3.9).

In order to switch off this cascade, a negative-feedback signal is required in the bone marrow to inhibit IL-4/IL-13-mediated up-regulation of FcεR1 expression, and based on the available in vitro data this signal can be provided via the build-up of type 1 IFN itself. Under such circumstances, any deficiency in capacity to generate type 1 IFN in response to virus (which has been suggested to be a hallmark of adult asthmatics) may increase risk for severe symptoms following infection. Related to this, a recent study profiling sputum-derived cells from children collected during acute severe asthma exacerbations has demonstrated that reduced type 1 IFN production is associated with increased risk for chronic airways obstruction following exacerbation.

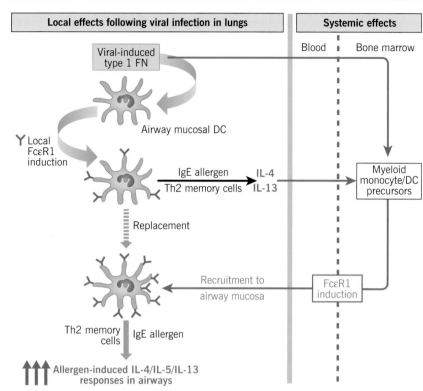

Local effects following viral infection in lungs	Systemic effects

Fig. 3.9 The lung:bone marrow 'axis' in atopics during respiratory viral infection. Th2 cytokines produced via FcεR1-facilitated allergen presentation to Th2 memory cells in airway tissue are sensed by cytokine-receptor-bearing myeloid precursors in the bone marrow, triggering expression of chemokine receptors and FcεR1 prior to their release into blood as replacements for airway mucosal DC. This further enhances Th2 cytokine production in the airway.

Summary of important messages

- The development of the persistent asthma phenotype is in many cases initiated during the first few years of life
- Intrauterine factors appear to 'prime' for early asthma development, but the mechanisms involved are poorly characterized
- The major risk factors operative during early postnatal life are respiratory infections and atopic sensitization
- These can operate independently, or can interact to maximize asthma risk
- Delayed postnatal maturation of immune competence, both innate and adaptive, is a key feature of the 'high-risk' phenotype
- Respiratory viral infections in atopic children trigger rapid up-regulation of FcER1-dependent effector mechanisms

Further reading

Calogero C, Sly PD. Developmental Physiology: lung function during growth and development from birth to old age. In: Frey U, Mercus P, eds. Paediatric lung function. European Respiratory Monograph 47. Lausanne: European Respiratory Society; 2010:1–15.

Holt P, Rowe J, Kusel M, et al. Towards improved prediction of risk for atopy and asthma amongst preschoolers: A prospective cohort study. J Allergy Clin Immunol 2010; 125:645–651.

Holt PG, Strickland DH, Bosco A, et al. Pathogenic mechanisms of allergic inflammation: Atopic asthma as a paradigm. In: Alt FW, ed. Advances in immunology 1. London: Elsevier; 2009:51–113.

Holt PG, Strickland DH, Wikstrom ME, et al. Regulation of immunological homeostasis in the respiratory tract. Nat Rev Immunol 2008; 8:142–152.

Holt PG, Upham JW, Sly PD. Contemporaneous maturation of immunologic and respiratory functions during early childhood: Implications for development of asthma prevention strategies. J Allergy Clin Immunol 2005; 116:16–24.

Latzin P, Roosli M, Huss A, et al. Air pollution during pregnancy and lung function in newborns: a birth cohort study. Eur Respir J 2009; 33:594–603.

Martino D, Prescott SL. Silent mysteries: epigenetic paradigms could hold the key to conquering the epidemic of allergy and immune disease. Allergy 2010; 65(1):7–15.

Prescott SL, Clifton VL. Asthma and pregnancy: emerging evidence of epigenetic interactions in utero. Curr Opin Allergy Clin Immunol 2009; 9 (5):417–426.

Sly PD, Boner AL, Björksten B, et al. Early identification of atopy in the prediction of persistent asthma in children. Lancet 2008; 372:1100–1106.

West CE, Videky D, Prescott SL. Role of diet in the development of immune tolerance in the context of allergic disease. Curr Opin Pediatrics 2010; 22(5):635–641.

Epidemiology of allergy and asthma

Rebecca S Gruchalla, Adnan Custovic and Erika von Mutius

DEFINITION

The epidemiology of allergy and asthma is concerned with the definitions, determinants, and distribution of allergic disease and their prevention, management, morbidity, and mortality.

Atopy, asthma, and allergy

There is a marked variability in the strength of the association between atopy and symptomatic allergic disease in different parts of the world. In addition, although a series of epidemiological studies have suggested that atopy is the strongest risk factor for asthma, most atopic subjects (i.e. those producing IgE antibodies towards common inhalant and food allergens) are not sick and do not have symptoms of asthma or other allergic disease. Whilst these subjects may be at risk of developing allergic diseases such as eczema, food allergy, allergic rhinoconjunctivitis or asthma, many atopic individuals remain asymptomatic throughout their lives. It is largely unknown which factors drive the onset of disease among atopic subjects. One of the reasons for the inconsistency of the findings on the association between atopy and asthma may be phenotypic heterogeneity. Thus, before reviewing the epidemiology of allergy and asthma and the relationship between atopy and symptoms of allergic disease, it is important to discuss the meaning of the diagnostic labels of 'atopy', 'asthma', and 'allergy'.

Most epidemiological studies define atopy as a positive allergen-specific serum IgE (i.e. specific IgE level >0.35 kU_A/L) or positive skin prick test (wheal diameter ≥ 3 mm) to any common food or inhalant allergen. However, when positive, these tests indicate only the presence of allergen-specific IgE, either in serum or bound to the membrane of mast cells in the skin; a sizeable proportion of individuals with positive allergy tests have no evidence of allergic disease. Atopy may not be a simple yes/no phenomenon in relation to onset and progression of allergic disease, and several studies have demonstrated that the level of specific IgE antibodies offers more information than the presence of IgE. It is now recognized that, amongst young wheezy children, quantification of allergen-specific serum IgE may help identify those who are at high risk of subsequent development of persistent asthma. In addition, the level of IgE antibodies to inhalant allergens is associated with an increased risk of hospital admission with acute asthma in childhood, and quantification of specific IgE gives more accurate prediction of hospitalization risk than 'atopy' defined using standard diagnostic criteria. One of the reasons for the inconsistency of findings on the association between atopy and symptomatic allergic disease in epidemiological studies may be phenotypic heterogeneity within the current diagnostic label of 'atopy'. Standard definition of atopy may encompass several different phenotypes that differ in their association with clinical expression of symptomatic disease. In this conceptual framework, detectable serum IgE or positive skin tests alone do not define

DOI: 10.1016/B978-0-7234-3658-4.00005-6

atopy. Rather, they should be viewed as intermediate phenotypes of a true allergic vulnerability – that is, atopy may not be a single phenotype, but rather a sum of many atopic vulnerabilities that differ in their relationship with clinical allergy.

Similarly, one of the difficulties when studying the epidemiology of asthma may arise from the fact that asthma is not a single disease entity, but a collection of diseases presenting as a single syndrome or collection of symptoms. Thus, wheezing may be just a final common pathway of expression of several diseases with different aetiologies, environmental triggers, and genetic associates. This needs to be taken into account when interpreting studies on epidemiology of allergy and asthma.

Worldwide prevalence of allergy and asthma

Across the world there is large variability in the prevalence of asthma, allergic disease, and atopy (Fig. 4.1). Generally low rates have been reported from developing countries and an elevated prevalence in western countries. Within the same ethnic group there is variation in the prevalence of allergic disease and atopy over time and across geographical areas. Such observations suggest an environmental component to the causation of these conditions. Conversely, there is clear familial aggregation and several genetic loci have been linked to asthma, atopy, and total IgE in genome-wide and linkage analyses. These findings strongly suggest an additional genetic component, which is discussed in depth in Chapter 2.

There has been a rise in the prevalence of asthma and allergic diseases in the last century, as documented in many repeated cross-sectional surveys over time (Fig. 4.2). This increasing prevalence has been accompanied by rising trends in allergic sensitization. Since the 1990s the prevalence of allergic diseases has peaked in regions with previously documented high prevalence, whereas an increase was recorded in several centres, mostly in low- and mid-income countries.

In general, allergic sensitization increases with affluence, both on the country and the individual level. The first medical reports described hay fever in the British aristocracy which then spread into less affluent classes of the population. Today high socioeconomic status as assessed by parental education is still a risk factor for atopy, even in affluent countries such as Germany. In contrast, in inner-city areas of the USA poverty is related to increased rates of allergic sensitization and asthma.

The 'hygiene hypothesis'

Family size, crowding, and sibship size are markers of affluence. Several reports had pointed to an inverse relation between crowding and allergic sensitization, before

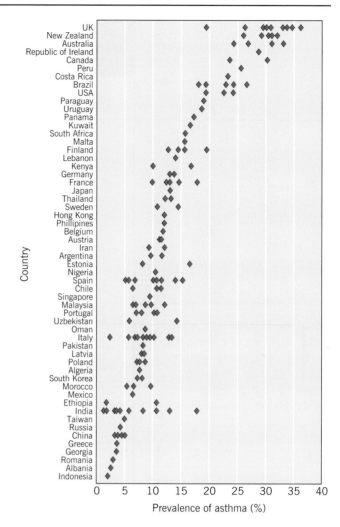

Fig. 4.1 Variation in self-reported wheeze by country. (From: Worldwide variation in prevalence of symptoms of asthma, allergic rhinoconjunctivitis, and atopic eczema: ISAAC. The International Study of Asthma and Allergies in Childhood (ISAAC) Steering Committee. Lancet 1998; 351(9111):1225–1232, with permission.)

Strachan showed that the risk of allergic sensitization and hay fever decreased with increasing numbers of siblings. This observation has been replicated in many populations around the world, but underlying mechanisms have not been elucidated. The original suggestion that infection or unhygienic contact from older siblings to the index child or the mother explains the observation has not been substantiated with respect to overt infections such as hepatitis A, *Helicobacter pylori*, or by counts of infections or antibiotic prescriptions in early life. The reverse notion that maternal atopy may result in reduced fertility and thus lower numbers of offspring has not been confirmed. The temporal changes in atopy prevalence since the 1960s are only marginally attributable to changes in family size.

Effects of contact with other children have been studied using daycare as proxy of exposure. Entry to daycare in

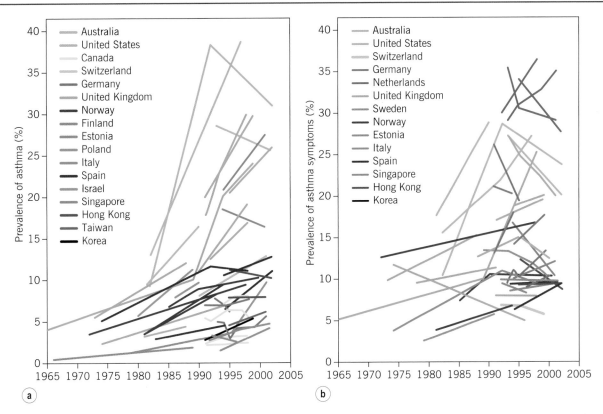

Fig. 4.2 Changes in the prevalence of diagnosed asthma and asthma symptoms over time in children and young adults. (From: Eder W, Ege MJ, von Mutius E. The asthma epidemic. N Engl J Med 2006; 355(21):2226–2235, with permission.)

the first year of life has been shown to decrease rates of allergic sensitization and asthma in Europe, Canada, and the USA. Contact with other living creatures, in particular dogs, early in life has been shown in a number of prospective birth cohort studies to protect from the development of allergic sensitization. All of these factors (crowding, daycare facilities, and dog ownership) have been associated with increased levels of environmental exposure to microbial compounds (endotoxin) and exposure to microbial diversity in the environment. Whether such exposures account for the protective effect associated with crowding, large sibship size, daycare, and dog exposure remains to be determined.

There is some evidence that infections with pathogens such as hepatitis A, salmonella, measles, *Helicobacter pylori*, *Toxoplasma gondii*, herpesvirus, and mycobacteria may be inversely related to the development of allergic sensitization. However, these mostly serological assessments may reflect unhygienic living conditions rather than protective effects of infectious illnesses per se, as these diseases are more easily spread under crowded and more unhygienic conditions. Many but not all of these infectious illnesses invade the host through the gastrointestinal tract, and this route of exposure may be particularly important. Moreover, infestation with parasites through the gastrointestinal tract has been related to decreased risk of allergic sensitization in developing

countries, though its role in the development of asthma, eczema, and allergic rhinitis is less clear.

The microbiome of the intestine and the subjacent immunological organ may play a pivotal role, as suggested by experimental animal studies. However, the evidence to support this notion in humans is still limited. The tools to assess the microbial diversity in the gut are just emerging and must be adapted to use in large-scale studies enrolling hundreds of subjects. Some studies have been based on cultures of faecal material that can detect only a minority of microbes residing in the gut. Significant differences in faecal colonization between areas of high and low prevalence of allergic disease have been found. Intervention studies using different combinations of probiotics and prebiotics have yielded conflicting results. Although some benefit may exist for the prevention of eczema, effects on allergic sensitization, asthma, and allergic rhinitis remain unclear. Finally, the administration of antibiotics may affect the gut microbiome, but in humans there is no clear evidence that the use of antibiotics antedates the new onset of allergic disease, in particular asthma. Prenatal maternal exposure to antibiotics may, however, affect the incidence of allergic disease in the offspring.

Whether other exposures related to unhygienic living conditions affect the production of IgE antibodies towards allergens has hardly been investigated. One study in Russian Karelia revealed that water contamination with mostly faecal bacteria was strongly inversely related to allergic sensitization. The impact of personal hygiene on the incidence of atopy and allergic disease in urban, westernized populations is unknown.

Virus infections

Over the last couple of decades there has been mounting evidence implicating viruses, especially rhinoviruses, as an important cause of asthma exacerbations in both children and adults. One of the earliest studies done in children to establish a link between asthma exacerbations and viral infections was performed by Johnston and colleagues in 1995 in the United Kingdom. In this study, upper respiratory viral infections were detected in 80–85% of asthma exacerbations and picornaviruses (mostly rhinoviruses) accounted for the majority of the infections. A strong correlation was observed between upper respiratory viral infections and hospital admissions for asthma, adding evidence that viral infections play a role not only in causing asthma exacerbations, but also in causing exacerbations severe enough to warrant hospitalization.

In addition to the finding that viruses are a major cause of asthma exacerbations is the one that allergic sensitization may be a risk factor for lower respiratory tract symptoms with these infections. This relationship was initially demonstrated by Duff and colleagues, who found that the presence of IgE antibodies to inhalant allergens was a significant risk factor for wheezing with viral infection in children presenting to an emergency department because of wheezing. A synergistic effect of allergen sensitization, high-level exposure to sensitizing allergen, and respiratory virus infection in increasing the risk of severe asthma exacerbations resulting in hospital admission has been demonstrated both amongst adults and amongst children, which suggests that there may be a combined effect of natural virus infection and real life allergen exposure in allergic asthmatics in inducing severe asthma exacerbations.

Urban lifestyle and air pollution

Other environmental exposures associated with urban residence such as air pollution and sedentary lifestyle have been scrutinized over the last decades. There is an ongoing debate about potential association of increasing body mass index, sedentary lifestyle, and asthma, but most studies have not found an effect on atopy. The data relating obesity and asthma are also conflicting. Although some studies have shown a positive correlation, others have not. The finding by Kattan and colleagues that obesity was associated with increased asthma symptoms and exacerbations only in females suggests that gender-specific factors may need to be considered when examining the asthma–obesity relationship.

Some types of air pollution, but not others have been related to the development of allergic sensitization. In urban areas in former East Germany with high levels of SO_2 and total suspended particles emanating from coal burning and industry, the prevalence of allergic sensitization was lower than in less-polluted urban areas in West Germany. In turn, exposure to traffic has been related to the development of sensitization, in particular pollen sensitization, but not all surveys have confirmed these effects. Overall, the adverse effect of traffic exposure seems to be more pronounced for the incidence of asthma than for allergic sensitization.

Numerous cross-sectional and time-series studies have demonstrated acute changes in lung function, respiratory symptoms, and/or medication/healthcare use after short-term exposure to elevated levels of O_3, particulate matter, NO_2, SO_2, and CO.

Although short-term exposures are probably important, it is essential to look at more chronic pollutant exposures, since longer exposure periods are likely to be more relevant to the development of long-term adverse airway effects. Akinbami and colleagues evaluated the association between chronic outdoor air pollutant exposure, using 12-month average levels, and asthma outcomes in a large national sample of US children (34 073, ages 3–17) living in metropolitan areas. Using continuous models, a 5-unit increase in O_3 exposure was significantly associated with both having current asthma (adjusted odds ratio of 1.08; CI 1.02, 1.14) and of having at least one asthma attack in the previous 12 months (1.07; 1.00, 1.13). Although significant associations were not demonstrated with other pollutants using continuous models, when pollutant values were divided into quartiles, children residing in counties with the highest ozone and particulate matter (PM_{10}) levels were more likely to have current asthma and/or a recent asthma attack than children living in counties with the lowest pollution levels.

In addition to outdoor pollutants, indoor particulate matter, especially indoor environmental tobacco smoke (ETS), also contributes to asthma-associated morbidity. However, as recently pointed out by McCormack and colleagues, there are other sources of particulate matter indoors besides ETS. Common cooking and cleaning activities are important sources of particulate matter, as is traffic-related particulate matter that seeps indoors.

Allergens

Whilst high allergen exposure amongst sensitized individuals is associated with more severe disease, the relationship between allergen exposure and development of sensitization and asthma is much more complex. Most, but not all, studies investigating the relationship between dust mite allergen exposure and development of sensitization to mites have demonstrated increases in the risk of sensitization with increasing allergen exposure. Some studies have suggested that dust mite allergen exposure may play a role in the development of asthma, but others have not been able to confirm this. For cockroach allergens, the prevalence of sensitization is associated with the levels of exposure, and cockroach infestation is a strong risk factor for cockroach sensitization (especially in US inner-city homes).

Contradictory findings have been reported with respect to exposure to domestic pets and pet allergens. Clearly, pet sensitization is a strong risk factor for asthma, and patients with established asthma who are pet sensitized and exposed to high levels of pet allergen tend to have more severe asthma than those who are not exposed. However, it is unclear whether pet ownership is a risk factor for sensitization or is protective. Numerous studies have been published, with some suggesting that exposure to pet allergens may be protective against sensitization or development of asthma, whereas others show that cat exposure may increase the risk of sensitization. The effects of exposure to cats may differ from that to dogs (e.g. no studies have shown an increase in risk associated with dog exposure).

Clinical outcomes reported from intervention studies which aimed to reduce allergen exposure in early life in order to prevent allergic sensitization and asthma appear inconsistent and often confusing. Ongoing prevention cohorts have provided us with a wealth of information, but much longer follow-up is required before we can be sure that the interventions do not cause any harm, and can confidently give any advice within the public health context.

On balance, the evidence suggests that the relationship between allergen exposure and the development of sensitization and asthma is likely to be determined by the type of allergen, timing, pattern, dose and type of exposure, and other interacting factors (including genetic).

Protective exposures in rural areas

A number of studies have addressed differences in the prevalence of allergic diseases and atopy between urban and rural areas within one country. In China and Mongolia, allergic sensitization rates were below or around 10% in rural areas, whereas in the big megacities Hong Kong and Ulaanbaatar atopy rates were comparable to western countries. In Europe similar strong gradients from rural to urban areas have been found in Greece and Poland. Similar urban–rural differences have been reported in Canada. Subjects moving from rural areas into cities retain in part their protection.

Numerous studies have been performed in rural areas in Europe to contrast prevalence of asthma and allergic diseases in children and adults living on farms as compared with subjects living in rural areas, but not on farms.

Almost all studies reported a decreased prevalence of hay fever and allergic rhinoconjunctivitis among farm children compared with non-farm children; studies that included objective measures of specific IgE antibodies (by skin prick tests or serum measurements) corroborated the findings.

Results relating to asthma and wheeze are less consistent. Only few studies included measures of airway hyperresponsiveness. In the Danish and the German study the prevalence of airway hyperresponsiveness was significantly reduced among farm children. A Canadian survey confirmed these findings, with no studies showing an increased prevalence of airway hyperresponsiveness among children raised on farms.

Looking at adult farming populations, similar figures have been observed. In the European farmers study, the prevalence of allergic rhinitis was 14.0% in 20–44-year-old animal farmers compared with 20.7% among the participants in the European Community Respiratory Health Survey. Likewise, the prevalence of asthma was significantly lower among animal farmers compared with the general population. For asthma, these findings have been confirmed in Norway, the Netherlands, Denmark, and Canada. Only the Norwegian study could not confirm a protective association between working on a farm and allergic rhinitis.

The studies cited above were based on a cross-sectional design. Only two studies have used a prospective, longitudinal approach. In Canada, over 13 000 asthma-free children aged 0–11 years were surveyed and the incidence of physician-diagnosed asthma was determined prospectively 2 years later. The 2-year cumulative incidence of asthma was 2.3%, 5.3%, and 5.7% among children living in farming, rural non-farming, and non-rural environments respectively. From the multivariate analysis with adjustment for confounders, children from a farming environment had a reduced risk of asthma compared with children from rural non-farming environment, with odds ratios of 0.22 (95% CI: 0.07–0.74) and 0.39 (0.24–0.65) for children with and without parental history of asthma respectively. In Austria, 1150 elementary school children were recruited from nine different areas in 1994 and followed for 3 years. Adjusting for potential confounders, parental farming was inversely related to the prevalence and new occurrence of atopy. Furthermore, children living in a farming environment were more likely to lose their positive skin prick test during follow-up.

Sources of protective exposures in farming environments

Farming practices vary between farms and between countries. Some investigators have attempted to identify individual exposures in farm surroundings contributing to the reduction in risk of asthma and allergic diseases. Initial observations from Germany and Switzerland reported that children from full-time farmers had lower risk of atopic disease than children of part-time farmers, suggesting a dose–response effect. Two recent studies conducted outside Europe suggest that an important component of the farm environment is livestock exposure, since no protective effect of farming was observed among children living in a primarily crop-farming region. This notion is supported by the finding of the European studies, where exposure to livestock has been identified as an important contributor to the protective farm effect. Interestingly, in the Austrian study children who did not live on a farm but had regular contact with farm animals also had less allergic sensitization (13.5 % versus 34.8%). Consumption of unpasteurized milk has been identified as a protective factor in a number of studies. As with livestock exposure, this effect was not restricted to children living on a farm, but was also seen among non-farm populations consuming unpasteurized milk. A recent in-depth analysis of the multicentre PARSIFAL study in rural areas in Europe has also shown significant inverse relations of asthma with keeping pigs in addition to dairy farming and the contact with fodder for the animals (such as silage and hay).

European studies among adult farmers also provide some evidence that the protective effect of farming on atopic diseases might be more pronounced among animal farmers, with the strongest effect among pig and cattle farmers. However, recent studies outside Europe were less consistent. In Canada, living on a farm had an overall protective effect on asthma and allergic rhinitis. Taking intensity of livestock contact into account did not make a difference with respect to prevalence of asthma or allergic rhinitis. Likewise, US farm women who worked with animals had the same prevalence of atopic and non-atopic asthma as those not working with animals. Therefore, the size and extent of industrialization of farming and other differences in farming practices have to be taken into account when studying the effect of different types of farming exposure on allergies and asthma.

Timing of farming exposures

There is increasing evidence to suggest that the effect of environmental exposures strongly depends on the timing. Throughout infancy, childhood, and adolescence, the human organism is in a constant process of development and maturation. It is conceivable that there are windows of accessibility and vulnerability towards extrinsic influences during certain stages of development. Prenatal factors may play a significant role either through mechanisms acting in utero, or as epigenetic modulation of subsequent developmental trajectories. In the PARSIFAL study, the risk of atopic sensitization was not only influenced by a child's exposure to the farming environment, but also strongly determined by maternal exposure to stables during pregnancy.

A number of studies have addressed the association between childhood contact to farming environments and the prevalence of asthma and allergies during adulthood. All of them found an inverse association between being raised on a farm and the prevalence of allergic sensitization and allergic rhinitis during adulthood. To analyse further the relevance of timing of exposure, several studies have assessed the potential interaction between childhood and adulthood exposure to farming environments and the prevalence of allergies and asthma during adulthood. Across these studies, the protective effect of farming environments on respiratory allergies was largest when farm contact started during childhood and was sustained until adulthood.

Overall, the protective effect of regular visits to animal houses on respiratory allergy was largest when these visits started during the first 6 years of life. Therefore, childhood exposure seems to be of uppermost importance in the life course of allergic sensitization.

Assuming that farm contact during childhood is also a proxy for prenatal and infant exposure provides additional evidence for the importance of prenatal factors on the development of asthma and allergies. One recent study among 137 university employees, of whom 36% were working with laboratory animals, indicated that those with farm contact during infancy were protected from sensitization to occupational allergens later in life. Likewise, among adults living in a rural agricultural area of Germany, occupational exposure to high-molecular-weight agents did not increase the risk of allergic sensitization – on the contrary, such exposure was inversely related to allergic sensitization to common allergens.

It is unclear why individuals who stopped contact with farming environments do not encounter the same protection as those with continuous exposure. This may be an indication of a 'healthy worker bias', meaning that those with symptoms leave the farming environment. Although this might partly explain the effect, the strengths of the relationship and the consistency of the association across studies cannot be explained by a self-selection into farming alone. Another possibility is that farmers tend to underreport symptoms. However, as the findings are evident not only for self-reported symptoms but also for objective markers (e.g. allergic sensitization assessed by skin prick test or specific IgE), underreporting is not a plausible explanation. It is more likely that the underlying cause of the observed interaction is a complex interplay between prenatal factors, early childhood exposures and events encountered over the life course.

Within childhood years the timing of exposures also plays a role. The paediatric farm studies have clearly shown that infant and prenatal exposures matter. In the PARSIFAL study, the risk of atopic sensitization was influenced not only by a child's exposure to the farming environment, but also by maternal exposure to stables during pregnancy. Moreover, immune responses in cord blood were influenced by maternal farm exposures during pregnancy.

Microbial exposures

Children exposed to livestock are likely to encounter higher levels of allergens, bacteria, and fungi than children without such exposure. Yet to date only few out of the many microbial exposures have been measured in farming environments. Bacterial substances such as endotoxin from gram-negative species and muramic acid, a component of peptidoglycan from the cell wall of all types of bacteria, have been found to be more abundant in mattress dust from farm children than non-farm children. Likewise, extracellular polysaccharide (EPS) from *Penicillium* and *Aspergillus spp.* is more prevalent in farming than non-farming households.

Endotoxin levels in dust samples from the children's mattresses have been shown to inversely relate to the occurrence of hay fever, atopic asthma, and atopic sensitization in rural but also in urban populations. Independently of endotoxin concentrations, increasing levels of muramic acid and a marker of fungal exposure (EPS) were associated with a lower frequency of wheezing and asthma among rural school children. Thus exposures not only to environmental bacteria but also to moulds might modulate immune responses and thereby protect against allergic diseases.

This concept is in line with a study on the effects of endotoxin and fungal spores on atopy and asthma in adult farmers in which fungal spores, rather than endotoxin, were inversely related to atopic wheeze. Another study among Dutch adult farmers designed a job exposure matrix (JEM) to assign individual occupational exposure to endotoxins. Using this JEM, endotoxin exposure was inversely related to self-reported symptoms of allergic rhinitis among the farmers. However, the prevalence of asthma symptoms augmented with increasing exposure, as seen with non-atopic wheeze among school-age children. This study confirms an earlier case-control study among Dutch pig farmers. Although higher endotoxin levels were associated with a reduced risk of sensitization to common allergens, farmers with higher levels of endotoxin exposure were more likely to have airway hyper-responsiveness and reduced lung function. These studies give further evidence that farming exposure might have differing effects on different phenotypes: while protecting from respiratory allergies and atopic asthma, such exposure may pose a risk for non-atopic asthma.

As discussed above, foodborne and orofaecal infections like *Helicobacter pylori*, *Toxoplasma gondii*, and hepatitis A virus might also protect from respiratory allergy. Therefore, one explanation for the protective effect of the farming environment might be that exposure to microbial agents in the farm environment is a proxy for such infections. A study analysing the association between farm animal contact, serological markers of foodborne and orofaecally transmitted infections, and atopy provided evidence that these mechanisms act independently. It was shown that early contact to animals increases the likelihood of *Toxoplasma gondii* seropositivity. However, early contact to farm animals was still the strongest predictor of atopy.

Racial disparities and asthma prevalence and morbidity in the USA

A recent National Health Interview Survey (NHIS), which included questions about asthma prevalence, asthma exacerbations, and asthma-related healthcare use during the period 1980–2004, found that the estimated number of persons with self-reported asthma during the previous 12 months had increased significantly from approximately 6.8 million (3.1%) in 1980 to 14.9 million (5.6%) in 1995 (Fig. 4.3). Even after 1995, it appeared that prevalence rates continued to rise. However, this is probably not the case since in 1997 the NHIS questionnaire was redesigned and this redesign made it difficult to compare post-1997 data with those obtained before 1997. Despite this problem of comparing previous data with current data, the fact remained that, although overall prevalence did not increase from 2001 to 2004, it remained high during this time period (2001: 7.3%; 2002: 7.2%; 2003: 6.9%; 2004: 7.1%).

Although the asthma prevalence rates increased in both adults and children from 1980 to 1995, the rise was more pronounced in children. During this time period, the rate for adults increased from 2.9% to 5.0%, while

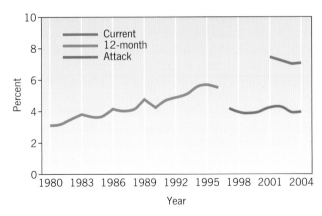

Source: National Health Interview Survey; National Center for Health Statistics

Fig. 4.3 Estimated prevalence of asthma, by persons who reported an asthma attack during the preceding 12 months, persons who reported having asthma during the preceding 12 months, and persons who reported current asthma – United States, 1980–2004. (From: National Health Interview Survey; National Center for Health Statistics.)

the rate for children more than doubled (3.5% to 7.5%). From 2001 to 2003, while there was no further significant rate increase in either group, prevalence rates remained high, especially in children (8.5% versus 6.7% in adults). The most recent measurement, which is from 2007, indicates that 9.1% or 6.7 million children in the USA have asthma.

Epidemiological studies done in the 1980s revealed not only that asthma and its associated morbidity were increasing in the USA, but also that they were increasing disproportionately in specific populations. Using national population-based data systems of the National Center for Health Statistics, it was found that hospitalization rates for asthma between 1965 and 1983 increased by 50% in adults and by over 200% in children, particularly in black adults and children. A study done in Maryland for the time period 1979–1982 found that the asthma hospital discharge rate for black children was three times greater than that for white children. Although this study did not specifically address the possible reasons for this disproportionate distribution, it appeared it was due to a greater prevalence of poverty among Maryland's black population. Similarly, another study done in New York City in the early 1980s found that hospitalization and death rates among blacks and Hispanics were 3–5.5 times those seen for whites and that asthma-associated morbidity and mortality rates were highest in low-income neighbourhoods that were predominately black or Hispanic.

The most recent figures available through the Centers for Disease Control and Prevention indicate that asthma-associated morbidity remains a serious health concern in US cities. In 2004, not only was the asthma death rate found to be over five-fold higher in black children compared with white children, but also this group of children, as well as Hispanic children, was found to have more indicators of poorer asthma control. More specifically, data obtained from the 2003–2004 four-state sample of the National Asthma Survey indicated that twice as many black children had asthma-related emergency department visits and hospitalizations compared with white children during that time period. Moreover, data from the same survey indicated that black children had greater short-acting β-agonist use compared with white children and that significantly fewer black and Hispanic children reported using inhaled corticosteroids in the past 3 months compared with white children.

Multiple factors are responsible for the high asthma-associated morbidity of children living in inner cities. These include poor access to quality care, psychological issues, poor understanding of the importance of controller medications and low adherence to these medications. In addition to these, another critical factor shown to be a major contributor to asthma-associated morbidity in this population is exposure and sensitization to cockroach allergen, an allergen often present in inner-city residences.

The relationship between cockroach allergy and asthma-associated morbidity was confirmed in the late 1990s. In a large study that evaluated US inner city children with asthma, Rosenstreich and colleagues found that the majority of these children were poor, primarily black or Hispanic, had a number of psychosocial problems, and had a high degree of environmental allergen reactivity. Most importantly, however, was the finding that, of the allergen sensitivities evaluated, only one, cockroach allergy, was related to asthma-associated morbidity. In addition, and as importantly, was the finding that sensitivity alone was not sufficient. Children had to be both cockroach-allergic and exposed to high levels of cockroach allergen (greater than 8 U/gram of dust). These children, unlike children who were not cockroach-allergic or children who were allergic but not exposed, had significantly greater unscheduled visits for asthma, days of wheezing, nights of disrupted sleep and school days missed (Fig. 4.4). Thus, the results of this study confirmed that cockroach allergy plays a central role in asthma, especially asthma in inner-city residents.

Fungal allergens have long been thought to be associated with asthma morbidity. In a study done in children and young adults with asthma in the early 1990s, *Alternaria* skin-test reactivity was associated with a 200-fold increased risk of respiratory arrest. This initial finding, that there may be a link between asthma and fungal allergy, was subsequently corroborated by the Childhood Asthma Management Program (CAMP). In this study, a direct correlation between increased sensitivity to inhaled methacholine and skin-test sensitivity to *Alternaria* was demonstrated. In inner-city children also, a similar relationship between fungal allergy and asthma-associated morbidity has been shown to exist.

Sensitivity to indoor mammalian allergens has also been associated with asthma-associated morbidity in US populations. However, while sensitivity to cat or dog dander has been associated with increased bronchial responsiveness in some children, mouse and rat allergy appears to play a more important role in children with asthma who live in the inner city. These allergens are prevalent in inner-city homes, and sensitization and exposure to them have been associated with increased asthma symptoms and asthma-associated unscheduled visits and hospitalizations.

In addition to allergen sensitivity and exposure, other factors that have been associated with asthma morbidity in inner-city US populations include indoor and outdoor air pollution, viral infections, access to care issues, and possibly obesity.

Although the first study to suggest a link between asthma exacerbations and viral infections was done by Johnson and colleagues in the UK (see Section on virus infections), there has also been evidence in the US to suggest a link between respiratory viral infections and

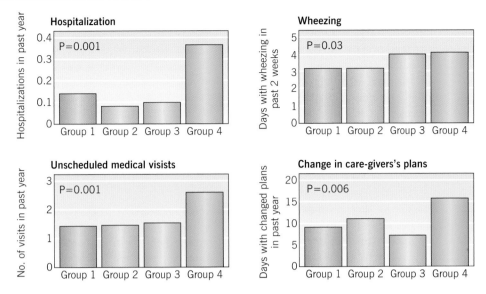

Fig. 4.4 Morbidity among children with asthma, according to the presence or absence of allergy to cockroach allergen and the degree of exposure. The values shown are the means for each measure of morbidity. Group 1 is made up of children without allergy to cockroach allergen and with low levels of exposure to the allergen; group 2, children without allergy to cockroach allergen and with high levels of exposure; group 3, children with allergy to cockroach allergen and with low levels of exposure; and group 4, children with allergy to cockroach allergen and with high levels of exposure. The p values are for the comparison between group 4 and groups 1, 2, and 3 combined.

asthma. In 2002, Gergen and colleagues found that asthma symptoms and healthcare utilization in inner-city children with asthma were more pronounced in the autumn–winter season. While outdoor levels of SO_2 were found to be correlated with this increased asthma-associated morbidity, the authors thought, but did not prove (due to absence of data), that the more likely explanation for this observation was the increased presence of viral infections in these children during this time period. Indeed, subsequently it was shown that respiratory viruses, especially rhinoviruses, were associated with asthma exacerbations.

In addition to the finding that viruses are a major cause of asthma exacerbation is the finding that allergic sensitization may be a risk factor for lower respiratory tract symptoms with these infections. This relationship was initially demonstrated by Duff and colleagues who found that the presence of IgE antibodies to inhalant allergens was a significant risk factor for wheezing with viral infection in children presenting to an emergency department because of wheezing. Subsequently, Green and colleagues were able to demonstrate a similar synergism between allergen sensitivity and viral infections in adults with acute asthma that resulted in hospitalization.

The finding that asthmatics, especially atopic asthmatics, have increased airway symptoms during respiratory viral illnesses has generated much research. Studies have been focused on not only why this happens, but also how (i.e. the mechanisms responsible). Although few data exist to answer these questions clearly, recent work reveals that there may be a synergistic relationship between allergic sensitization and viral infections, and that this synergism leads to a loss of asthma control (i.e. increased exacerbations).

Another very important factor that contributes to asthma-associated morbidity, especially for those living in inner-city environments is access to quality health care. To analyse this issue in more detail, Flores and colleagues examined 220 minority children who had an emergency department or inpatient ward admission for asthma. Of these children, 92% had a primary care provider, 96% had either public or private insurance and 95% had prescription medications for their asthma. Despite this, only 44% of children had asthma action plans, only 17% had an asthma specialist and almost two-thirds of parents indicated that they used the emergency department for their usual source of asthma care. When multivariate analyses were performed, two important things were noted: one, having an asthma care plan was associated with a reduced risk of asthma exacerbations and, two, having an asthma specialist was associated with a five-fold increased likelihood of having an asthma care plan.

Another study, which was conducted in the Denver Public Schools, found that the majority (90%) of children with asthma had health insurance and 92% had a physician caring for their asthma. However, this study too found that having a medical provider did not have a major impact on asthma control. Students who had medical providers were as likely as those who did not have providers to report a hospitalization or emergency department visit for asthma, daytime and nighttime asthma symptoms and rescue inhaler use.

A possible explanation for the findings of these two groups is that, although inner-city children with asthma appear to have both insurance and primary care providers, they do not seek regular medical care for their disease. Since asthma is an episodic disease with long asymptomatic periods, not having daily reminders of the disease may cause families not to seek regular medical care but rather to seek care only during asthma crises. Since inner-city families are known to have numerous stressors in their lives, it is indeed possible that obtaining regular care for a chronic disease such as asthma takes a back seat to more pressing family needs. If further studies confirm this possibility, then implementation of disease management programmes that focus on daily reinforcement of self-management practices may lead to significantly reduced asthma-associated morbidity in inner-city populations.

Conclusions

There has been a marked increase in the prevalence of allergy and asthma in the latter part of the 20th century, seen across all ages and ranges of severity. More recent evidence suggests that this increase may have now reversed in some developed countries and in some age groups. The prevalence rates vary throughout the world, being the highest in English-speaking nations, higher in western than in eastern parts of Europe, and higher in urban than in rural parts of Africa. In developing parts of the world the prevalence continues to increase, and global differences may be getting smaller.

The fundamental role of the environment is emphasized by the short time frame within which the increase in allergies and asthma occurred. The environmental changes that have occurred contemporaneously with the increase in allergies include changes in patterns of microbial exposure in early life, family size and childcare arrangements, housing design, exposure to a number of pollutants, diet, and exercise. The increase in prevalence of allergies and asthma is probably a consequence of environmental factors increasing the risk in genetically susceptible individuals mediated through gene–environment interactions.

In addition to the rise in prevalence, the increased asthma-associated morbidity that has been seen, especially in US inner cities, is also due to multiple factors. Most importantly, exposures to environmental allergens such as cockroach and rodent allergens, exposure to indoor and outdoor pollutants, and poor access to quality healthcare are leading factors responsible for this continuing severe healthcare issue.

Summary of important messages

- Across the world there is large variability in the prevalence of allergic illnesses and asthma. Whereas in some affluent areas almost half the population is sensitized to common aeroallergens, in other parts these diseases are almost non-existent
- Both environmental exposures and genetic factors play an important role in the new onset of these conditions, but their roles differ for asthma and atopy
- There is not a single gene for asthma or allergy; rather, many genetic factors contribute to the manifestation of disease
- There are a number of environmental risk factors that have been associated with asthma and allergies such as inner city environments in the US, active and passive smoking, air pollution, indoor environment, diet, and exercise
- Environmental exposures protecting from allergy and asthma have also been identified, for example farming environments, microbial exposure in early life, family size, and childcare arrangements
- A complex interplay of environmental and genetic factors results in the new onset of allergy and asthma

Further reading

Asher MI, Montefort S, Bjorksten B, et al. Worldwide time trends in the prevalence of symptoms of asthma, allergic rhinoconjunctivitis, and eczema in childhood: ISAAC Phases One and Three repeat multicountry cross-sectional surveys. Lancet 2006; 368:733–743.

Braun-Fahrlander C, Riedler J, Herz U, et al. Environmental exposure to endotoxin and its relation to asthma in school-age children. N Engl J Med 2002; 347:869–877.

Ede MJ, Mayer M, Normand AC, et al. Exposure to environmental microorganisms and childhood asthma. N Engl J Med 2011; 364(8):701–709.

Eder W, Ege MJ, von Mutius E. The asthma epidemic. N Engl J Med 2006; 355:2226–2235.

Ginde AA, Espinola JA, Camargo CA Jr. Improved overall trends but persistent racial disparities in emergency department visits for acute asthma, 1993–2005. J Allergy Clin Immunol 2008; 122:313–318.

Gruchalla RS, Pongracic J, Plaut M, et al. Inner City Asthma Study: relationships among sensitivity, allergen exposure, and asthma morbidity. J Allergy Clin Immunol 2005; 115:478–485.

Moorman JE, Rudd RA, Johnson CA, et al. National surveillance for asthma-United States, 1980–2004. MMWR Surveill Summ 2007; 56:1–54.

Rosenstreich DL, Eggleston P, Kattan M, et al. The role of cockroach allergy and exposure to cockroach allergen in causing morbidity among inner-city children with asthma. N Engl J Med 1997; 336:1356–1363.

Simpson A, John SL, Jury F, et al. Endotoxin exposure, CD14, and allergic disease: an interaction between genes and the environment. Am J Respir Crit Care Med 2006; 174:386–392.

von Mutius E, Vercelli D. Farm living: effects on childhood asthma and allergy. Nat Rev Immunol 2010; 10(12):861–868.

5

Allergens and air pollutants

Geoffrey A Stewart, David B Peden,
Philip J Thompson and Martha Ludwig

DEFINITION

Allergens are antigens, usually proteinaceous in nature, that sensitize the host for allergic reactions involving specific IgE and mast cells. Their sources are diverse and include house dust mite products, pollens, fungal spores, animals, drugs, and foods.

Air pollutants are chemicals, gases and dusts that contaminate the air we breathe. They usually arise from human activity, and have the potential to damage health. In general, they are non-allergenic but they may contribute to allergic sensitization and/or exacerbate allergic diseases. Major pollutants arise from both outdoor and indoor sources and include both gases and non-biological and biological particulates such as ozone, nitrogen dioxide, diesel fumes, cigarette smoke, and microbial- and plant-derived products.

Allergens

Introduction

Humans are exposed to a variety of environmental, non-pathogen-associated antigens that may induce the production of IgE, the antibody isotype associated with Type-1-mediated diseases, in about up to 30% of Western populations. Originally thought to have evolved to combat metazoan parasite infection caused by helminthic worms and ectoparasites by activating the T-helper-2 (Th2) arm of the adaptive immune response (IgE production, basophilia, eosinophilia, mast cell degranulation, IL-4 and IL-5 cytokine production), this system is capable of being activated by supposedly innocuous proteins in genetically predisposed, non-parasitized individuals. Those substances that stimulate the production of, and bind to, IgE are usually referred to as allergens rather than antigens (*anti*body *gen*erator) to distinguish them from those routinely associated with IgA, IgG, and IgM production, and the capacity of a protein to stimulate an IgE response is referred to as allergenicity rather than immunogenicity. The host may come into contact with allergens in either domestic or occupational settings via a number of routes, but inhalation represents the most important, although exposure due to ingestion, injection, and absorption through the skin and gut frequently occurs. The sequelae resulting from the interaction between allergens and IgE bound to mast cells and basophils via these portals underlie diseases such as rhinitis, sinusitis, asthma, conjunctivitis, urticaria, eczema, atopic dermatitis, anaphylaxis and angioedema, allergic and migraine headache, and certain gastrointestinal disorders (Box 5.1). As they result from the activation of the adaptive immune system, Type-1-mediated allergic diseases result from two temporally distinct stages. In the first (also known as the sensitization or antibody-induction) stage, inhaled, injected, or ingested allergen is presented to the immune system by professional antigen-presenting cells (e.g. dendritic cells, B cells, basophils, and macrophages) and this, in susceptible individuals, causes plasma cells to produce IgE, which then binds to mast cells and basophils via specific receptors that interact with the Fc region of IgE such as the high-affinity FcεRI. In the second (effector) phase, allergen interacts with receptor-bound IgE to cause mast cell degranulation, which clinically manifests within 5–15 minutes after the sensitized host is re-exposed. The degranulation process results in the release of various inflammatory mediators

Box 5.1 Allergen sources and allergic diseases

Asthma and/or rhinitis	Anaphylaxis	Atopic dermatitis
Animal danders	Biologicals	Bacteria
Cockroaches	Food allergens	Dust mites
Dust mites	Insect venoms	Food allergens
Food allergens	Low-molecular-weight drugs	Human autoallergen
Fungi	Biologicals	Occupational allergens
Grass pollen		
Latex		
Occupational allergens		
Tree pollen		
Weed pollen		

(see elsewhere in this book) that give rise to the characteristic features of Type-1-mediated allergic disease. At both stages, it is assumed that allergens breach innate defence barriers such as skin and internal gut and respiratory epithelial layers to facilitate interaction with IgE-sensitized mast cells and thus initiate disease.

Most of the clinically important allergens have now been cloned and several genomes of allergen sources sequenced, and thus their biological function within a source determined. Many are hydrolytic enzymes such as proteases, carbohydrases, ribonucleases, and enzymes involved in pectin degradation from mites, fungi, and pollens, or non-hydrolytic enzymes such as pectin lyase from herbaceous dicotyledon and tree pollen, the glycolytic enzymes from fungi such as enolase, alcohol dehydrogenase, aldolase and phosphoglycerate kinase, and glutathione transferases from cockroach and dust mites. Similarly, many show enzyme-inhibitory activity or demonstrate marked sequence homology to known inhibitors, and are commonly found in seeds, potatoes, pollens, and hen's egg white. Many others are proteins involved in the transport of ligands such as lipids, pheromones, electrons, oxygen, and iron, particularly the lipocalin allergens from animals such as rodents, dogs, cows, and horses. Some allergens have been shown to be similar to a disparate but ubiquitous group of proteins known or considered to possess regulatory properties. These proteins are also encountered as allergens in pollinosis, parasite infection, and autoimmunity, and include profilins, the EF-hand calcium-binding proteins, the cytoskeletal protein tropomyosin, and heat-shock proteins. Although their regulatory properties are varied, many appear to be associated with actin biology such as is seen with pollen tube growth. The production of these proteins by recombinant technologies has now made it possible to determine the three-dimensional structures of a large number of clinically important allergens as well as determine the structure and location of B-cell and T-cell epitopes (Fig. 5.1).

Allergen nomenclature

The Allergen Nomenclature Subcommittee of the International Union of Immunological Societies (IUIS) (http://www.allergen.org) first introduced guidelines in 1986 to facilitate the consistent naming of purified allergens from complex sources prior to the emergence of data about their true function and structure. This committee is responsible for denominating allergens as long as they are recognized by more than 5% of an allergic population using a panel of more than five individual patients, and it also maintains an allergen reference database. With regard to denominating allergens, specific guidelines must be adhered to and details of a novel allergen must be submitted to the committee for naming. For example, using the published guidelines, the designation for the cysteine protease allergen Der p 1, from the house dust mite *Dermatophagoides pteronyssinus*, is constructed by taking the first three letters of the genus (i.e. *Dermatophagoides*) together with the first letter of the species (i.e. *pteronyssinus*) and combining them with an arabic numeral that reflects the order in which the allergen was isolated or its clinical importance. In the case of Der p 1, this was the first mite allergen to be isolated and characterized, as well as cloned. If there is likely to be confusion with a previously named allergen, an additional letter may be used from either the genus or species name to avoid such a possibility. For example, the fungal alkaline serine protease allergen from *Penicillium chrysogenum* is designated Pen ch 13 to distinguish it from the related allergen Pen c 13 from *Penicillium citrinum*. Similarly, the allergen from *Candida albicans* is designated Cand a 1 to differentiate it from the dog allergen Can d 1. Allergens from different species within a genus or across genera use the same numbering arrangement. For example, the related mite cysteine protease allergens from the species *D. farinae* and *Euroglyphus maynei* are referred to as Der f 1 and Eur m 1, respectively. Collectively, such related allergens are often referred to as belonging to a particular group (e.g. the 'Group 1 mite allergens'). With the significant increase in the amount of sequence data generated owing to the adoption of cloning and whole-genome sequencing technologies, it is apparent that a particular allergen source may contain a number of allergens with sequences that are very similar (>67% sequence identity using the IUIS Allergen Nomenclature Subcommittee guidelines). In this case, such allergens are described as isoallergens and are given a suffix ranging from 00 to 99 (e.g. Amb a 1.01, Amb a 1.02). In situations where similar allergens are described but differ only in the occasional residue (polymorphism), these are described as variants, and an additional two digits are used in the description (e.g. Amb a 1.0101 – the first variant of the isoallergen Amb a 1.01).

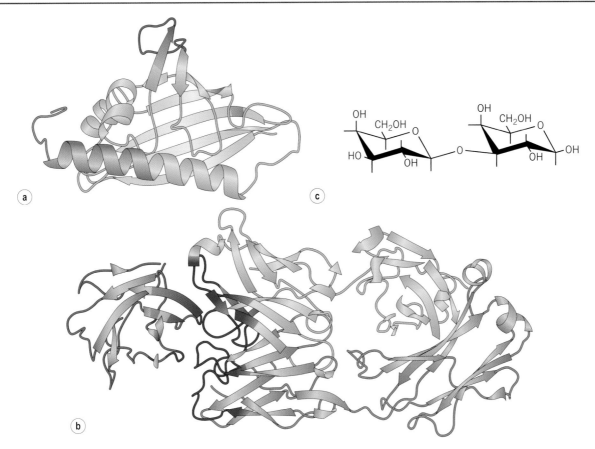

Fig. 5.1 Allergenic B-cell and T-cell epitopes on allergens. (a) The location of a B-cell (blue) and a T-cell (red) epitope superimposed on the three-dimensional structure of the major Birch pollen allergen Bet v I. (b) The binding of the Fab portion of a genetically engineered IgE antibody molecule to a conformational B-cell epitope of the Timothy grass pollen allergen, *Phl p 2*. The Phl p 2 allergen is shown in red, whereas the light and heavy chains of the Fab portion of the IgE molecule are shown in blue and green, respectively. The actual amino acid residues of the allergenic epitope of Phl p 2 are shown in grey, as are the interacting amino acid residues of the hypervariable regions of the antibody-combining site in the Fab fragments. The figures were constructed with PyMol using PDB entries 1BV1 and 2VXQ. (c) A schematic representation of the terminal disaccharide epitope galactose-α-1,3-galactose found on many glycoprotein allergens (Figure courtesy of Dr Brian Skelton, University of Western Australia).

Factors influencing allergenicity

Intrinsic factors

So far, there does not appear to be any one inherent molecular or biological characteristic that determines whether a protein is destined to be allergenic. Most allergens are proteins or glycoproteins with molecular masses in the range 5000–100000 Da and are derived from sources such as arthropod faeces, foods, parasite secretions, fungal spores, and plant pollens. Interestingly, few allergens from commonly encountered bacteria have been described apart from the enterotoxins produced by staphylococcal species associated with atopic dermatitis, although this might reflect a special case as they are superantigens and capable of non-specifically activating adaptive immune responses including those involving IgE. The reason for the dearth of bacterial or viral allergens is

thought to be related to the fact that the human immune system has evolved a specific set of innate immune recognition receptors that respond to unique pathogen-associated molecular patterns (PAMPs, e.g. peptidoglycan, lipopolysaccharide, DNA, RNA). These PAMPs tend to stimulate Th1 rather than Th2 responses via the stimulation of dendritic cell IL-12 production and thus drive an adaptive immune response down a non-IgE-producing pathway. Alternatively, it is possible that early life exposure to bacteria results in immune tolerance to associated proteins. The capacity of allergens to stimulate IgE in humans is influenced by properties that will also influence the production of IgG, IgA, and IgM to any immunogen. These include size, solubility, foreignness (i.e. amino acid sequence dissimilarity with human homologues), concentration, and route of exposure (Box 5.2). In addition, data are now acumulating that suggest intrinsic factors other than those described above may influence allergenicity

Box 5.2 Factors that influence allergenicity

Intrinsic	Extrinsic
Biochemical activity	Adjuvants
Concentration*	Birth weight
Foreignness	Cigarette smoke
Glycosylation	Genetic predisposition
Molecular complexity (size)	and gender
Resistance to cooking	Hygiene
Resistance to digestion	Pollutants**
Route of exposure	Season of birth
Solubility	Viral infection

*Allergen concentration may influence sensitization or tolerization.
**See later section for the influence of pollutants on allergens and allergenicity.

such as biochemical properties (Table 5.1). Some of these properties, particularly physicochemical, may also influence the site at which an allergic reaction will manifest. For example, some individuals may be allergic to specific food components, but do not manifest symptoms when the food is cooked because the IgE-binding (B-cell) epitopes are dependent on a precise conformational arrangement of amino acids (conformational epitopes), which are altered by heat. However, if the epitopes are resistant (non-conformation-dependent, linear epitopes) or uncooked foods are ingested, then symptoms may be manifest in the oral cavity and/or the gut. Although the majority of allergens are proteinaceous, glycan moieties, for example, the terminal disaccharide galactose-α-1,3-galactose structure (see Fig. 5.1), commonly found on some non-primate glycoprotein allergens, may also stimulate the production of specific IgE, particularly those

Table 5.1 A summary of the potential consequences of the intrinsic and extrinsic factors and properties of allergens/allergen sources

Property	Cell/molecular interaction	Possible consequence
Extrinsic		
High focal allergen	Epithelium	Increased permeability due to osmotic shock, concentration influencing allergen entry and presentation
Pollen lipid	Epithelium	Adjuvant activity, increased allergen mediators presentation due to effects on dendritic cells (DC), eosinophils and polymorphonuclear cells
Pollutants such as diesel exhaust particulates and environmental tobacco smoke	Epithelium	Carrier of allergen into lower lung, adjuvant properties, epigenetic effects
Reactive oxygen species	Epithelium	Increased permeability, influencing allergen entry
Intrinsic		
Glycosylation	Macrophages, DC, surfactant proteins A, D	Increased antigen presentation, DC activation and T-cell polarization
Oligomerization	Antigen-presenting cells such as DC and macrophages	Increased allergenicity
Protease activity	Epithelium	Increased permeability, influencing allergen entry due to apoptosis, mast cell degranulation, kinin production and tight junction protein degradation Proinflammatory cytokine release (IL-6, IL-8, GM-CSF) due to interaction with protease activated receptors (PAR) Up-regulation of cell surface molecules, increasing cell recruitment/decreasing activation potential
	Basophil	Activation and presentation of allergen

from seafood, plant- and animal-derived foods, and insects. Interestingly, IgG antibodies to this epitope are present at high concentration in most humans owing to its ubiquitous presence on glycoproteins from foods and microbes. In addition to the above, data are emerging that suggest that the propensity of an allergen to form dimers or oligomers may also determine how effectively allergens interact with IgE bound to mast cells, thus triggering degranulation. This might be an important characteristic of relatively low-molecular-weight allergens, where the small number of potential epitopes may limit the capacity of a monomeric allergen to cross-link the two or more allergen-specific IgE molecules necessary for the mast cell activation process. In this regard, multimers of various allergens from pollen, mites, foods, and danders have been described (Table 5.2). Finally, data suggest that allergens possessing glycan moieties may be taken up specifically by dendritic cells in the respiratory mucosa either directly via C-type lectins such as the mannose receptor and the dendritic cell-specific 1CAM3-grabbing non-integrin (DC-SIGN) receptor or indirectly via their interaction with surfactant protein D present in respiratory fluids (see Table 5.1). Such interactions may bias allergen-specific T cells towards a Th2 phenotype.

Extrinsic factors

A number of extrinsic factors, both endogenous and exogenous, may also contribute to the recognition of potential allergens by the immune system by altering normal homeostatic defence mechanisms, for example, genetic factors, climate change, industrial pollutants, cigarette smoke, or viral infections (see subsequent sections in this chapter; Table 5.3). For initial sensitization to occur, the genetic characteristics of the host are important, not only in influencing clinical progression but also in influencing the induction of IgE *per se* as well as allergic responses to specific allergens. For example, genes associated with innate immunity and immunoregulation are likely to play very important roles owing to their ability to influence allergen entry, recognition, presentation, and IgE induction. With regard to allergen entry, the innate immune function of the epithelial barrier is emerging as being particularly important in sensitization, given recent findings showing loss-of-function mutations in the filaggrin protein in patients with atopic dermatitis. This protein plays an important role in the stratum corneum, particularly in the formation of microfibrils comprising the keratin cytoskeleton. Originally described as playing a significant role in skin lesions, mutations associated with allergic sensitization and asthma in this group of patients have been identified, suggesting a role for percutaneous allergen exposure. In addition to genes associated with barrier function, genes encoding the highly polymorphic major histocompatibility class (MHC) II complex proteins also play a role. These cell surface proteins present allergen-derived peptides (about 13–24 amino acids) to T-helper cells to initiate IgE production and they have been shown to influence the presentation of allergens derived from a number of sources including pollens and low-molecular-weight occupational allergens such as the polyisocyanates (see elsewhere in this book). For example, IgE production to the olive pollen allergens Ole e 2 (profilin) and Ole e 10 (1,3-β-glucanase) in certain individuals is associated with the expression of HLA DR7 and DP2, and HLA-DR2 on their antigen-presenting cells. As the size of an allergen increases, however, and therefore the number of potential epitopes increases, such associations becomes difficult to discern. Information on regions of the allergen (agretope) which bind to the class II molecule and the region (epitope) which binds to the T-cell receptor or IgE-combining site (paratope) is increasing rapidly owing to their potential usefulness in the development of novel immunotherapeutic regimens. With regard to epitopes, data indicate that allergen-specific IgE binds to epitopes that are located on the surface of an allergen, in contrast to that seen with MHC and T-cell receptor interactions, where T-cell epitopes may be located either on the surface or buried inside the protein (see Fig. 5.1).

Extrinsic factors may also influence the spectrum of allergens or concentration of individual allergens present within a particular source or, indeed, the sources themselves. For example, climate change involving rising temperature and atmospheric CO_2 concentrations (in the case of pollen allergens), environmental factors influencing available food sources for arthropods (mite and insect allergens), and pollution (pollen allergens) (see later

Table 5.2 Allergens known to exist as multimers in nature

Source	Allergen
Invertebrates	
Bee	Api m 4
Cockroach	Per a 3
Fire ant	Sol i 2
House dust mite	Der p 1, Der p 5
Wasp venom	Ves v 5
Plants	
Pollens	Phl p 1, Phl p 5b, Phl p 7, Phl p 11 sa, BGP-2, Bet v 1
Seeds	Ara h 1, Ara h 2
Vertebrates	
Danders	Fel d 1, Equ c 1
Milk	Bos d 5

Table 5.3 Examples of allergen sources

Allergen group	Examples	Seasonality
Airborne		
Animal dander and urine	Cat, dog, horse, rabbit, guinea pig, hamster, mouse, rat, cow	Perennial
Bird feathers	Budgerigar, parrot, pigeon, duck, chicken	Perennial
Cereal flours	Wheat, rye, oat	Perennial
Pollens		
Grasses	Rye, couch, wild oat, Timothy, Bermuda, Kentucky blue, cocksfoot	Spring/early summer
Herbaceous dicotyledonous species	Ragweed, *Parietaria* spp., plantain, mugwort	Summer/autumn
Trees	Alder, birch, hazel, beech, oak, olive, cyprus, cedar	Winter/spring
House dust and storage mites	*Dermatophagoides pteronyssinus, D. farinae, Euroglyphus maynei, Blomia tropocalis, Acaris siro, Tyrophagus putrescentiae*	Perennial
Insects	Cockroach, fly, locust, midge	Perennial/seasonal
Fungi	*Aspergillus* spp., *Cladosporium* spp., *Alternaria* spp., *Candida* spp. *Pencillium* spp., *Malassezia* spp.	Perennial/variable
Plant products	Latex, papain, bromelain	Perennial
Envenomated		
Insects	Bee and wasp stings, ant and mosquito bites	Summer
Orally administered and injectable		
Drugs	Penicillins, sulphonamides and other antibiotics, sulphasalazine (sulfasalazine), carbamazepine, chimeric (human/mouse) monoclonal antibodies	Non-seasonal
Food	Seafood, legumes, tree nuts, sesame, cereals, milk, eggs, fruits, mushrooms, alcoholic beverages, coffee, chocolate	Non-seasonal

sections of this chapter) have all been shown to influence the spectrum of allergens to which individuals might be exposed. Similarly, concentrations of plant-derived allergens within a particular cultivar may be influenced by environmental or cultivation conditions. Such changes have the potential to influence whether an allergen manifests as 'major' or 'minor' in a population, although not diagnostically problematic as long as all relevant allergens are represented in any reagent used to detect allergy. In addition to these extrinsic factors, others derived from the allergen sources themselves may act as adjuvants or proinflammatory agents. For example, pollen-associated lipid mediators (PALM), NADPH oxidases and cysteine and serine proteases may contribute to allergenicity. In this regard, PALM (e.g. phytoprostanes) may modulate dendritic cell function whereas the oxidases and proteases may influence epithelial integrity or stimulate the production of proinflammatory cytokines (see Table 5.1).

Origins of allergens

Most individuals are exposed to mixtures of allergens rather than to single proteins. This is because they most often come into contact with allergen-rich 'containers', in contrast to the animal danders, pollen submicronic particles, and occupational allergens. Such 'containers' include arthropod faeces (enclosed by a peritrophic membrane), and pollen grains and fungal spores, where the complex array of allergens contained therein play major physiological roles such as in digestion (faeces) and somatic growth and fertilization (fungal spores and pollen). Reflecting their role in the natural environment, many of the allergens in these containers rapidly leach out of their particulate structures when they become hydrated on contact with mucosal surfaces. The most complex sources of allergens are domestic, and include fungi, pollen, and mites, with the least complex being animal dander and urine extracts, as are the occupational sources (see Tables 5.4 and 5.5). Up to 60% of the proteins from a given source are allergenic and a sensitized patient may recognize more than one allergen from within a source as well as allergens from multiple sources. With regard to source, patients are described as being mono- or polysensitized, and there are data suggesting that monosensitization is more frequent with house dust mite allergy than with pollen, food, and animal danders, and with milk rather than hen's egg, nuts, and wheat. Furthermore, cosensitization to airborne sources appears more frequently in patients with cow's milk and soy allergy, and cosensitization to food is relatively infrequent in those with allergy to house dust mites and dog dander. The precise number of allergens recognized within a source reflects both the genetic capability of the host, the complexity, and concentration of the source, and the assay used to determine allergenicity. The more frequently recognized proteins (>50%) within an allergic population exposed to the same source are termed 'major allergens', in contrast to 'minor allergens'. However, these arbitrary divisions do not necessarily indicate that minor allergens will be clinically insignificant in certain individuals. Allergens in domestic settings are sometimes referred to as 'indoor' or 'outdoor' allergens to reflect the origin of the allergen source. Typical outdoor allergens include pollens and fungi, whereas indoor allergens include animal dander, fungi, and mite and insect faeces (see Table 5.3). Exposure to an allergen source may result in the production of allergen-specific IgE in genetically predisposed people, but it is also possible for such individuals to manifest allergic reactions to either similar (e.g. pollen versus pollen) or dissimilar (e.g. snail versus house dust mite) sources to which they have been exposed. This occurs because both the similar and/or the dissimilar sources contain allergens that are structurally and functionally similar and thus share a high degree of amino acid sequence homology or, in the case of the carbohydrate epitope galactose-α-1,3-galactose, are present in the glycan component of dissimilar glycoproteins. This sequence similarity will increase the likelihood of allergen-specific IgE produced against one allergen recognizing the

Table 5.4 Examples of occupational allergens

Source	Examples	Industry
Bacteria		
Enzymes	Alcalase and esperase (serine proteases), amylase, empynase	Detergents
Drugs		
Antibiotics	Penicillin, tetracycline, cephalosporin	Manufacture, domestic use
Miscellaneous	Albuterol, methyldopa, opiates	Manufacture, domestic use
Fungi		
Enzymes	Protease, pectinase, cellulase, glucoamylase, β-xylosidase	Food processing
Invertebrates		
Miscellaneous	Scales, somatic debris, body fluids, faecal pellets	Research, breeding
Low-molecular-weight substances		
Organic compounds	Chloramine-T, polycolophony (pine rosin), polyvinyl chloride, polyisocyanates, anhydrides, wrapping plastics and ethylenediamine, plicatic acid	Brewing, soldering, meat chemical processing, wood processing
Metals and their salts	Platinum, aluminium, vanadium, nickel and chromium salts	Metal refining, plating, boiler cleaning, welding
Plants		
Enzymes	Papain, bromelain, pectinase, cellulase, amylase	Pharmaceuticals, food processing
Latex	Rubber plant	Healthcare workers, spina bifida patients
Vegetable dusts	Wood, cereals, legumes	Carpentry, baking, milling, processing
Vertebrates		
Enzymes	Trypsin, pepsin, amylase, lysozyme, lipase	Manufacture, domestic use
Miscellaneous	Danders, urine, serum, feathers, droppings	Research, breeding

same epitope in the other source. This phenomenon is known as 'allergenic cross-reactivity', and such cross-reactivity may be extensive, particularly in small but physiologically essential allergens, where extensive genetic mutations in the encoding genes cannot be tolerated. This type of extensive cross-reactivity between allergens from diverse sources gives rise to the term 'pan-allergen' and is usually associated with low-moleculer-weight, relatively minor allergens such as the profilins, polycalcins, and non-specific lipid transfer proteins found in pollens and fruit sources.

Airborne allergens

Plant allergens

Pollens (from the Greek for 'fine flour') are the male gametophytes of flowering plants and gymnosperms, and represent some of the more clinically important allergen sources (10–20% of community allergic disease); the most common disease presentation is rhinitis. The major allergenic pollens (grasses, herbaceous dicotyledons, and trees) are derived from wind-pollinated (anemophilous) rather than insect-pollinated (entomophilous) plants, and pollen seasons may last for several months. The anemophilous pollens, in contrast to those from insect-pollinated plants, possess a thin, complex and chemically resistant exterior cell wall that has two main layers: the inner intine layer lying next to the plasma membrane and the outer exine layer, which may be highly sculptured. An additional layer, the Z-layer, lies between the intine and exine and is thickest at the germination pore – the opening through which the pollen tube extends during pollen germination. The exine is constructed from sporopollenin over which lies the pollen coat comprising lipids and proteins. Inside the pollen grain is the cytoplasm that contains various structures including nuclei, mitochondria, plastids containing starch granules (amyloplasts), and P (polysaccharide) particles. The clinically important pollens will vary according to geographical location, as well as season and microclimatic conditions, and may be indigenous or introduced (Fig. 5.2). Pollens from anemophilous plants are also characterized by their buoyant density, which contributes to their ease of dispersion and profusion, and grains from individual species may vary in size, ranging from 5 to over 200 µm. Pollen release is usually seasonal, with late spring and summer representing the most important pollination seasons (Fig. 5.3), and the temporal sequence of pollination is usually trees, grasses, and herbaceous dicotyledons. The daily atmospheric concentration of pollen will vary during the pollen season and may be reduced by rain and falls in ambient temperature. The number of pollen grains required to provoke disease will vary from species to species but that required to initiate symptoms at the beginning of the hay-fever season is likely to be greater than at the end owing to stimulation of the immune system, and may range from 20 pollen grains/m³ upward. For example, for grass pollen sensitivity, 50 grains/m³ may be sufficient but 400 grains/m³ may be required for olive-pollen-allergic patients. In addition to pollen grains per se, some plants also produce pollen-related orbicules (0.2–1 µm), which arise from the pollen-forming process in the anther and consist of exine material and possibly allergens. For example, gymnospermous trees such as *Crypotomeria* species and *Cupressus* species, and the herbaceous

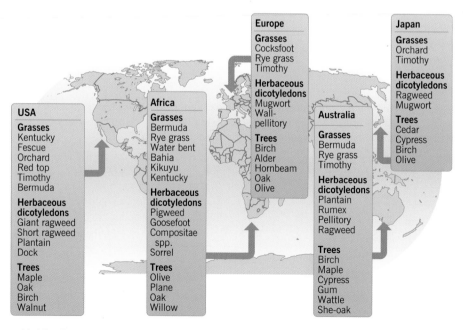

Fig. 5.2 Selected worldwide distribution of clinically important pollen allergens.

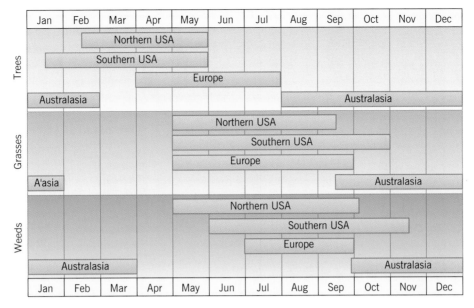

Fig. 5.3 Pollen seasons in USA, Australasia, and Europe. (Adapted from Sicherer SH, Eggleston PA. In: Lieberman P, Anderson J, eds. Environmental allergens in allergic diseases: diagnosis and treatment. Totowa, NJ: Humana Press; 2000.)

dicotyledonous *Parietaria* species, produce orbicules that contain allergen but the angiosperm tree species *Betula verrucosa* does not. Pollen allergens may be found in the pollen coat associated with the exine, but the majority reside within the cytoplasm per se or are associated with specific structures therein, such as the starch granules or P particles. These particles are released through the germination pore (Fig. 5.4) when whole pollen lands on mucosal surfaces in humans. Allergens may also leach out through microchannels in the exine. A significant number of the allergenic proteins released from the pollen coat and cytoplasm are hydrolases involved in cell wall synthesis and pollen tube growth as well as helping the pollen tube breach the cell wall of the ovule so that fertilization may occur (see Appendices 5.1 to 5.3). The pollen grain and the orbicules are considered the primary sources of allergen, but studies show that individuals may be exposed to submicronic particles (0.5–2 μm in diameter) derived from the grains themselves. For example starch grains and P particles are released from pollen after rain and then become airborne as the environment dries out, and therefore become capable of triggering allergic disease. As pollen grains are too large to penetrate into the deeper airways, it is likely that submicronic particles carrying allergens infiltrate the lower bronchi, consequently provoking asthma in 2.5–10% of susceptible individuals.

Grass pollen

Grasses, which comprise part of the major plant group, the monocotyledons, are significant contributors to pollinosis globally because of their wide distribution and propensity to produce large amounts of airborne pollen. Allergens from a variety of grass pollens from species belonging to the clinically important subfamilies Pooideae (e.g. *Lolium* and *Phleum* species, found in temperate climes), Chloridoideae (e.g. *Cynodon* species, found in warmer climes) and Panicoideae (e.g. *Paspalum* species, found in more tropical climes) have been described. The pollen allergens from the different grass species were originally divided into groups on the basis of marked physicochemical and immunochemical similarities, and this scheme has now been adopted for similar allergens derived from sources other than grass pollen. Grass pollen allergens demonstrate various functions associated with cell wall synthesis/remodelling, fertilization, and pollen tube growth and include expansins, extensins, ribonucleases, glucosidases, protease inhibitor-like proteins, calcium-binding proteins, and profilins (Appendix 5.1). In addition, enzymes involved in the breakdown of the plant cell wall necessary for pollen tube growth, such as pecate lysase and polygalacturonase, are also allergenic. Pectin degradation involves a number of enzymes working in concert and the grass pollen allergen types, together with the pectin methylesterases, are also significant allergens in herbaceous dicotyledons and tree pollens.

Herbaceous dicotyledonous species pollen

The principal allergenic herbaceous dicotyledons (sometimes referred to as weeds because they represent unwanted plants within a garden or field) are those belonging to the Asteraceae, such as ragweed, mugwort, sunflower, and feverfew, as well as wall pellitory belonging to the Urticaceae. Several allergens from each of

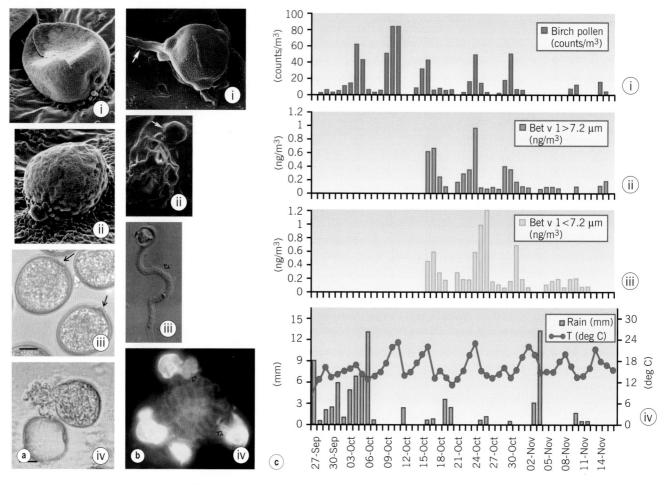

Fig. 5.4 (a) Scanning electron and light micrographs of rye grass *(Lolium perenne)* pollen. (i,iii) The aperture through which the pollen tube grows and; (ii,iv) pollen extruding its starch granules. (Electron micrographs courtesy of Professor Frank Murray, Murdoch University, Perth, Western Australia; light micrographs courtesy of Ms Cecilia Tong, University of Western Australia, scale bars; 10 μm).

(b) Micrographs of germinating birch pollen and bursting pollen tubes. (i) Scanning electron micrograph (SEM) of a triporate birch *(Betula verrucosa)* pollen grain on a birch leaf. The pollen grain has germinated, producing a pollen tube (see arrow). (ii) SEM of birch leaf gland with one birch pollen grain nearby (see arrow). (iii) A germinated birch pollen grain with a pollen tube (see arrow) of about 90 μm showing dense cytoplasmic contents. This was viewed with Nomarski optics after being washed off a birch leaf. (iv) Germinating pollen accumulates around the birch leaf gland. Each grain produces a pollen tube (see arrows). Within hours of germinating, the pollen tube tips rupture releasing the cytoplasmic contents. Prominent amongst this discharged cytoplasm are numerous starch granules. Scale bars represent 10 μm.

(c) (i) Birch pollen (counts/m^3); (ii) Bet v 1 concentrations (ng/m^3) in particles greater than 7.2 μm in diameter; (iii) Bet v 1 concentrations (ng/m^3) in inhalable particles less than 7.2 μm in diameter; (iv) rainfall (mm) and temperature (°C) in the atmosphere of Melbourne during the 1996 birch pollen season. Bet v 1 concentrations were determined from 16 October to 15 November 1996. Bet v 1 data for 20 October and 3 November are not available. (b & c reproduced from Schäppi GF et al. Sex Plant Reprod 1997; 10:315-323, with permission of Springer-Verlag.)

these species have been identified. The major allergens include pectate lyases, polygalacturonases, calcium-binding proteins, polycalcins, profilins, and lipid transfer proteins. The latter proteins are common allergens found in other sources such as seeds and belong to the prolamin superfamily (Appendix 5.2). Interestingly, the major Group 1 β-expansin allergens found in grasses do not appear to be prominent allergens in the pollen of herbaceous dicotyledon or tree pollen (see below).

Tree pollen

Pollen from several tree species belonging to both the angiosperms (flowering) and the gymnosperms (non-flowering) are associated with allergic diseases and include species in the Orders Fagales, Scrophulariales, and Pinales. In this regard, birch, hazel, olive, and ash (angiosperms), and the conifers, cypress, cedar, and juniper (gymnosperms) are particularly important sources of allergen. It is clear that, in general, pollen allergens from species within the same order and/or family are related; for example, in the Scrophulariales species olive, lilac, ash, and privet, the major allergens are proteins showing limited homology with known seed-derived protease inhibitors, polycalcins, and 1,3-β-glucanase (Appendix 5.3); in the Fagales species birch, hazel, and ash, the major allergens belong to or show homology with members of a diverse group of proteins known as pathogenesis-related proteins (Table 5.5). These proteins, as the name suggests, are either constitutively produced or are expressed when plants are exposed to microbial attack or abiotic stresses. They comprise proteins with varied activities and, in this regard, the Fagales group 1 (e.g. Bet v 1) allergens belong to the PR10 family, members of which are likely to be involved in the transport of plant steroids such as the brassinosteroids found in pollens and play a role in pollen tube growth. Both the Fagales and Scrophulariales species produce allergenic enzymes involved in pectin degradation. Interestingly, there is limited similarity in the spectrum of allergens found in angiospermous species, compared with gymnospermous species. In the latter, enzymes involved in pectin degradation dominate (Appendix 5.3), and these differences are likely to reflect the proteins and enzymes important in the fertilization process. For example, in angiospermous trees, the pollination process is similar to that seen with the grasses and herbaceous dicotyledons, but in conifer species associated with allergy it is different. Here, the erect ovule within the cone exudes a drop of fluid, known as the pollen drop, through the micropyle. When the pollen grains land on the drop, it quickly recedes into the ovule and the process of fertilization begins. Inside the ovule, the pollen grain exine bursts, and the intine then elongates along the micropyle canal. This may take several weeks, in contrast to the short time taken for pollen tube growth in the woody and herbaceous angiosperms, and once in contact with the nucellus a small pollen tube is formed, which then penetrates the ovule.

Non-pollen, plant-derived aeroallergens

A number of aeroallergens have been described that are derived from non-pollen plant tissue such as seeds and latex (Appendices 5.4 and 5.6). They are a significant source of allergens in occupational settings in industries such as baking and include flours prepared from wheat, barley, castor beans, mustard seed, green coffee beans, rice, cotton seed, Ispaghula, and soybeans. The major seed-derived allergens usually belong to one of several types of storage proteins, which account for about 75%

Table 5.5 The relationship between plant pathogenesis-related proteins and allergens

Family	Description or characteristics	Examples
PR-1	Antifungal, mechanism unknown	Cum c 3
PR-2	Endo-β-1,3-glucanase	Hev b 2, Ole e 4/9
PR-3	Chitinases (type I, II)	Pers a 1, Hev b 11
PR-4	Chitinases (type I, II)	Turnip prohevein, Hev b 6, wheat germ agglutinin
PR-5	Thaumatin-like proteins, antifungal, may have endo-β-1,3-glucanase activity	Pru av 2, Mal d 2, Jun a 3
PR-6	Protease inhibitor	Soybean, wheat, barley, rice allergens
PR-7	Protease	?
PR-8	Chitinase (type III)	Latex hevamine
PR-9	Peroxidase	Wheat, barley allergens
PR-10	Plant steroid carrier	Bet v 1, Mal d 1, Pru av 1, Pyr c 1, Api g 1, Dau c 1, etc.
PR-11	Chitinase (type I)	?
PR-12	Plant defensins	?
PR-13	Plant defensins	?
PR-14	Lipid transfer proteins	Pru p 3, Mal d 3, Gly m 1
PR-15	Oxalate oxidase	?
PR-16	Oxalate oxidase-like	?
PR-17	Unknown	?

? indicates that allergens belonging to a particular group have yet to be described.

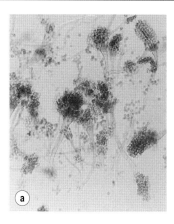 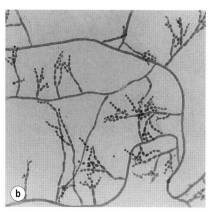 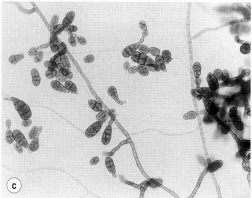

Fig. 5.5 Fungi commonly involved in allergic disease. (a) *Aspergillus fumigatus*. (b) *Cladosporium*. (c) *Alternaria*. (Photographs courtesy of Ms Rose McAleer, PathCentre, Western Australia.)

of total seed protein or proteins involved in protection against insects due to antimicrobial or enzyme-inhibitory activities and are often denominated by their sedimentation coefficients (e.g. 2S, 7S, and 11S). These groupings include the cupin (vicilins and legumins) and prolamin (2S albumins) superfamilies, lipid transfer proteins, and the pathogenesis-related proteins. Some of the food allergens such as the lipid transfer proteins appear to be highly resistant to digestion and heating, which is thought to enable them to cross epithelial barriers in relatively intact form. In addition to seeds, allergens may also be derived from other plant tissues including fruit, vegetables, and latex, which are generally important in occupational settings. Of significance are the latex allergens, which may become absorbed into the starch powder used as a lubricant in latex gloves, and become aerosolized. This results in a high prevalence of allergy in healthcare workers (20%) and patients with spina bifida (50%) who are exposed to latex products during surgical manipulations. Latex, a suspension of proteins in a water phase, is produced in response to deliberate cutting of the bark of the rubber tree and contains a variety of enzymes, proteins, and lectins for defensive purposes (cf. the pathogenesis-related proteins). At least 13 latex allergens have now been described and include a rubber elongation factor, chitin-binding lectin, chitinase, profilin, and endo-1,3-β glucosidase as well as proteins of unknown function (Appendix 5.4).

Fungal allergens

Fungi may be broadly divided into two groups based on their structure and include the unicellular yeasts, and the multicellular fungi that produce hyphae and spores. Although allergen-producing yeasts have been identified (e.g. *Candida* species, *Malassezia* species), most of the clinically important allergen-producing species are multicellular. Fungi are further subdivided according to their means of reproduction and morphology. The allergenicity

(and pathogenicity) of several fungal species has been studied in detail, and those belonging to the Ascomycota (*Aspergillus*, *Cladosporium*, *Penicillium*, *Candida*, and *Alternaria* species) are important sources of allergen worldwide (Fig. 5.5). However, Basidiomycota species (*Malassezia* species, mushrooms, puffballs, rusts, smuts, and bracket fungi) are also thought to represent significant allergen sources in certain situations. Multicellular fungi in both phyla produce spores that are often found in very large quantities in the air. The size of spores will vary between species, ranging from 1 to >100 μm although, in general, most of the clinically important species produce spores in the range 7–12 μm. Theoretically, fungal allergens should be more clinically significant because spores containing them are the most abundant airborne particles (e.g. >5,000 spores/m³) and are small enough to penetrate deep into the respiratory tree, in contrast to pollen grains. Meteorological studies reveal that atmospheric conditions such as wind speed, temperature, and humidity influence the release of spores. For example, ascospores may be released after rainfall (*Didymella exitialis*) or hot dry conditions (*Cladosporium*), and basidiospores may be released due to humidity. *Aspergillus* and *Alternaria* spores appear to be particularly significant in asthma, but those from *Cladosporium herbarum* and *Penicillium* species may also be important. Spore concentrations required to provoke symptoms will depend on the species (e.g. 50–100/m³ for *Alternaria* and 3,000/m³ for *Cladosporium*). Fungal allergens are thought to be produced by both spores and/or hyphae as they develop, and are then released into the environment (Appendix 5.5). In addition to natural exposure, individual fungal allergens (often hydrolytic enzymes used in a variety of industries) have been shown to be allergenic (Appendix 5.6).

Several allergens from non-occupationally important fungal species including *Alternaria alternata*, *Cladosporium herbarum*, *Aspergillus fumigatus*, *Penicillium* species, and *Candida albicans* have been characterized because of their association with allergic disease as well as with aspergillosis and candidiasis. Occupationally important fungal enzymes such as amylase from *A. oryzae*, which is added to dough, have been shown to be potent allergens in the baking industry. In contrast to the occupational fungal allergens, the domestic fungal allergens are often enzymes associated with glycolysis or are of unknown function (Appendices 5.5 and 5.6).

Occupational allergens

Occupational allergens range from low-molecular-weight chemicals of relatively simple structure through to complex proteins and glycoproteins derived from a variety of animal, arthropod, bacterial, fungal, and plant sources. Allergy may affect only a few individuals in the workforce or up to 30% of exposed workers. The response time between exposure and symptoms may be delayed by many hours, with the consequence that the affected individual may not be in the workplace when symptoms occur, thus complicating the diagnosis. Recurrent exposure may lead to chronic disease with little variability being discernible, making it difficult to associate disease with exposure. A number of predisposing factors for occupational allergy have been demonstrated including prior atopic status, duration of exposure, and smoking history. Most high-molecular-weight occupational allergens are hydrolytic enzymes, and include the bacterial subtilisins (serine proteases) and amylases used in the detergent industry, and the fungal enzymes and egg proteins used in the baking industry (Appendix 5.6).

Vertebrate-derived allergens

Vertebrate-derived allergens are of major clinical significance in domestic and occupational settings, and the incidence of positive skin tests to such proteins in an unselected population is approximately 5%, which rises to over 30% in allergic populations. In domestic situations, allergy to cats and dogs is particularly common, whereas in occupational settings, allergy to rats, horses, rabbits, mice, gerbils, and guinea pigs may be prevalent. The allergens are found in dander, epithelium, fur, urine, and saliva, and originate from sebaceous glands, lacrimal glands, salivary glands, anal sacks, and urine, which then accumulate on fur (Appendix 5.7). Many of the major dander allergens belong to the lipocalin superfamily, members of which are involved in the transport of low-molecular-weight hydrophobic substances in hydrophilic environments. The major cat allergen Fel d 1 may also be a ligand-binding protein but its true function remains unclear despite its three-dimensional structure being available. It is a non-convalent bond tetramer comprising two covalently linked heterodimers, and has been shown to exist in proteolytically truncated forms ranging in size

from 7 to 40 kDa. In addition to the lipocalins, serum proteins such as albumin and the immunoglobulins (IgG, IgA and IgM) may also be allergenic, but data suggest that allergenicity to the latter is associated with the galactose-α-1,3-galactose epitope (Appendix 5.7) present in the glycan moiety of each.

Invertebrate-derived allergens

Allergy to invertebrates may arise either through domestic or occupational contact in scientific institutions where they are reared for study, and cause allergic disease in up to a third of workers. The main arthropod allergen sources are found in the classes Insecta and Arachnida, and include chironomid midges, moths, butterflies, locusts, cockroaches, and house dust and storage mites, respectively (Fig. 5.6). However, house dust mites and cockroaches represent two of the most clinically important allergen sources worldwide owing to their ubiquity (Fig. 5.7). The clinically important species are the German (*Blatela germanica*) and American (*Periplaneta americana*) cockroaches, and the house dust mite species *Dermatophagoides pteronyssinus*, *D. farinae*, *Blomia tropicalis*, and *Euroglyphus maynei*. Both mites and cockroaches prefer the warm environment and food sources provided by domestic dwellings, with mites preferring to live in carpets, soft furnishings, and mattresses, and growth being dependent on temperature and humidity. The major mite and cockroach allergens are gut-derived and hence are found in faecal material (Appendix 5.8). The spectra of allergens found in mites and insects, whilst demonstrating some overlap (e.g. the tropomyosins, troponin C, glutathione transferases, arginine kinases, and trypsins) also reveal marked differences. For example, in the cockroach, inactive aspartate proteases, lipocalins, and insect haemolymph-related proteins (Appendix 5.8) are prominent, with mite allergenic homologues yet to be described. Similarly, many of the major mite allergens are hydrolytic enzymes involved in digestion, and include cysteine proteases, serine proteases, and amylase, whereas others are non-enzymatic with homologues in insects yet to be described (Appendix 5.8). Allergy to mites may also occur in occupational settings where foods are stored; in these circumstances, mite species such as *Acarus siro* and *A. farris*, *Tyrophagus putrescentiae*, *T. longior*, *Glycyphagus domesticus*, and *Lepidoglyphus destructor* are significant. However, the spectra of allergens produced by storage and house dust mites are similar. These mite species may also be found in house dust. In addition to mites and cockroaches, a number of other invertebrate-derived aeroallergens may be found in house dust and occupational settings including, for example, those from midges such as the bloodworms (*Chironomus thummi thummi*) and the green nimitti midge (*Cladotanytarsus lewisi*), and the Indianmeal moth. The major midge allergens are the haemoglobins and tropomyosins, whereas

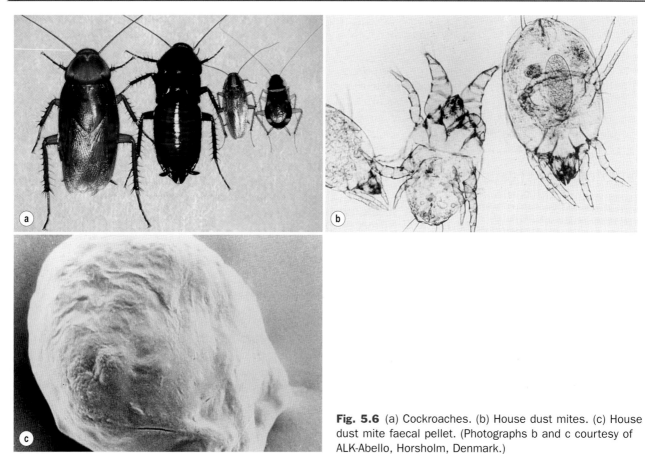

Fig. 5.6 (a) Cockroaches. (b) House dust mites. (c) House dust mite faecal pellet. (Photographs b and c courtesy of ALK-Abello, Horsholm, Denmark.)

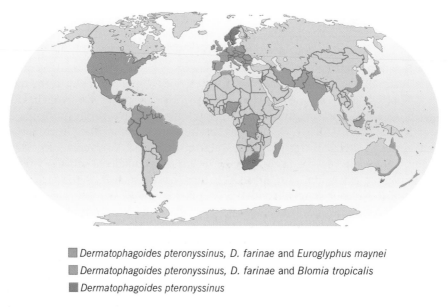

■ *Dermatophagoides pteronyssinus, D. farinae* and *Euroglyphus maynei*
■ *Dermatophagoides pteronyssinus, D. farinae* and *Blomia tropicalis*
■ *Dermatophagoides pteronyssinus*

Fig. 5.7 Reported worldwide distribution of the major house dust mite species. (Modified from Colloff MJ. Dust Mites, CSIRO Publishing, Dordrecht: Melbourne and Springer; 2009 and van Bronswijk JEMH, Sinha RN. J Allergy 1971; 47:31–52.)

the only Indianmeal moth allergen described so far is an arginine kinase.

Oral and injected allergens

Food allergens

The frequency, severity, and variety of diseases caused by exposure to foods may be associated with a number of pathological mechanisms, not all of which are IgE mediated. However, those that are may manifest not only as gastrointestinal disease but also as neurological, cutaneous, or respiratory disorders. In addition, IgE-mediated food allergies may also be clinically important because of their potential to induce fatal anaphylaxis. Prevalence data suggest that about 2% of adults and between 4 and 8% of children may be allergic to food, and, of the >160 estimated foods linked to IgE-mediated food allergy, eight appear to be the most clinically important in that they account for >90% of all food-induced allergic reactions. It has been estimated that food allergy, in the USA alone, accounts for 30,000 emergency room visits and 150 deaths per year. IgE-mediated food allergy is diagnosed on the basis of the presence of food-specific IgE and on documented adverse reactions in double-blind placebo-controlled food challenges (which are regarded as the definitive diagnostic tests). Although there will be regional and age-related effects due to diet, the most frequently occuring food allergen sources include milk, eggs, wheat, peanut, tree nuts, soy, fish, and shellfish (both crustacean and molluscan) (Table 5.6). Most children allergic to milk, eggs, and wheat become tolerized to these allergenic sources by the time they reach 5 years

of age although, with regard to the remaining food groups, allergies may continue through to adulthood. This differential tolerance is thought to be related to the presence of conformational epitopes within milk, eggs, and wheat sources that are more tolerizable than the linear epitope forms associated with the latter food groups.

The major shellfish/fish/amphibian, bird, and mammal-derived allergens are the parvalbumins and tropomyosins, the α-livetin and ovotransferrin, and immunoglobulin and casein, respectively. The plant-derived food allergens include the cupins, prolamins, profilins, and pathogenesis-related proteins (Appendices 5.9 and 5.10). In addition to food allergens being responsible for direct sensitization and provocation, they may also provoke symptoms in individuals who have become sensitized to aeroallergens from a variety of sources, in particular pollens (Table 5.7). Such diseases are referred to as 'oral allergy syndromes' (OAS, or pollen-food syndromes) and result from allergenic cross-reactivity (sequence similarity) between allergens within the food and those in the aeroallergen source. OAS are usually associated with uncooked foods rather than cooked (as cooking would denature the allergens) and exposure may precipitate local (oral) or systemic reactions.

The major cross-reacting plant food allergens have been shown to correspond to the Fagales tree pollen Group 1 and 2 allergens, although other allergens such as the latex allergens chitinase, hevein, profilin, and Hev b 5 also cross-react. The major invertebrate cross-reacting allergens are the tropomyosins (Appendices 5.12 and 5.13).

Orally administered and injectable drug allergens

IgE-mediated allergy to orally administered drugs is reported to occur in about 3% of the general population and is of concern, as with food, because of the possibility of anaphylaxis. It can occur with both low- and high-molecular weight drugs, although it is most frequently associated with the former. These drugs are generally characterized by the presence of a chemically reactive group enabling them to interact with host proteins to create novel epitopes that render them allergenic in susceptible individuals. These compounds, which on their own are neither allergenic nor immunogenic, are known as haptens, and typical drugs involved in type 1 hypersensitivity include the β-lactam antibiotics (e.g. penicillins and cephalosporins), anaesthetics, and muscle relaxants (see elsewhere in this book). With regard to the antibiotics, the β-lactam ring is central as it is chemically unstable and reacts with lysyl residues to form the penicilloyl epitope on cell membrane proteins. Allergic reactions may manifest as urticaria or anaphylaxis, although the latter is usually associated with injected drugs. The frequency of sensitivity to drugs such as the antibiotics

Table 5.6 Common sources of food allergens

Source	Common name
Bird derived	
	Chicken egg (white and yolk)
Fish and crustacean derived	
Bony fish	Salmon, cod
Crustaceans	Crab, lobster, shrimp, prawn
Mammal derived	
	Milk, meat
Plant derived	
Fruits	Apple, cherry, peach, melon, tomato
Seeds	Buckwheat, sunflower, peanut, soybean, lupins
Tree nuts	Brazil nut, walnut
Vegetables	Celery, carrot, potato

Table 5.7 Allergens involved in cross-reactivity syndromes

Syndromes sensitizing source	Syndromes sensitizing source	Cross-reacting allergen(s)
INVERTEBRATE AND VERTEBRATE DERIVED		
Arthropod–shellfish		
Mites	Shellfish, snails	Tropomyosin
Mites	*Anisakis simplex*	Tropomyosin
Cockroach	Shellfish, snails	Tropomyosin
Bird–egg		
Bird material	Egg yolk	Serum albumin (Gal d 5)
Egg–egg		
Egg white powder	Egg-containing foods	Lysozyme (Gal d 4)
Pork–cat		
Animal meat	Animal danders	Serum albumin
PLANT DERIVED		
Latex–fruit/vegetable/nut		
Latex	Avocado, potato, banana, tomato, chestnut, kiwifruit, herbs, carrot	Patatin (e.g. Sol t 1), profilin, Class I chitinases, Hev b 6, Per a 1
Latex–mould		
Latex	*Aspergillus* spp.	Manganese superoxide dismutase
Pollen–fruit/vegetable/nut/seed/honey		
Birch pollen	Apple, carrot, cherry, pear, peach, plum, fennel, walnut, potato, spinach, wheat, buckwheat, peanut, honey, celery, kiwifruit, persimmon	Profilin, Bet v 1 and Bet v 6 analogues
Grass pollen	Melon, tomato, watermelon, orange, cherry, potato	Profilin
Japanese cedar pollen	Melon, apple, peach, kiwifruit	Pectate lyase
Mugwort pollen	Celery, carrot, spices, melon, watermelon, apple, camomile, hazelnut, chestnut	Lipid transfer proteins, profilins, 34 and 60 kDa allergens, Art v 1 analogues
Ragweed pollen	Melon, camomile, honey, banana, sunflower seeds	Pectate lyase

may vary from 0.7 to 10% of the general population. Allergy to high-molecular-weight drugs, usually proteins and referred to as 'biologicals' (e.g. antibodies targeted to specific host proteins, receptor antagonists) occurs with low frequency. For example, cetuximab, an intravenously delivered chimeric mouse–human monoclonal antibody specific for the epidermal growth factor receptor and used in the treatment of certain cancers, has been shown to induce IgE-mediated sequelae. Interestingly, most reactions occur on first exposure, suggesting prior sensitivity. In this regard, it has been shown that the responsible epitope is the galactose-α-1,3-galactose epitope associated with the mouse Fab region of the molecule. This epitope does not usually stimulate the production of the IgE in these situations; rather it is formed prior to drug delivery owing to the exposure of patients to glycoproteins containing this disaccharide in its glycan structure (e.g. foods). Similar results have been observed with the chimeric monoclonal antibody, omalizumab, which was engineered to bind human IgE and used to treat patients with allergic disease.

Envenomated and salivary allergens

Allergen exposure via envenomation and saliva results from the bites and stings of certain insects. The major stinging insects associated with allergic disease include bees, wasps, hornets, and ants, which may inject many micrograms of venom at any one time. About 3% of the general population may experience systemic reactions after envenomation, and about 15–30% of individuals become sensitized after being stung, and predisposing factors may include prior allergy to inhalant allergens. Of the stinging insects, allergens from the honey bee appear to be the most clinically important, and anaphylaxis is not uncommon. The venoms from bees, wasps, hornets, and paper wasps are similar in that they contain vasoactive amines in addition to peptides and enzymes, and extensive allergenic cross-reactivity may occur amongst the vespid species. The most important stinging-insect allergens are those associated with the venom from bees (*Apis* species), wasps (yellow jackets; *Vespula* species), hornets (*Dolichovespula* species), paper wasps (*Polistes* species) and ants (*Solenopsis* species) (Appendix 5.11). The venoms contain a number of allergens that show homology with proteins associated with mammalian reproduction and it has been suggested that, since the allergens are derived from stingers that represent modified ovipositors, it is feasible that the allergens may have played some ancestral role in insect reproduction. The allergens derived from stinging insects belonging to different families are structurally similar and include enzymes such as phospholipase, hyaluronidase, and acid phosphatase as well as proteins of unknown function. Although the function of the vespid Group 5 allergens is unclear, they demonstrate sequence similarity with the plant pathogenesis-related proteins (Appendix 5.11). With regard to biting insects, the major allergenic species are ticks, triatomines, ants, horsefly, and mosquitoes. Here, the major allergenic proteins are calycin, procalin, an 80K allergen of unknown function, an Ag5 homologue and hyaluronidase, and apyrase, respectively.

Human and parasite allergens

Human autoallergens

Autoallergy was first recognized phenomenologically in the first half of the last century when immediate wheal and flare reactions resulted from the introduction of human dander extracts into the skin of allergic individuals, although the nature of the autoallergens was unclear. The concept of autoallergy was later invigorated when autoallergens were subsequently identified using recombinant DNA technologies. Autoallergens are usually found in patients with atopic dermatitis and may be divided into two categories. In the first, the human autoallergens (MnSOD, ribosomal P2 protein, and profilin) (Appendix 5.12) share significant homology with environmental allergens from pollen and fungal sources and are thus thought to be cross-reactive allergens. Allergens in the second (Hom s 1 to 5) category do not have environmental analogues, indicating they are likely to be genuine autoallergens. Most of the autoallergens are intracellular proteins and often restricted to skin, but can be found in sera complexed with IgE suggesting that they may be released – presumably due to tissue damage resulting from the disease process.

Parasite allergens

Parasite allergens have been demonstrated in a variety of helminthic parasites; the most studied are those from the fish parasite *Anisakis simplex* and the human parasite *Ascaris lumbricoides*. Allergy to the former parasite occurs because it is found in edible fish species and thus manifests as a food allergy, and to the latter because of infestation. The major allergens include a variety of proteases and protease inhibitors, lipid-binding polyproteins and tropomyosins, which show amino acid sequence homology with tropomyosin allergens from cockroach and house dust mites (Appendix 5.13).

Detection of allergen or allergen-specific IgE

Several techniques have been developed to determine whether an individual is allergic to a particular allergenic source and are thus useful as diagnostic tools, in contrast to others that have been developed for academic purposes to determine whether a protein isolated from a source is allergenic or to characterize IgE and T-cell epitopes; yet others have been developed for environmental-monitoring purposes.

In vivo diagnostic tests

Before the discovery of IgE and the subsequent development of serum-based immunochemical assays, the skin prick test was the principle means of determining the allergenic status of an individual. It remains a useful diagnostic tool that is robust and easy to administer and interpret. In this assay, an aliquot of allergenic material is placed onto the forearm of the patient under investigation, and a needle is used to prick the skin directly below the solution such that a small amount of allergenic material is introduced. Alternatively, allergen solution may be injected intradermally, although the risk of anaphylaxis is greater. In both, if allergen-specific IgE bound to mast cells is present below the epidermis, a wheal-and-flare reaction results owing to the degranulation process and appears within 5–15 minutes of allergen introduction.

In vitro diagnostic tests

The direct demonstration of IgE binding to a particular allergen using immunochemical methods offers some advantages over skin tests because of the ease of automation, standardization, and efficiency. All such assays use immobilized allergens and sensitive methods for detecting IgE that has bound, and are known collectively as allergosorbent tests (AST). In these assays, allergen is immobilized on an insoluble matrix such as plastic, cellulose nitrate, cellulose (paper), or agarose beads and incubated with sera from patients under investigation. Any specific IgE antibody present will bind to the immobilized allergen and, after washing away non-bound serum proteins, can be detected by antibody directed against human IgE. The first tracer used to detect IgE was ^{125}I but this has now been replaced by enzyme tracers such as β-galactosidase and alkaline phosphatase. The amount of IgE binding with the latter is then determined by measuring the amount of chromogenic product released (Fig. 5.8) using an appropriate, colourless substrate system. Clearly, the quality of the allergen used to attach to the matrix will be important and either whole extracts or single, purified allergens (the latter tests are known as component-resolved assays) can be used. ASTs may be easily converted to inhibition assays, where varying concentrations of allergens are mixed with aliquots of an allergic serum before incubation with the matrix-bound allergen. If the soluble allergen has bound IgE in the serum, this is reflected in decreased IgE binding to the matrix. The results are expressed as the amount of allergen required to give 50% inhibition of maximum binding and, when comparing similar extracts, the lower the concentration required the more potent it is. In addition, the slope of the inhibition curve obtained gives information regarding the range of allergens contained within an extract and this technique is regularly used in allergen standardization.

Quicker and more efficient variants of ASTs have emerged and include, for example, biochips based on microarray protein technology. Here, small spots of allergen are bound to activated glass slides and then treated with sera as described above, and bound IgE is detected using fluorescent-dye-labelled anti-IgE. The advantage of this technique lies in its ability to determine whether a patient is allergic to one or more sources using single chips containing a large panel of individual allergens with minimal amounts of serum (20 µL). Whilst these AST

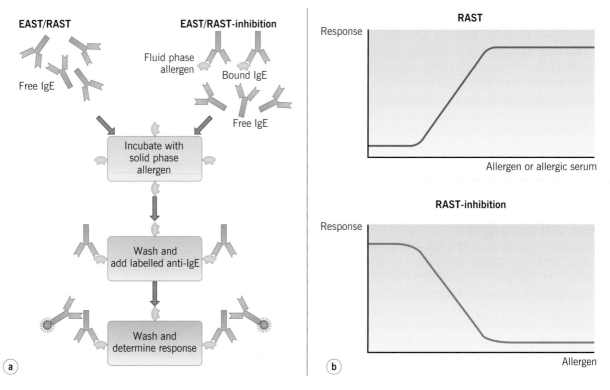

Fig. 5.8 Outline of the steps involved in allergosorbent and allergosorbent-inhibition assays (a). In enzyme-linked and radioallergosorbent assays (EAST/RAST) used for allergen characterization purposes, increasing concentrations of allergen are coupled to a solid phase and then incubated with a constant volume of serum from an allergic donor. For diagnostic purposes, a constant amount of allergen is coupled to the solid phase and varying dilutions of serum are then added. The amount of IgE bound is detected using a labelled anti-IgE. In each case, a positive dose response curve is obtained (b). In EAST/RAST-inhibition, allergic serum is incubated with fluid phase allergen prior to incubation with solid phase allergen (a). The more potent the fluid phase allergen, the less free IgE is available to bind to the solid phase allergen. This gives rise to a negative dose response curve, which can then be converted to a percent inhibition dose responsive curve (b).

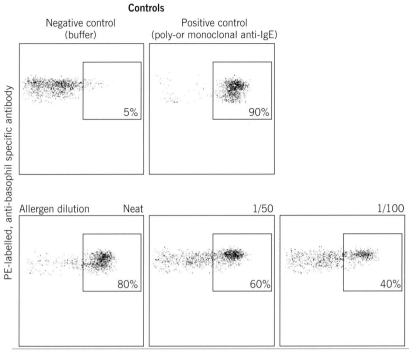

Controls

Negative control (buffer)

Positive control (poly-or monoclonal anti-IgE)

5%

90%

Allergen dilution   Neat   1/50   1/100

80%   60%   40%

PE-labelled, anti-basophil specific antibody

FITC-labelled, anti-granule associated protein antibodies

Fig. 5.9 Basophil activation assay for the detection of allergen-specific IgE. The set of panels in this figure show the flow cytometric data obtained using blood samples from the same allergic individual. The blood samples were mixed with dilutions of allergen and then with fluorescein iso-thiocyanate (FITC)-labelled anti-granule-associated protein and phycoerythin (PE) labelled anti-basophil antibodies. The boxes show the basophil activation obtained using different concentrations of allergen. Note that as the allergen is diluted, fewer cells are stained. (Modified from Boumiza R, Debard A-L, Monneret G. The basophil activation test by flow cytometry: recent developments in clinical studies, standardization and emerging perspectives. Clin Mol Allergy 2005; 3:9.)

assays are quantitative, semiquantitative assays are available, in particular those based on lateral flow technology. Here, allergen(s) is conjugated to a cellulose nitrate strip as a band upstream of an application point comprising an absorbent pad fixed at one end of the strip. This pad also contains an anti-IgE antibody conjugated with colloidal gold and when a liquid sample (e.g. blood) under investigation is applied to the pad, this reagent is solubilized and any IgE (or IgG) in the sample will bind to the anti-IgE colloidal gold conjugate. Both will then move up the strip by capilliary action. As the complex moves up the strip, it will come into contact with the immobilized band of allergen and any IgE specific for the allergen will become immobilized at this point, while any other IgE will continue to move along the strip. With time, the accumulated complex of IgE bound to allergen becomes visible owing to the pink colour of the colloidal gold attached to the anti-IgE. Such assays usually include a control band of antibody situated above the original capture antibody that recognizes excess anti-IgE-colloidal gold conjugate. In addition to being used diagnostically, this assay may also be modified to detect allergen in dust (e.g. from house dust mite) or in foods (e.g. soybean). In such situations, the anti-IgE-colloidal gold conjugate is replaced by an anti-allergen conjugate and the capture reagent is an antibody directed against the antibody raised against the allergen in question. In addition to these immunochemical assays, it is also possible to detect allergen-specific IgE using an in vitro cell-based assay based on the degranulation of basophils in whole blood. Here, whole blood is incubated with putative allergen, which will activate any allergen-specific IgE bound to the surface of basophils. This binding will then cause granules from within the cytoplasm to fuse with the basophil plasma membrane and release their contents. The whole blood is then treated with two or more different fluorescently labelled antibodies, one of which will identify the basophil [often an anti-IgE or a specific basophil cell surface molecule such as chemoattractant receptor homologous molecule expressed on Th2 cells/DP2 (CRTH2)] and the other that will recognize a granule-associated protein (such as CD63 or CD203c) that is expressed on the basophil surface when activated by allergen. The percentage of activated cells is then determined by flow cytometry (Fig. 5.9), and a reaction is classified as positive (binding both types of antibody) if more than 15% of basophils are activated after exposure to allergen.

One- and two-dimensional SDS-PAGE and immunoblotting

In the one-dimensional sodium dodecyl sulphate polyacrylamide gel electrophoretic (SDS-PAGE) analysis of allergens, individual protein components in an allergen extract are separated after denaturation and reduction of both intra- and interchain disulphide bonds. The proteins, which separate on the basis of their molecular weight in descending order, are then transferred electrophoretically or by capillary action to a cellulose nitrate or nylon membrane. After washing, the membranes are blocked with an extraneous, non-allergenic protein to reduce non-specific effects and then incubated with

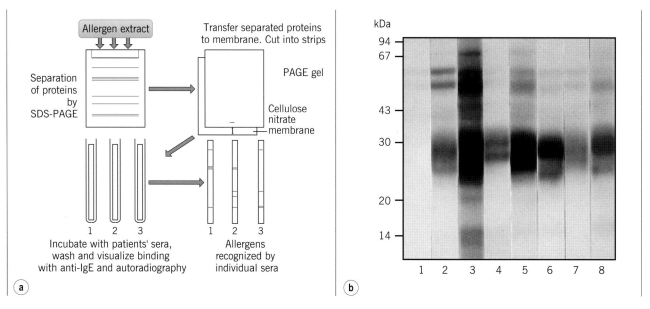

Fig. 5.10 SDS-PAGE and immunoblotting analysis of allergen extracts (a). SDS-PAGE-IgE immunoblot of *Lolium perenne* pollen extracts (b), demonstrating the responses obtained with sera from a non-atopic (lane 1) and seven atopic individuals (lanes 2–8).

allergic serum. IgE binding to individual allergens is then visualized using a labelled anti-IgE reagent (Fig. 5.10). Immunoblotting provides information about the total number of allergens in an extract recognized by a sensitized individual as well as their apparent molecular weights. This technique is often used to determine the frequency of reactivities to allergenic components within an allergen extract. If this is the desired outcome, aliquots of the extract are separated in each lane of the gel and, following immunoblotting, each lane is incubated with serum from a different individual in the study population. In two-dimensional electrophoresis, the allergen extract is first subjected to isoelectric focusing in polyacrylamide gels containing ampholines, which separate proteins on the basis of their isoelectric point (pI). The separated proteins within the gel are then subjected to SDS-PAGE at right angles to the isoelectric focusing step. The resulting gels may then be immunoblotted as described above. This technique is superior to the one-dimensional approach in its resolving ability, and has been particularly useful in separating and characterizing allergens. In either one- or two-dimensional SDS-PAGE, protein allergens of interest may be digested in situ using trypsin and the resulting peptides identified by mass spectroscopy.

B-cell and T-cell allergenic epitope determination

B-cell epitopes and T-cell epitopes may be identified once the amino acid sequence of an allergen is known and, if the three-dimensional structure has been determined,

they can be visualized (see Fig. 5.1). In this regard, B-cell epitopes are detected by synthesizing small, overlapping peptides representing the entire length of an allergen and attaching them to a matrix and incubating them with sera from an allergic individual as described above in the AST section. In this way, it is possible to 'map' potential epitopes and determine whether they are major (recognized by most allergic individuals). It is also possible to use phage expression libraries in a similar fashion and these have the additional advantage that it is possible to express longer epitopes, which may enable conformational epitopes to be expressed and detected. To detect T-cell epitopes, use is made of the proliferative capacity of T cells bearing the appropriate cell surface T-cell receptor. Here, overlapping peptides are incubated with antigen-presenting cells and T cells, and cell proliferation is then determined.

Allergen isolation

Individual allergens are usually isolated from aqueous extracts prepared from the original allergenic source material. As most allergens are protein or glycoprotein, any of the physicochemical techniques available for isolating proteins in general (e.g. gel filtration, ion exchange, reverse phase chromatography) can be used, including monoclonal antibody technology. More recently, recombinant DNA technology has become the method of choice for the characterization and production of allergens for diagnostic, structural, and functional studies and, in this regard, many of the clinically important allergens have now been cloned.

Cloning of allergens

In this technique, messenger (m)RNA is isolated from the allergen source, and complementary (c)DNA prepared by transcribing the RNA using the enzyme reverse transcriptase (Fig. 5.11). The single-stranded cDNA produced is then converted into double-stranded DNA with a DNA polymerase and the resulting material inserted into appropriate vectors such as plasmids using restriction endonucleases, and the genetic material amplified and cloned. The array of cDNA reflecting the starting mRNA represents the library, which is then screened to isolate the cDNA coding for the allergens of interest. Screening may be accomplished by hybridization using oligonucleotide probes synthesized on the basis of amino acid sequences obtained by conventional protein sequencing of known allergens or, alternatively, using sera from individuals allergic to the allergen source being cloned. The latter technique is used when direct sequence information of the allergens is unavailable. Here, use is made of expression vectors that facilitate the synthesis of the recombinant allergen. Once cloned, the cDNA is sequenced and the putative amino acid data checked to see if the allergen shows homology with any protein so far sequenced. Using a variety of sequence databases, such information identifies the protein and helps determine the role played by the allergen within the original source. These techniques are also used to prepare purified allergen for diagnostic purposes or to generate allergy vaccines based on reduced IgE reactivity but possessing relevant T-cell reactivity. This process has the potential to produce conformationally altered mutants that are unlikely to induce adverse reactions in sensitized individuals yet be capable of modulating specific T-cell responses during immunotherapy. The Allergen Nomenclature Subcommittee guidelines indicate that such recombinant allergens should be identified by placing the letter 'r' in front of the allergen designation, e.g. rDer p 1 for the recombinant form of the mite cysteine protease allergen. If allergens are chemically synthesized, then the letter 's' must be used, e.g. sDer p 1.

Monoclonal antibody techniques

In monoclonal antibody (mAb) techniques, mice are immunized with the purified allergen and spleen cells, obtained a few weeks after primary and secondary immunization, are subsequently fused with plasmacytoma cells using a fusogenic agent. Antibody-producing hybridomas that result are screened using appropriate selection chemicals and those possessing the appropriate specificity are isolated, cloned, and then used to produce antibody in large quantities. Such hybridomas represent a potentially immortal supply of antibody that may be used to purify allergens, map epitopes, determine allergen concentrations in the environment, and standardize the concentration of allergens within extracts (Fig. 5.12).

Allergen usage and standardization

Allergens, usually in the form of aqueous extracts prepared from individual sources (whole pollen, mites, fungi, etc.), are used diagnostically and to desensitize patients (termed 'allergen vaccines'). Most of the available extracts used for these purposes are crude in that they contain not only allergens of interest but also irrelevant antigens. They have a finite shelf-life, and there may be wide variation in potency between the same types of extract produced by different manufacturers. However, a number of standardized allergen extracts (Timothy grass pollen, birch pollen, dog hair/dander, *Dermatophagoides pteronyssinus*, and short ragweed) have been prepared under the auspices of the World Health Organization that meet appropriate requirements of potency and reproducibility for both diagnostic and immunotherapeutic purposes, and contain defined concentrations of specific allergens. Recombinant allergens are now available and are giving rise to the concept of 'component-resolved' diagnosis, in contrast to 'extract-based' diagnosis. It has been shown, for example, that tests performed using a single or a combination of a limited number of recombinant allergens are sufficient to identify most, if not all, patients allergic to a particular source. Although recombinant allergens are available, they are not without potential problems such as poor stability, aggregation, incorrent folding, and reduced allergenicity and/or biochemical activity.

Monitoring allergen exposure or allergen content

Monitoring the environment for the presence of an allergen source or individual allergen (as a surrogate for the source per se), or determination of allergen concentrations in food, can prove useful in a variety of situations. For example, monitoring atmospheric whole pollen concentrations (by counting grains) can warn people at risk of seasonal allergies, as long as it is possible to distinguish between allergy-associated and non-allergy-associated species. Similarly, determining the concentration of whole mites in house dust may also be used to assess potential exposure risks. However, these approaches are not necessarily quick, or technologically simple to perform. On this basis, various immunoassays have been developed (see earlier) for domestic or occupational allergen exposure. Such assays have been useful for developing an understanding of threshold concentrations either beyond which sensitization and/or precipitation of

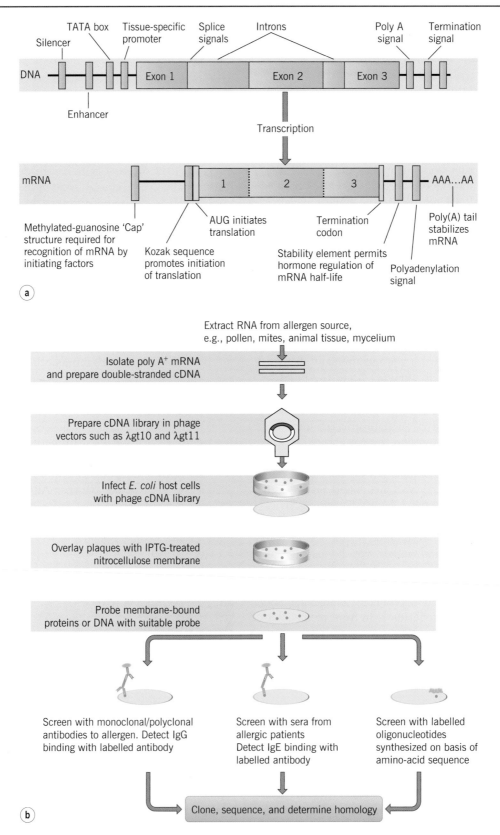

Fig. 5.11 (a) Schematic representation of the structure of a typical eukaryotic gene coding for an allergen. (b) Schematic representation of the steps involved in cloning allergen specific cDNA into phage for subsequent expression as protein. (Modified from Stewart GA. Molecular biology of allergens. In: Busse WW, Holgate ST, eds. Asthma and rhinitis. Oxford: Blackwell Scientific.)

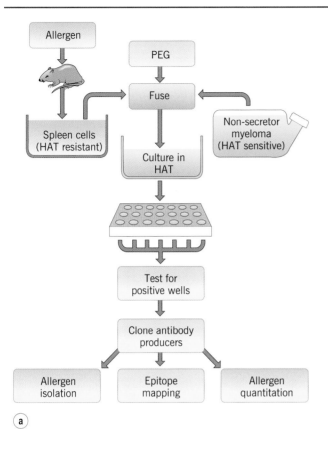

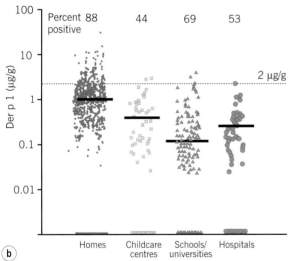

Fig. 5.12 (a) The production of monoclonal antibodies to allergens. (b) The determination of the house dust mite allergen Der p 1 in dust obtained from various locations. The bars represent geometric means and the dashed lines indicate currently accepted threshold levels. The mean levels of allergen in the home are significantly higher than elsewhere. (Modified from Zhang L, Chew FT, Soh SY, et al. Prevalence and distribution of indoor allergens in Singapore. Clin Exp Allergy 1997; 27:876-885.)

Table 5.8 Proposed allergen threshold concentrations

Allergen source	Specific allergen	Threshold concentration
Air		ng/m^3
Detergent enzymes	Subtilisin	15–60
Flour mixture	Asp o 2	0.25
Latex	—	0.6
Dust		µg/g
Cat dander	Fel d 1	8
Cow dander	Bos d 2	1–20
Dog dander	Can f 1	10
House dust mite	Der p 1	<2–10

adverse reactions may occur or, conversely, below which neither occurs. Determination of the concentrations of particular allergens with specific assays may also be useful to resolve the atmospheric (for respiratory exposure) or food (for gastrointestinal exposure) concentrations that either sensitize an individual or constitute a risk in the workplace or in the home. Because occupational exposure is usually restricted to a single allergen or simple allergenic mixtures, it has proved relatively easy to monitor airborne concentrations, but in the home the allergen content of settled dust is usually sampled. Here, mAb assays have proved very useful and commercial kits are available to measure mite, cockroach, and cat allergens. These assays have helped in determining the concentrations of allergen associated with sensitization and provocation (Table 5.8). Such assays for measuring allergen concentrations are useful for assessing the effectiveness and timing of avoidance or intervention measures.

Allergen avoidance and immunotherapy

One approach to reducing allergen-induced disease is to avoid the allergen source. This has had some success but, in many instances, total avoidance proves to be impossible. The simplest strategy may be to change jobs or move residence, but this is not often practical because of social and financial implications as well as the possibility that other allergens in the new location may show cross-reactivity with the allergen being avoided. It is also possible to remove the source completely (e.g. by relinquishing the family pet, killing mites with acaricides, or installing high-efficiency filters to remove allergens from the atmosphere). A more recent approach has been to modify the allergen itself in situ so as to render it

Table 5.9 Possible novel allergen-specific immunotherapeutic approaches to the treatment of allergy

Modality*	Allergen	Comment
Allergen DNA or mRNA	rPhl p 5, rDer p 1, rFel d 1	Direct injection of plasmids or genetically engineered live vectors such as *Salmonella typhimurium* or *Bacillus Calmette-Guerin* containing DNA encoding allergen or portion of allergen Self-replicating mRNA vaccines
Chimeric allergens	rFel d 1	Variable region of anti-CD64 (FcγRI) monoclonal antibody grafted to Fel d 1, targets allergen to dendritic cells and up-regulates thymic stromal lymphopoietin with Th2-promoting effect Fc region of IgG grafted to allergen, Fc fragment targets complex to FcγRIIb and allergen cross-links with the FcεRI, inhibiting mast cell degranulation
Hypoallergens	rBet v 1, rFel d 1	Reduced allergenicity but retaining T-cell stimulatory activity, naturally occurring or modified recombinant allergens
High-density allergen-containing particles	rFel d 1	Attachment of multiple allergenic proteins to surface of bacteriophage or agarose beads, directs complex to antigen-presenting cells and increases production of allergen-specific IgG
Peptide based	rFel d 1	Cocktail of peptides representing known T-cell epitopes
Allergen–toll-like receptor (TLR) agonist conjugates	rAmb a 1	Attachment of TLR agonists such as cytosine phosphorothioate guanosine (CpG) motifs, or lipopolysaccharide to allergen, targets allergen to TLR-9 and TLR-4, respectively, on antigen presenting cells, and redirect Th2 responses to Th1

*Modalities are mainly experimental at present.

non-allergenic [e.g. by chemically modifying allergens such as those from the mite, with tannic acid or genetically engineering hypoallergenic sources of allergen (pets and plants)]. With regard to immunotherapy, the availability of recombinant allergens has now made it possible to develop novel allergen-specific modalities, particularly with patients who are monosensitized. Despite our lack of understanding of the underlying mechanisms of clinical success, most have been developed on the basis that activating T cells (Th1 or regulatory T cells) without activating mast cells, or inducing allergen-specific IgG at the expense of IgE, is essential (Table 5.9). These modalities include the intradermal, subcutaneous, or sublingual administration of naturally occuring or genetically engineered hypoallergenic variants, DNA vaccines, T-cell epitope peptide cocktails, chimeric molecules comprising allergen and ligand for the FcεRI, and high-density allergen particles.

Conclusions

Over the last few years, progress in allergen research has been considerable and the majority of the clinically important allergens have now been characterized. All these developments should contribute significantly to our understanding of the nature of allergens and how they interact with the mechanisms involved in the disease process and, ultimately, result in better management of allergic conditions.

Air pollutants

Introduction

The air that we breathe, whether indoors or outdoors, is universally contaminated by particles and gases emanating from both natural and artificial sources that can reach the eyes, the nose, the upper and lower airways, and the lung parenchyma (Fig. 5.13). Airborne allergens arising from natural sources of course have a prominent role in causing and exacerbating allergic diseases, including hay fever and asthma, but the effects of pollutants resulting from human activity may also be relevant in allergy. For example, some of these pollutants may augment responses to allergens, and people with allergic diseases tend to be more susceptible to a number of key indoor and outdoor pollutants. Symptoms caused by air pollutants, particularly at high levels of exposure, tend to mimic symptoms of allergic diseases and, because of this, patients with atopic diseases may turn to allergists for guidance concerning the self-management of their susceptibility to air pollution, particularly at a time when air pollution warnings are issued.

People with allergic diseases can be exposed to air pollutants in diverse indoor and outdoor environments that may constitute either global or microenvironments (Fig. 5.14). The latter term is used for specific locations that have unique air quality characteristics and, for a typical adult, these may vary according to the time of the day and might include, for example, the home, vehicles, office, factory floor, city streets, and various public places such as restaurants, bars, sports facilities, and shopping areas. For children, school and childcare facilities might be relevant microenvironments in addition to the home and its environs. Exposure in any of these microenvironments may be clinically relevant, and a detailed, systematic history is needed to uncover the contributing pollutants in each.

Outdoor air pollutants

Non-biological pollutants

Pollutants in outdoor air can arise from natural sources such as vegetation, the sea, and volcanoes; however, the most relevant with regard to health are those arising from artificial sources contaminating not only urban environments but broader regions of entire countries–including, for example, the central and eastern portions of the USA and many countries of the former Soviet Republic such as Estonia and Poland. The artificial sources of outdoor pollutants can be broadly grouped as either stationary or mobile. The major stationary sources include power-generating stations, which may burn coal, natural gas, or petroleum; fossil-fuel-burning industrial plants; and various additional manufacturing facilities. In contrast, mobile sources will include the major gasoline- and diesel-fuelled vehicles.

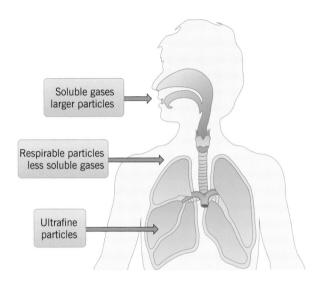

Fig. 5.13 Sites of absorption and deposition of inhaled particles and gases.

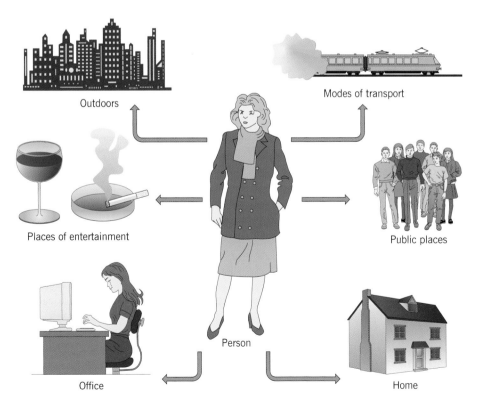

Fig. 5.14 Principal microenvironments for the average adult.

The principal outdoor non-biological air pollutants relevant to people with allergic diseases are typically present in complex mixtures, and evidence for the toxicity of the individual pollutants may not fully reflect the synergistic effects of the mixture. Fossil-fuel combustion typically generates particulate matter (PM) of varying sizes, some of which will be small enough to enter the lung. It also generates gases, including oxides of sulphur and nitrogen as well as carbon monoxide. The last of these impairs oxygen transport by binding to haemoglobin, although not specifically affecting people with allergic diseases. Sulphur oxides and nitrogen oxides undergo chemical transformation to form respirable secondary pollutants such as sulphate- and nitrate-containing particles, some of which are acidic. These small particles may also possess heavy metals and organic chemicals on their surfaces, which can leach out in the airways to produce toxic effects. Sulphur dioxide, a highly water soluble gas, is efficiently absorbed in the nose and upper airways whereas nitrogen dioxide, a less soluble one, may reach the smaller airways of the lung.

In areas with both heavy vehicle traffic and high levels of sunlight, photochemical pollution or smog is generated. This type of pollution is a rich mixture of oxidative chemicals, generally indexed by the level of ozone (O_3). First identified in Los Angeles about 50 years ago, ozone pollution may become an increasingly widespread problem as urbanization increases, and cities become progressively choked by vehicle traffic. In the USA, the problem of ozone pollution extends across the eastern portions of the country in the summer, and elsewhere affects many of the world's 'mega-cities'.

Various point sources of pollution may also affect people with allergic diseases. For example, volatile organic compounds (VOCs), which exist as gases at typical ambient temperatures, and other respiratory irritants may contaminate air in communities.

Biological pollutants

Outdoor biological pollution occurs where more specific sensitizing agents are released into the environment as a result of faulty workplace processes or marked, but transient, climatic changes. The best-known examples of biological contamination of the outdoor environment that has impacted on allergic disease are the epidemics of asthma resulting from exposure to soybeans in various port cities in the USA and Spain. All appear to be associated with exposure to dusts resulting from the unloading of soybeans from ships and their transfer to silos. However, due to faulty equipment, people were exposed to high concentrations of soybean allergens, in particular the 8 kDa Gly m 1 and 2 allergen (see Appendix 5.6). These exposures gave rise to sporadically occurring days of endemic asthma in New Orleans in the 1950s and 60s, in Barcelona in the 80s, and in Cartagena in the 90s. With regard to the Barcelona outbreak, the installation of filters on the storage silos ended the epidemic, although only after some detective work. With regard to climatic influences generating biological pollution, thunderstorm activity has been associated with epidemics of asthma, in both the United Kingdom and Australia. Although the precise mechanism(s) involved remain unclear, it has been proposed that the storm conditions promoted the release of spores from fungi such as *Aspergillus* species, *Didymella exitialis* and *Sporobolomyces* species or the generation of submicronic grass pollen material (e.g. starch granules, see earlier in this chapter) could be involved.

Indoor air pollutants

Non-biological pollutants

Indoor air pollutants, both non-biological and biological, are even more diverse than outdoor air pollutants – although, of course, many outdoor pollutants may ultimately permeate indoors. Such indoor pollutants can arise domestically or in the workplace, and are broadly grouped by source and type (Table 5.10). Indoor environments are, of course, the principal microenvironments where exposure to biological pollutants such as microbes and allergens and non-biological pollutants from sources such as gas-fired ranges, space-heating devices, tobacco smoke, and various VOCs will commonly occur. With regard to gas-fired ranges, ovens, and space-heating devices, all can emit nitrogen dioxide, particularly if they have continuously burning pilot lights. In addition, space-heating devices using kerosene combustion may also generate acids from sulphur present in the fuel. In the developing world, smoke from the burning of biomass fuels is a dominant contributor to personal exposure, although in developed countries properly operated woodstoves and fireplaces have little impact on indoor air quality.

With regard to non-biological pollutant exposure, tobacco smoking, which will create a mixture of exhaled smoke and smoke released by smouldering cigarettes, may be significant. This mixture, referred to as environmental tobacco smoke (ETS) will contain a range of pollutants including fine particles, gases (including nicotine), irritants such as acrolein, and various aldehydes. Homes with smokers tend to have much higher levels of respirable particles than do those without smokers, and there is little debate that burning cigarettes significantly increase particulate matter levels in indoor airspaces. For example, a comparison of fine-mode particulates in smoking and non-smoking sections of 11 restaurants revealed that areas in which smoking was permitted contained 177 μg/m^3 of PM versus 87 μg/m^3 in areas in which smoking did not occur. As the smoking and non-smoking sections of these establishments were generally separate areas of one large indoor space, even the non-smoking section was

Table 5.10 Sources of common indoor contaminants

Contaminant	Source
Asbestos	
Chrysotile, crocidolite, amosite, tremolite	Some wall and ceiling insulation installed between 1930 and 1950; old insulation on heating pipes and equipment; old woodstove door gaskets; some vinyl floor tiles; drywall joint-finishing material and textured paint purchased before 1977; cement asbestos millboard and exterior wall shingles; some sprayed and trowelled ceiling finish plaster installed between 1945 and 1973; fire-retardant sprayed into some structural steel beams
Combustion by-products	
Carbon monoxide, nitrogen dioxide and sulphur dioxide	Gas ranges, wood and coal stoves, fireplaces, backdraft of exhaust flues, particulate soot, nitrogenated compounds candles and incense
Formaldehyde	
	Some particleboard, plywood, pressboard, paneling, some carpeting and carpet backing, some furniture and dyed materials, UFFI, some household cleaners and deodorizers, combustion gas, tobacco, wood, some glues and resins, tobacco smoke, cosmetics, permanent-press textiles
Biologicals	
Fungal spores, bacteria, viruses, pollens	Mould, mildew, and other fungi, humidifiers with stagnant water, water-damaged surfaces and materials, condensing coils and drip pans in HVAC systems, refrigerator drainage pans, some thermophilics on dirty heating coils, animals, rodents, insects, humans
Radon	
Radon gas, 210Bi, 218Po, 210Po, 210Pb	Soil, rocks, water (gas diffuses through cracks and holes in the foundation and floor), well water, natural gas used near the source wells, some building material such as granite
Tobacco smoke	
Carbon monoxide, nitrogen and carbon dioxide, hydrogen cyanide, nitrosamines, aromatic hydrocarbons, benzo[a]pyrene, particles, benzene, formaldehyde, nicotine	Cigarettes, pipes, cigars
Volatile organic compounds (VOE)	
Alkanes, aromatic hydrocarbons, esters, alcohols, aldehydes, ketones	Solvents and cleaning compounds, paints, glue and resins, spray propellants, fabric softeners and deodorizers, combustion, dry-cleaning fluids, some fabrics and furnishings, store gasoline, out-gassing from water, some building materials, waxes and polishing compounds, pens and markers, binders and plasticizers

Modified from Samet JM, et al. Indoor air pollution. In: Rom WN, ed. Environmental and occupational medicine. Philadelphia: Lippincott–Raven; 1998:1523–1537.
HVAC, heating ventilation and air conditioning; UFFI, urea-formaldehyde foam insulation.

significantly polluted, with PM levels that were 29-fold greater than smoke-free air and 6-fold higher than outdoor air.

The observation that secondhand smoke increases indoor PM correlates with the clear observations that such exposure contributes to airway disease. These effects include exacerbation of asthma and development of allergic sensitization. Indeed, tobacco smoke is increasingly recognized to have immunomodulatory effects. Animal studies have shown that tobacco smoke exposure enhances development of Th2 responses to allergen, and examination of systemic IL-13 levels (a key cytokine involved in IgE induction) in samples collected from identical twins with discordant smoking histories reveals increased IL-13 levels in smokers compared with non-smokers. Experimental in vivo nasal challenge of human volunteers with allergic airway disease with secondhand tobacco smoke also demonstrates increased IgE-mediated response to allergen. Recent studies using both in vitro and in vivo challenge of nasal epithelial cells suggest that tobacco smoke may modify type I interferon response to viral infection. Nasal epithelial cells from smokers that were experimentally infected with influenza were found to have increased cytotoxicity, IL-6, and viral shedding compared with cells from non-smokers. Cells from smokers also produced less INF-α and IRF7 (a key transcription factor for the production of INF-α) than those from non-smokers. Analysis of nasal epithelial cell production of IRF7 in smokers and non-smokers of cells recovered after in vivo inoculation with live attenuated influenza virus confirmed that smokers produce less IRF7 following influenza infection. In sum, there is increasing appreciation that tobacco smoke modifies IgE-mediated response and probably decreases host defences against airway viral infection. As viral infections are the leading immediate cause of asthma exacerbation, this is an important mechanism by which tobacco smoke impacts on asthma.

Many different non-cigarette smoking-related VOCs may also be found in indoor air and arise from building materials, furnishings, household products, office equipment, and other sources. The best known of this group of relatively low-molecular-weight chemicals is formaldehyde and, by definition, all VOCs are gaseous at room temperature. Concentrations of VOCs are typically highest when a building is new and then decline as materials age, but renovations and installation of new processes or equipment such as printers and copiers may increase their emission. Two other indoor pollutants, namely radon and asbestos, are carcinogens but are of no direct relevance to allergic diseases.

Biological pollutants

Biological contaminants are important components of respirable particulates, and most derive from a variety of microbial sources such as bacteria and fungi. Many of these microbial agents are characterized by the presence of cell wall components (PAMPs) such as lipopolysaccharide (LPS) and peptidoglycan. Importantly, PAMPs may evoke potent inflammatory responses in an exposed host since they are ligands for a number of receptors on host cells including airway epithelial cells, and circulating monocytes, macrophages, and granulocytes, which mediate a wide variety of immunomodulatory processes. The most notable of these receptors are the Toll-like receptors (TLRs), and, although a full review of the TLRs is beyond the scope of this chapter, the role of TLR2 and TLR4 in mediating responses to inhaled environmental contaminants will be highlighted.

Among the ligands for TLR2 are lipoteichoic acid and peptidoglycans from Gram-positive bacteria as well as agents derived from fungi. TLR4 is a receptor for LPS derived from Gram-negative bacteria, as well as a number of host-derived molecules such as fibronectin, fibrinogen, heat-shock proteins, and hyaluronic acid generated by host cells after injury by inhaled agents, for example ozone. Recent studies demonstrate that hyaluronic acid, in part, via TLR4 signalling, can mediate host response to ozone.

The role of an innate immune response to bioaerosols on asthma pathogenesis has been avidly studied over the past two decades. Several studies have suggested that responses to biological agents in indoor settings protects against development of atopy and asthma. However, other equally compelling studies have shown that indoor LPS levels are linked to increased airway disease in domestic and occupational settings. Further complicating this debate are reports that genetic variation in LPS response genes (CD14 and TLR4 alleles), coupled with differences in domestic or occupational endotoxin levels, result in either protection from or increased risk for airway disease.

Overall, it appears that domestic LPS and Gram-positive microbial exposure generally protect infants from development of atopic disease. However, in persons who have developed allergic airway disease, exposure to LPS exacerbates asthma. Likewise, people working in or living near hog-farming operations are exposed to bioaerosols, which contain Gram-positive and -negative flora and are associated with respiratory disease over time. In domestic settings, the number of animals (dogs, cats, and evidence of rodents) and people living in the home correlate with the amount of LPS present and has been shown to enhance responses to inhaled allergens. In addition, dog owners also appear to have increased responses to other non-biogenic ambient air pollutants. Taken together, these observations suggest that PAMP exposure may directly induce disease or prime enhanced response to other pollutants or allergens.

Humidity

Indoor relative humidity is increasingly recognized as an important factor in determining asthma severity. Decreased levels of humidity are associated with decreased severity of asthma. A large cross-sectional study of fourth-grade schoolchildren in Munich, Germany identified 234 children with active asthma, with 155 of these children undergoing lung function and non-specific airway reactivity tests within a 3-year span. Dampness was associated with increased night time wheeze and shortness of breath, but not with persisting asthma. Risk factors for bronchial hyperreactivity in adolescence included allergen exposure and damp housing conditions.

Mite allergen levels were examined from homes of 70% of the asthma cohort and found to significantly correlate with dampness and bronchial hyperreactivity. However, the effect of dampness was not due to mite allergen alone because bronchial hyperreactivity remained significantly correlated with humidity, even when adjusting for mite allergen levels.

Mechanisms of toxicity

The toxicity of the various air pollutants depends on the site of deposition and the specific chemical properties of the pollutants (Table 5.11). The site of particle deposition depends largely on the size of the particles, which is usually expressed as the aerodynamic diameter (Fig. 5.15). The larger airborne particles – those above approximately 10 μm in aerodynamic diameter and referred to as PM10 – do not penetrate into the respiratory tract, and particles of size PM10 down to PM2.5 are filtered in the upper airway. Particles less than 2.5 μm in diameter can enter the lower respiratory tract, whereas the smaller particles – those under 1 μm in diameter – deposit in the small airways and alveoli.

With regard to chemical properties, the more water-soluble pollutants affect the mucous membranes of the eyes and upper airway and do not reach the lower airways and alveoli without the increased ventilation that results from exercise; less soluble gases, including nitrogen dioxide and ozone, can reach the lungs, where absorption from the airways is greatest.

Inflammation is central to the response of the respiratory tract, and probably also the eye, to non-allergenic pollutants. Although specific mechanisms of action may differ, all these pollutants initiate inflammation at the sites of deposition. In experimental studies, pollution exposure has been shown to induce cytokine release and neutrophil influx. The effects of prolonged exposures to most pollutants are not yet well characterized, although experimental and epidemiological evidence indicates the possibility of airways fibrosis and narrowing and air-space enlargement, which leads to reduced ventilatory function and thus to increased frequency of respiratory symptoms.

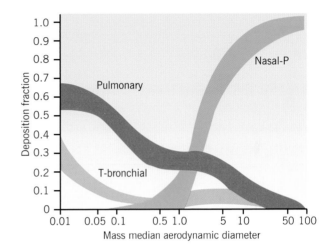

Fig. 5.15 Regional deposition predictions based on the model proposed by the International Commission on Radiological Protection Task Group on Lung Dynamics. (Modified from Wilson R, Spengler JD, eds. Particles in our air. Concentrations and health effects. Cambridge, MA: Harvard University Press; 1996.)

Table 5.11 Pathophysiological responses of respiratory tract to environmental particles and gases

Site	Agent	Response	Comments
Airways	Aeroallergens	Asthma	Immunological reaction
	Formaldehyde	Nasal cancer	Not conclusively established
	Formaldehyde, wood smoke	Irritation, cough	Immunological/non-immunological mechanisms
	Nitrogen dioxide, sulphur dioxide	Bronchoconstriction	Reflex, irritant
	Radon, asbestos	Cancer	Relationship between environmental asbestos exposure and lung cancer uncertain
None	Pollen	Hay fever, rhinitis	Immunological/non-immunological mechanisms
Parenchyma	Thermophilic actinomycetes, fungi	Hypersensitivity, pneumoconiosis	Immunological mechanisms
	Inorganic dust	Pneumoconiosis	Unrelated to environmental exposure

Modified from Utell MJ, Samet JM. Environmentally mediated disorders of the respiratory tract. Med Clin North Am 1990; 74:291–306.

The inflammation resulting from exposure to pollutants may be of consequence to the allergic disorders through several pathways. For example, the presence of non-specific inflammation may enhance responses to allergens such as the facilitation of allergen penetration as a result of increased permeability of the respiratory epithelium. In experimental exposures of volunteers with asthma, both ozone and nitrogen dioxide enhance the response to subsequent allergen challenge. There is also the possibility of synergism between inflammation caused by air pollution and that provoked by allergens. With regard to asthma, heightened airway responsiveness secondary to pollutant exposure might augment the response to allergens and make clinically relevant effects more frequent.

Air pollution, allergic diseases, and allergens

Allergic diseases

The nose acts as a filter, removing larger particles and soluble gases from inhaled air, and inflammatory responses of the nose following inhalation of various pollutants have been well described. Ozone characteristically causes burning and irritation of the eyes and upper airway including the nose, and other pollutant gases have been shown to behave similarly. However, clinically relevant consequences of air pollution exposure for persons with allergic rhinitis have received little attention.

In contrast, the role of air pollution in causing and exacerbating asthma has been investigated extensively. Many of the relevant data come from epidemiological studies that have been directed at either assessing risk factors for disease or determining if the status of people with asthma varies in relation to air pollution exposure. Additional data come from controlled air pollution exposures of volunteers with asthma in a variety of clinical studies where, of necessity, exposures are brief and limited to lower levels of pollutants, and the protocols generally exclude people with more severe disease.

There is little indication that the general types of air pollution found in urban and industrialised areas contribute to the production of asthma. Some reports describe a higher prevalence of non-specific bronchial hyperresponsiveness in more polluted areas, but definitive links to asthma have not been made. As indicated earlier, some outbreaks of asthma have been linked to specific agents, such as the problem of soybean-dust-induced asthma in Barcelona, but such episodes appear to be infrequent.

Indoor air pollutants have been identified as causes of asthma, although it is still not known whether onset of asthma is a reflection of environmental and genetic interaction or if some patients develop asthma solely because

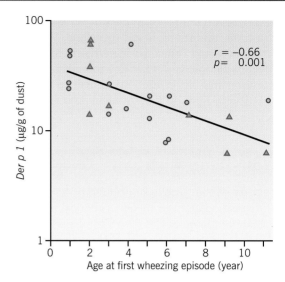

Fig. 5.16 Relationship between the age at the onset of the first wheezing episode in 21 atopic children and the highest level of Der p 1 in house dust in 1979. (From Sporik R, Holgate ST, Platts-Mills TAE, et al. Exposure to house-dust mite allergen (Der p 1) and the development of asthma in childhood. A prospective study. N Engl J Med 1990; 323:502–507, with permission of Massachusetts Medical Society.)

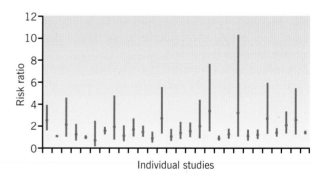

Fig. 5.17 Reported risk ratios (95% confidence intervals) in young children exposed to environmental tobacco smoke in studies that used clinically recognized asthma as an outcome. (From Office of Environmental Health Hazard Assessment, 1997.)

of environmental factors. The level of house dust mite exposure predicts the age of initial wheezing in children at risk of asthma (Fig. 5.16). Of the many indoor air pollutants other than indoor allergens, passive exposure to tobacco smoke is most firmly established as a cause of asthma in young children (Fig. 5.17). Mounting evidence shows that children of mothers who smoke are at increased risk, which may partially reflect the consequences of in utero exposure to tobacco smoke components from maternal smoking during pregnancy.

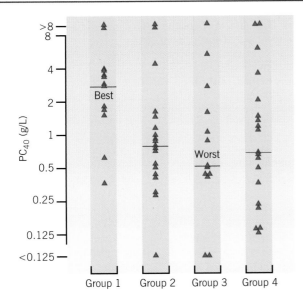

Fig. 5.18 Individual values for the histamine concentrations that provoked a decrease of 40% in maximal flow at functional residual capacity [VmaxFRC (PC40)]. Group 1: no family history of asthma, both parents non-smokers; group 2: family history of asthma, both parents non-smokers; group 3: no family history of asthma, one or both parents smokers; group 4: family history of asthma, one or both parents smokers. The horizontal lines show the median PC40 for each group. Two infants in group 2 had baseline flow limitation and therefore could not be challenged with histamine. No PC40 value could be determined for one infant in group 4, in whom excessive upper-airway noise developed, necessitating discontinuation of the challenge. (From Young S, Le Souf PN, Geelhoed GC, et al. The influence of a family history of asthma and parental smoking on airway responsiveness in early infancy. N Engl J Med 1991; 324:1168–1173, with permission of Massachusetts Medical Society.)

Physiological testing shortly after birth shows that infants of smoking mothers have reduced airway function and a higher level of non-specific bronchial hyperresponsiveness compared with infants of non-smoking mothers (Fig. 5.18). Formaldehyde, a common indoor exposure, is infrequently found to be a cause of asthma.

Both indoor and outdoor air pollutants can, however, adversely affect people with asthma. Indoor allergen exposure is, of course, tightly linked to the clinical status of asthmatics. For children, exposure to tobacco smoke increases the level of non-specific bronchial hyperresponsiveness and exposed children tend to use medical resources more often than non-exposed children. Some clinical studies indicate that nitrogen dioxide, another prevalent indoor gaseous agent, increases airway responsiveness and also the degree of response to inhaled allergens. Epidemiological data on indoor nitrogen dioxide and exacerbation of asthma are limited.

Outdoor pollutants that may exacerbate asthma include particulate matter, sulphur dioxide, nitrogen dioxide, and

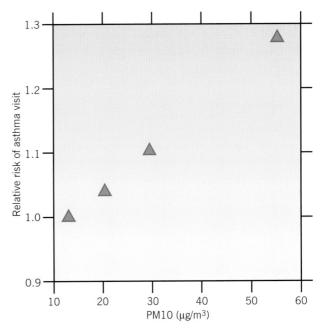

Fig. 5.19 Relative risk of asthma visits by quartile of airborne particles with aerodynamic diameter above approximately 10 μm (PM10) concentration, plotted against the mean PM10 concentration in the quartile. The relative risks are adjusted for temperature, season, day of week, hospital, time trends, age, and September peak. (From Schwartz J, Slater D, Larson TV, et al. Particulate air pollution and hospital emergency room visits for asthma in Seattle. Am Rev Respir Dis 1993; 147:826–831. Reprinted with permission of the American Thoracic Society. Copyright © 1993 American Thoracic Society.)

ozone. Data on these pollutants have been gained from clinical studies, follow-up studies of people with asthma, and studies on rates of clinic and emergency room visits and hospitalization. Evidence from throughout the world indicates that these pollutants can exacerbate asthma. Particulate air pollution of diverse composition, including wood smoke particles and acidic particles, has been associated with measures of exacerbation (Fig. 5.19). Clinical studies show that some asthmatics have exquisite sensitivity to sulphur dioxide, particularly when the dose delivered to the lungs is increased by exercise. The evidence from clinical studies that nitrogen dioxide can increase airway responsiveness is less clear. Extensive epidemiological data show that ozone exposure can adversely affect people with asthma, although asthmatics are not more sensitive than non-asthmatics to the reduction of lung function that follows ozone exposure.

Allergens

Several comparative and in vitro studies have shown that pollutants, both in the air (e.g. SO_2, O_3, NO_2) and soil (e.g. heavy metals such as cadmium) may have a variety of effects on allergens, particularly those of pollens, because many are pathogenesis-related proteins (see Table 5.5). Although the presence of some allergens is constitutive, increases are likely because such proteins are produced in response to a variety of abiotic stressors, including pollutants. In this regard, allergen production per se, concentration and releasability may all be influenced by pollutants. For example, the concentration of some pollen allergens may be higher in urban environments (e.g. Lol p 5, Cup a 3), others may be higher in rural environments (Phl p 5), and others may not be influenced (e.g. Bet v 1, 2 and 3) by environment. In addition, pollen extracts (e.g. birch) obtained from pollen derived from urban environments may demonstrate enhanced proinflammatory properties, indicating that pollutants act on proteins other than allergens. Other studies have shown that cadmium-polluted soils, whilst not necessarily influencing certain known pollen allergens (e.g. Poa a 1, 5), may cause the up-regulation of stress-related proteins with allergenic potential, given their sequence homology with allergens from other plant sources such as the pectin methyl esterase allergen Act d 7. With regard to releasability, both airborne and soil pollutants have been shown to damage pollen grains and/or increase the rate of release of allergen-containing starch granules. In addition to these effects, exposure of pollen to pollutants has been shown to alter their allergenicity by a process of post-translational modification such as nitration due to exposure to NO_2, which may enhance or decrease allergenicity.

Climate change and allergic disease

In early considerations of the impact of climate change on human health due to pollution, allergy-based diseases received far less attention than infectious diseases. However, with the mounting awareness within the scientific and medical communities of the connections between epidemiological, aerobiological, and phenomenological data with respect to aeroallergen sources, in particular pollens, and climate change, there is growing recognition that allergic disease will have an increased impact on future public health. Currently, there is a scarcity of information regarding the impacts of increased CO_2 and/or temperature on pollen allergen production, despite the fact that pollens contribute significantly to airborne allergen loads and are the major cause of aeroallergen-related allergy in about 30% of the population in temperate regions. Because of the reproductive role of pollen, changes to number, structure, and/or biochemistry may have significant impacts on plant fitness, which then has implications for species occurrence, biodiversity, and ecosystem dynamics. The prevalence of pollinosis has increased in recent decades and accumulating evidence indicates that some of this increase is a consequence of

Box 5.3 Effects of pollution and climate change on allergens and allergenicity of pollen

Pollutants (particulates, heavy metals, DEP, ETS, NO_2, SO_2, O_3)	Climate change (temperatures, CO_2)
Enhanced allergenicity due to adjuvant properties of particulates	Extended pollen seasons – earlier start, later finish
Differential expression of allergens in pollen grains	Increased allergen expression in pollen grains
Increased allergen content in pollen grain	Increased allergen content in pollen grains
Increase in pollen protein expression with possibility of creating new allergens	Increase in pollen protein expression with possibility of creating new allergens
Increased releasability of cytoplasmic allergens from pollen grains	Change in distribution of pollen-producing plants
Post-translational modification of pollen allergens	Increased pollen grain diameter
	Variation in pollen distribution range due to air current change

climate changes with the potential to influence a variety of pollen parameters (Box 5.3). In this regard, earlier and extended pollen seasons have been positively correlated with climate warming in Europe, North America, and Asia for a number of allergen-producing species, for example *Parietaria*, olive, and cypress. Increased concentrations of airborne pollen have also been shown to be a function of climate warming and modelling studies predict future increases. Increased airborne pollen concentrations and warming temperatures have been linked with both the prevalence of pollinosis and increases in allergen amounts in pollen.

In addition to a projected rise in global surface temperature of 1.4 °C to 5.8 °C by 2100, climate change scenarios predict atmospheric CO_2 levels will at least double in the twenty-first century from the preindustrial level of 280 $\mu mol\ mol^{-1}$. However, there is a scarcity of data on the effect(s) of CO_2 enrichment alone, or in combination with temperature, on allergenic pollen-producing species and pollinosis. The few studies that do exist have focused on ragweed (*Ambrosia artemisiifolia*) where an increase in pollen number was found when it was grown at 600–700 $\mu mol\ mol^{-1}$ CO_2, compared with growth at ambient levels of about 370 $\mu mol\ mol^{-1}$. In addition, increased atmospheric CO_2 concentrations led to an increase in the content of Amb a 1, a major allergen, of ragweed pollen. A positive correlation between ragweed

Table 5.12 Expected performance ratings for different filter types

Filter types	Filter media	Weight arrestance (%)	Atmospheric dust spot efficiency (%)	DOP efficiency (%)
Extended-area pleated HEPA-type filters	Wet-laid ultrafine glass fibre paper	99.99		99.7–99.99
Extended surface-type supported or non-supported	Fine glass fibres, fine electret synthetic fibres, or wet-laid paper of cellulose glass or all-glass fibres	95–99.7	30–98	0-90
Panel-type filter	Spun-glass, open cell foam, expanded metals and screen, synthetics, textile denier woven and non-woven, or animal hair	50–85		
Pleated panel-type filter	Fine denier non-woven synthetic and synthetic-natural fibre blends, or all natural fibre	85–90	20–30	

From Am J Respir Crit Care Med 1997; 156:S31–S64, ©American Thoracic Society.
DOP, dioctyl phthalate; HEPA, high-efficiency particulate air.

pollen production and increased CO_2 and temperature was also found along a CO_2/temperature gradient between rural and urban areas. Taken together, these results and the above temperature data indicate that climate change has significantly affected, and will continue to affect, the prevalence and intensity of pollen-related allergy, with a likely concomitant effect on allergenic disease.

Clinical implications

The evidence for the link between indoor and outdoor air pollution and asthma has implications for the prevention of asthma and the management of patients with asthma. With regard to prevention, the damning evidence on maternal smoking during pregnancy and early childhood is sufficient to warrant educational intervention, particularly if parental history of allergic disease indicates that the child is at high risk of asthma. Reduction of allergen exposure would also be prudent for such children.

Exposures in both indoor and outdoor environments have been linked to exacerbation of asthma. For the indoor environment, source control can be recommended as a prudent strategy. Tobacco smoking in the home can be limited and many countries are implementing workplace regulations to prohibit or limit smoking.

Increasingly, products are being manufactured with low emission rates of various VOCs. Proper venting of combustion appliances and use of gas cookers and ranges without pilot lights further reduce exposure to combustion gases.

Air-cleaning devices can remove both particles and gases. The most up-to-date devices incorporate high-efficiency particulate air filters for particles and a sorbent for gases. Table 5.12 reviews the principal types of filters and their performances. These devices can clean pollutants from air but the volumes handled are limited in relation to room size. Clinically relevant effects have not been shown and most clinical trials on air cleaners have not had sufficiently large sample sizes.

Exposures to most outdoor pollutants can be reduced by staying indoors. The concentration of ozone, a reactive gas, is typically much lower indoors than outdoors. Small particles do penetrate indoors, but concentrations are generally lower than outdoors. At times when pollutant levels are high, people with asthma can be counselled to stay indoors and, in particular, to avoid vigorous exercise. The response to air pollutants may be blunted by inhaled sympathomimetics and cromolin sodium. Air pollution regulations in many countries have been devised to control adverse health effects for everyone, including those with asthma. However, protecting the most susceptible people may not be possible.

Summary of important messages

- Atopic individuals produce IgE when exposed to complex mixtures of proteins contained within structures such as pollens, spores, and faecal pellets or when exposed to simpler mixtures such as food, animal danders, occupational allergens, and venoms. Exposure may occur via the respiratory route through breathing, via the skin through direct surface contact or injection, or via the gut through ingestion. Proteins stimulating an atopic reaction are termed allergens, which are denominated (separate from their trivial or systematic names) according to their genus and species, and order of identification within a source
- Not all proteins in these sources will stimulate IgE production in all atopic individuals under normal conditions of exposure, as allergenicity will be influenced by the genetic make-up of the host as well as factors associated with the proteins themselves such as size, foreignness, solubility, concentration, the presence of adjuvant factors, and biochemical properties. This gives rise to an operational definition of a protein as being a major (stimulation in more than 50% of individuals) or minor (less than 50%) allergen
- The primary structures and functions (within the originating source) of most, if not all, of the clinically important allergens are now known, and this information is now being exploited in the development of more precise diagnostic and therapeutic options in the treatment of allergic diseases, as well as understanding their genesis
- Atopic individuals are also exposed to biological and non-biological pollutants arising from human activity and contaminate the air, both inside and outside the home. The most important non-biologicals are the gases ozone, sulphur dioxide, and nitrogen dioxide, vapours such as volatile organic compounds and water, and particulates such as environmental tobacco smoke and fuel combustion products. The major biologicals are bacterial and fungal cell wall components such as lipopolysaccharide and peptidoglycan, occupational allergens such as industrial enzymes, and seed flours and debri
- Exposure to these pollutants can give rise to direct toxic reactions, initiation of allergic diseases per se, or exacerbation of existing allergic diseases, all of which are likely to be related to the generation of inflammatory responses (e.g. cytokine release, cellular influx) initiated at the sites of deposition due to cell damage or recognition of microbial components via Toll-like receptors and other innate immune receptors. Sites of deposition will be influenced by the size of the inhaled particle. Given the link with pollutants and allergic disease, management of exposure has implications for both prevention and control of clinical disease
- Pollutants also influence allergen production as well as allergen concentration, since many of the pollen allergens belong to the group of proteins known as pathogenesis-related proteins, which have evolved to deal with abiotic stressors. Pollution may also influence climate change and, thus, pollination per se with consequent effects on the start and finish of pollen seasons and rates of pollinosis

Further reading

Alexis N, Barnes C, Bernstein I, et al. Rostrum article: Health effects of air pollution. What the allergist needs to know. J Allergy Clin Immunol 2004; 114:1116–1123.

Alexis N, Lay JC, Almond M, et al. Inhalation of low dose endotoxin by human volunteers favors a local TH2 response profile and primes airway phagocytes in vivo. J Allergy Clin Immunol 2004; 114:1325–1331.

Breiteneder H, Mills EN. Molecular properties of food allergens. J Allergy Clin Immunol. 2005; 115:14–23.

Chapman MD, Ferreira F, Villalba M, et al. The European Union CREATE Project: a model for international standardization of allergy diagnostics and vaccines. J Allergy Clin Immunol 2008; 122:882–889.

Chen LL, Tager IB, Peden DB, et al. Effect of ozone exposure on airway responses to inhaled allergen in asthmatic subjects. Chest 2004; 125:2328–2335.

Douwes J, Le Gros G, Gibson P, et al. Can bacterial endotoxin exposure reverse atopy and atopic disease? J Allergy Clin Immunol 2004; 114:1051–1054.

Eggleston PA. Improving indoor environments: reducing allergen exposures. J Allergy Clin Immunol 2005; 116:122–126.

Fitzsimmons CM, Dunne DW. Survival of the fittest: allergology or parasitology? Trends Parasitol 2009; 25:447-451.

Lockey RF, Ledford DK, eds. Allergen and allergen immunotherapy, 4th edn. New York: Informa Healthcare USA; 2008.

Peden DB. Effect of pollutants in rhinitis. Curr Allergy Asthma Rep 2001; 1:242–246.

Peden DB. Influences on the development of allergy and asthma. Toxicology 2002; Dec 27:181–182, 323–328.

Stewart GA, Zhang J, Robinson C. The structure and function of allergens. In: Adkinson NFJ, Bochner BS, Yunginger JW, et al, eds. Middleton's allergy: principles and practice, 7th edn. Philadelphia: Mosby; 2009: 585–609

Traidl-Hoffman C, Jakob T, Bohrendt H. Determinants of allergenicity. J Allergy Clin Immunology 2009; 123:558–566.

Valenata R, Ferreira F, Focke-Tejkl M, et al. From allergen genes to allergy vaccines. Annu Rev Immunol 2010; 28:211–241.

Appendices

Appendix 5.1 Physicochemical and biochemical characteristics of grass pollen aeroallergens

Allergen	Frequency of reactivity (%)*	Mol. weight (K)	Function
Poaceae (e.g. *Phleum pratense, Lolium perenne, Cynodon dactylon*)			
Group 1 (e.g. Lol p 1)	>90	30	β-Expansins involved in cell wall loosening, shows homology with Groups 2 and 3 allergens
Group 2 (e.g. Lol p 2)	>60	11	Shows homology with Groups 1 and 3 allergens
Group 3 (e.g. Lol p 3)	70	11	Shows homology with Groups 1 and 2 allergens
Group 4 (e.g. Lol p 4)	50–88	57	Pectate lyase
Group 5 (e.g. Lol p 5)	>90	29–31	Ribonuclease
Group 6 (e.g. Phl p 6)	76	12	Shows homology with Group 5 allergens, associated with P particles
Group 7 (e.g. Cyn d 7)	10	9	Calcium-binding protein, polycalcin, shows homology with Bet v 4
Group 10 (e.g. Lol p 10)	0–?	12	Cytochrome C
Group 11 (e.g. Lol p 11)	65	15	Function unknown, shows homology with tree allergen Ole e 1 and soybean trypsin inhibitor
Group 12 (e.g. Phl p 12)	20–36	12	Profilin
Group 13 (e.g. Phl p 13)	50	55–60	Polygalacturonase
Group 15 (e.g. Phl p 15)	?	9	Function unknown
Group 22 (e.g. Phl p 22)	?	?	Enolase
Group 23 (e.g. Phl p 23)	?	9	Function unknown
Group 24 (e.g. Phl p 24)	?	21	Pathogenesis-related protein PR-1
Cyn d Bd46K	64	46	Shows homology with cytochrome c oxidase III from corn pollen
Cyn d BG60	?	60	Berberine bridge enzyme

*Frequency data presented in each of these tables have been derived from many sources and may vary with population studied. In addition, the data presented may reflect immediate hypersensitivity diseases including atopic dermatitis and allergic bronchopulmonary aspergillosis as well as delayed type hypersensitivity disease.? indicates lack of data. Tables modified from Stewart GA, Zhang J, Robinson C. The structure and function of allergens. In: Adkinson, NFJ, Bochner BS, Yunginger, JW, et al, eds. Middleton's allergy: principles and practice, 7th edn. Philadelphia: Mosby: 2008; 585-609; see also http://www.allergen.org and http://www.allergome.org. Classification of species throughout is derived from the Catalogue of Life (www.catalogueoflife.org). Some allergens may not be listed in these tables.

Appendix 5.2 Physicochemical and biochemical characteristics of pollen-derived aeroallergens from herbaceous dicotyledons

Allergen	Frequency of reactivity (%)	Mol. weight (K)	Function
ASTERACEAE			
Short ragweed (*Ambrosia artemisiifolia*)			
Amb a 1	>90	40	Pectate lyase
Amb a 2	>90	41	Pectate lyase
Amb a 3	51	11	Plastocyanine

Appendix 5.2 Continued

Allergen	Frequency of reactivity (%)	Mol. weight (K)	Function
Amb a 4	30	30	Defensin-like protein, shows homology with Art v 1
Amb a 5	17	5	Function unknown
Amb a 6	21	11	Lipid transfer protein
Amb a 7	20	12	Plastocyanin
Amb a 8	26	14	Profilin
Amb a 9	11	10	Polycalcin
Amb a 10	10	8	Polycalcin-like protein
Cystatin	30	10	Cysteine protease inhibitor
Mugwort (*Artemisia vulgaris*)			
Art v 1	>90	28	Function unknown; contains antifungal plant defensin-like domain and a hydroxyproline/proline-rich domain
Art v 2	33	20	Pathogenesis-related protein PR-1
Art v 3	?	12	Non-specific lipid transfer protein
Art v 4	36	14	Profilin
Art v 5	?	10	Polcalcin
Art v 6	?	44	Pectate lyase
Feverfew (*Parthenium hysterophorus*)			
Par h 1	>90	31	Extensin
Sunflower (*Helianthus annuus*)			
Hel a 1	57	34	Function unknown
Hel a 2	31	15	Profilin
Hel a 3	?	9	Lipid transfer protein
URTICACEAE			
Wall pellitory (*Parietaria judaica/officinalis*)			
Group 1 (e.g. Par o 1)	100	15	Lipid transfer protein
Group 2 (e.g. Par o 2)	82	10–14	Lipid transfer protein
Group 3 (e.g. Par j 3)	?	14	Profilin
Group 4 (e.g. Par j 4)	?	9	Polycalcin
BRASSICACEAE			
Oilseed rape (*Brassica napus*)			
6/8 kDa protein	50	6/8	Calcium-binding protein
14 kDa protein	34	14	Profilin
27–69 kDa cluster	80	27–69	Shows homology with grass pollen Group 4 allergens, pectate lyase
40 kDa protein	?	40	Receptor-like protein kinase
43 kDa protein	28–56	43	Polygalacturonase
70 kDa protein	?	70	Berberine bridge protein

Appendix 5.2 Continued

Allergen	Frequency of reactivity (%)	Mol. weight (K)	Function
80 kDa protein	?	80	Cobalamin-independent methionine synthetase
TRX-H-1	?	14	Thioredoxin
PCP-1	?	9	Pollen coat protein
Turnip (*Brassica rapa*)			
PEC-1	>30	13	Lipid transfer protein
PEC-2	?	14	Thioredoxin
PCP-3	?	9	Pollen coat protein
EUPHORBIACEAE			
Mercurialis annua			
Mer a 1	>59	14	Profilin
CHENOPODIACEAE			
Chenopodium album			
Che a 1	77	17	Shows homology with Ole e 1
Che a 2	55	14	Profilin
Che a 3	46	10	Polycalcin

Appendix 5.3 Physicochemical and biochemical characteristics of tree pollen aeroallergens

Allergen	Frequency of reactivity (%)	Mol. weight (K)	Function
ANGIOSPERMS			
Fagales: Birch (*Betula verrucosa*), Alder (*Alnus glutinosa*), Hornbeam (*Carpinus betulus*), Oak (*Quercus alba*), Chestnut (*Castanea sativa*), Hazel (*Corylus avellana*)			
Group 1 (e.g. Bet v 1)	>95	17	Plant steroid carrier, shows homology with pathogenesis-related proteins (PR-10)
Group 2 (e.g. Bet v 2)	20	15	Profilin
Group 3 (e.g. Bet v 3)	<10	24	Calcium-binding protein, polycalcin
Group 4 (e.g. Bet v 4)	20	9	EF hand calcium-binding protein, a polycalcin, shows homology with Aln g 4, Ole e 3, Syr v 3
Group 6 (e.g. Bet v 6)	32	35	Isoflavone reductase
Group 7 (e.g. Bet v 7)	21	18	Peptidyl-prolyl isomerase (cyclophilin)
Group 8 (e.g. Bet v 8?)	66	65	Pectin methylesterase
Scrophulariales: Olive (*Olea europaea*), Lilac (*Syringa vulgaris*), Privet (*Ligustrum vulgare*), Ash (*Fraxinus excelsior*)			
Group 1 (e.g. Ole e 1)	>90	20	Shows limited homology with soybean trypsin inhibitor and Lol p 11
Group 2 (e.g. Ole e 2)	24–75	15	Profilin

Appendix 5.3 Continued

Allergen	Frequency of reactivity (%)	Mol. weight (K)	Function
Group 3 (e.g. Ole e 3)	20–>50	15	Polycalcin
Group 4 (e.g. Ole e 4/9)	65–80	32–46	1,3-β-glucanase
Group 5 (e.g. Ole e 5)	35	16	Cu/Zn superoxide dismutase
Group 6 (e.g. Ole e 6)	5–20	10	Cysteine-rich protein
Group 7 (e.g. Ole e 7)	>60	10	Lipid transfer protein
Group 8 (e.g. Ole e 8)	3–4	21	Polycalcin-like protein
Group 9 (e.g. Ole e 9)	65	45	1,3 β-Glucanase
Group 10 (e.g. Ole e 10)	55	11	Shows homology with the C-terminal domain of Ole e 9, carbohydrate-binding module CBM 43
Group 11 (e.g. Ole e 11)	56–76	39	Pectin methylesterase
Hamamelidales London plane tree (*Platanus acerifolia*)			
Pla a 1	84	18	Invertase inhibitor
Pla a 2	83	43	Polygalacturonase
GYMNOSPERMS (CONIFERS)			
Cupressaceae Japanese cedar (*Cryptomeria japonica*)			
Cry j 1	>85	41–45	Pectate lyase, shows homology with bacterial pectate lyase and Amb a 1 and 2
Cry j 2	76	45	Polymethylgalacturonase
Cry j 3	27	27	Shows homology with thaumatin, osmotin and amylase/trypsin inhibitor, PR-5 related
CPA63	58	52	Aspartate protease
CJP	76	34	Isoflavone reductase, shows homology with Bet v 5 and Pyr c 5
Juniper species (e.g. *Juniperus ashei*, *J. rigida*, *J. virginiana*, *J. oxycedrus*)			
Group 1 (e.g. Jun a 1)	71	43	Pectate lyase
Group 2 (e.g. Jun a 2)	100	43	Polymethylgalacturonase
Group 3 (e.g. Jun a 3)	33	30	Shows homology with thaumatin, osmotin and amylase/trypsin inhibitor, PR-5 related
Group 4 (e.g. Jun v 4)	?	29	Calmodulin
70 kDa allergen	100	70	Function unknown
Cypress (*Cupressus sempervirens*, *C. arizonica*, *Chamaecyparis obtusa*)			
Group 1 (e.g. Cup s 1)	50–81	38–42	Pectate lyase
Group 2 (e.g. Cha o 2)	83	45	Polymethylgalacturonase
Group 3 (e.g. Cup a 3)	?	34	Shows homology with thaumatin, osmotin and amylase/trypsin inhibitor, PR-5 related

Appendix 5.4 Physicochemical and biochemical characteristics of latex aeroallergens

Allergen	Frequency of reactivity (%)	Mol. weight (K)	Function
EUPHORBIACEAE			
Rubber tree (latex; *Hevea brasiliensis*)			
Hev b 1	50–82	14	Rubber elongation factor, exists as homotetramer with mol wt of 58K and pI of 8.5
Hev b 2	20–61	34	Endo-1,3-β-glucosidase
Hev b 3	79	24	Shows some homology with rubber elongation factor, Hev b 1
Hev b 4	65–77	53–55	Microhelix component
Hev b 5	56–92	*16	Shows homology with an acidic protein from kiwifruit and potato
Hev b 6	83	20	Prohevein; chitin-binding lectin, causes latex agglutination; native hevein exists as 5 kDa protein
Hev b 7	8–49	42	A patatin-like protein with lipid acyl-hydrolase and PLA$_2$ activity; shows cross-reactivity with Sol t 1
Hev b 8	24	15	Profilin
Hev b 9	15	51	Enolase
Hev b 10	4	26	Manganese superoxide dismutase, shows homology with Asp f 6
Hev b 11	3	30	Class I chitinase
Hev b 12	24	9	Lipid transfer protein
Hev b 13	78	42–46	Esterase, shows homology with early nodule-specific protein from legumes

*Hevein is a 4.7 K chitin-binding domain from this precursor.

Appendix 5.5 Physicochemical and biochemical characteristics of domestic fungal aeroallergens

Allergen	Frequency of reactivity (%)	Mol. weight (K)	Function
ASCOMYCOTA			
Alternaria alternata			
Alt a 1	>80	14	Function unknown
Alt a 2	61	20	EIF-2 α-kinase
Alt a 3	?	70	Heat-shock protein 70
Alt a 4	?	57	Protein disulphide isomerase
Alt a 5	8	11	Ribosomal P2 protein, shows homology with Cla h 4
Alt a 6	50	45	Enolase
Alt a 7	7	22	1,4-benzoquinone reductase, shows homology with Cla h 5
Alt a 8	?	29	Mannitol dehydrogenase
Alt a 10	2	54	Aldehyde dehydrogenase, shows homology with Cla h 3
Alt a 12	?	11	Ribosomal P1 protein
Alt a 13	?	26	Glutathione S-transferase

Appendix 5.5 Continued

Allergen	Frequency of reactivity (%)	Mol. weight (K)	Function
Aspergillus fumigatus			
Asp f 1	85	17	Ribonuclease; ribotoxin shows homology with mitogillin
Asp f 2	96	37	Shows homology with *Candida albicans* fibrinogen-binding protein
Asp f 3	84	19	Peroxisomal membrane protein; belongs to the peroxiredoxin family, thiol-dependent peroxidase
Asp f 4	*78–83	30	Shows homology with bacterial ABC transporter binding protein, associated with peroxisome
Asp f 5	74	40	Metalloprotease
Asp f 6	*42–56	27	Manganese superoxide dismutase, shows homology with Mal s 11 and Hev b 10
Asp f 7	29	12	Shows homology with fungal riboflavin, aldehyde-forming enzyme
Asp f 8	8–15	11	Ribosomal P2 protein
Asp f 9	31	34	Shows homology with plant and bacterial endo-β-1,3(4) glucanases
Asp f 10	3	34	Aspartic protease
Asp f 11	?	24	Peptidyl-prolyl isomerase (cyclophilin)
Asp f 12	?	90	Heat-shock protein 90
Asp f 13	79	34	Alkaline serine protease
Asp f 15	?	16	Shows homology with a serine protease antigen from *Coccidioides immitis*, also designated Asp f 13
Asp f 16	70	43	Shows homology with Asp f 9
Asp f 18	79	34	Vacuolar serine protease
Asp f 22	30	46	Enolase, shows homology with Pen c 22
Asp f 23	?	44	L3 ribosomal protein
Asp f 27	?	18	Cyclophilin
Asp f 28	?	13	Thioredoxin
Asp f 29	?	13	Thioredoxin
Asp f 34	?	20	Phi A cell wall protein
Cladosporium herbarum			
Cla h 2	43	45	Function unknown
Cla h 5	22	11	Ribosomal P2 protein
Cla h 6	20	46	Enolase
Cla h 7	22	22	Function unknown
Cla h 8	57	28	NADP-dependent mannitol dehydrogenase
Cla h 9	16	38	Vacuolar serine protease, shows homology with Pen ch 18 and Asp f 18

Appendix 5.5 Continued

Allergen	Frequency of reactivity (%)	Mol. weight (K)	Function
Cla h 10	36	53	Aldehyde dehydrogenase
Cla h 12	?	11	Ribosomal P1 protein
HSP 70	?	70	Heat-shock protein, also denominated Cla h 4
TCTP 50	50	19	Shows homology to human transitionally controlled tumor protein (TCTP)
Penicillium chrysogenum/notatum			
Pen ch 13	>80	34	Alkaline serine protease
Pen ch 18	77	32	Vacuolar serine protease
Pen ch 20	56	68	β-N-acetylglucosaminidase from *Candida albicans*
Penicillium citrinum			
Pen c 3	46	18	Peroxisomal membrane protein, belongs to the peroxiredoxin family, thiol-dependent peroxidase
Pen c 13	100	33	Alkaline serine protease
Pen c 19	41	70	Show homology with hsp 70 heat-shock protein
Pen c 22	?	46	Enolase
Pen c 30	?	97	Catalase
Pen c 32	?	40	Pectate lyase
Penicillium oxalicum			
Pen a 18	89	34	Vacuolar serine protease
Candida albicans			
Cand a 1	?	40	Alcohol dehydrogenase
Cand a 3	?	20	Peroxisomal protein
37 kDa allergen	?	37	Aldolase
43 kDa allergen	?	43	Phosphoglycerate kinase
48 kDa allergen	50	46	Enolase
Acid protease	75	35	Aspartate protease
Trichophyton tonsurans			
Tri t 1	54	30	Function unknown
Tri t 2	42	30	Subtilisin-like protease, shows homology with Pen ch 13, Pen c 13
Tri t 4	61	83	Dipeptidyl peptidase
Trichophyton rubrum			
Tri r 1/2	?	30	Subtilisin-like protease, shows homology with Pen ch 13, Pen c 13
Tri r 4	?	83	Dipeptidyl peptidase

Appendix 5.5 Continued

Allergen	Frequency of reactivity (%)	Mol. weight (K)	Function
BASIDIOMYCOTA			
Malassezia furfur			
Mala f 1	61	35	Function unknown, cell wall protein
Mala f 2	72	21	Peroxisomal membrane protein, belongs to the peroxiredoxin family, thiol-dependent peroxidase, shows homology with Asp f 3
Mala f 3	70	20	Peroxisomal membrane protein, belongs to the peroxiredoxin family, thiol-dependent peroxidase, shows homology with Asp f 3 and Mala f 2
Mala f 4	?	35	Mitochondrial malate dehydrogenase
Mala f 5	?	18	Peroxisomal membrane protein, belongs to the peroxiredoxin family, thiol-dependent peroxidase, shows homology with Mala f 2/3 and Asp f 3
Mala f 6	?	17	Peptidyl-prolyl isomerase (cyclophilin)
Mala f 7	89	16	Function unknown
Mala f 8	?	19	Shows homology with immunoreactive mannoprotein from *Cryptococcus neoformans*
Mala f 9	44	14	Function unknown
Malassezia sympodialis			
Mala s 10	?	86	Heat-shock protein 70
Mala s 11	?	23	Manganese superoxide dismutase, homology with Asp f 6
Mala s 12	?	67	Glucose-methanol-choline (GMC) oxidoreductase
Mala s 13	?	13	Thioredoxin
Coprinus comatus			
Cop c 1	25	9	Leucine zipper protein
Cop c 2	19	12	Thioredoxin
Cop c 3	?	37	Function unknown
Cop c 5	?	16	Function unknown
Cop c 7	?	16	Function unknown
Psilocybe cubensis			
Psi c 1	>50	46	Function unknown
Psi c 2	>50	16	Peptidyl-prolyl isomerase (cyclophilin)
Rhodotorula mucilaginosa			
Rho m 1	21	47	Enolase
Rho m 2	?	31	Vacuolar serine protease

*Frequency determined in allergic bronchopulmonary aspergillosis.

Appendix 5.6 Physicochemical and biochemical characteristics of occupational aeroallergens

Allergen	Frequency of reactivity (%)	Mol. weight (K)	Function
FUNGAL SOURCES			
Aspergillus niger			
Asp n 14	14	105	β-Xylosidase
Asp n 18	?	34	Vacuolar serine protease
Asp n 25	>50	66–100	Histidine acid phosphatase (phytase)
Pectinase	?	35	Poly(1,4)-α-D-galacturonidase
Cellulase	8	26	1,4-β-D-Glucan 4-glucanohydrolase
Glucoamylase	5	66	Glucan 1,4-α-glucosidase
Aspergillus oryzae			
Asp o 13	?	34	Alkaline serine protease, belongs to subtilase family
Asp o 21	56	53	α-Amylase
Lactase	?	?	1,4-β-D-Galactoside galactohydrolase
Cryphonectira parasitica			
Renin	?	34	Aspartate protease, shows homology with mammalian and cockroach pepsins
BACTERIAL SOURCES			
Bacillus subtilis			
Alcalase	>50	28	Subtilisin serine protease
Bacillus licheniformis			
Esperase	>50	28	Subtilisin serine protease
Clostridium histolyticum			
Collagenase*	>50	68–125	Metalloprotease
Streptomyces griseus			
Empynase	19–32	20–60	Pronase B, a mixture of proteases
MAMMALIAN SOURCES			
Trypsin (porcine)	?	24	Serine protease, shows homology with mite Groups 3, 6 and 9 allergens
Chymotrypsin (bovine)	?	25	Serine protease, shows homology with mite Groups 3, 6 and 9 allergens
Pepsin (porcine)	?	35	Aspartate protease, shows homology with Bla g 2 and renin
CHICKEN (*Gallus domesticus*)			
Egg white			
Gal d 1	34–38	20	Ovomucoid, protease inhibitor
Gal d 2	32	43	Ovalbumin, function unknown but protein shows homology with serine protease inhibitors
Gal d 3	47–53	76	Conalbumin (ovotransferrin), iron transport protein
Gal d 4	15	14	1, 4-β-N-acetylmuramidase (lysozyme)
Egg yolk			
Gal d 5	>50	65–70	Serum albumin (α-livetin)

Appendix 5.6 Continued

Allergen	Frequency of reactivity (%)	Mol. weight (K)	Function
PLANT SOURCES			
Pawpaw (*Carica papaya*)			
Car p 1	?	23	Papain, cysteine protease
Kiwifruit (*Actinidia chinensis/deliciosa*)			
Act c 1	100	30	Actinidin, cysteine protease
Act c 2	100	24	Thaumatin-like protein, possesses antifungal activity
Pineapple (*Ananas comosus*)			
Ana c 1	?	23	Bromelain, cysteine protease
Mustard seed (*Sinapis alba* L., *Brassica junceae*, *Brassica napus*)			
Group 1 (e.g. Sin a 1)	?	14	Mustard seed (*Sinapis alba* L., *Brassica junceae*, *B. napus*)
Group 2 (e.g. Sin a 2)	?	51	11S globulin
Group 3 (e.g. Sin a 3)	?	12	Non-specific lipid transfer protein
Group 4 (e.g. Sin a 4)	?	13	Profilin
Castorbean (*Ricinus communis*)			
Ric c 1	96	14	2S albumin
Ric c 2	?	47	11S crystalloid protein
Ric c 3	?	47–51	Function unknown
Soybean (*Glycine max*) seed allergens			
Gly m 1[+]	95	7	Cysteine-rich, hydrophobic seed protein, member of lipid transfer protein family
Gly m 2	95	8	Defensin
Soybean flour allergens*			
Trypsin-inhibitor (B)	86	20	Kunitz protease inhibitor
Lipoxygenase	?	94	Lipoxygenase
Barley (*Hordeum vulgare*)			
Hor v 15	?	14	α-Amylase/trypsin inhibitor, shows homology with wheat allergens and 2S albumin allergens (BMAI-1)
Hor v 16	>96	64	α-Amylase (1,4,-α-D-glucan glucanohydrolase)
Hor v 17	>96	60	β-Amylase (1,4-α-D-glucan maltohydrolase)
Hor v 21	[a]91	34	Hordein, shows homology with rye secalins and wheat gliadins
Rice (*Oryza sativa*)			
Ory s 1	>90	15	α-Amylase inhibitor, shows homology with wheat and barley α-amylase/trypsin inhibitor allergens
Ory s 12	?	14	Profilin
33 kDa protein	?	33	Glyoxalase I
Amylase inhibitor	>90	15	α-Amylase inhibitor, shows homology with wheat and barley α-amylase/trypsin inhibitor allergens

Appendix 5.6 Continued

Allergen	Frequency of reactivity (%)	Mol. weight (K)	Function
Wheat (*Triticum* species)			
Tri a 3	?	?	Function unknown, found in wheat ovaries, shows homology with pollen allergens
Tri a 18	?	17	Lectin
Tri a 19	100	65	ω-Gliadin, shows homology with rye secalins and barley hordein
Tri a Bd 17K	>50	13	Wheat α-amylase/trypsin inhibitor, shows homology with barley allergens and 2S albumin allergens
Tri a 27	?	27	γ-Interferon inducible thiol reductase
CM16	>50	13	
WMAI-1	?	13	Wheat α-amylase/trypsin inhibitor, shows homology with barley allergens and 2S albumin allergens
27 kDa allergen	?	27	Shows homology with acyl-CoA oxidase from barley and rice
Tri a Bd 36K	60	36	Peroxidase
Gliadin	72	40	α-Gliadin
37 kDa allergen	?	37	Fructose bisphosphate-aldolase
Rye (*Secale cereale*)			
Sec c 1	>50	14	α-Amylase/trypsin inhibitor, shows homology with wheat allergens and 2S albumin allergens
Sec c 20	91	20	Secalin
34 kDa protein	83[a]	34	Rye γ-35 secalin, shows homology with wheat gliadins and barley hordeins
70 kDa protein	91[a]	70	Rye γ-70 secalin, shows homology with wheat gliadins and barley hordeins

*Represents a mixture of proteases.
[a]Frequency based on patients with wheat-dependent, exercise-induced anaphylaxis. Note that the rye and wheat proteins may also be food allergens (see Appendix 5.10).

Appendix 5.7 Physicochemical and biochemical characteristics of vertebrate aeroallergens

Allergen	Frequency of reactivity (%)	Mol. weight (K)	Function
Cat (*Felis domesticus*)			
Fel d 1	95	33–39*	Tetramer of two heterodimers (α and β chains), a possible ligand-binding molecule; α chain shows homology with 10 kDa secretory protein from human Clara cells, mouse salivary androgen-binding protein subunit, rabbit uteroglobin and a Syrian hamster protein
Fel d 2	20–35	69	Serum albumin
Fel d 3	10	11	Cystatin
Fel d 4	60	20	Lipocalin
Fel d 5	38	400	Immunoglobulin A, IgE is directed against the galactose-α-1,3-galactose moiety which is also found on the heavy chain of IgM

Appendix 5.7 Continued

Allergen	Frequency of reactivity (%)	Mol. weight (K)	Function
Fel d 6	?	900	IgM
Fel d 7	?	18	von Ebner's gland protein
Dog (*Canis familiaris*)			
Can f 1	50	19–25	Lipocalin, shows homology with Von Ebner's gland protein which has cysteine protease inhibitory activity
Can f 2	20–22	27	Lipocalin, shows homology with Can f 1 and Fel d 4 and with other lipocalin allergens
Can f 3	16–40	69	Serum albumin
Can f 4	35	23	Shows homology with bovine odorant binding protein
Can f 5	70	28	Prostatic kallikrein, shows homology with human prostate specific antigen PSA, which is allergenic
IgG	88	150	Immunoglobulin G
Horse (*Equus caballus*)			
Equ c 1	100	25	Lipocalin, shows homology with rodent urinary proteins
Equ c 2	100	17	Lipocalin, shows homology with rodent urinary proteins
Equ c 3	?	67	Serum albumin
Equ c 4	?	17	Shows homology with rat mandibular gland protein A
Equ c 5	?	21	Function unknown
Cow (*Bos taurus*)			
Bos d 2	97	20	Lipocalin
Bos d 3	?	11	S100 calcium-binding protein
AS1	31	21	Oligomycin sensitivity-conferring protein of the mitochondrial adenosine triphosphate synthase complex
BDA 11	?	12	Shows homology with human calcium-binding psoriasin protein
Guinea pig (*Cavia porcellus*)			
Cav p 1	70	20	Lipocalin, shows homology with Cav p 2
Cav p 2	55	17	Lipocalin, shows homology with Bos d 2
Mouse (*Mus musculus*)			
Mus m 1	>80	17	Major urinary protein, shows homology with lipocalins such as β-lactoglobulin, odorant-binding proteins, Rat n 2
Rat (*Rattus novegicus*)			
Rat n 1	>80	17	Lipocalin, shows homology with lipocalins such as β-lactoglobulin Bos d 5, odorant-binding proteins, Mus m 1
Albumin	24	69	Serum albumin
Rabbit (*Oryctolagus cuniculus*)			
Ory c 1	?	18	Odorant-binding protein, lipocalin, shows homology with Ory c 2
Ory c 2	?	21	Odorant-binding protein
8kDa allergen	?	8	Shows homology with rabbit uteroglobin
Albumin	<50	69	Serum albumin

*Mol wt given represents dimer; each chain approx 18 K.

Appendix 5.8 Physicochemical and biochemical characteristics of invertebrate aeroallergens

Allergen	Frequency of reactivity (%)	Mol. weight (K)	Function
CHIRONOMIDAE (MIDGES)			
Chironomus thummi thummi			
Chi t 1 to Chi t 9	>50	15	Haemoglobin
Cladotanytarsus lewisi			
Cla l 1	>50	17	Haemoglobin
Polypedilum nubifer			
Pol n 1	>50	17	Haemoglobin
Chironomus kiiensis			
Chi k 10	81	31	Tropomyosin
BLATTIDAE AND BLATTELLIDAE			
German cockroach (*Blattella germanica*), American cockroach (*Periplaneta americana*)			
Group 1 (e.g. Bla g 1)	50	46	Shows homology with ANG12 secretory mosquito protein
Group 2 (e.g. Bla g 2)	58	36	Aspartate protease (inactive), shows homology with pepsin
Group 3 (e.g. Per a 3)	83	78	Hexamerin, subunit showing homology with larval insect storage proteins
Group 4 (e.g. Bla g 4)	40–60	21	Calycin
Group 5 (e.g. Bla g 5)	70	23	Glutathione S-transferase
Group 6 (e.g. Bla g 6)	50	21	Troponin C
Group 7 (e.g. Per a 7)	57	31	Tropomyosin
Group 8 (e.g. Bla g 8)	?	20	Myosin
Group 9 (e.g. Per a 9)	100	45	Arginine kinase
Group 10 (e.g. Per a 10)	28	80	Trypsin
PYRALIDAE			
Indianmeal moth (*Plodia interpunctella*)			
Plo i 1	25	40	Arginine kinase
BOMBYCIDAE			
Silkworm larvae (*Bombyx mori*)			
Bom m 1	>90	42	Arginine kinase, shows homology with cockroach enzyme, Per a 9
Pyroglyphidae/glycyphagidae/acaridae/echimyopodidae			
Group 1 (e.g. Der p 1)	>90	25	Cysteine protease

Appendix 5.8 Continued

Allergen	Frequency of reactivity (%)	Mol. weight (K)	Function
Group 2 (e.g. Der p 2)	>90	14	Shows homology with putative human epididymal protein, possible cholesterol binding protein, belongs to NPC2 family
Group 3 (e.g. Der p 3)	90	25	Trypsin
Group 4 (e.g. Der p 4)	25–46	60	Amylase
Group 5 (e.g. Der p 5)	9-70	14	Function unknown, possible ligand-binding protein
Group 6 (e.g. Der p 6)	39	25	Chymotrypsin
Group 7 (e.g. Der p 7)	53–62	26–31	Function unknown, possible pathogen-associated molecular pattern-binding protein
Group 8 (e.g. Der p 8)	40	27	Glutathione S-transferase
Group 9 (e.g. Der p 9)	>90	29	Collagenase-like serine protease
Group 10 (e.g. Der p 10)	81	36	Tropomyosin
Group 11 (e.g. Der f 11)	82	103	Paramyosin
Group 12 (e.g. Blo t 12)	50	16	May be a chitinase, shows homology with Der f 15
Group 13 (e.g. Lep d 13)	11–23	15	Fatty-acid-binding protein
Group 14 (e.g. Der f 14)	84	177	Vitellogenin or lipophorin
Group 15 (e.g. Der f 15)	95	63/98*	Chitinase, shows homology with Blo t 12 allergen
Group 16 (e.g. Der f 16)	50–62	53	Gelsolin
Group 17 (e.g. Der f 17)	35	30	Calcium-binding protein
Group 18 (e.g. Der f 18)	63	60	Chitinase
Group 19 (e.g. Blo t 19)	10	7	Antimicrobial peptide homology
Group 20 (e.g. Der p 20)	?	?	Arginine kinase
Group 21 (e.g. Der p 21)	26	15	Function unknown, shows homology with Group 5 allergens
Group 22 (e.g. Der p 22)	?	?	Shows homology with Group 2 mite allergen, belongs to ML domain family, implicated in lipid binding
Group 23 (e.g. Der p 23)	?	14	Unknown function, shows homology with peritrophin-A domain
Group 24 (e.g. Tyr p 24)	11	18	Troponin C, shows homology with Bla g 6
Mag29	?	67	Heat-shock protein, found in *D. farinae*
α-Tubulin	29	56	Found in *T. putrescentiae*

*Non-glycosylated and glycosylated forms. Frequency determined in dogs with atopic dermatitis.

Appendix 5.9 Physicochemical and biochemical characteristics of ingested, vertebrate-derived food allergens

Allergen	Frequency of reactivity (%)	Mol. weight (K)	Function
MAMMALIAN DERIVED			
Cow (*Bos taurus*)			
Bos d 4	6	14	α-Lactalbumin, lactose synthase
Bos d 5	13	18	β-Lactoglobulin, lipocalin
Bos d 6	29	67	Serum albumin
Bos d 7	83	160	Immunoglobulin
Bos d 8	>90	20–30	Caseins
75 kDa allergen	16	75	Transferrin
Chicken (*Gallus domesticus*)			
Egg white			
Gal d 1	34-38	28	Ovomucoid, a Kazal-type serine protease inhibitor
Gal d 2	32	43	Ovalbumin, serine protease inhibitor
Gal d 3	47–53	78	Ovotransferrin
Gal d 4	15	14	Lysozyme
Egg yolk			
Gal d 5	>50	64–70	α-Livetin, a serum albumin
Gal d 6	18	35	YGP42, fragment of vitellogenin-1 precursor
FISH/SHELLFISH/AMPHIBIAN DERIVED			
Bony fish, e.g. Atlantic salmon (*Salmo salar*), Cod (*Gadus callarias*), Tuna (*Thunnus albacares*)			
Group 1 (e.g. Gad c 1)	100	12	Parvalbumin, calcium-binding protein
Shrimp/prawn (*Metapenaeus* spp., *Penaeus* spp., *Litopenaeus* spp.)			
Group 1 (e.g. Met p 1)	>50	34–36	Tropomyosin
Group 2 (e.g. Pen m 2)	70	39	Arginine kinase
Group 3 (e.g. Lit v 3)	55	20	Myosin light chain
Group 4 (e.g. Lit v 4)	38	22	Sarcoplasmic E F-hand calcium-binding protein
Crab (*Charybdis feriatus*)			
Group 1 (e.g. Cha f 1)	>50	34	Tropomyosin
Squid (*Todarodes pacificus*)			
Group 1 (e.g. Tod p 1)	>50	38	Tropomyosin
Edible frog (*Rana esculenta*)			
Rana e 1	?	12	α-Parvalbumin
Rana e 2	?	12	β-Parvalbumin

Appendix 5.10 Physicochemical and biochemical characteristics of ingested seed and fruit allergens

Allergen	Frequency of reactivity (%)	Mol. weight (K)	Function
FABACEAE			
Peanut (*Arachis hypogaea*)			
Ara h 1	>90	64	Cupin (Vicilin type), 7S seed storage protein
Ara h 2	>90	17	Conglutin, 2S albumin seed storage protein
Ara h 3	35–53	14–60	Glycinin, 11S seed storage protein
Ara h 4	43	37	Cupin, seed storage protein
Ara h 5	16	14	Profilin
Ara h 6	38	15	Conglutin (2S albumin)
Ara h 7	43	15	Conglutin (2S albumin)
Ara h 8	85	17	Pathogenesis-related protein, PR-10 shows homology with Bet v 1
Ara h 9	91	10	Non-specific lipid transfer protein
Ara h 10	?	16	Oleosin
Ara h 11	?	14	Oleosin
Peanut agglutinin	50	27	Lectin
Soybean (*Glycine max*)			
Gly m 3	69	14	Profilin
Gly m 4	?	17	Pathogenesis-related protein PR-10
Gly m 25	?	?	Albumin
Gly m Bd 30K/P34	90	34	Syringolide receptor, seed vacuolar protein, shows homology with mite Group 1 allergen, papain and bromelain but not active
Gly m Bd 28K	>50	22	Vicilin-like glycoprotein, shows homology with Ara h 1
21 kDa allergen	?	22	A member of the G2 glycinin family
G1 glycinin	?	40	A member of the G1 glycinin family, shows homology with Ara h 3
Gly m Bd 60K	25	60	β-Gonglycinin
LECYTHIDACEAE			
Brazil nut (*Bertholletia excelsa*)			
Ber e 1	100	9	2S Albumin
Ber e 2	?	29	11S Globulin
JUGLANDACEAE			
English walnut (*Juglans regia, J. nigra*)			
Jug r 1	?	15–16	2S Albumin
Jug r 2	60	44	Vicilin-like glycoprotein
Jug r 3	80	9	Non-specific lipid transfer protein 1
Jug r 4	57	50–60	11S Globulin seed storage protein

Appendix 5.10 Continued

Allergen	Frequency of reactivity (%)	Mol. weight (K)	Function
POLYGONACEAE			
Buckwheat (*Fagopyrum esculentum Moench*)			
Fag e 1	>50	26	13S Seed storage protein
Fag e 2	78	16	2S Albumin
ASTERACEAE			
Sunflower (*Helianthus annuus*)			
Hel a 3	?	9	Lipid transfer protein
16 kDa allergen	66	16/17	2S Albumin
APIACEAE			
Celery (*Apium graveolens*)			
Api g 1	100	15	Pathogenesis-related protein, PR-10
Api g 2	?	9	Lipid transfer protein
Api g 4	?	14	Profilin
Api g 5	?	58	Flavin adenine dinucleotide-dependent oxidase
ROSACEAE			
Apple, cherry, peach, plum, almond, apricot			
Group 1 (e.g. Pru av 1)	89	9	Pathogenesis related protein; PR-10
Group 2 (e.g. Pru av 2)	100	23–30	Thaumatin-like protein
Group 3 (e.g. Pru av 3)	?	10	Non-specific lipid transfer protein
Group 4 (e.g. Pru av 4)	?	14	Profilin
Group 5 (e.g. Pru av 5)	?	10	60S Acidic ribosomal protein P2
Group 6 (e.g. Pru av 6)	?	360	Amandin, 11S globulin
60 kDa apple allergen	?	60	Phosphoglyceromutase
SOLANACEAE			
Potato (*Solanum tuberosum*)			
Sol t 1	74	43	Patatin, defence-related storage protein, has PLA$_2$ activity
Sol t 2	51	21	Cathepsin D protease inhibitor
Sol t 3	43	21	Cysteine protease inhibitor
Sol t 4	58	16	Aspartate protease inhibitor
CUCURBITACEAE			
Melon (*Cucumis melo*)			
Cuc m 1	100	67	Cucumisin, subtilisin serine protease
Cuc m 2	?	14	Profilin
Cuc m 3	71	16	Pathogenesis-related protein, shows homology with the vespid group 5 allergens

Appendix 5.10 Continued

Allergen	Frequency of reactivity (%)	Mol. weight (K)	Function
ACTINIDIACEAE			
Kiwifruit (*Actinidia chinensis/deliciosa*)			
Group 1 (e.g. Act d 1)	100	27	Cysteine protease, actinidin
Group 2 (e.g. Act d 2)	10	24	Thaumatin-like protein
Group 3 (e.g. Act d 3)	33	42	Unknown function
Group 4 (e.g. Act d 4)	20	11	Phytocystatin
Group 5 (e.g. Act c 5)	?	26	Kiwellin
Group 6 (e.g. Act c 6)	72	18	Pectin methylesterase inhibitor
Group 7 (e.g. Act d 7)	32	50	Pectin methylesterase
Group 8 (e.g. Act c 8)	43	17	Pathogenesis-related protein PR-10
Group 9 (e.g. Act d 9)	20	14	Profilin
Group 10 (e.g. Act c 10)	33	10	Lipid transfer protein
Group 11 (e.g. Act d 11)	22	17	Member of the Major latex/Ripening related subfamily, shows homology with *Act* group 8 allergens and birch Bet v 1
BRASSICACEAE			
Oilseed rape (*Brassica napus*) and turnip (*Brassica rapa*)			
Group 1 (e.g. Bra n 1)	?	10–14	2S Albumin
Group 2 (e.g. Bra r 2)	82	25	Prohevein homologue

See also Appendix 5.6 for ingested wheat and rye allergens.

Appendix 5.11 Physicochemical and biochemical characteristics of envenomated and salivary invertebrate allergens

Allergen	Frequency of reactivity (%)	Mol. weight (K)	Function
VENOM ALLERGENS			
Apidae			
Honey bee (*Apis mellifera*)			
Api m 1	>90	16	Phospholipase A$_2$
Api m 2	95	39	Hyaluronidase
Api m 3	>50	43	Acid phosphatase prostatic
Api m 4	<50	3	Melittin
Api m 5	60	100	Dipeptidyl peptidase IV
Api m 6	>42	8	Function unknown
Api m 7	?	39	CUB serine protease
Api m 8	?	70	Carboxylesterase

Appendix 5.11 Continued

Allergen	Frequency of reactivity (%)	Mol. weight (K)	Function
Api m 9	?	60	Serine carboxypeptidase
Api m 10	?	50–55	Icarapin variant 2
Bumble bee (*Bombus pennsylvanicus/terrestris*)			
Bom p 1	?	16	Phospholipase A$_2$
Bom p 4	?	27	Protease
Bom t 1	?	49	Acid phosphatase
Vespidae			
White-faced and yellow hornets (*Dolichovespula* spp.), paper wasps (*Polistes* spp.) and yellow jackets (*Vespula* spp.)			
Group 1 (e.g. Pol a 1)	46	34	Phospholipase A$_1$
Group 2 (e.g. Pol a 2)	26	39	Hyaluronidase
Group 3 (e.g. Ves v 3)	57	?	Shows homology with Api m 5
Group 4 (e.g. Pol a 4)	?	32–34	Serine protease
Group 5 (e.g. Pol a 5)	8	23	Shows homology with cysteine rich secretory protein found in epididymis, testis and salivary gland, and pathogenesis-related proteins, also known as antigen 5
Formicidae			
Fire ant (*Solenopsis invicta*)			
Sol i 1	26	18	Phospholipase A$_1$
Sol i 2	87	14	Function unknown
Sol i 3	17	26	Shows homology with the vespid group 5 allergens
Sol i 4	26	12	Shows homology with Sol i 2
Australian jumper ant (*Myrmecia pilosula*)			
Myr p 1	>50	9	Pilosulin 1, function unknown
Myr p 2	35	5	Function unknown
SALIVARY ALLERGENS			
Culicidae			
Mosquito (*Aedes aegypti*, *A. vexans, A. albopictus*)			
Group 1 (e.g. Aed a 1)	29–65	68	Apyrase
Group 2 (e.g. Aed a 2)	11–32	37	Female-specific protein D7
Group 3 (e.g. Aed a 3)	32	30	Function unknown
Group 4 (e.g. Aed a 4)	47	67	α-Glucosidase

Appendix 5.11 Continued

Allergen	Frequency of reactivity (%)	Mol. weight (K)	Function
Pulicidae			
Flea (*Ctenocephalides felis*)			
Cte f 1	80	18	Function unknown
Cte f 2	?	27	Salivary protein, shows homology with ant Sol i 3 allergen, and vespid group 5 allergens
Cte f 3	?	25	Function unknown
Reduviidae			
Kissing bug (*Triatoma protracta*)			
Tria p 1	89	19	Procalin, a member of the lipocalin family, shows homology with triabin, a thrombin inhibitor
Tabanidae			
Horse fly (*Tabanidae yao*)			
Tab a 1	87	26	Shows homology with the vespid group 5 allergens
Tab a 2	92	35	Hyaluronidase
Argasidae			
Pigeon tick (*Argas reflexus*)			
Arg r 1	100	17	Calycin

Appendix 5.12 Physicochemical and biochemical characteristics of human autoallergens

Allergen	Frequency of reactivity (%)	Mol. weight (K)	Function
Humans (*Homo sapiens*)			
Hom s 1	?	55–60	Squamous cell carcinoma antigen SART-1
Hom s 2	?	10	Nascent polypeptide-associated complex alpha subunit (NAC)
Hom s 3	?	22–23	BCL7B protein
Hom s 4	10	36	Atopy related autoantigen, a calcium-binding protein cross-reacting with Phl p 7 and Cyp c 1 (Carp parvalbumin)
Hom s 5	?	43	Cytokeratin, type II cytoskeletal 6A
MnSOD	?	27	Manganese superoxide dismutase, shows homology with Asp f 6, Hev b 10 and Mala s 11
Profilin	?	14	Shows homology with Bet v 2
P2 protein	?	11	Ribosomal P2 protein, shows homology with Asp f 8

Autoallergens Hom s 1 to 5 associated with atopic dermatitis patients.

Appendix 5.13 Physicochemical and biochemical characteristics of parasite allergens

Allergen	Frequency of reactivity (%)	Mol. weight (K)	Function
ASCARIDIDA			
Anisakis simplex			
Ani s 1	14–86	24	Shows homology with Kunitz-type serine protease inhibitors
Ani s 2	88	97	Paramyosin
Ani s 3	13	41	Tropomyosin
Ani s 4	30–75	9	Cysteine protease inhibitor
Ani s 5	25–49	15	Member of the SXP/RAL family
Ani s 6	18	7	Serine protease inhibitor
Ani s 7	100	139	Function unknown
Ani s 8	25	15	SXP/RAL family
Ani s 9	14	14	SXP/RAL family
Ani s 10	?	21	Function unknown
Ascaris suum/lumbricoides			
Asc l 3	42–78	40	Tropomyosin
ABA-1	>80	14	Polyprotein, lipid-binding protein
AS 14	?	?	Shows homology with Ani s 5, 8, 9
CYCLOPHYLLIDAE			
Echinococcus granulosus			
EA21	80	17	Peptidyl-prolyl isomerase, cyclophilin, shows homology with Mal f 6 and Asp f 11
EgEF-1 beta/delta	56–90	14	Elongation factor
EgHSP70	57	70	Heat-shock protein
AgB	?	12	Protease inhibitor
Antigen 5	?	67	Dimer, 22 kDa chain and 38 kDa chain with tryspin-like similarity although not active
SPIRURIDA			
Brugia malayi			
58 kDa allergen	100	58	γ-Glutamyl transpeptidase
Bm 23-25	?	23–25	Function unknown
Dirofilaria immitis			
DiAg	?	15	Polyprotein, function unknown
TRICHURIDA			
Trichinella spiralis			
Serine proteases	?	18, 40, 50	Serine proteases
STRONGYLIDA			
Trichostrongylus coubriformis (Sheep parasite)			
31 kDa allergen	?	31	Aspartyl protease inhibitor homologue (Aspin)

Appendix 5.13 Continued

Allergen	Frequency of reactivity (%)	Mol. weight (K)	Function
Necator americanus			
60 kDa protein	?	60	Calreticulin
STRIGEATIDA			
Schistosoma mansoni, S. japonicum, S. haematobium			
Group 1	>50	23	Calmodulin-like, shows homology with the Gad c 1 parvalbumin fish allergen and to Bra n 1
Schistosoma haematobium			
Serpin	>90	54	Serine protease inhibitor

6

Principles of allergy diagnosis

R Stokes Peebles, Martin K Church and
Stephen R Durham

DEFINITION

Successful management of allergic disease is dependent on the accurate diagnosis of the problem and its likely causes. This chapter describes allergy diagnosis from taking a history to specific allergy tests.

Introduction

Allergy is a disease of our modern civilized society. One hundred and fifty years ago asthma was considered rare and allergic rhinitis was almost unheard of. Today in Europe, it is estimated that over 80 million persons have some manifestation of allergic disease. In the United States some 50 million persons, approximately 20% of the population, suffer from at least one form of allergy; it is the fifth leading chronic disease for all ages, and the third most common chronic disorder for children under 18 years of age. Allergic disease can take many different forms (Box 6.1), but three of the most common manifestations of allergy include atopic dermatitis or eczema, allergic rhino-conjunctivitis or hay fever, and allergic asthma. In Europe, approximately 10% of infants suffer from eczema, while amongst teenagers one in four experience allergic rhinoconjunctivitis symptoms and 20% will develop asthma. In population studies, allergic diseases peak at different ages – food allergy and atopic dermatitis predominate in early childhood, whereas allergic rhinitis peaks in the second or third decade, and asthma shows a biphasic peak (Fig. 6.1).

Although the main consequence of allergic diseases is the suffering they cause the patients who have these conditions, there are also substantial monetary costs. In Europe, direct medical costs for asthma are estimated to be €17.7 billion per year, while the loss in productivity because of poor asthma control is approximately €9.8 billion annually. In the USA, the annual total cost associated with rhinitis alone is approximately $11.5 billion – that is, $7.3 billion in direct costs including medication and doctor office visits and $4.28 billion for lost productivity. It is estimated that allergic rhinitis accounts for nearly 4 million missed or lost workdays each year in the USA. Some diseases, such as cancer and heart disease, have higher annual health utilization costs while affecting persons near the end of life; allergic disease, however, often start early in life and continue throughout it, resulting in a greater cumulative health cost that is not apparent when viewing annual healthcare expenditures.

Much of this suffering and many of these costs could be greatly reduced, as effective treatments exist for the majority of allergic conditions. However, allergy often remains undiagnosed and inadequately treated, despite clear diagnostic and therapeutic guidelines. Patients often wait too long to seek medical evaluation and instead take inappropriate over-the-counter remedies.

© 2012 Elsevier Ltd
DOI: 10.1016/B978-0-7234-3658-4.00005-6

Box 6.1 Spectrum of allergic diseases

- Anaphylaxis
- Asthma
- Atopic dermatitis
- Drug allergy
- Food allergy
- Insect venom allergy
- Rhinoconjunctivitis
- Urticaria

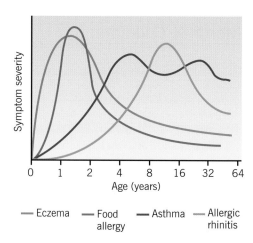

Fig. 6.1 Manifestations of allergy differ with age.

Also, many clinicians treat allergies as trivial and do not explore properly the medical basis of the disease and its effect on the quality of life of individuals. Because of this, appropriate management and therapy are often not put in place.

Definitions and basic pathophysiology

Allergies are a family of diseases with complex and differing genetic underlying components that predispose allergy-prone individuals to mount symptoms in response to specific environmental stimuli, such as high house dust mite and pollen loads and pollution. Although the genetic basis, development, and epidemiology of allergy are reviewed in depth in Chapters 2, 3, and 4 respectively, it is necessary to mention some aspects of these within the following definitions so that the reader can understand the concepts of allergy diagnosis. In simple terms, an allergic individual must have 'allergy genes' and 'allergy facilitatory genes'. 'Allergy genes' predispose individuals to produce IgE in response to exposure to allergens. This does not mean that they will express clinically demonstrable allergies. Approximately 40% of the population has raised IgE levels, while in only 20% are there symptoms of allergy. To express disease, individuals must also

have 'allergy facilitatory genes'. For example, in atopic dermatitis the primary defect is poor epidermal integrity, which allows penetration of allergens through the skin and the subsequent development of allergy. In allergic rhinoconjunctivitis and allergic asthma, poor epithelial defence again allows entry to cause stimulation of IgE synthesis and, on re-exposure, clinical disease. In asthma, both allergic and non-allergic, there are also 'lung genes', which are described elsewhere.

Among healthcare professionals, even in the same country, the vocabulary of allergic diseases can be quite varied. As a result, the World Allergy Organization (WAO) has published a glossary of terminology to help healthcare professionals standardize communication with one another.

- **Atopy** is defined as a personal and/or familial tendency, usually in childhood or adolescence, to become sensitized and produce IgE antibodies in response to ordinary exposure to allergens, usually proteins. Atopy, therefore, is a definition of an IgE antibody high-responder who *may* or *may not* have clinical symptoms. Therefore, in practical terms 'atopy' may be defined as the presence of a positive skin test and/or elevated serum allergen-specific IgE to one or more common inhaled allergens.

- **Allergy** is defined as 'a hypersensitivity reaction initiated by immunologic mechanisms' which can be either antibody or cell mediated. In other words, allergic individuals have symptoms of asthma, rhinoconjunctivitis, or eczema. The antibody isotype most commonly responsible for allergic reactions is IgE. However, it is important to recognize that not all hypersensitivity reactions that appear to be allergic in nature are necessarily caused by IgE. For example, systemic reactions to dextran, although they mimic anaphylaxis, result from IgG immune complexes. Other allergic reactions seem not to be mediated by antibodies at all. For instance, the pathogenesis of allergic contact dermatitis is attributed to activated antigen-specific lymphocytes.

- **Allergens** are antigens that lead to one of the allergic phenotypes when a person sensitized to that antigen is subsequently exposed to that antigen. The majority of allergens are protein antigens, sometimes with carbohydrate side chains; however, there are instances in which carbohydrates themselves are likely to be allergens. One example may be delayed anaphylaxis to mammalian meats which appears to be related to IgE binding to the carbohydrate moiety galactose-α-1,3-galactose. Reactivity to this allergen has implications for hypersensitivity to murine monoclonal antibody therapeutics containing this oligosaccharide. Low-molecular-weight chemicals including medications such as penicillin that are not antigenic in isolation can act as haptens and bind to host 'carrier' proteins to become allergenic and stimulate IgE responses. Additionally, other low-molecular-weight chemicals, of which chromium, nickel, and formaldehyde are examples, can induce T-cell-mediated hypersensitivity reactions.

Allergy history

Before taking an allergy history, adopting a professional but friendly manner, the early establishment of eye contact, and the avoidance of extraneous distractions by interviewers should put patients at their ease. The history need not be time consuming, although patients should be allowed to give their own accounts of symptoms followed by structured prompts or questions to cover points listed below. A recent study showed that standardized questions put to the parents of children (aged 1–17 years) by a trained interviewer were highly predictive of answers obtained by an experienced paediatric allergist (Table 6.1).

Table 6.1 Accuracy of standardized questions put to the parents of children (aged 1–17 years) by a trained interviewer, used for predicting answers obtained by an experienced paediatric allergist

Questions	Accuracy (%)*
Months when symptoms are worse	94
Worse in bed at night	95
Worse in morning when awakening	96
Better when outside	95
Better when in dry area of the country	96
Worse when with dogs	97
Worse when with cats	97
Worse when vacuuming or dusting	93
Worse when blankets are shaken	96
Worse when among trees in March and April	85
Worse when in grass	97
Number of patients interviewed: 151	

*Accuracy (%) (true positive + true negative) × 100. (True positive + true negative + false positive + false negative.)
Data modified from Murray AB, Milner RA. The accuracy of features in the clinical history for predicting atopic sensitization to airborne allergens in children. J Allergy Clin Immunol 1995; 96:588–596.

Personal history – the patient's account

Obtaining an accurate patient history is crucial in diagnosing allergic disease. Initially, patients should be allowed to give their own account of symptoms followed by structured prompts or questions to cover the given points.

- Listen to the patient's account of the symptoms. Patients often have their own way of describing symptoms. Some disease-related symptoms are listed in Box 6.2.
- Determine the frequency and/or severity of the symptoms
- Establish whether there **is** a personal or family history of asthma, rhinitis, and eczema. If one parent has allergic disease, then there is an approximate 40% likelihood that each of the offspring will have symptoms of allergy. If both parents have allergic disease, then the likelihood that a child has an allergic condition increases to roughly 80–85%.
- Ask whether the symptoms are seasonal or perennial. Symptoms of aeroallergen-induced rhinitis and asthma may be seasonal if caused by trees, grasses, weeds, or moulds. It is helpful for the evaluating physician to understand the general timing of the pollen seasons in the community in which the patient lives. Figure 6.2 shows examples of the seasonal variations in outdoor allergens in the United Kingdom and USA. Not all allergic manifestations caused by aeroallergens are necessarily seasonal in nature; allergy symptoms may be year round or perennial if they are caused by

Box 6.2 Symptoms of allergic conditions

Allergic rhinitis
- Nasal congestion; rhinorrhoea; sneezing; itching

Asthma
- Wheezing; dyspnoea; chest tightness; cough

Anaphylaxis
- Flushing; urticaria; pruritus of lips, tongue, palms, and soles; gastrointestinal cramping, nausea, vomiting, and diarrhoea; dyspnoea, chest tightness and wheezing; palpitations, tachycardia and chest pain; syncope or near syncope, altered mental status or dizziness; uterine contractions in women

Atopic dermatitis
- Itching; red and patchy rash; fluid filled sores that can ooze or crust over tough, thick skin that results from constant scratching (lichenification)

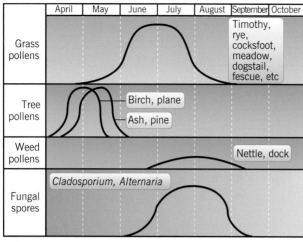

(a)

Seasonal allergens in the mid-Atlantic region of the US

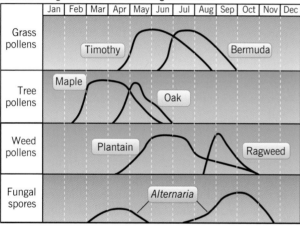

(b)

Fig. 6.2 Seasonal allergens in (a) the UK and (b) the USA. In general, the order of appearance of allergens is tree pollens before grass pollens and then weed pollens and fungal spores. The timing, which is usually evident from the clinical history, will vary according to geographic areas.

dust mites, indoor moulds, cockroaches, or animals that live in the home.

- Ask about possible allergens in the home. Establishing the environmental conditions in the home is often essential in obtaining a correct diagnosis. Some critical factors that may be taken into consideration are listed in Box 6.3.
- Ask about the patient's occupation and hobbies particularly in relation to the presence of possible allergens.
- Ask about food allergies and any adverse reactions to drugs.
- Enquire about possible trigger factors (allergic or non-allergic). It is important to recognize that some patients experience symptoms identical to those caused by allergic mechanisms, but for which testing

Box 6.3 Environmental factors that modulate rhinitis and asthma symptoms

- **High humidity (55–75%):** conducive to dust mite and mould growth
- **Leftover food that is unsealed:** attractive to cockroaches and mice
- **High-density living:** cockroaches
- **Cats and dogs in the home or in the community:** allergens from these animals are detected in the dust of homes with and without pets
- **Woodstoves and fireplaces:** produces particulates and oxidant gases
- **Cigarette smoke:** contributes to exacerbations of asthma and rhinitis, and may advance allergic sensitization
- **Natural gas appliances:** source of nitrogen dioxide, which can increase respiratory symptoms of cough and sputum
- **Living at elevations greater than 1700 metres (5000 feet):** dust mites do not thrive in this situation
- **Scratching sounds in the home:** presence of mice living in the walls or squirrels living in attics
- **Presence of fungus on caulking between tiles, dry wall, or on floors:** clear evidence of moulds
- **Homes that have plumbing leaks, flooding, or demonstration of water damage:** confirmation of risk of moulds

does not reveal any allergic cause. In this situation, either the testing to the allergen causing disease has not been performed, and therefore a diagnosis of allergy cannot be made, or those symptoms are caused by non-allergic mechanisms. This has an impact on response to therapy as symptoms caused by allergic diseases are more likely to respond to some therapies (e.g. corticosteroids) than the same symptoms elicited by non-allergic mechanisms.

- Ask about any previous treatments the patient may have received. Establish its efficacy, whether it had any adverse effects, whether the patient was compliant, and whether the person had concerns about the treatment.
- Ask about any impact on lifestyle (i.e. work or school, leisure time, and sleep). This will be dealt with more deeply in the next section.
- Finally, ask the patient again what the main problem is. You may get a different answer at this point, after the patient has learned more about the disease during the interview.

Measuring disease control and quality of life

There is increasing focus on how allergic disease affects patients' quality of life. Questionnaires to assess health related quality of life examine how patients perceive the impact of their illness on sleep, functioning at work or school, interpersonal relationships, and other features of daily life. For instance, children with asthma and allergy have greater rates of absence from school, whereas those with symptomatic allergic rhinitis have more difficulty in learning and may achieve lower grades in examinations. Therefore recognition of the severity of symptoms and intervention with appropriate disease-specific therapy will improve performance of both children at school and adults at work.

Questionnaires that assess health-related quality of life can be segregated into those that are generic or disease specific. Generic questionnaires are pertinent for all persons and permit comparison of disease burden for a variety of medical conditions. Since generic questionnaires can be used for any disease state, they may not have the specificity to discern between small changes in one parameter of quality of life for a certain disease that is meaningful to the individual patient. Disease-specific quality of life questionnaires are programmed to assess a particular patient demographic, an individual disease, or a particular symptom or function. These qualities of disease-specific questionnaires are designed to be more sensitive for changes in health status as they apply criteria that are relevant only to a particular condition.

There are now many disease-specific questionnaires that measure health-related quality of life for allergic conditions, which are listed in Appendix 6.1. It is beyond the scope of this chapter to detail these questionnaires.

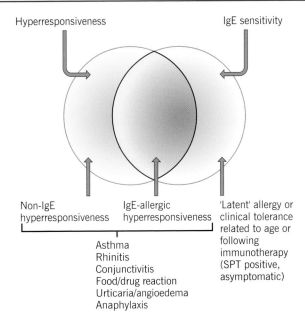

Fig. 6.3 Interrelationships between allergy and hyperresponsiveness, including features suggesting an allergic or non-allergic trigger as the cause of symptoms.

Special cases

Allergic versus non-allergic triggers

Patients with inhalant allergies from whatever cause develop hyperresponsiveness in the target organ. Certain features in the history may point to either allergic or non-allergic triggers as of an immediate response following either natural or experimental allergen exposure. Irritant-induced symptoms tend to be solely immediate, resolving within minutes or hours, to provoke symptoms on first exposure, to require high exposure concentrations, and to affect the majority of exposed subjects to a lesser or greater extent (Fig. 6.3). A good example is the patient with non-allergic, non-infective rhinitis who typically complains of symptoms on exposure to changes in temperature, tobacco smoke, pollutants, perfumes, domestic sprays, bleach, and stressful circumstances. However, these distinctions should be regarded as only a guide since there is considerable overlap. There is no doubt that perennial allergens – resulting in repeated early and late symptoms – result in increased target organ hyperresponsiveness with heightened sensitivity to non-specific

triggers. In these circumstances, symptoms may become continuous and a causal relationship between allergen exposure and symptoms may not be evident to either the patient or the clinician.

Occupational allergy

An occupational history should be obtained in all patients with asthma, rhinitis, and eczema. In contrast to occupational asthma (OA) (Table 6.2), occupational rhinitis is less well documented although likely to be very common, with or without associated asthma. Knowledge of potential occupational causes is important. Symptoms tend to occur within the workplace or during the evening following work; they may improve at weekends and during holiday periods. OA, at least within the UK, is a registered and compensatable industrial disease – 5% of adult onset asthma may be attributed to an occupational cause. The associated loss of self-esteem, together with financial and social difficulties, may provoke symptoms of depressive illness and even suicidal tendencies. Moreover, in up to 50% of cases symptoms may persist for months or even years following termination of the occupational exposure. For these reasons an occupational cause should be established early and certainly not missed. A history of all occupations since leaving school should be obtained if a critical timing of exposure to a potential occupational sensitizer and onset of symptoms is not to be missed. Allergic contact eczema (Table 6.3) may also result from common sensitizers in the home and workplace.

Table 6.2 Common examples of causes of occupational asthma

Agent	At-risk employment
Laboratory animals	Scientific, animal-house work, etc.
Flour	Baking
Biological enzymes	Soap powder industry work
Wood dusts	Saw milling, furniture manufacture
Latex rubber gloves	Health workers
Bleaching agents, hair dyes	Hairdressing
Isocyanates	Paint spraying, printing industry
Colophony (solder fumes)	Electronics industry

Table 6.3 Examples of allergic contact eczema

Agent	Source
Nickel	Coins, watches, jewellery
Cobalt	Metal-plated objects, wet cement
Fragrances	Cosmetics
Lanolin	Cosmetics, moisturizing creams
p-Phenylenediamine	Hair dye, fur dye
Epoxy resins	Adhesives

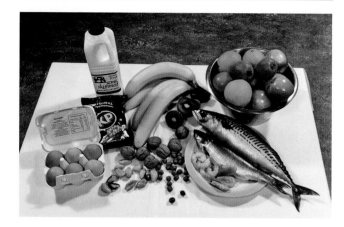

Fig 6.4 Common allergenic foods.

Food allergy and intolerance

Up to 20% of the population perceive food as a cause of their allergy-like symptoms, whereas the prevalence of true food allergy is around 3–4% in adults and up to 6% in children. Food allergens may be split into two major classes: class 1, the major food allergens, and class 2, the indirect food allergens.

Class 1 allergens comprise the classical food allergens to which patients become sensitized by the oral route or, possibly, through the skin. For these allergens, there is a clear association between ingestion (or contact) with the food and the onset of symptoms. In children the primary allergens are eggs, milk, and peanuts whereas in adults they are fish, shellfish, peanuts, tree nuts, soybean, and some fruits (Fig. 6.4). Usually the allergens are heat stable; therefore both uncooked and cooked foods are problematical. Frequently, more than one organ system is involved. For example, true food allergy is a rare cause of isolated asthma in adults, although severe food-induced allergy may provoke asthma associated with other typical organ involvement, e.g. lip tingling, angioedema, nettle rash, nausea, and vomiting.

Although obtaining a detailed history is absolutely necessary in diagnosing food allergy, it is sometimes difficult because patients often have difficulty in dissociating symptoms provoked by food from other causes. In order to obtain information that will be useful for defining skin tests and oral food challenge tests, the following structured approach to questioning may be adopted:

1. What food do you believe caused the reaction?
2. How much of the food did you eat?
3. How long after eating the food did symptoms start to develop?
4. Have you had the same symptoms when eating the food on previous occasions?
5. Are other factors, such as exercise, necessary to cause the symptoms?
6. How long is it since you had the last reaction to this food?

To obtain a definitive diagnosis, the history should be backed up by a skin test, patch testing, a diet diary, elimination diets, and/or a double-blind placebo-controlled food challenge. More information about these will be found in Chapter 14.

Class 2 allergens comprise mainly pollen-derived allergens with cross-reactivity to foods (Table 6.4) and are often associated with oral allergy syndrome, sometimes called pollen-food allergy syndrome. Most commonly, sensitization is through the respiratory tract following pollen inhalation. The primary allergens are highly conserved proteins or carbohydrates present within the pollen and fruits of a wide variety of plants. They include pathogenesis-related proteins (PRP), profilins,

Table 6.4 Some clinically relevant cross-reactions between inhalant allergens and foods

Plant	Pollen allergen	Fruits	Vegetables
Birch	Bet v1 (PR 10)	Apple, cherry, apricot, pear, peach, plum, almond, hazelnut, mango, kiwi, strawberry	Carrot, celery, parsley, chilli pepper, soybean, peanut
	Bet v2 (profilins) (celery–mugwort–spice syndrome)	Cherry, pear	Latex, celery, potato, peanut, soybean
Mugwort		Mango	Celery, carrot, spices
Grass		Melon, watermelon, kiwi, orange	Tomato, potato, peanut
Ragweed		Melon, watermelon, cantaloupe, banana	Courgette, cucumber
Latex	PR2	Avocado, banana, chestnut, kiwi, fig	

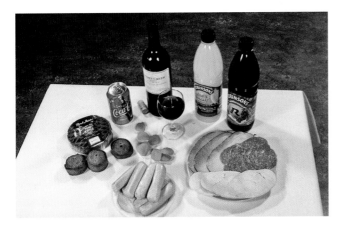

Fig. 6.5 Common food and drink products containing preservatives.

cross-reactive carbohydrate determinants (CCD) and lipid transfer proteins (LTP). Because class 2 allergens are usually heat labile and destroyed in the gastrointestinal tract, symptoms occur *immediately* following eating *raw* fruit or vegetables. The most common symptoms are tingling of the lips, erythema or angioedema of the lips, tongue, and oropharynx, and itching or tightness of the throat.

Diagnosis is similar to class 1 food allergens with the exception that positive skin or provocation tests will be seen with raw fruits or vegetables. Results will be negative with cooked fruits or vegetables.

Non-IgE-mediated food-induced reactions may occur following the ingestion of preservatives such as salicylates, benzoates, and tartrazine. Common products containing preservatives include meat pies, sausages, cooked ham and salami, coloured fruit drinks, confectionery, and wine (Fig. 6.5). No diagnostic tests are available and diagnosis depends upon the history and observation of the effect of exclusion diets and, where necessary, blinded food challenges.

Box 6.4 Anaphylaxis

The presence of one major and two minor features (arbitrarily) may be regarded as diagnostic. If in doubt, give adrenaline!

Major features of anaphylaxis

- Respiratory difficulty (either severe asthma or stridor due to laryngeal oedema)
- Hypotension (fainting, collapse, loss of consciousness)

Minor features of anaphylaxis

- Itching (particularly the hands, feet, groin, and scalp)
- Erythema
- Urticaria
- Angioedema
- Asthma (mild or moderate)
- Rhinoconjunctivitis
- Nausea, vomiting, abdominal pain
- Palpitations
- Sense of impending doom

Anaphylaxis

Anaphylaxis by definition (Box 6.4) may be life threatening. The differential diagnosis depends upon the history of provoking factors; where possible, an eyewitness account should always be obtained. The differential diagnosis includes anaphylactoid reactions, syncope, and psychogenic reactions, as well as other medical conditions such as myocardial infarction, epilepsy, and metabolic or other causes of loss of consciousness. Also, airway obstruction due to a foreign body could be the cause.

Physical examination

A physical examination is required for all patients, although the extent will be guided by the history (Table 6.5).

Table 6.5 Examination of the allergic patient

Organ	Technique	Comments
General	Appearance	Does patient look well or ill, mood, attitude to interview?
	Height, weight	Failure to thrive?
	Inspection of skin including scalp, hair, nails, and buccal mucosa	Dry skin, excoriations? Flexural eczema? Infection? Urticaria or angioedema? Drug rash?
	Look for evidence of corticosteroid side effects	Striae, truncal obesity, bruising, proximal myopathy, hypertension, cataracts?
Eyes	Inspection of eyes and/or eversion of upper lid	Presence of allergic 'shiners'. Conjunctiva in allergic conjunctivitis often appears normal
Nose	External inspection of nose and use of auroscope	Deformity?
	Attachment with ophthalmoscope	Transverse skin creases?
	Ideally, use of head mirror or flexible or rigid endoscopy	Nasal mucosa may appear normal or pale bluish, swollen with watery secretions but only if patient is symptomatic. Exclude structural problems (polyps, deflected nasal septum)
Chest	Inspection	Hyperinflation? Pigeon chest deformity?
	Auscultation	Presence of stridor? Wheeze?

Physical examination is required for all patients although the extent will be guided by the history.

Skin

When rash is the presenting symptom the entire skin, including hair and nails, should be examined. Individual lesions of urticaria may coalesce, are intensely itchy, and characteristically last for several hours (though generally less than 24 hours).

Urticarial lesions that remain fixed, persist for longer than 24 to 48 hours, or leave a residual bruise should raise the possibility of an underlying vasculitic cause. Dermographism is a common accompaniment of urticaria, or it may be the only manifestation, and may confound the interpretation of skin prick tests. Urticaria is evident as raised irregular wheals usually on a red base; there may be associated subcutaneous swellings (angioedema). In view of the episodic nature of urticaria, examination results may be entirely normal.

The distribution of eczema varies with age. Eczema during infancy is prominent on the face and trunk, whereas later in childhood the typical flexural distribution develops. This is frequently associated with artefactual excoriation, sometimes with associated bleeding, and there may be evidence of secondary infection. The skin is dry and in chronic cases may be thickened owing to hyperkeratinization.

Nose

External examination of the nose may reveal a transverse skin crease, which is rare. Internal inspection of the nasal mucosa may reveal the typical appearance of a pale, watery swollen bluish mucosa in allergic patients, but only if they are symptomatic at the time of examination. Structural causes of obstruction should be excluded. Oropharyngeal candidiasis may occasionally be evident in patients using inhaled corticosteroids. The larynx should be examined in cases where there is associated hoarseness – although this will usually be due to concomitant inhaled corticosteroid therapy for asthma when the larynx appears normal, though occasionally a 'midline chink' on adduction of the cords may be evident.

Chest

In patients with asthma the shape of the chest (pigeon chest deformity) may indicate chronic, poorly controlled asthma. There may be a barrel chest with hyperresonance on percussion, diminished breath sounds, and an audible wheeze.

Rarely, rhinitis and asthma or urticaria may be a presenting feature of underlying systemic vasculitic illness such as Churg–Strauss syndrome when purpura, other vasculitic rash, cardiomegaly, pericardial rub, peripheral neuropathy, proteinuria or hematuria, and the presence of casts on routine urine testing, may be evident. Generally these patients are ill, have weight loss and recurrent fevers, and there is leukocytosis, a raised eosinophil count, and considerable elevation of the erythrocyte sedimentation rate.

Clinical and laboratory evaluation of allergy

Treatment for allergic diseases is often initiated based on the patient's history alone. Symptoms of type I hypersensitivity that begin after a clearly defined environmental exposure should prompt institution of environmental controls to eliminate future exposure to the suspected allergen. Pharmacotherapy may also be started if environmental controls are not able to eliminate the allergen to levels that do not precipitate symptoms (for instance, in the case of ubiquitous pollens). However, many patients will continue to have symptoms despite these initial therapeutic manoeuvres. In such cases, the allergen may not have been correctly identified by history, prompting a more comprehensive search to identify the relevant allergen to institute more aggressive and definitive (as well as expensive!) environmental controls. In other instances, pharmacotherapy may either not be providing sufficient relief from the symptoms, or side effects or toxicity may be limiting the use of these agents. In these cases, testing to confirm that allergic disease is indeed causing the patient's symptoms is important to reassure the patient and physician that the therapeutic plan is indeed on target to mitigate the patient's suffering, and whether pharmacotherapy should be continued or increased. In cases where the maximal pharmacological therapy that the patient desires or can tolerate has been reached, then allergen testing is critical to decide whether specific immunotherapy or anti-IgE therapy should be considered. This section reviews the in vivo and in vitro tests that have evidence-based utility in allergic disease diagnosis, as well as tests that are used by some practitioners in diagnosing allergy, but have unproven effectiveness.

Lung function tests

Peak flow monitoring and spirometry, together with an assessment of reversibility (either before or after a bronchodilator), or repeated peak flow measurements at home in order to detect diurnal variation, will confirm or exclude the reversibility of airflow obstruction (i.e. asthma) in the majority of cases. Measurements of airway hyperresponsiveness by means of histamine or methacholine inhalation testing may be helpful, particularly in mild cases where lung function may be normal and response to a bronchodilator is absent. In these circumstances, a low-histamine PC_{20} [i.e. a provocation concentration that causes a 20% reduction in FEV_1 (forced expiratory volume in 1 second)] within the asthmatic range (less than 8 mg/mL) would confirm the need for a trial of bronchodilator therapy and further peak flow monitoring.

Assessment of IgE

The heart of the allergic response lies in the quantity and specificity of IgE production of patients to allergens. IgE levels are low in the fetus and newborn because these molecules do not readily cross the placenta. In general, serum IgE increases with age until the first half of the second decade of life, whereupon they begin to decrease proportionately with age. Therefore, it is important to examine total IgE levels in the framework of age-adjusted reference values for non-allergic persons. Allowing for these caveats, measuring total IgE can be useful as shown by the fact that total serum IgE >100 IU/mL before age 6 is a well-recognized risk factor for allergic rhinitis. However, it must also be emphasized that the presence or absence of IgE antibodies alone is not conclusive of disease. For example, smokers often have high IgE levels in the absence of demonstrable allergic disease. Therefore, IgE levels may be used only as supportive information in the diagnosis of allergy and not in isolation.

Testing for allergen-specific IgE may be done in two ways: in vivo tests such as skin testing and in vitro measurement in blood samples. In general, skin testing tends to be more sensitive whereas allergen-specific IgE measurements in vitro may be more specific. Skin testing is usually performed first for evaluation of sensitization to aeroallergens. However, there are other instances, such as in evaluation of sensitivity to hymenoptera, where determination of allergen-specific IgE can be an important adjunct to skin testing, especially when skin-testing results are negative. Both skin testing and in vitro determination of allergen-specific IgE are generally used before direct allergen provocation as this testing has the risk of inciting significant allergic reactions.

Skin testing

Skin testing can take one of two forms: epicutaneous (more usually known as skin prick testing, or SPT) or intradermal testing. A summary of the uses of skin prick testing is shown in Box 6.5.

Skin prick testing usually has sufficient sensitivity and specificity to be the sole method of skin testing necessary for most clinical scenarios. In allergic rhinitis, the sensitivity of SPT is 85–87% and its specificity 79–86%, while in allergic asthma the sensitivity of SPT has been reported to be as high as 91–98%. There are some situations, however, such as testing for penicillin allergy or venom hypersensitivity, in which intradermal testing is warranted because of its increased sensitivity. However, for safety reasons, SPT should be the only skin testing procedure performed in the diagnosis of food allergy.

Skin prick tests are usually performed either on the volar aspect of the patient's forearm or on the back. Whereas the back is considered to be more reactive, the forearm is more convenient. A drop of an allergen extract

Box 6.5 Uses of skin prick testing – a particular advantage is their educational value for patients

- Allows diagnosis (or exclusion) of atopy
- Provide supportive evidence (with clinical history) for diagnosis (or exclusion) of allergy
- Educational value, providing a clear illustration for patients that may reinforce verbal advice
- Essential when expensive or time-consuming allergen avoidance measures, removal of a family pet, or immunotherapy, are being considered
- Serum allergen-specific IgE concentrations generally provide the same information if skin tests are unavailable

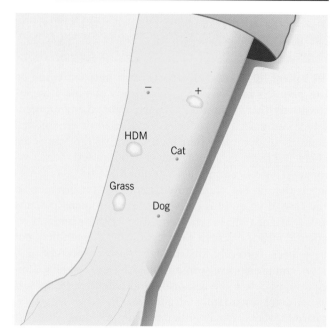

Fig. 6.7 Skin prick tests to common allergens on the forearm. Compared with the negative control, results indicate the presence of allergen-specific IgE to house dust mite (HDM) and grass pollen (grass). + is positive control (histamine) and − is negative control (saline or vehicle).

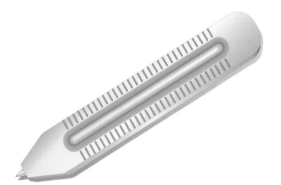

Fig. 6.6 A standard lancet used for skin prick testing.

Box 6.6 Practical points for skin prick tests

- Skin prick testing requires training, both for performance and interpretation of results
- Check that patient is not taking antihistamines
- Oral corticosteroids do not (significantly) inhibit skin prick tests
- Include positive (histamine) and negative (saline or allergen diluent) controls
- Skin prick tests may be performed on the flexor aspect of the forearm (or back) using sterile lancets
- The procedure should be painless and not draw blood
- The wheal diameter is recorded as the mean of the longest diameter and the diameter at right angles to this
- A positive test (arbitrarily) is 2 mm or more greater than negative control; a positive skin prick test is usually at least 6 mm when concordant with clinical history of sensitivity
- Demographism may confound results (although it is evident as a positive response with the negative control solution)
- Skin tests should not be performed in the presence of severe eczema

is placed on a previously cleaned area of skin surface; a sharp instrument, either a needle or a lancet (Fig. 6.6), is then passed through the extract drop at a 45° to 60° angle to the skin and the skin is lifted gently to create a small break in the epidermis to enable allergen penetration into the skin. Test sites, which should be 2–2.5 cm apart to avoid overlapping reactions from occurring, should be marked for allergen identification (Fig. 6.7) and the excess allergen extract carefully wiped away to avoid contamination with other test sites. For routine clinical use, wheal size should be measured at 15–20 minutes and recorded as the mean of the longest diameter and the orthogonal diameter (i.e. the diameter at 90° to the midpoint of the longest diameter, excluding pseudopodia). A summary of the procedure is shown in Box 6.6.

The possibility of either false negative or false positive results in skin testing should always be considered and appropriate controls be placed to evaluate these situations. False negative results can occur when a patient has taken an antihistamine, or a drug with antihistaminic properties such as a tricyclic antidepressant, before skin testing. The recommended times when such medications should be discontinued prior to skin testing are shown in Table 6.6. To assess the potential for a false negative result, a positive control with histamine (10 mg/mL) should be used at one skin-testing site. False positive

results may occur if the skin test extract unknowingly contains histamine or causes an irritant reaction. The most common cause of a false positive skin test is dermographism, which is experienced by 2–5% of the population. To assess the potential for this aetiology of false

Table 6.6 Days that specific pharmacological agents should be discontinued prior to skin testing

Agent	Period to be discontinued prior to skin testing
First-generation antihistamine	
Chlorpheniramine (chlorphenamine)	3 days
Clemastine	5 days
Cyproheptidine	9 days
Dexchlorpheniramine (polaramine)	4 days
Diphenhydramine	2 days
Hydroxyzine	5 days
Promethazine	3 days
Tripelennamine	3 days
Second-generation antihistamine	
Azelastine nasal spray	2 days
Cetirizine	3 days
Fexofenadine	2 days
Loratadine	7 days
Levocabastine nasal and ophthalmic	0 day
Tricyclic antidepressants	
Desipramine	2 days
Imipramine	>10 days
Doxepin	6 days
Doxepin Topical	11 days
Histamine H_2 antagonists	1 day
Cysteinyl leukotriene antagonists	0 day
Corticosteroids	
Prednisone 30 mg for 1 week	0 day
Topical corticosteroids >3 weeks	Avoid testing at this site for 3 weeks after steroids discontinued

The data in this table have been modified from Joint Task Force on Practice Parameters, Allergy diagnostic testing: an updated practice parameter. Ann Allergy Asthma Immunol 2008; 100:S1–148.

positive test, a drop of saline or vehicle instead of allergen extract should be used at one skin-testing site. To be deemed as positive, allergen-induced wheals should have a maximum diameter at least 3 mm greater than the appropriate negative control.

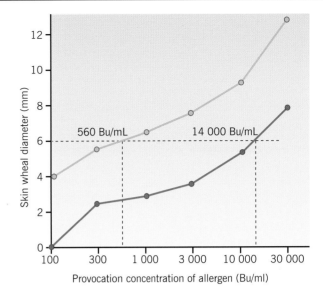

Fig. 6.8 Log dose–response curve illustrating allergen PC6, i.e. the provocation concentration of allergen causing a 6 mm skin wheal. The choice of wheal sizes is arbitrary and, ideally, should lie on the linear part of the curve. The results are from two patients following skin prick tests with grass pollen extract.

Intradermal skin testing is performed by injecting sufficient allergen to produce a 2–3 mm bleb in the dermis (usually 0.02–0.05 mL) using a disposable 1mL syringe with a 26 to 30 gauge needle. Because of the larger volume injected, allergen extracts for intradermal injection are usually 100–1000-fold less concentrated than those used for skin prick testing. The maximum wheal diameter should be measured at 10–15 minutes. Intradermal testing is usually performed on the volar aspect of the forearm, rather than the patient's back, so that a tourniquet can be placed in the event of a systemic reaction to the skin test. While life-threatening reactions are rare with skin testing, immediate systemic reactions are more common with intradermal testing than with skin prick tests. The appropriate negative controls, as detailed above, should again be used for accurate test interpretation. For a positive control intradermal skin test, 0.10 mg/mL of histamine base should be utilized. It is important to recognize that subcutaneous administration of the extract may result in a false positive result, so care must be taken in ensuring intradermal administration of the skin-testing material.

For research purposes, particularly when changes in immediate cutaneous allergen sensitivity may be important, more precision is required. In these circumstances a dose–response curve using half-log or log allergen concentrations may be constructed and the result expressed as the provocation concentration of allergen to cause a skin wheal of a given size, generally 4–6 mm, since this represents the linear portion of the dose–response curve for many subjects. An example is given in Figure 6.8.

There are specific circumstances regarding skin test that deserve special notice, particularly anaphylaxis and food allergy. Following anaphylaxis, skin testing should be delayed for at least 4 weeks as testing following may give a false negative result to the allergen that actually caused the anaphylactic episode. This situation often arises in situations where anaphylaxis has occurred to foods, insect venom, or medications. Investigation of possible allergic reactions to food also warrants special mention as extensive research has been performed in this field that has been further evaluated by double-blind, placebo-controlled food challenges. Such studies reveal that a negative skin prick test has a negative predicative accuracy of greater than 90%, essentially ruling out an IgE-mediated reaction to the food being tested. Using fresh fruit and vegetables in skin testing increases the diagnosis yield as commercially prepared extracts may not be as stable as the fresh food. In the situation where a patient has symptoms of allergy to a certain food, the size of a positive skin test to a food does correspond with the likelihood of allergy to that food, but the size does not correspond to the severity of the clinical reaction when the food is ingested. Intradermal skin testing should not be performed with foods because of poor specificity with positive results from this form of testing. Finally, skin testing should not be performed in the absence of a clinical history suggesting food allergy because a positive skin test may reveal the presence of allergen-specific IgE, but may not mean the patient is allergic to the food giving the positive skin test. Similarly, testing to venom in the absence of a positive history is not recommended because it is estimated that one-quarter of people without history of systemic reaction may have positive skin tests to these allergen extracts.

In vitro laboratory tests

In vitro measurement of allergen-specific IgE is the laboratory equivalent of clinical skin testing. Formerly, measurement of allergen-specific IgE was performed using the radioallergosorbent test (RAST); however, new tools have been developed that supersede this method. Although there is some variation among different proprietary methods for measurement of allergen-specific IgE, the basic concept is that an allergen is linked to a solid phase to which a patient's serum is added. With incubation, the patient's allergen-specific IgE binds to the allergen-linked solid phase (Fig. 6.9). After washing of unbound patient antibody from the allergen-linked solid phase, a labelled human anti-IgE antibody is added; this will then bind to the patient's IgE that is bound to the allergen-linked solid phase. Detection of this human anti-IgE antibody bound to the patient's allergen-specific IgE provides the readout for this assay. It is important to note that, although this general scheme is used to detect allergen-specific IgE, there are substantial differences among the

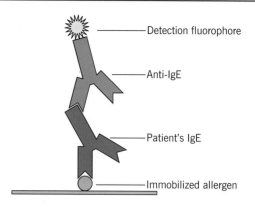

Fig. 6.9 Principles of immunoassay for measuring allergen-specific IgE in serum.

manufacturers of these assays, which does not allow for complete interchangeability of results. For instance, these differences include variations in the different solid phases to which allergen is bound, as well as in the composition, concentration, and potency of the specific allergen linked to the solid phase. Variations in the allergen used result in different populations of a patient's IgE that are detected in the assay.

More recently the advent of chip technology has improved allergen-specific IgE detection, as a single chip is able to identify multiple allergens in as little as 20 μL of serum. This system has the major benefit of allowing the recognition of cross-reactivity of a patient's IgE against structurally similar antigens from different sources. This test is currently available in Europe and will soon be available in the USA.

Many clinical studies have been performed to evaluate the reliability of in vitro testing for food-specific IgE to clinical food allergy. Using the ImmunoCAP system, threshold levels of allergen-specific IgE to egg (6 kUa/L), peanut (15 kUa/L), fish (20 kUa/L), and milk (32 kUa/L) have been shown to portend positive food challenge results with greater than 95% accuracy. Therefore, evaluation of allergen-specific IgE could possibly obviate the need for potentially life-threatening reactions to foods during challenge tests. Just as in skin testing, where the size of the test corresponds to the likelihood that a patient has allergy to that allergen but does not reflect the severity of the clinical reaction, it is important to note that the levels of allergen-specific IgE have also not been shown to correlate with the severity of a clinical allergen reaction for either food or insect venoms. A comparison of skin prick testing and in vitro tests is shown in Box 6.7.

Basophil histamine release test

Allergy screening may also be performed by assessing histamine released from blood basophils after the addition of allergen extract. In this test, blood samples, which may be as small as 20 μL for each allergen, are pipetted into the wells of an ELISA plate precoated with the suspected allergens. The plate is then incubated at 37°C for up to 1 hour and the resultant histamine release estimated. Basophil histamine release, which is usually performed by specialist laboratories, takes only a few hours to perform. This test, which has a sensitivity and specificity similar to that of RAST, is semiquantified on the basis of the concentration of the allergen extract that gives rise to a certain amount of histamine released. As the basophils of about 5% of the population do not release histamine in vitro, a positive response to anti-IgE, used as a positive control, is absolutely necessary to validate a negative result. Furthermore, as the majority of the population has some circulating IgE, a positive result to anti-IgE is not indicative of the presence of allergy in the absence of a corroborative history.

A second use of the basophil degranulation test is in the investigation of chronic spontaneous urticaria. At least 30% of patients with this condition have histamine-releasing autoantibodies directed to either IgE or FcεR1, the high-affinity receptor for IgE. Evidence for these antibodies comes from in vivo studies of autoreactivity with the autologous serum skin test (ASST) in which autologous intradermal injection of serum causes a wheal and flare response. In vitro detection of these antibodies is performed by incubation of 40 μl of patient's serum with white blood cells, containing 1–2% basophils, from a healthy non-atopic donor for 1 hour in the presence of IL-3.

Measurement of environmental allergens

A number of naturally occurring protein antigens in the patient's environment may give rise to sensitization and stimulation of IgE production. Many of these allergens are well known or visible; others are hidden and have to be determined by a thorough medical history and analysis of the environment. Different biological and immuno-chemical methods are presently available for the demonstration of allergens in air and in dust sampling (Table 6.7). Determining the relationship between symptoms and allergens and the decrease in symptoms during allergen reduction makes up a part of the testing for allergy.

A simple technique for sampling dust is to use a vacuum cleaner with a special filter that retains small particles found in the dust. The dust is extracted 1:3 (w/v) in saline for an hour; the presence of a detergent in the buffer may be required for optimal extraction and the allergen content is identified and quantified by immuno-chemical techniques. For some purified allergens, mono-clonal antibodies have been produced, thereby enabling quantification (in nanograms of major allergen per gram

Box 6.7 Advantages of skin prick tests compared with serum allergen-specific IgE tests

Both have a high sensitivity but low specificity, i.e. a negative test is more effective for excluding the clinical relevance of a particular allergen than a positive test for confirming clinical relevance.

Skin prick test	Serum-specific IgE test
Inexpensive	Not affected by concurrent drugs
Immediate results	Not influenced by skin disease
Educational value	Completely safe
Mostly more sensitive	Testing for wide range of possible allergens

Table 6.7 Measurement of environmental allergens

Measurement	Allergens	Detection
Pollen, spore counts in relation to diary symptom/medications	Grass, trees, weeds, moulds	Burkard spore trap (or other device) followed by microscopy; counts expressed as particles per cubic metre
Dust sampling and allergen detection	House dust mite, laboratory animals, domestic pets, cockroaches	Vacuum cleaning or collection of settled dust, followed by allergen extraction and detection using RAST inhibition or specific immunoassay
Air sampling and allergen detection	House dust mites, laboratory animals, domestic pets	Personal air sampler, followed by allergen extraction from air filter and detection using RAST inhibition or specific immunoassay
Culture for mould identification	Molds such as *Aspergillus cladosporium* and *Alternaria*	Specialized microbiological culture techniques
Occupational agents, RAST test	Isocyanates	Isocyanate meter

of dust). Other devices for collecting airborne allergens are available (e.g. stationary high volume air samplers and portable air samplers). Mould spores can be identified and quantified in the home, the working place of the patient, or the outdoor air.

Mast cell tryptase

The measurement of serum tryptase is used to diagnosis conditions where mast cell activation occurs either acutely, such as in anaphylaxis, or in situations of ongoing mast cell activation, such as in systemic mastocytosis. Mast cells contain approximately 300–700 times more tryptase than do basophils, and consequently serum tryptase is more reflective of a mast cell source. There are two forms of mast-cell-derived tryptase: α-tryptase and β-tryptase. The concentration of serum α-tryptase is considered to be reflective of the number of mast cells, while serum β-tryptase is a marker of mast cell activation. Levels of α-tryptase are obtained by subtracting the concentration of β-tryptase from the total tryptase concentration. In healthy subjects, total serum tryptase levels range between 1 and 10 ng/mL while serum β-tryptase levels are less than 1 ng/mL. In contrast, if baseline serum total tryptase levels are greater than 20 ng/mL and serum β-tryptase levels are greater than 1 ng/mL, systemic mastocytosis should be strongly considered. If an anaphylactic event is suspected, blood for total and β-tryptase should be obtained from 30 minutes to 4 hours after the episode occurs. Although because of ethnic differences there is no absolute cut-off level for diagnosing anaphylaxis, levels above 12–14 ng/mL are generally accepted as indicative of anaphylaxis.

Interpretation of specific IgE/skin tests

The sensitivity and specificity of diagnostic cut-points for clinical relevance for either skin testing and/or serum allergen-specific IgE will depend on a number of factors. These include the quality of extracts used and the experience of the operator (or laboratory). Geographic location and variation of the prevalence of environmental allergens will have an enormous impact. Similarly, the predictive value of tests will be influenced by the prevalence of the suspected allergy in the population studied. For example the prevalence of 'true' allergy in relation to positive IgE tests is likely to be higher in referrals to a specialist allergy clinic compared with those screened in primary care.

Whereas it is true that the negative predictive value of skin tests and specific IgE is far more robust, the phenomenon of local IgE synthesis and expression has been increasingly recognized. Again this illustrates the importance of re-evaluation of the history in the interpretation of discordant IgE/skin tests, whether positive or negative. The presence of a negative test in the face of a strong positive history on re-evaluation is an indication for provocation testing in the target organ, whether food challenge or nasal or bronchial inhalation challenge.

In vivo provocation tests

The clinical history may occasionally not provide a clear diagnosis, such as when a patient's shortness of breath has some but not all of the features of asthma. Additionally, there will be instances when the clinical history of manifestations of allergic disease does not match skin testing or in vitro assays assessing antigen-specific IgE. In these situations, in vivo provocation testing can be considered to assess further the relationship between symptoms and physiological end points. Such tests may use pharmacological agents and therefore not be allergen specific, for instance inhaled methacholine or histamine challenges used in asthma assessment, or the presumed allergen may be used in certain in vivo diagnostic assessment such as double-blind, placebo-controlled food challenges (DBPCFC) utilized to evaluate symptoms presumed to be caused by ingestion of foods or other substances via the gastrointestinal tract.

Organ challenge tests can be performed to assess whether or not a specific allergen is definitively causing a specific constellation of symptoms suggestive of an allergic reaction. The site of organ challenge is based on the patient's history and may include the conjunctiva, upper or lower respiratory tract, or skin for allergic contact dermatitis or insect sting. These tests are usually reserved for the situation where skin test or in vitro allergen IgE results do not correspond to patient history or clinical situation. Most often, these tests are performed in a controlled research setting because of the possible risk of severe, life-threatening reactions to direct organ allergen challenge. Details of specific in vivo provocation tests will be found in later chapters on individual diseases.

Unproven tests

There are many unproven 'diagnostic' tests performed by 'food ecologists' and alternative practitioners. These tests are of unproven diagnostic validity, are often time consuming and expensive, and are therefore not to be recommended (Box 6.8).

Golden rules of allergy diagnosis

(Box 6.9)

In this chapter, the importance, first, of taking a careful history in accurate allergy diagnosis has been emphasized. Furthermore, the importance of using specific IgE/skin tests as confirmation, and interpreting them *only* in

Box 6.8 Tests for which there is no diagnostic validity in allergic disorders

- Cytotoxic tests
- Provocation–neutralization tests
- Vega testing (a 'black box' electrical test); test is based on the addition of food extracts to a chamber contained within an electrical circuit completed by the patient
- Applied kinesiology
- Iridology
- Chemical analysis of body fluids, hair, or other tissue
- Food-specific IgG, IgG4, and IgG/IgG4 antibody tests
- Auricular cardiac reflex testing (based on pulse rate)

Box 6.9 Golden rules of allergy diagnosis

1. An accurate clinical history is the mainstay of allergy diagnosis
2. Skin prick/serum IgE tests provide objective confirmation of IgE sensitivity
3. Skin prick/serum IgE tests must *always* be interpreted in the context of the history
4. If you do not need the result of a test then don't do the test. Indiscriminate skin prick/serum IgE 'panels' are more likely to confuse rather than inform diagnosis and should be avoided*

*Multiple IgE-testing panels may occasionally be indicated, e.g. evaluation of exercise-induced anaphylaxis where food may be an important cofactor and in paediatric practice where the history may be less discriminating.

the context of the clinical history has been repeatedly highlighted.

A fourth 'golden rule' in allergy diagnosis is that if you do not want to know the result of a test then don't do the test! Allergists are frequently confronted by patients referred to them who have a 'panel' of allergy tests in their possession with multiple positives that do not coincide with symptoms on exposure. This is particularly problematic for indiscriminate food allergy panels where patients are concerned whether or not they should avoid foods to which they may have positive IgE/skin tests, but which they tolerate perfectly well. This requires much consultation time to unravel, and may require performance of otherwise unnecessary provocation tests in order to exclude allergy and/or to reassure an understandably anxious patient. There are also medicolegal implications as to whether verbal reassurance in the absence of provocation testing is sufficient in such a setting.

It follows naturally from the foregoing that there is almost no place for indiscriminate 'allergy-screening panels'. This is particularly relevant in adult allergy practice where the perception of food allergy in the general population is high and 'food allergy panels' are increasingly available on the high street or the internet. Like all rules, however, there are exceptions, such as exercise-induced anaphylaxis where 'latent ' allergy to foods such as wheat, peanut, or fish may represent cofactors that manifest only after exercise. In paediatric practice there is also a legitimate lower threshold for multiple IgE testing in the presence of potentially allergic clinical manifestations where the history may be less discriminating – although in the authors' view, to avoid confusion and anxiety, 'paediatric panels' should be initiated only by practitioners with considerable experience and skill in the diagnosis and management of paediatric allergy.

Conclusion – diagnostic approach

Allergy diagnosis depends primarily on the clinical history. This history, aided by a physical examination and objective tests of IgE sensitivity (either skin tests or serum IgE measurements), is used to focus on the following questions:

- Is the patient atopic?
- Does allergy contribute to the patient's symptoms?
- What are the clinically relevant allergens?

A simple diagnostic approach, including points when patients should be referred to an allergy specialist is presented in Figure 6.10. There should be a high index of suspicion for allergy in patients presenting with symptoms of asthma, rhinitis, or eczema, particularly if there is an associated personal or family history of other atopic disease. Whether or not allergy is suspected on the basis of the initial history, a limited number of skin prick tests or in vitro tests for specific IgE, to a limited number of common aeroallergens should be performed in the majority of patients to confirm or exclude atopy; a physical examination should also be included. Only when both the clinical history and other investigations are negative can allergy be excluded with a high degree of confidence. Conversely, only when the history and tests are both positive should allergy management or pharmacotherapy be instituted. Where there is discordance, above all, the history should be reassessed. Specialist referral and, occasionally, more sophisticated tests or specific provocation testing may be required. However, it should be emphasized that results of clinical investigations, even when combined with a careful history, will not confirm or exclude absolutely relevant allergy in every individual case.

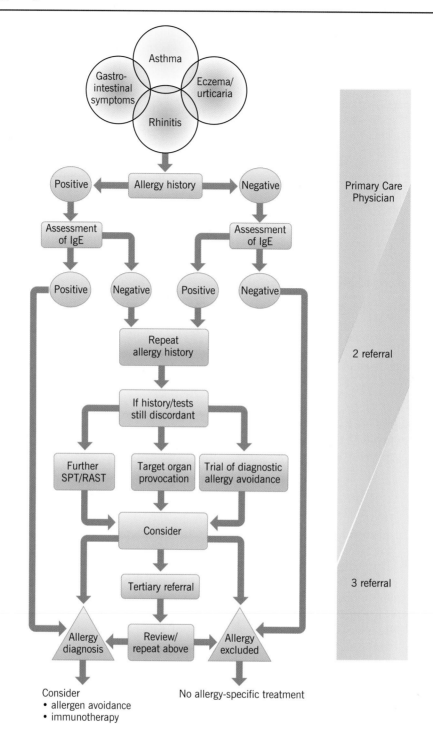

Fig. 6.10 Diagnostic approach to allergy.

Summary of important messages

- Allergy diagnosis depends primarily on the clinical history. This history, aided by a physical examination and objective tests of IgE sensitivity (either skin tests or serum IgE measurements), is used to focus on the following questions:
  - Is the patient atopic?
  - Does allergy contribute to the patient's symptoms?
  - What are the clinically relevant allergens?
- There should be a high index of suspicion for allergy in patients presenting with symptoms of asthma, rhinitis, or eczema, particularly if there is an associated personal or family history of other atopic disease
- Skin prick tests or in vitro tests for specific IgE, to a limited number of common aeroallergens, should be performed in the majority of patients to confirm or exclude atopy
- Only when both the clinical history and other investigations agree can either allergy be excluded with a high degree of confidence or allergy management or pharmacotherapy be instituted
- Where there is discordance, the history should be reassessed and specialist referral and, occasionally, more sophisticated tests or specific provocation testing may be required
- It should be emphasized that results of clinical investigations, even when combined with a careful history, will not always confirm allergy or exclude it absolutely in every individual case

Further reading

Cockcroft D, Davis B. Direct and indirect challenges in the clinical assessment of asthma. Ann Allergy Asthma Immunol 2009; 103:363–370.

Eckman J, Saini SS, Hamilton RG. Diagnostic evaluation of food-related allergic diseases. Allergy, Asthma, and Clinical Immunology 2009; 5:2.

Halbert RJ, Tinkelman DG, Globe DR, et al. Measuring asthma control is the first step to patient management: a literature review. J Asthma 2009; 46:659–664.

Hamilton RG. Clinical laboratory assessment of immediate-type hypersensitivity. J Allergy Clin Immunol 2010; 125:S284–296.

Joint Task Force on Practice Parameters. The diagnosis and management of rhinitis: an updated practice parameter. J Allergy Clin Immunol 2008; 122:S1–84.

Joint Task Force on Practice Parameters. Allergy diagnostic testing: an updated practice parameter. Ann Allergy Asthma Immunol 2008; 100:S1–148.

Khan DA, Solensky R. Drug allergy. J Allergy Clin Immunol 2010; 125:S126–137.

Peden D, Reed CE. Environmental and occupational allergies. J Allergy Clin Immunol 2010; 125:S150–160.

Sicherer SH, Sampson HA. Food allergy. J Allergy Clin Immunol 2010; 125:S116–125.

Simons FER. Anaphylaxis: recent advances in assessment and treatment. J Allergy Clin Immunol 2009; 124:625–636.

Appendix 6.1 Allergy-specific health related quality of life measures

Instrument	Reference
Asthma	
Asthma Control Questionnaire (ACQ)*	Eur Respir J 1999; 14:902
Asthma Control Scoring System (ACSS)	Chest 2002; 122:2217
Asthma Control Test (ACT)	J Allergy Clin Immunol 2004; 113:59
Childhood Asthma Control Test (C-ACT)	J Allergy Clin Immunol 2007; 119:817
Asthma Therapy Assessment Questionnaire (ATAQ)	Am J Respir Crit Care Med 1999; 160:1647
Lara Asthma Symptom Scale (LASS)	J Allergy Clin Immunol 2007; 120:1368
Asthma Quality of Life Questionnaire (AQLQ)*	Thorax 1992; 47:76
Asthma Quality of Life Questionnaire-standardized version (AQLQ(S))*	Chest 1999; 115:1265
Mini Asthma Quality of Life Questionnaire (MiniAQLQ)*	Eur Respir J 1999; 14:32
Paediatric Asthma Quality of Life Questionnaire (PAQLQ)*	Qual Life Res 1996; 5:35
Allergic rhinoconjunctivitis	
Rhinoconjunctivitis Quality of Life Questionnaire (RQLQ)*	Clin Exp Allergy 1991; 21:77
Rhinoconjunctivitis Quality of Life Questionnaire-standardized version (RQLQ(S))*	J Allergy Clin Immunol 1991; 104:77
Mini Rhinoconjunctivitis Quality of Life Questionnaire (MiniRQLQ)*	Clin Exp Allergy 2000; 30:132
Adolescent Rhinoconjunctivitis Quality of Life Questionnaire (AdolRQLQ)*	J Allergy Clin Immunol 1994; 93:413
Paediatric Rhinoconjunctivitis Quality of Life Questionnaire (PRQLQ)*	J Allergy Clin Immunol 1998; 101:163
Chronic Sinusitis Survey	Laryngoscope 1995; 105:387
Rhinosinusitis Outcome Measure (RSOM-31)	Am J Rhinol 1995; 9:297
Rhinosinusitis Disability Index (RSDI)	Arch Otolaryngol Head Neck Surg 1997; 123:1175
Rhinitis Symptom Utility Index (RSUI)	Qual Life Res 1997; 7:693
Sino-Nasal Outcome Test (SNOT-20)	Clin Exp Allergy 2000; 30:132
Rhinasthma	Allergy 2003; 58:289
Rhinitis Outcomes Questionnaire (ROQ)	Ann Allergy Asthma Immunol 2001; 86:222–5
Urticaria	
Chronic Urticaria Quality of Life Questionnaire (CU-Q$_2$oL)	Allergy 2005; 60:1073
Dermatology Life Quality Index (DLQI)	Clin Exp Dermatol 1994; 19:210
Atopic dermatitis	
Scoring Atopic Dermatitis (SCORAD)	Dermatology 1993; 186:23
Eczema Area and Severity Index (EASI)	Exp Dermatol 2001; 10:11
Family Dermatitis Index (FDI)	Br J Dermatol 2001; 144:104
Infants' Dermatitis Quality of Life Index (IDQOL)	Br J Dermatol 2001; 144:104
Dermatology Life Quality Index (DLQI)	Clin Exp Dermatol 1994; 19:210

*This questionnaire may be obtained online, together with instructions for administration, analysis, and interpretation, from www.qoltech.co.uk.

Principles of pharmacotherapy

Martin K Church and Thomas B Casale

DEFINITION

The principles of pharmacotherapy are to relieve symptoms and to treat underlying inflammation in order to reduce the progression of the disease.

Introduction

Allergy comprises a wide spectrum of conditions affecting many organs, each of which requires treatment with different drugs. The principles, however, are the same. In its early stages, allergy may present as isolated episodes of asthma, rhinitis, or urticaria. However, as the condition progresses, an underlying pathology of allergic inflammation develops leading to chronic disease in which the episodic exacerbations, or attacks, can become more severe. The drugs used to treat allergy may, therefore, be classified into two groups: those aimed primarily at the relief of the symptoms of the acute exacerbations and those primarily for treatment of the underlying inflammation. These categories are not completely watertight as some drugs aimed principally at providing relief from immediate symptoms may also influence the underlying inflammation. It should be stressed, however, that the treatment strategies outlined in this chapter are primarily aimed at relieving symptoms and controlling the progression of the allergic condition rather than curing it as, to date, this has not been possible.

Adrenaline (US epinephrine) and adrenoceptor stimulants

The use of adrenaline in the relief of asthma symptoms and as a life-saving drug in systemic anaphylaxis has been established for almost 100 years. Chemical modification of adrenaline to improve receptor selectivity has yielded α- and β-adrenoceptor stimulants for the treatment of nasal congestion and asthma respectively.

Adrenaline

For the treatment of systemic anaphylaxis, the ability of adrenaline to stimulate both α- and β-receptors, as illustrated in Figure 7.1, contributes to its beneficial effects. Of particular note are its bronchodilator properties, its capacity to inhibit mast-cell-mediator secretion, and its restoration of a satisfactory circulation by its action on the heart, blood vessels, and renin–angiotensin system and its constriction of the vascular beds in the

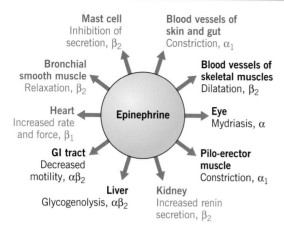

Fig. 7.1 Actions of adrenaline (epinephrine).

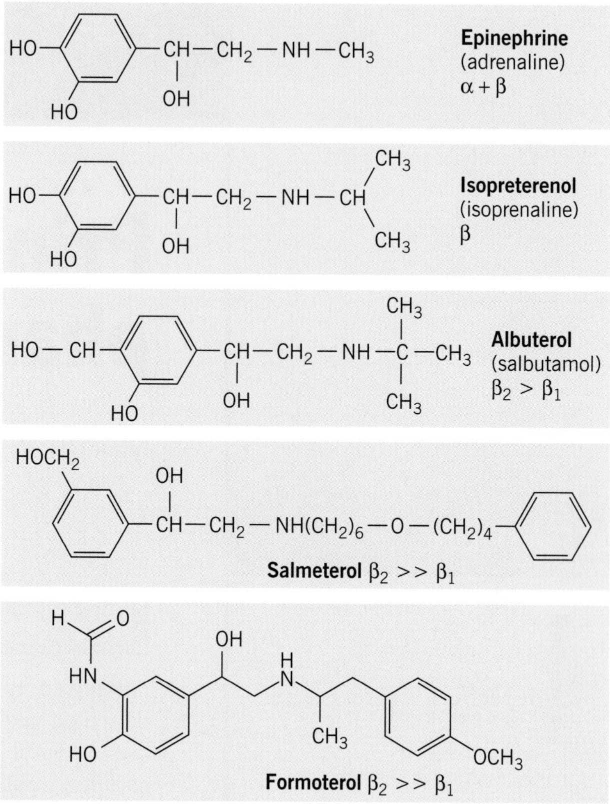

Mast cell
Inhibition of secretion, β_2

Blood vessels of skin and gut
Constriction, α_1

Bronchial smooth muscle
Relaxation, β_2

Blood vessels of skeletal muscles
Dilatation, β_2

Heart
Increased rate and force, β_1

Eye
Mydriasis, α

GI tract
Decreased motility, $\alpha\beta_2$

Pilo-erector muscle
Constriction, α_1

Liver
Glycogenolysis, $\alpha\beta_2$

Kidney
Increased renin secretion, β_2

Epinephrine

Fig. 7.2 Chemical development of β_2-adrenoceptor agonists.

Epinephrine (adrenaline) $\alpha + \beta$

Isopreterenol (isoprenaline) β

Albuterol (salbutamol) $\beta_2 > \beta_1$

Salmeterol $\beta_2 >> \beta_1$

Formoterol $\beta_2 >> \beta_1$

skin and viscera. Adrenaline is rapidly inactivated by two enzymatic processes: by monoamine oxidase (MAO) in neuronal tissue and by catechol-O-methyltransferase (COMT) in extraneuronal tissues. This means that is has a short duration of action and may have to be given repeatedly as described below.

Uses and administration

Anaphylaxis

Adrenaline is the drug of choice for the management of anaphylaxis. The sooner adrenaline is administered after the diagnosis of anaphylaxis the better is the prognosis. Underprescribing or delayed prescribing results in a poorer prognosis and an increased frequency of emergency admissions and death. Physicians treating patients with anaphylaxis should administer adrenaline into the muscle of the lateral thigh (vastus lateralis) since this results in faster rises in blood levels and higher concentrations compared with administration subcutaneously or into the muscle of the arm.

The dose of adrenaline in adults is 0.3–0.5 mL of a 1 in 1000 solution (0.3–0.5 mg). In children, the dose of adrenaline is 0.01 mg per kilogram of body weight. The administration of adrenaline can be repeated every 5–15 minutes as needed. In adult patients who do not respond to intramuscular adrenaline and have shock with cardiovascular collapse, intravenous adrenaline can be administered at a starting rate of 1–4 μg per minute. In children, this dose is typically 0.1 μg per kilogram of body weight. It is imperative that intravenous injection of adrenaline be given slowly so as to avoid the possibility of causing a cardiac arrhythmia.

Self-administration of adrenaline by patients can be lifesaving. Patients at risk should carry a preloaded syringe of adrenaline (EpiPen, Twinject, or the equivalent) with them at all times and be taught the appropriate use with administration into the lateral thigh. Even if patients feel better after administration of adrenaline, they should see a physician immediately or go to the nearest emergency department as anaphylaxis can sometimes recur and be protracted. It is therefore essential that prompt follow-up care is given.

β_2-Adrenoceptor stimulants

For the treatment of bronchial asthma, many of the effects of adrenaline are undesirable; the cardiovascular effects, particularly stimulation of cardiac arrhythmias, are of particular concern. Many of those problems have now been overcome by chemical modifications of the adrenaline molecule and by developing preparations with a satisfactory pharmacokinetic profile when administered to the lung by inhalation.

The chemical modification of adrenaline in 1941 was to replace the terminal methyl group on the side chain by an isopropyl group (Fig. 7.2). This increase in the bulk of the side-chain produced isoprenaline (US isoproterenol), a drug that acts almost exclusively at β-receptors. Further increases in the bulk of this substituent produced drugs that, although having decreased absolute potency, have an increased degree of selectivity for β_2-receptors over β_1-receptors. Further chemical modifications to reduce metabolism have lengthened their duration of action up to ≈4 hours for salbutamol (US albuterol) and terbutaline, in excess of 12 hours for salmeterol and formoterol, and up to 24 hours in newer formulations undergoing clinical trials. Examples of such drugs are shown in Figure 7.2. It should be emphasized, however, that such chemical manoeuvres do not confer an absolute specificity for β_2-receptors but only selectivity. Thus, with high systemic concentrations, β_1-receptor-mediated effects on the heart may become apparent.

Mechanism of action

More is probably known about the biochemical mechanism of action of β_2-adrenoceptor stimulants than any of the other drugs used in the treatment of allergic diseases. The actions of β_2-adrenoceptor stimulants are summarized in Figure 7.3. Briefly, interaction of a β_2-stimulant with its receptor unit initiates the binding of guanosine triphosphate (GTP) to the α-subunit of the regulatory G protein leading to its dissociation from the G-protein complex. This subunit then complexes with adenylate cyclase (AC), the catalytic unit of the complex, activating it to generate cyclic adenosine monophosphate (cAMP) from adenosine triphosphate (ATP). cAMP then acts as a second or intracellular messenger to activate a series of cAMP-dependent protein kinases (cAMP-dPK), which phosphorylate a number of proteins crucial to many intracellular biochemical events.

By these mechanisms, β_2-stimulants cause potent relaxation of bronchial smooth muscle, from which the term 'bronchodilator' is derived. As this is a direct action, β_2-agonists are able to relax bronchial smooth muscle regardless of the contractile stimulus, thus giving rise to the term 'functional antagonists'. Similarly, β_2-adrenoceptor stimulants prevent the activation of mast cells, but not basophils, to release their mediators. In this respect, β_2-stimulants are considerably more effective than the archetypal mast cell stabilizer, cromolyn sodium. As the highest concentration of β_2-receptors in the lung is found on the luminal aspect of bronchial epithelial cells, it is postulated that β_2-agonists stimulate these cells to release their bronchorelaxant factors. β_2-Receptors are also present on ganglia of vagal efferent nerves and inhibit the release of acetylcholine. It is for this reason that β-antagonist-induced bronchoconstriction responds to anticholinergics.

Uses and administration

Asthma

Dose-dependent side effects such as tachycardia, palpitations, and tremor occur at higher rates in oral versus

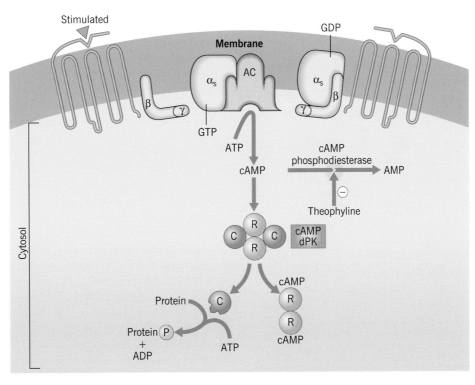

Fig. 7.3 Activation of adenylyl cyclase and protein kinases. The diagram shows two β-adrenoceptor molecules, each of which is composed of three transmembrane loops. Stimulation of the receptor (left) causes its activation, in which the α_s unit of the heterotrimeric Gs protein binds GTP and dissociates from the complex to the adenylyl cyclase catalytic unit (AC). Activated AC catalyses the formation of cyclic adenosine monophosphate (cAMP), which binds to the regulatory units (R) of cAMP-dependent protein kinases (cAMP-dPK) thus freeing the catalytic units (C) to phosphorylate-specific proteins. The activated state exists only transiently, ATP hydrolysis to ADP leading to reassociation of the $\alpha s\beta\gamma$ complex of Gs, inactivation of AC, receptor regeneration, and the breakdown of AMP by phosphodiesterases.

inhaled β_2-agonist formulations limiting their utility. Although oral β_2-agonists may have a role in some children, metered dose inhalers with appropriate spacer devices are preferred. Similarly, the inhaled route is also preferred over parenteral administration since the onset of action is quicker and the degree of bronchodilatation equivalent or greater with fewer side effects. Proper metered-dose inhaler technique results in rapid and high dose delivery of β_2-agonists. Used with a holding chamber, metered dose inhalers require less patient coordination and reduce oropharyngeal deposition. In the emergency management of asthma exacerbations, metered dose inhalers with or without a spacer device can be administered every 20–30 minutes. Nebulizer therapy may be preferred for patients who are uncooperative or severely obstructed and unable to appropriately use a metered dose inhaler. However, the routine use of nebulizers for delivery of short acting β_2-agonists is generally unnecessary. Dry-powder inhalers are breath actuated and also require less patient coordination. Because they typically require a rapid deep inhalation, their use is best reserved for children at least 4 years of age and adults, and not during an exacerbation.

Short-acting β_2-agonists have an onset of action within 5 minutes and a typical duration of action of 4–6 hours (Table 7.1). These agents are now designated 'quick relief medications' and they are the drug of choice for treating acute asthma symptoms and exacerbations as well as for preventing exercise-induced bronchospasm. The use of short acting β_2-agonists more than twice per week indicates inadequate asthma control and the need for initiation or intensification of anti-inflammatory controller medications. Regularly scheduled daily chronic use of short acting β_2-agonists is not recommended.

There are currently two available long-acting β_2-agonists (LABA): salmeterol and formoterol, which have onsets of action in approximately 30 minutes and less than 5 minutes respectively. Both agents have duration of action of greater than 12 hours (see Table 7.1). Because formoterol has an onset of action similar to short-acting β_2-agonists, it has been used as a rescue medication with and without inhaled corticosteroids. There are several longer-acting formulations with onset of action in less than 5

minutes and duration of approximately 24 hours undergoing clinical trials.

Guideline-driven asthma care does not support the use of LABA as monotherapy or for the treatment of acute symptoms or exacerbations. They can, however, be used for prevention of exercise-induced bronchospasm. LABA are most appropriately used in a combination inhaler with corticosteroids for the management of chronic persistent asthma in patients not adequately controlled on inhaled corticosteroids alone.

Recently, the United States Food and Drug Administration (FDA) raised concerns about the potential adverse consequences of LABA, including death. The FDA made two controversial recommendations: to stop the use of LABA if possible once asthma control is achieved, stepping the dose down, and to use LABA only in patients whose asthma is not well controlled with low or medium doses of inhaled corticosteroid, stepping it up. However, there is a large body of evidence suggesting that the addition of a LABA to inhaled corticosteroids improves asthma control and quality of life. Asthma deaths have declined since LABA have become available. At present, we recommend following evidence-based guidelines for the appropriate use of LABA unless new data confirm a potential increased risk to benefit ratio than currently reported.

α-Adrenoceptor stimulants

The nasal mucosa is highly vascular, containing an extensive capillary network and large cavernous vascular sinusoids. The tone of these vessels is largely maintained by sympathetic nervous system fibres, which release noradrenaline (US norepinephrine) and neuropeptide Y to cause vasoconstriction. Nasal decongestants, such as ephedrine, oxymetazoline, and xylometazoline, are α-adrenoceptor stimulants that mimic the vasoconstrictor effects of noradrenaline to reduce nasal blockage by decreasing nasal blood flow and reducing mucosal oedema.

A major problem with the use of topical nasal decongestants, particularly with the more potent agents such as oxymetazoline and xylometazoline, is that they cause a reduction in the number of α-adrenoceptors – which occurs over just a few days. Thus when intranasal decongestants are used for more than 3–5 days they may lead to rebound swelling of the nasal mucosa. This may tempt the further use of the decongestant, leading to a vicious cycle of events with possible long-term consequences.

Uses and administration

Allergic rhinitis

There are very few data supporting the clinical efficacy of oral decongestants for the treatment of allergic rhinitis and nasal congestion. Due to side effects, including insomnia, irritability, anxiety, tremors, palpitations,

Table 7.1 Duration of action of β_2-stimulants

β_2-stimulant	Onset of action	Duration of action
Salbutamol (albuterol)	<5 min	4–6 h
Terbutaline	<5 min	4–6 h
Formoterol	<5 min	>12 h
Salmeterol	~30 min	>12 h

tachycardia, and dizziness, they are not recommended for use as monotherapy. However, some patients may benefit from their use on an as-needed basis for the acute management of nasal congestion. Oral decongestants should not be used by the elderly, during pregnancy and by patients with underlying cardiovascular disorders including hypertension. Furthermore, sympathomimetics may cause a hypertensive crisis if used during treatment with MAO inhibitor drugs.

Intranasal decongestants are much more effective in relieving nasal obstruction. They have a rapid onset of action and can improve nasal obstruction when used for 3–5 days. However, they do not improve other symptoms of rhinitis. Intranasal decongestants may have the same systemic side effects as oral decongestants, but typically the scope and severity are less. However, the use of intranasal decongestants should be limited to no more than 3–5 days because of the concern that prolonged use may lead to rebound swelling of the nasal mucosa and to drug-induced rhinitis (rhinitis medicamentosa).

There is a net clinical benefit from regular use of a combination of oral H_1-antihistamine and oral decongestant compared with oral H_1-antihistamine alone in allergic rhinitis. However, the small improvement in nasal symptoms seems to be counterbalanced by the increased risk of adverse effects. Although there are no published reports supporting the use of a combination of oral H_1-antihistamine and oral decongestant as a rescue or as-needed medication, it may be of benefit for some patients.

Methylxanthines

Methylxanthines, in the form of coffee and extracts from the tea plant, have been used for the treatment of bronchial asthma for almost 700 years. Today the predominant methylxanthine in clinical use is theophylline, given either as the native drug, as its water-soluble ethylene diamine salt, aminophylline, or as a long-acting conjugate, such as choline theophyllinate. The use of these drugs has markedly diminished with the availability of long acting β_2-agonists.

Theophylline

Mechanism of action

The precise mechanism by which theophylline acts as an antiasthma drug is still somewhat obscure. Clearly it has the potential to inhibit cAMP phosphodiesterase (PDE), thus causing the elevation of intracellular levels of cAMP by preventing its breakdown (see Fig. 7.3). The theory for this mechanism of action in asthma has been based on biochemical and in vitro studies that use theophylline at concentrations which would be toxic in vivo.

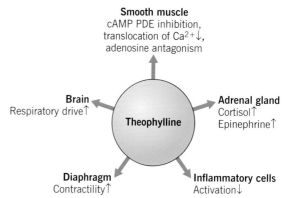

Fig. 7.4 Proposed mechanisms of action of theophylline. cAMP, cyclic adenosine monophosphate; PDE, phosphodiesterase.

Consequently, a variety of alternative mechanisms have been proposed, which are summarized in Figure 7.4. However, the PDE inhibition theory has recently gained more credence from two lines of evidence. First is the observation that, at therapeutic doses, there is evidence in leukocytes in vivo of increased levels of cAMP, which suggests that even a small and subtle action on PDE at these concentrations may be sufficient to confer clinical activity. Second is the identification of seven families of PDE isoenzymes, many of which contain multiple subtypes that are encoded by distinct genes, and the synthesis of specific inhibitors for them. Of particular note is the finding that bronchial smooth muscle and inflammatory cells, including mast cells, have type 4 PDE (PDE4). Initial studies with inhibitors of this isoenzyme indicate that they carry the beneficial actions of theophylline while being devoid of some of the side effects. Drugs of this class are undergoing intense clinical trial at present and are described later.

The major disadvantage with theophylline is its narrow therapeutic window (Fig. 7.5). The beneficial effects of the drug in long-term management are usually observed only with plasma levels in the range of 5–15 mg/mL. Below 5 mg/mL, the drug is comparatively ineffective and, above 20 mg/mL, toxic effects are observed that increase in number and in severity with increasing plasma concentrations. Because of this relationship, the prudent physician will regularly monitor serum theophylline levels and adjust the dose so that possible life-threatening toxicity is avoided.

Uses and administration

Asthma

Methylxanthines can be administered intravenously, orally, or rectally. Intravenous aminophylline is rarely used since there is no significant benefit over inhaled β_2-agonists for the management of acute severe asthma. The

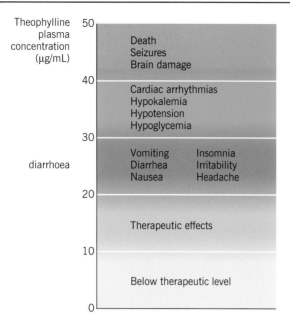

Fig. 7.5 Dose-related therapeutic and toxic effects of theophylline.

only currently recommended route of administration is orally. Oral theophylline is recommended in patients who are not well controlled on inhaled corticosteroids. Theophylline and aminophylline are rapidly and completely absorbed from the intestinal tract. Theophylline is metabolized in the liver with a half-life of approximately 6 hours in normal individuals. Because of this relatively short duration of action, many slow-release preparations have been formulated to extend its duration to 8–24 hours. However, care must be taken with such preparations, as fluctuations in plasma concentrations may occur, bringing with them either lack of efficacy or potential toxicity. The main limitation of the use of theophylline has been related to side effects especially when plasma levels exceed 20 mg/L. At high plasma concentrations, cardiac arrhythmias, seizures, nausea and vomiting, headache, and restlessness can occur. Most of the side effects can be avoided without compromising efficacy when plasma levels are maintained between 5 and 10 mg/L,. Theophylline interacts with a number of other drugs affecting blood levels, which also limits its utility.

Adding low-dose theophylline results in better asthma control than doubling the dose of inhaled corticosteroid. Theophylline improves lung functions and has anti-inflammatory effects that contribute to its efficacy. Theophylline can be used for the management of nocturnal asthma when given at night. However, long acting β_2-agonists are as effective without compromising the quality of sleep.

Phosphodiesterase 4 inhibitors

Phosphodiesterase 4 inhibitors have a broad spectrum of anti-inflammatory effects important in asthma. Several phosphodiesterase 4 inhibitors have been tested in COPD and asthma. Although having some therapeutic effectiveness, their side effects, especially nausea and vomiting, have thus far limited their development for asthma.

Anticholinergic agents

Antimuscarinic agents, particularly from the smoking of leaves of stramonium, belladonna, and hyoscyamus, have been used for the treatment of asthma for centuries. Today, chemically modified derivatives of atropine are used as bronchodilator drugs.

Mechanism of action

Stimulation by acetylcholine of muscarinic M_3-receptors on bronchial smooth muscle initiates its contraction by a cyclic guanosine monophosphate (cGMP)-mediated pathway. Atropine and related drugs are competitive and reversible antagonists of this effect of acetylcholine, thereby producing a dose-related inhibition of smooth muscle contraction (Fig. 7.6).

Uses and administration

Asthma and chronic obstructive pulmonary disease (COPD)

Atropine is well absorbed, even following inhalation, and produces systemic inhibition of parasympathetic nervous system activity. This severely limits its use as a bronchodilator. However, ipratropium bromide and oxitropium bromide, both of which are potent topical anticholinergics and bronchodilators with poor systemic absorption and hence few systemic side effects, are widely available. In adults, the routine use of topical anticholinergics is primarily reserved for the treatment of COPD. These agents have found little place in the chronic management of asthma. Anticholinergics in combination with short acting β_2-agonists are recommended for the acute management of moderate to severe asthma exacerbations in both children and adults. The usual dose of ipratropium bromide nebulizer solution is 0.25–0.5 mg every 20 minutes for three doses, then as needed. Alternatively, four to eight puffs from a metered dose inhaler can be used. Anticholinergics can also be used to manage beta blocker-induced asthma exacerbations and as a quick reliever in patients that cannot tolerate short-acting β_2-agonists. Longer-acting inhaled anticholinergic preparations (e.g. tiotropium) can be used once daily for the management of COPD, but have only recently been shown to possibly be of benefit in asthma.

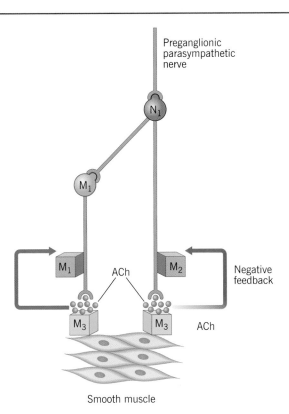

Fig. 7.6 Muscarinic cholinergic receptors in the airways. Postganglionic fibres are excited by the action of ACh at N1 receptors. These fibres go directly to smooth muscle where the ACh released interacts with M3 receptors to cause contraction. ACh also feeds back to stimulate M2 receptors on the nerves and to reduce ACh release. The site of M1 receptors is speculative but they are thought to be present as secondary stimulant nerves that augment parasympathetic stimulation in the airways. ACh, acetylcholine.

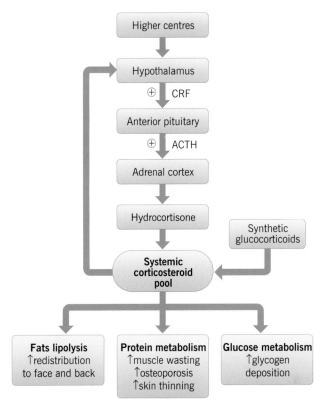

Fig. 7.7 Control of secretion and metabolic effects of glucocorticosteroids. In normal individuals, the positive signals of corticotropin-releasing factor (CRF) and adrenocorticotropic hormone (ACTH) from the hypothalamus and pituitary gland, respectively, induce the secretion of hydrocortisone from the adrenal cortex. Both hydrocortisone and exogenous glucocorticoids exert a negative effect on the hypothalamus to reduce natural hydrocortisone secretion.

Allergic rhinitis

Intranasal anticholinergic preparations are effective in decreasing mucus production in upper respiratory tract infections and rhinitis. They do not affect other symptoms of rhinitis.

Corticosteroids

Corticosteroids, or steroids as they are often loosely termed, have been the drugs of choice for the treatment of chronic severe asthma since their introduction in 1950. More recently it has been recognized that the treatment of milder asthma with steroids may also help to reduce bronchial inflammation and positively affect both the impairment and risk domains. In addition, their ability to reduce allergic inflammation has led to the widespread use of steroids in all allergic diseases, including those of the nose, eye, skin, and gastrointestinal tract. However,

it must be stressed that steroids have potentially debilitating, unwanted effects when used systemically in a chronic fashion, incorrectly or inappropriately.

The natural glucocorticoid released from the zona fasciularis of the human adrenal cortex is hydrocortisone. While possessing potent anti-inflammatory effects, hydrocortisone also carries with it considerable glucocorticoid (Fig. 7.7) and mineralocorticoid effects. Chemical manipulation of the steroid molecule has essentially removed the mineralocorticoid action but, to date, has been unable to separate anti-inflammatory and glucocorticoid effects – the latter causing the major unwanted effects with systemic therapy. Further chemical manipulation has led to an optimization of the pharmacokinetic profile of synthetic steroids. For systemic activity, this increases potency and extends duration of action (e.g. prednisolone and dexamethasone). For topical administration, a different pharmacokinetic profile is required, viz. slow absorption from the site of delivery and rapid

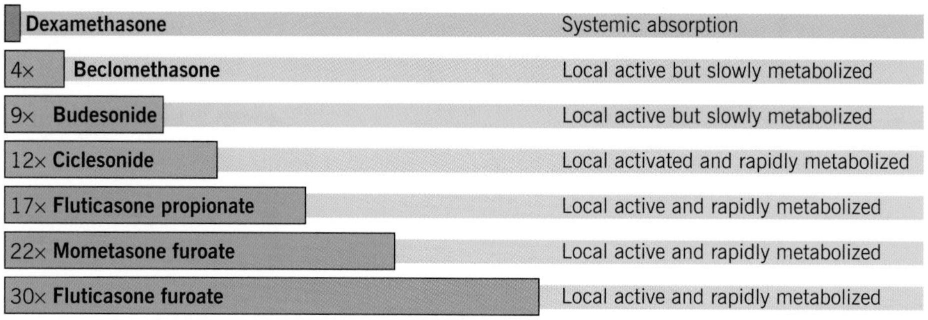

Dexamethasone		Systemic absorption
4×	Beclomethasone	Local active but slowly metabolized
9×	Budesonide	Local active but slowly metabolized
12× Ciclesonide		Local activated and rapidly metabolized
17× Fluticasone propionate		Local active and rapidly metabolized
22× Mometasone furoate		Local active and rapidly metabolized
30× Fluticasone furoate		Local active and rapidly metabolized

Fig. 7.8 Relative affinity of corticosteroids for the glucocorticoid receptor versus dexamethasone (=1).

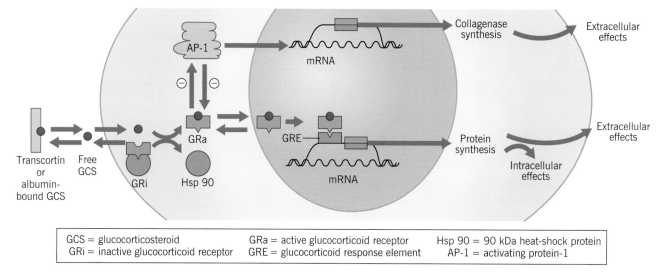

GCS = glucocorticosteroid GRa = active glucocorticoid receptor Hsp 90 = 90 kDa heat-shock protein
GRi = inactive glucocorticoid receptor GRE = glucocorticoid response element AP-1 = activating protein-1

Fig. 7.9 Intracellular mechanisms of action of corticosteroids (for details see text).

metabolism once the drug enters the systemic circulation. The first of these criteria was met with the introduction of the dipropionate ester of beclomethasone (Fig. 7.8), which has been used in aerosol form for several years with few overt systemic effects especially at low to medium doses. The second of these criteria is now being achieved with the introduction of many newer formulations including fluticasone propionate and furoate, mometasone, and ciclesonide (see Fig. 7.8). Ciclesonide also has the unique feature of being a relatively weak prodrug that is converted to its active form by lung esterases.

Delivery devices for corticosteroid metered dose inhalers (MDIs) are changing. Inhalers using chlorofluorocarbon (CFC) as propellant were banned in many countries, including the USA, in 2009 because of their ability to deplete the Earth's ozone layer. In most cases, propellant has been replaced by hydroflouroalkane (HFA), which is more environmentally friendly. In addition, some manufacturers have taken advantage of this enforced change to develop preparations (e.g. beclomethasone (Qvar) and ciclesonide) with a smaller particle size that penetrate deeper into the lung.

Mechanism of action

Both natural and synthetic steroids are highly lipophilic and largely bound to one of two plasma proteins: transcortin, a specific corticosteroid-binding globulin that binds glucocorticoids with high affinity, and albumin, which binds all steroids with low affinity. Free steroid molecules diffuse across the cell membrane where they interact with glucocorticoid receptors (GR) in the cytoplasm (Fig. 7.9). In the absence of glucocorticoids, inactive glucocorticoid receptors (GRi) are maintained in their resting state by being bound to a 90 kDa heat-shock protein. Interaction with a glucocorticoid molecule leads to shedding of the heat-shock protein to expose the active site. The resultant activated receptor (GRa) then diffuses into the nucleus where it interacts with a specific glucocorticoid response element (GRE) on the chromatin of the DNA to influence transcription and, consequently, de novo synthesis of steroid-susceptible proteins. Two examples of proteins whose synthesis are up-regulated are lipomodulin, which exerts an anti-inflammatory activity by inhibiting the activity of phospholipase A_2 and inhibitory factor κB (IκB), the inhibitory factor of nuclear factor κB (NF-κB), which is the transcription factor responsible for the synthesis of many proinflammatory cytokines and adhesion proteins. Glucocorticoids may also down-regulate transcription. An example of this is the inhibition of transcription of activating protein-1 (AP-1), a factor responsible for the synthesis of many proinflammatory cytokines and growth factors. In addition, corticosteroids may reduce the stability of messenger RNA for cytokines such as IL-4. The complexities of these processes account for the considerable time delay of 6–12 hours, even after intravenous administration, before the beneficial effects of corticosteroids begin to be observed.

At the cellular level, glucocorticoids suppress both acute and chronic inflammation, irrespective of cause, by inhibiting many steps in the inflammatory process. Some cellular actions pertinent to allergy are shown in Figure 7.10. Of these, corticosteroid reduction of proinflammatory cytokine production from many cells, including Th2 lymphocytes, mast cells, and eosinophils, reduction of eosinophil and mast cell influx and maturation, and promotion of apoptosis in inflammatory cells are likely to be the mechanisms by which corticosteroids achieve their long-term anti-inflammatory effects in chronic allergic disease (Fig. 7.11). Their therapeutic benefits are apparent within 6–12 hours of intravenous injection in acute severe asthma, and are more likely to be due to the ability of the drugs to reduce odema, reduce the local generation of ecosanoids following lipomodulin generation, reduce inflammatory cell influx and activation, and reverse adrenoceptor down-regulation.

The intracellular events that are responsible for the anti-inflammatory effects of glucocorticoids cannot be separated from their effects on glucose, protein, and lipid metabolism and their suppressive effects on the hypothalamus–pituitary–adrenal (HPA) axis. These effects are summarized in Figure 7.7. It should be noted that all glucocorticoids, whether natural or synthetic, will exert these effects when present in the systemic circulation. Furthermore, the magnitude of the side effects is dependent on:

- the dose of the drug absorbed systemically
- the presence of active metabolites
- the potency and duration of the systemic effect
- the duration of treatment.

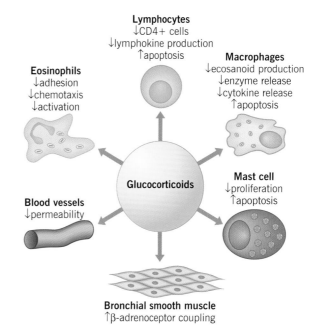

Fig. 7.10 Possible mechanisms by which corticosteroids reduce allergic diseases.

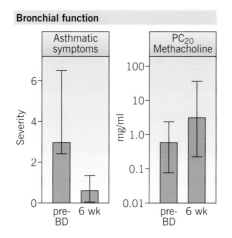

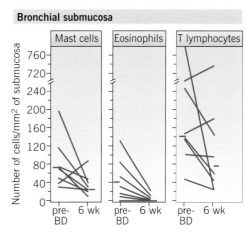

Fig. 7.11 The effect of beclomethasone dipropionate in asthma. Patients were examined before and after treatment with beclomethasone dipropionate (BD), 1000 μg a day by inhalation. Improvements were observed in subjective symptoms and bronchial hyperresponsiveness to methacholine. These were paralleled by significant falls in submucosal mast cell and eosinophil numbers as assessed in bronchial biopsies.

Thus, instigation of systemic treatment should begin only when bearing in mind the balance between beneficial and harmful effects of corticosteroids and with the knowledge that suppression of the HPA axis is likely to lead to adrenocortical atrophy, particularly with prolonged parenteral treatment. Although adrenocortical atrophy is reversible, this occurs only slowly, thus making it potentially dangerous to withdraw corticosteroids abruptly from a chronically treated patient.

Uses and administration

Asthma

The choice of an individual corticosteroid for the treatment of allergic disease depends on the route of administration. For oral use or for intravenous use, as in acute severe asthma, the drug should be rapidly absorbed and slowly metabolized, have a high affinity for the receptor, and be devoid of mineralocorticoid actions. These criteria are best met by prednisolone, prednisone, and dexamethasone. To minimize unwanted side effects, short duration of parenteral therapy, generally less than 48 hours, is recommended. This is typically followed by oral dosages of 0.5 to 1 mg per kilogram per day for up to 14 days. Neither the optimal dose nor the duration of treatment has been defined by evidence based guidelines and treatment should be tailored to the individual patient. It is not necessary to taper oral corticosteroids and they can be abruptly stopped if given for less than 2 weeks. With the advent of newer and more potent topical preparations, it is rare for patients to be on chronic oral steroid treatment. To minimize side effects of oral steroid treatment, lower doses given on an every-other-day schedule should be tried. The number of courses of systemic steroids an individual patient receives over the course of 6–12 months is a good indication of asthma control.

In patients with chronic persistent asthma, regardless of severity, the initial best treatment is an inhaled corticosteroid. Based on the patient's presentation, a low, medium or high daily dose should be started as recommended by evidence-based guidelines. Differences between individual steroid preparations should be taken into account when prescribing. The ideal pharmacokinetic properties of such a drug are slow absorption from the site of deposition and rapid metabolism once absorbed systemically. Beclomethasone has the potential for more adverse affects owing to active metabolites and is typically avoided in young children because of the possibility of impaired growth rates. Systemic adverse affects of newer inhaled corticosteroids are rarely seen unless the doses exceed the recommended high daily dose in evidence-based guidelines. However, individual patients should be monitored for cataracts, oral thrush, skin thinning, easy bruisability, and other potential adverse effects. It is also important to consider the concomitant use of other steroid preparations such as those for the skin and nose when assessing possible adverse consequences. In addition, frequent oral corticosteroid 'bursts' in patients receiving chronic high-dose topical corticosteroids increase the risk of adverse events such as osteoporosis. Clinically important adrenal insufficiency is extremely rare in patients receiving topical corticosteroids alone. In addition to adverse consequences of an individual corticosteroid, another major consideration in choosing a particular formulation is the delivery system. For example, the HFA preparations of beclomethasone and ciclesonide have smaller particle sizes that translate into better delivery into the distal lung. In younger children and the elderly, metered-dose inhalers are sometimes difficult to use and dry-powder inhalers can be a better choice providing the patients have an adequate inspiratory flow rate to actuate the device and achieve good drug delivery.

Guidelines for the appropriate use of steroids in asthma have been formulated in many countries. Briefly, they suggest the introduction of inhaled preparations even in relatively mild asthma, increased inhaled doses as asthma becomes more severe/less controlled, and the use of oral therapy only when the disease cannot be controlled satisfactorily by inhaled therapy. It is important to recognize that the dose–response effect of inhaled corticosteroids is relatively steep, so that more may not necessarily improve efficacy but could lead to more side effects.

Many important questions involving the use of inhaled corticosteroids for asthma have recently been investigated. Although inhaled corticosteroids improve symptoms, improve lung function, reduce airway hyper-responsiveness, reduce the need for rescue inhaler, and decrease overall morbidity and mortality, there is little evidence to support their effects on preventing the development or significantly altering the course of asthma.

In summary, inhaled corticosteroids are the best treatment for chronic persistent asthma, but have little in the way of disease-modifying effects. As with other therapies, not everyone responds to corticosteroids. Preliminary data suggest that risk factors for unresponsiveness include cigarette smoking and possibly obesity.

Allergic rhinitis

In allergic rhinitis, steroid nasal sprays are used particularly to relieve nasal blockage. They reduce the influx of mast cells and other inflammatory cells into the nasal mucosa, but, as they do not inhibit mast cell degranulation or inhibit the effects of histamine, they do not provide immediate relief. However, some symptom improvement has been demonstrated in less than 12 hours. Intranasal corticosteroids are the single most effective therapy for allergic rhinitis and should be used unless symptoms are mild and intermittent. Although there is less evidence to support the use of intranasal corticosteroids for other types of rhinitis, they are frequently the drug of choice especially for patients that have nasal polyps or non-allergic rhinitis with eosinophilia. Systemic therapy should be used only in extremely debilitating conditions and for a short period of time, typically less than 1 week.

Allergic conjunctivitis

Steroid eye drops are very effective in the treatment of many forms of conjunctivitis, including allergic conjunctivitis. In extreme conditions, the drug may also be given systemically. In eye disease, however, steroids should be used only under expert medical supervision because of their local unwanted effects. The most potentially dangerous of these are as follows.

- Aggravation of 'red eye', a condition of dendritic ulceration caused by the herpes simplex virus, may occur. The local immunosuppressive effects of steroids worsen this condition and may lead to loss of sight, or even of the eye.

- In persons predisposed to chronic simple glaucoma, steroid eye drops may induce 'steroid glaucoma' after a few weeks' use. Again, this may be sight threatening.

- Use of high doses of steroids for conjunctival inflammation, particularly when given systemically, is associated with the development of 'steroid cataract'. This problem is both dose and duration related. For example, daily oral dosage with 15 mg of prednisolone (or equivalent with other steroids) for prolonged periods carries a risk of 'steroid cataract' of around 75%.

Urticaria and atopic dermatitis

In the skin, steroid creams and ointments are used for a wide variety of inflammatory conditions, including eczema and atopic dermatitis. They act to suppress symptoms and are in no sense curative, rebound exacerbations often occurring on cessation of treatment. They are not of value in urticaria (unless given systemically) and are contraindicated in rosacea and ulcerative conditions, which they worsen. Because of their local unwanted effects (Box 7.1) and their ability to be absorbed through the skin and cause systemic effects, steroids should not be the drugs of first choice but reserved for the more problematic conditions. Even then, the lowest strength of the least potent steroids should be used. Also, short courses are recommended wherever possible. The use of topical steroids in the skin of children is discouraged because of the systemic effects.

Conclusions

Corticosteroids afford effective therapy in allergic disease when the appropriate formulations are given and the physician observes with diligence the basic rules to avoid unwanted effects.

Box 7.1 Possible detrimental effects of steroids in the skin

- Spread and worsening of untreated infection
- Thinning of the skin, which may be only partially reversible
- Irreversible striae atrophicae
- Increased hair growth
- Perioral dermatitis
- Acne at the site of application
- Mild depigmentation of the skin

H$_1$-Antihistamines

Histamine, released from mast cells and basophils, plays a major role in the pathophysiology of all allergic diseases, including rhinitis, urticaria, asthma, and systemic anaphylaxis. Therefore, prevention of its ability to stimulate its target organs has presented an obvious goal in drug development. Today, we know that histamine has many biological actions mediated through four distinct receptors (Table 7.2). H$_1$-receptor stimulation activates phospholipase C and is responsible for most of the symptoms of the early phase allergic response including rhinorrhoea, itching and sneezing in allergic rhinitis, and whealing and pruritus in urticaria. The H$_2$-receptor stimulates cyclic AMP production and is primarily involved in gastric acid secretion, although it has some amelioratory actions on inflammatory leukocytes. The H$_3$- and H$_4$-receptors are Gi linked and inhibit cyclic AMP production. Whilst the H$_3$-receptor is primarily neuroprotective in the central nervous system, it has recently been demonstrated in human nasal tissue on sympathetic nerves and colocalized with H$_1$-receptors. The H$_4$-receptor is largely expressed on haemopoietic cells, particularly dendritic cells, eosinophils, and mast cells, stimulation of which leads to amplification of histamine-mediated immune responses. H$_4$-antihistamines have recently been shown to be particularly effective in models of pruritus, but whether this results from peripheral or central actions is not yet known. No H$_3$-antihistamines or H$_4$-antihistamines are available for clinical use at present, but are in clinical trials. The remainder of this chapter will focus on H$_1$-antihistamines.

H$_1$-antihistamines are usually classified into the older or first-generation antihistamines and the newer or second-generation antihistamines. The commonly used members of these drug classes are listed in Box 7.2 and the chemical structures of some of them shown in Figure 7.12. The main differences between the two generations of drugs are their propensity to cause central nervous system (CNS) sedation and their side effects. The first-generation antihistamines penetrate well into the CNS where they induce sedation. Although this sedative effect

Table 7.2 Receptor-mediated effects of histamine

Target tissue	Effect	Receptor
Airways		
Bronchial smooth muscle	Contraction	H_1
Bronchial epithelium	Increased permeability	H_1
Secretory glands	Increased glycoprotein secretion	H_1, H_2
	Secretion	H_1
Blood vessels		
Postcapillary venules	Dilatation	H_1
	Increased permeability	H_1
Nerves		
Sensory nerves	Stimulation	H_1
Central nervous system	Neuroregulation	H_3
Nose	Rhinorrhoea	H_1
	Oedema	H_1
Leukocytes	Modulation of lymphocyte function	H_2
	Chemotaxis of dendritic cells, mast cells and eosinophils	H_4

Box 7.2 Common H_1-receptor antagonists

First generation	Second generation
Hydroxyzine	Acrivastine
Diphenhydramine	Cetirizine
Chlorpheniramine	Desloratadine
	Fexofenadine
	Levocetirizine
	Loratadine
	Mequitazine
	Rupatadine

Mechanism of action

H_1-antihistamines are not receptor antagonists as previously thought, but are inverse agonists; therefore the preferred term for them today is 'H_1-antihistamines'. When neither histamine nor antihistamine is present, the active and inactive states of the H_1-receptor are in equilibrium or a balanced state. Histamine combines preferentially with the active form of the receptor to stabilize it and shift the balance towards the activated state and stimulate the cell (Fig. 7.13). In contrast, H_1-antihistamines stabilize the inactive form and shift the equilibrium in the opposite direction. Thus, the amount of histamine-induced stimulation of a cell or tissue depends on the balance between histamine and H_1-antihistamine.

Histamine effects stimulated through the H_1-receptor include: pruritus, pain, vasodilatation, vascular permeability, hypotension, flushing, headache, tachycardia, bronchoconstriction, and stimulation of airway vagal afferent nerves and cough receptors, and decreased atrioventricular-node conduction. Although most of the effects of histamine in allergic diseases are mediated by H_1-receptor stimulation, hypotension, tachycardia, flushing, and headache, cutaneous itching and nasal congestion have been suggested to have a minor component mediated through both H_1- and H_2-receptors.

Through H_1-receptors histamine has proinflammatory activity mediated by its ability to activate the transcription factor NF-κB and increase the synthesis of the adhesion molecules e-selectin, ICAM-1 and VCAM-1, and cytokines including IL-8, GM-CSF, and TNF. By reducing the production of these molecules, H_1-antihistamines reduce the accumulation of inflammatory cells, such as eosinophils and neutrophils, and ameliorate allergic inflammation. However, these effects are minor compared with intranasal corticosteroids.

There are approximately 64 000 histamine-producing neurons, located in the tuberomamillary nucleus of the human brain. The H_1-receptor mediated actions in the brain include arousal in the circadian sleep/wake cycle, reinforcement of learning and memory, fluid balance, suppression of feeding, control of body temperature, control of cardiovascular system, and mediation of stress-triggered release of ACTH and β-endorphin from the

may have some clinical benefit in the treatment of night-time exacerbations of allergy responses, especially in children, it severely compromises such drug use in ambulatory patients in whom doses capable of causing only a 3–5-fold shift of the histamine dose–response curve may be given. The potential to enhance the central effects of alcohol and other CNS sedatives further limits such use. In addition, many of these drugs also have actions that reflect their poor receptor selectivity, including an atropine-like effect and blockade of both α-adrenergic and 5-hydroxytryptamine receptors.

The second-generation H_1-antihistamines cause much-reduced CNS sedation and are essentially free of this effect at doses recommended for the treatment of rhinitis or urticaria. Consequently, the shift of the histamine dose–response curve that can be achieved with these drugs is much greater. Also, these drugs have little or no atropine-like activity or effects at other receptors. Some second-generation drugs have been suggested to have antiallergic and anti-inflammatory effects that may contribute to their therapeutic benefit.

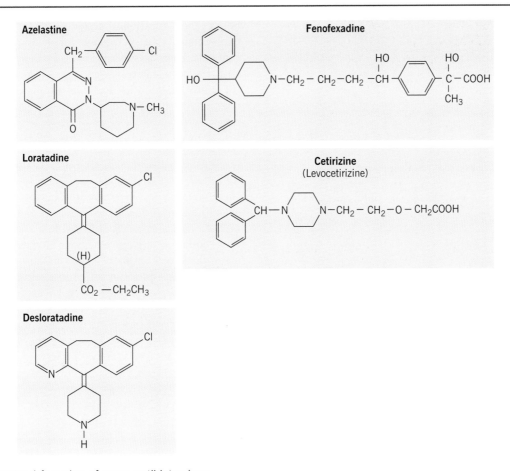

Fig. 7.12 Structural formulae of some antihistamines.

pituitary gland. First-generation H₁-antihistamines, such as chlorpheniramine, diphenhydramine, hydroxyzine, and promethazine, penetrate readily into the brain, in which they occupy 50–90% of the H₁-receptors, as shown by positron-emission tomography (PET). Even in recommended doses, H₁-antihistamines frequently lead to daytime somnolence, sedation, drowsiness, fatigue, and impaired concentration and memory. Consequently these drugs have been implicated in road traffic and airplane accidents and, in children, poor examination results. Furthermore, due to long half-lives, these agents can cause impairment the next morning even when used before sleep. It is for these reasons that the use of first-generation H₁-antihistamines should be discouraged.

On the other hand, second-generation H₁-antihistamines penetrate the CNS poorly, as they are actively pumped out by a number of organic anion-transporting protein pumps, such as P-glycoprotein, which is expressed on the luminal surface of vascular endothelial cells in the blood vessels that constitute the blood–brain barrier. The propensity of these drugs to occupy H₁-receptors in the CNS varies from 0% for fexofenadine to 30% for cetirizine. Thus, second-generation H₁-antihistamines are relatively

free of sedating effects and impairment of driving performance. Currently, desloratadine, fexofenadine, and loratadine are the H₁-antihistamines for which pilots can receive a waiver for use from the Federal Aviation Administration.

Cardiac toxic effects induced by H₁-antihistamines occur rarely and independently of the H₁- receptor. Two early second-generation H₁-antihistamines, astemizole and terfenadine, which are no longer marketed, potentially prolong the QT interval and have been shown to cause torsades de pointes. No such effects occur with new second-generation H₁-antihistamines.

All of the first-generation H₁-antihistamines and some of the second-generation antihistamines are oxidatively metabolized by the hepatic cytochrome P450 system, the main exceptions being levocetirizine, cetirizine, and fexofenadine. Levocetirizine and cetirizine are excreted largely unchanged in urine and fexofenadine is excreted largely in the faeces. Hepatic metabolism has several implications: prolongation of the serum half-life in patients with hepatic dysfunction and those receiving concomitant cytochrome P450 inhibitors, such as ketoconazole and erythromycin. Also, a longer duration of

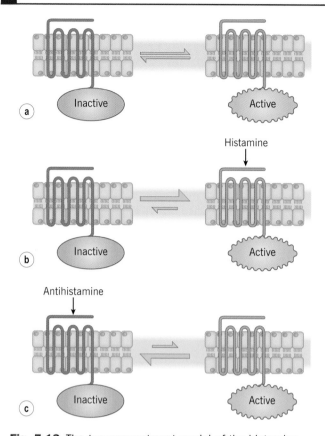

Fig. 7.13 The two-compartment model of the histamine receptor. The transmembrane histamine H_1-receptors are shown in their inactive (left) and active (right) forms. Panel (a) shows that the inactive and active conformations of the H_1-receptor are in equilibrium in the absence of either histamine or an H_1-antihistamine. In reality, the equilibrium would be very much in favour of the much more stable inactive form. Panel (b) shows the effect of histamine, which has a preferential affinity for the active conformation of the receptor. Histamine combines with the active form of the receptor to stabilize it and thus cause the equilibrium to shift in favour of the activated form. Panel (c) shows the effect of an antihistamine, which has a preferential affinity for the inactive conformation of the receptor. Consequentially, the antihistamine combines with the inactive form of the receptor to stabilize it and thus cause the equilibrium to shift in the opposite direction. (Adapted from Leurs R, Church MK, Taglialatela M. H1-antihistamines: inverse agonism, anti-inflammatory actions and cardiac effects. Clin Exp Allergy 2002; 32:489–498.)

action is found in elderly patients who have reduced liver function. Although these interactions have a theoretical possibility of precipitating unwanted effects, the safety margin of second-generation antihistamines in particular is so great that serious reactions are very rare.

Uses and administration

All H_1-antihistamines are well absorbed from the gastrointestinal tract after oral dosage. With most oral H_1-antihistamines, symptomatic relief is observed within 1–4 hours. Their duration of action varies from several hours to 24 hours, that of the second-generation drugs being generally around 24 hours. No tolerance to the suppressive effects on skin test reactivity to histamine is observed for at least 3 months. Residual suppression of skin test reactivity to allergens may last for up to 7 days after the discontinuation of an H_1-antihistamine.

Allergic rhinitis

In patients with allergic rhinitis, H_1-antihistamines are useful in ameliorating sneezes, itching, and nasal discharge but are less effective in relieving nasal blockage – even though studies have shown prolonged courses of H_1-antihistamines they do provide a statistically significant reduction in nasal blockage. However, reduction of nasal blockage is primarily the domain of the intranasal corticosteroids. In some patients, a combination of a leukotriene receptor antagonist with an H_1-antihistamine has been shown to reduce nasal symptoms more than monotherapy with each of the agents.

Topical nasal sprays of azelastine and olopatadine have a rapid onset of action, are well tolerated and have clinical efficacy for treating allergic rhinitis that is reported to be equal or superior to that of oral second-generation H_1-antihistamines. Nasal sprays have the advantage of not causing systemic effects, but have the disadvantages of having a bitter taste, especially azelastine, and having to be administered twice daily.

Allergic conjunctivitis

The ocular symptoms of allergic conjunctivitis or rhinoconjunctivitis such as itching, tearing, and reddening are reduced by administration of H_1-antihistamines either systemically or locally as eye drops. Topical H_1-antihistamines include azelastine, epinastine, ketotifen, and olopatadine. Some of these agents also inhibit mast cell degranulation.

Urticaria and atopic dermatitis

Histamine can reproduce all of the symptoms of urticaria, including wheal, flare, and itching. Consequently, the recent guideline on the management of urticaria from the European Academy of Allergy and Clinical Immunology (EAACI), the Global Allergy and Asthma European Network (GA$_2$LEN), the European Dermatology Forum (EDF) and the World Allergy Organization (WAO) recommend second-generation non-sedating H_1-antihistamines as the first-line medication in all types of acute and chronic urticaria. Furthermore, they recommend that, if standard dosing is not effective, the dosage may be increased up to four-fold.

In atopic dermatitis, itching is one of the major symptoms and scratching often causes a worsening of the lesion. Since histamine is a major pruritogen, the use of H_1-antihistamines may help to relieve pruritus, reduces scratching, and seems to have glucocorticoid-sparing effects.

Asthma

In chronic asthma, current evidence does not support the use of H_1-antihistamines for treatment. However, second-generation H_1-antihistamines, especially used in combination with intranasal corticosteroids, are reported to reduce symptoms of allergic asthma patients and exacerbation of asthma in adult patients with allergic rhinitis. The most likely explanation for this is that the nose warms, humidifies, and filters the air before it reaches the lung. If a patient's nose is blocked, this protective function is lost.

Anaphylaxis

Although most of the symptoms of anaphylaxis can be reproduced by histamine, the treatment of choice for this condition is injection of adrenaline. The use of an H_1-antihistamine, such as chlorpheniramine or diphenhydramine, given as an intramuscular injection or intravenous infusion, can be useful for adjunctive relief of pruritus, urticaria, rhinorrhoea, and other symptoms.

Conclusions

The most obvious adverse effects of first-generation H_1-antihistamines are those on the CNS, including drowsiness, impaired driving performance, fatigue, lassitude, and dizziness. In addition, dry mouth, urinary retention, gastrointestinal upset, and appetite stimulation may occur. Clinical tolerance to the sedating effects of first-generation H_1-antihistamines has been suggested but has not been found consistently in objective tests. If taken by mothers, first-generation drugs may cause irritability, drowsiness, or respiration suppression in nursing infants. The incidence of CNS sedation from second-generation H_1-antihistamines, when used at the manufacturers' recommended doses, is greatly reduced or absent.

Some first-generation H_1-antihistamines may cause sinus tachycardia, reflex tachycardia, and supraventricular arrhythmia, and prolongation of the QT interval in a dose-dependent manner. The potentially unwanted serious cardiac effects of astemizole and terfenadine, which are not marketed now, are described above.

Some of the oral H_1-antihistamines including cetirizine, levocetirizine, and loratadine, are considered relatively safe for use during pregnancy (FDA category B: no adverse effect in animals, but no data in humans, or adverse effects in animals but no adverse effects in humans).

Leukotriene synthesis inhibitors and receptor antagonists

Leukotrienes (LTs) are important inflammatory lipid mediators derived from arachidonic acid following its oxidation by 5-lipoxygenase (5-LO) on the nuclear envelope. There are two types of LTs: the dihydroxy acid LTB4 and the cysteinyl LTs (CysLT: LTC_4, LTD_4, LTE_4).

5-LO mediates the conversion of arachidonic acid into the unstable epoxide LTA_4, which is converted by LTA4 hydrolase into LTB_4 or by LTC_4 synthase into LTC4, depending on cell type; eosinophils predominantly produce CysLTs, whereas neutrophils mainly produce LTB_4. Once LTC_4 is released from inflammatory cells, it is converted into LTD_4 by γ-glutamyl transpeptidase and subsequently into stable LTE_4 by a dipeptidase. LTB4 has a specific LTB receptor and acts mainly as a neutrophil chemoattractant.

CysLTs show activities through two different receptors: $CysLT_1$ and $CysLT_2$ receptors (Table 7.3). The $CysLT_1$ receptor seems to be very important for the induction of asthmatic reaction as it induces constriction of airway smooth muscle, increases microvasculature leakage and secretion of bronchial mucosa, and induces the inflammation of the airways, including eosinophil infiltration, and finally hypertrophy of bronchial smooth muscle. Hypertrophy of smooth muscle is a component of airway remodelling seen in asthma (Fig. 7.14). In addition, the $CysLT_1$ receptor has important roles in allergic reactions, such as allergic rhinitis, atopic dermatitis, and chronic urticaria.

CysLTs are produced in response to allergic or other stimuli. Allergen-induced provocation of asthma is associated with the increased leukotriene levels in bronchoalveolar lavage fluids. Furthermore, increased urinary levels

Table 7.3 Summary of the properties of human CysLT receptors

	Receptor	
	Human CysLT1	Human CysLT2
Amino acid	337	346
Chromosome	Xq13-q21	13q14.2
Binding affinity	LTD4 >> LTC4 > LTE4	LTD4 = LTC4 > LTE4
Antagonist	Montelukast	
	Zafirlukast	
	Pranlukast	
Expression	Lung smooth muscle	Lung smooth muscle
	Eosinophils	Brain and Purkinje cells
	Mast cells	Macrophages
	B lymphocytes	Mast cells
	Monocytes/ macrophages	PBL

LTC4, D4, E4, leukotriene C4, D4, E4; PBL, peripheral blood lymphocyte. (From Evans JF. Cysteinyl leukotriene receptors. Prostaglandins Other Lipid Mediat 2002; 68–69:587–597.)

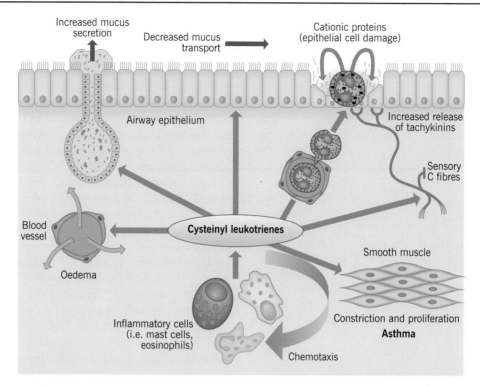

Increased mucus secretion

Decreased mucus transport

Cationic proteins (epithelial cell damage)

Airway epithelium

Increased release of tachykinins

Sensory C fibres

Cysteinyl leukotrienes

Blood vessel

Oedema

Smooth muscle

Constriction and proliferation
Asthma

Inflammatory cells (i.e. mast cells, eosinophils)

Chemotaxis

Fig. 7.14 The actions of cysteinyl leukotrienes in asthma.

of the stable leukotriene metabolite, LTE$_4$, are found in both allergen- and aspirin-induced asthma.

Importantly, CysLTs have been found in bronchoalveolar lavage fluids despite treatment with low to high doses of corticosteroids although corticosteroids are the most potent anti-inflammatory agents used in the treatment of asthma, supporting the theory that corticosteroids do not directly reduce the production of CysLTs. Consequently, drugs that interfere with either the synthesis of leukotrienes or their receptor actions are likely to be beneficial in asthma. Both of these have been successful, leading to the development of new drugs for the treatment of asthma.

The LT receptor antagonists (LTRAs), montelukast, zafirlukast, and pranlukast were approved in 1998, 1996 in the USA, and 1995 in Japan, respectively. Both montelukast and pranlukast are approved for the treatment of allergic rhinitis in adults. In 1996 the leukotriene synthesis inhibitor, zileuton, was approved for use in the USA.

Mechanism of action

The development of drugs to inhibit the synthesis of leukotrienes has been aimed at two targets, 5-LO and 5-LO-activating protein (FLAP). Zileuton is an antioxidant inhibitor of 5-LO. However, it is not entirely specific as it inhibits some other oxidizing enzymes, such as hepatic microsomal cytochrome enzyme, CYP3A4, involved in the metabolism of terfenadine, theophylline,

and warfarin. Following allergen challenge of atopic asthmatic subjects, zileuton produces inhibition of the early, but not the late asthmatic response. The degree of inhibition of bronchospasm is correlated with the reduction of urinary LTE$_4$. Zileuton also suppresses aspirin-induced asthma, in which a reduction of the urinary excretion of LTE$_4$ is also observed.

Although FLAP inhibitors have shown activity in experimental models and have been used to suppress early and late asthmatic response in humans, none has yet been marketed, largely because of their lack of potency.

LTRAs have been developed to prevent the interaction of LTC$_4$ and LTD$_4$ at the CysLT$_1$ receptor, which is responsible for many of the effects of asthma as described. The human CysLT1 receptors are expressed in peripheral blood leukocytes (eosinophils, subsets of monocytes, macrophages, basophils, and pregranulocytic CD34$^+$ cells), lung smooth muscle cells and interstitial macrophages, and spleen, and less strongly in the small intestine, pancreas, and placenta. Human CysLT$_2$ receptors are expressed in heart (myocytes, fibroblasts, and vascular smooth muscle cells), adrenal medulla, peripheral blood leukocytes, spleen, lymph nodes, CNS, interstitial macrophages, and smooth muscle cells in the lung. Because LTRAs have relatively high receptor selectivity and do not block the CysLT$_2$ receptor, they usually have fewer unwanted effects than do leukotriene synthesis inhibitors. LTRAs suppress airway inflammation including eosinophil infiltration. In sensitized experimental animals, LTRAs suppress antigen-induced early and late responses

Box 7.3 Effects of leukotriene antagonists (LTRAs) in the airways in asthma

Suppression of:

- constriction of bronchial smooth muscle
- increased vascular permeability
- increased mucus production
- increased airway hyperresponsiveness
- airway inflammation including eosinophil migration and activation
- airway remodelling including airway smooth muscle hyperplasia

and eosinophil infiltration in bronchoalveolar lavage fluid. In asthma patients, prolonged administration of LTRAs suppresses eosinophils in sputum and the airway wall. They also suppress allergen-induced early and late asthmatic responses.

In antigen-sensitized/challenged animal models, montelukast has been reported to have antiremodelling activities, such as reduction of smooth muscle hypertrophy and subepithelial fibrosis and pranlukast abolished LTD_4 epithelium growth factor-induced human airway smooth muscle proliferation in vitro (Box 7.3).

As enhanced leukotriene production is a primary feature in aspirin-induced asthma, it is hardly surprising that $CysLT_1$-receptor antagonists inhibit this response.

In chronic asthma, zafirlukast and intravenous/oral montelukast show a rapid increase of the forced expired volume in 1 second (FEV_1), suggesting that leukotrienes are continuously released in chronic asthma, thereby causing bronchoconstriction and enhancing non-specific airway hyperresponsiveness.

Uses and administration

Asthma

LTRAs (montelukast 10 mg once daily, zafirlukast 20 mg twice daily, and pranlukast 225 mg twice daily in adults) and zileuton 600 mg four times daily have shown to improve pulmonary function and symptoms in patients with mild-to-severe asthma. In children, montelukast (2 years of age or older), zafirlukast (5 years of age or older), and pranlukast (2 years of age or older) are indicated for asthma. In both adults and children, LTRAs provide significant protection against exercise- and antigen-induced bronchoconstriction as well as AIA. In addition to beneficial effects on pulmonary functions, LTRAs and zileuton decreased markers of airway inflammation. LTRAs are approved for treatment of allergic rhinitis. Moreover, LTRAs are generally safe and well tolerated.

Randomized, double-blind, placebo-controlled clinical trials have demonstrated the efficacies of LTRAs (montelukast 10 mg once daily, zafirlukast 20 mg twice daily, and pranlukast 225 mg twice daily) and zileuton 600 mg

four times daily in improving pulmonary function, symptoms, and quality of life and decreasing risk of asthma exacerbation in patients with mild-to-moderate asthma compared with placebo.

LTRAs or zileuton can be an alternative therapy to low-dose inhaled corticosteroids in mild persistent asthma, although they are less effective in most studies. Low-dose inhaled corticosteroids improve pulmonary functions to a greater degree than LTRAs or zileuton. However, the differences between low-dose inhaled corticosteroid and LTRAs are not as pronounced in the risk domain, asthma exacerbation. None the less, evidence-based guidelines recommend low-dose inhaled corticosteroid over LTRAs or zileuton for the management of mild persistent asthma. Typically, only 40–60% of patients respond to LTRAs, so physicians need to evaluate whether or not a given patient should remain on the treatment. If patients do not respond within 4–8 weeks, an alternative treatment such as inhaled corticosteroids should be used. Currently, there are no predictors or biomarkers to indicate who will respond to these agents. One caveat when considering which patients to place on LTRAs is ease of use. Patients unable to appropriately use inhalers, for example, very young children, would be candidates for LTRAs. In addition, some children are more susceptible to the adverse events related to inhaled corticosteroids, especially deleterious effects on growth rates, and LTRAs could be a suitable alternative. Finally, in patients that have concomitant allergic rhinitis, using a single agent that might treat both upper and lower airway symptoms can be an attractive alternative. In patients with moderate to severe asthma, LTRAs and zileuton can be used as an add-on therapy to inhaled corticosteroids. There is evidence that LTRAs, or zileuton. used in this way reduce the dose of inhaled corticosteroids required by patients with moderate-to-severe asthma, or improve asthma control in patients whose asthma is not controlled with low to high doses of inhaled corticosteroids. In patients inadequately controlled by low–medium dose inhaled corticosteroids, inhaled corticosteroids plus LTRAs or a double dose of inhaled corticosteroids showed similar progressive improvement in several measures of asthma control compared with baseline. Moreover LTRAs plus inhaled corticosteroids showed faster onset of action than a double dose of inhaled corticosteroids.

Evidence-based guidelines and Cochrane analysis indicate that long acting β-agonists (LABAs) are superior to LTRAs or zileuton as add-on therapy in patients uncontrolled with inhaled corticosteroids. A recently published study compared doubling the dose of inhaled corticosteroids against the addition of LABAs or montelukast in children not controlled on low-dose inhaled corticosteroids. The authors found that the addition of LABA was superior to either of the other two treatments and recommended LABAs as the preferred step-up therapy for the paediatric population.

LTRAs and zileuton have been used for the emergency management of acute asthma exacerbations. Intravenous LTRAs work rapidly, within 15 minutes, and result in added bronchodilatation to short-acting β-agonists. The peak effects of oral preparations are achieved later, approximately 2 hours, and result in additive bronchodilatation to short-acting β-agonist as well. These effects have been demonstrated both in adults and children and suggest that LTRAs could be useful in the management of acute severe asthma.

LTRAs decrease the number of eosinophils in sputum and peripheral blood suggesting that part of the effect of LTRAs is anti-inflammatory. LTRAs prevent exercised-induced asthma. No tolerance to the bronchoprotective effects has been observed with LTRAs.

Approximately 4–28% of adult patients have asthma exacerbation by taking aspirin or other NSAIDs with anticyclooxygenase activity. These patients show increased production of cysteinyl leukotrienes. Inhaled corticosteroids continue to be the mainstay of therapy, but LTRAs and zileuton are useful for additional control of underlying symptoms. We recommend that all patients with aspirin-induced asthma take LTRAs or zileuton.

Allergic rhinitis

In patients with seasonal and perennial rhinitis, with or without concomitant asthma, LTRAs improved nasal, eye, and throat symptoms as well as quality of life. However, the combination of an H_1-antihistamine plus LTRA does not consistently provide beneficial treatment effect over either agent alone. In addition, recent studies show that intranasal corticosteroids are more effective than LTRAs either alone or in combination with an antihistamine for the relief of seasonal allergic rhinitis.

Urticaria and atopic dermatitis

LTRAs and zileuton have had limited success in managing other allergic disorders including atopic dermatitis. In combination with H_1-antihistamines, LTRAs and zileuton might provide marginal beneficial effect over H_1-antihistamines alone for chronic urticaria.

Safety

LTRAs are generally safe and well tolerated. The incidence of adverse effects in asthma patients is similar to those seen in placebo in double-blind, placebo-controlled trials. To date, no specific adverse effects have been reported with these drugs. Zileuton and higher doses of zafirlukast can lead to elevations of liver enzymes and possible hepatitis. In patients on zileuton, alanine aminotransferase (ALT) levels should be monitored. Churg–Strauss syndrome (CSS), an eosinophilic vasculitis, has been reported with all three LTRAs and zileuton. It is speculated that they unmask an underlying vasculitic syndrome that was suppressed by previous corticosteroid therapy. Physicians should monitor complaints of neurological symptoms, new rashes, and worsening respiratory symptoms in patients on these agents, especially during corticosteroid tapering. Zileuton also inhibits the metabolism of other drugs that interact with the P450 system such as theophylline.

Conclusion

In summary, findings from many studies support the hypothesis that LTRAs and zileuton improve pulmonary functions and symptoms in patients with mild to moderate asthma, mediate anti-inflammatory effects, and complement the anti-inflammatory properties of corticosteroids. In patients with moderate-to-severe asthma, LTRAs or zileuton permit corticosteroid tapering. However, LABAs are the preferred add-on therapy according to evidence-based asthma treatment guidelines. In patients not controlled with inhaled corticosteroids and LABA, there is little evidence to support additive beneficial effects of LTRAs or zileuton. An advantage of LTRAs is their administration as a tablet rather than an inhaler, since compliance is an especially critical element in controlling asthma.

Cromolyn sodium and nedocromil sodium

The chromones, cromolyn sodium and nedocromil sodium (Fig. 7.15) are often termed 'antiallergic drugs'. Cromolyn sodium was originally introduced in the 1970s as a mast-cell stabilizer for the treatment of asthma while nedocromil sodium was marketed as a drug to reduce allergic inflammation. The similarity in the mechanisms of action of the two drugs indicates that they both have the two effects, the effect on the mast cell being

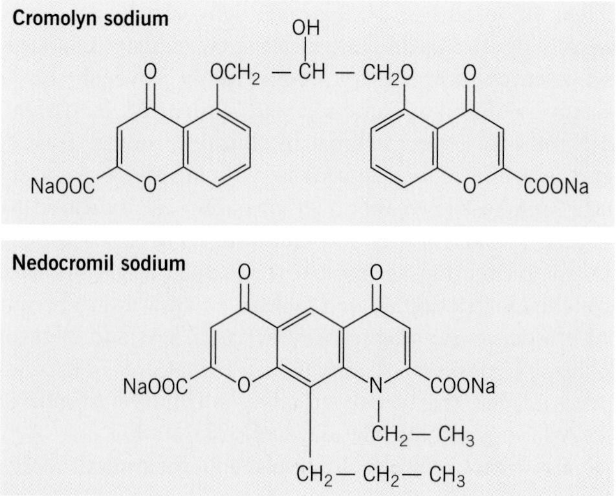

Fig. 7.15 Structures of cromolyn sodium and nedocromil sodium.

responsible for their ability to prevent and treat immediate hypersensitivity responses and the effect on allergic inflammation.

Both cromolin sodium and nedocromil sodium (see Fig. 7.15) are acidic drugs with pKa values of 1.0–2.5 and, consequently, exist almost exclusively in the ionized form at physiological pH (~7.4). These physicochemical characteristics mean that the drugs have negligible absorption from the gastrointestinal tract and must be given topically. Aerosols are available for asthma, both drops and sprays for rhinitis, and drops for conjunctivitis. In addition, oral solutions have been suggested for the topical treatment of gastrointestinal allergy. A major advantage of the drugs existing almost exclusively in the ionized form is that any drug absorbed systemically remains in the extracellular compartment, thus giving negligible toxicity.

Mechanism of action

The primary action of chromones is to inhibit a $Na^+/K^+/2Cl^-$ cotransporter involved in the activation of both mast cells and sensory neurons. This activity is shared with the loop diuretics, frusemide (US furosemide) and bumetanide. Although an action on mast cells may explain the action of the drugs on bronchoconstriction induced by allergen, exercise, and cold air, the effect induced by irritant agents, such as sulphur dioxide, is unlikely to be mast cell mediated. An effect on neuronal reflexes, possibly involving C-fibre sensory neurons, is more likely. The ability of nedocromil sodium to inhibit bronchoconstriction induced by bradykinin and capsaicin would support this theory. Thus, there are probably two complementary mechanisms by which chromones may exert their beneficial effects against the early phase of acute asthma attacks.

Uses and administration

Although cromolyn sodium and nedocromil sodium were both originally introduced for the treatment of asthma, they are now used widely as topical therapies for allergic rhinitis and conjunctivitis.

Asthma

Until the turn of the century, cromolyn sodium and nedocromil sodium had a well-established place in the control of mildly to moderately severe asthma, particularly in children. However, because of their relatively weak action and the fact that they are ineffective in approximately 30% of patients, a series of meta-analyses concluded that their effectiveness was no better than placebo. Guidelines now reflect this. However, many clinicians believe that, because of their freedom from toxicity, chromones may represent an appropriate therapy in children with mild asthma who are responsive to them.

Allergic rhinitis

Cromolyn sodium and nedocromil sodium drops and nasal sprays have found a place in the treatment of allergic rhinitis. For maximal effect, treatment should begin 2–3 weeks before the hay-fever season and continue throughout its duration. The only unwanted effect is local irritation of the nasal mucosa, very rarely associated with transient bronchospasm.

Allergic conjunctivitis

Cromolyn sodium and nedocromil sodium drops are also effective, particularly against the itch of allergic conjunctivitis. This is likely to result from the inhibition of activation of the sensory nerves transducing itch.

Conclusions

Because cromolyn sodium and nedocromil sodium have almost no systemic absorption they have negligible systemic adverse effects. This makes them particularly useful drugs for the treatment of allergic disease in patients, especially young children, where the unwanted effects of drugs of other classes may be a problem. The most common unwanted effects following inhalation are transient cough and mild wheezing. In the nose and the eye, they may cause transient stinging.

Non-steroidal anti-inflammatory drugs

Cyclooxygenase inhibition is the primary mechanism of action of all non-steroidal anti-inflammatory drugs (NSAIDs), such as aspirin, indomethacin (US indometacin), ibuprofen, or flurbiprofen. Consequently, they have the ability to cause a dose-related inhibition of the formation of all prostaglandins, whether potentially harmful or beneficial. In asthma, non-specific inhibition of the production of prostanoids, including the bronchoconstrictors PGD_2 and TXA_2, has some beneficial effects in acute allergen provocation but appears to have little benefit in clinical asthma. PGE_2 has been suggested to shift the balance of T cells in favour of a Th2 response in part by PGE_4-mediated mechanisms. However, NSAIDs may precipitate aspirin-induced asthma (AIA) in 4–28% of adult patients, a property that precludes their indiscriminate use in asthma. AIA is characterized by increased production of cysteinyl leukotrienes, although the exact mechanism by which aspirin acts on cylooxygenases to trigger bronchoconstriction remains unknown (Fig. 7.16).

PGD_2 mediates a number of proinflammatory effects through the interaction of two receptors: DP_1 and DP_2. The latter is a prime target for potential therapeutic agents for asthma and allergic diseases, and is reviewed later in this chapter.

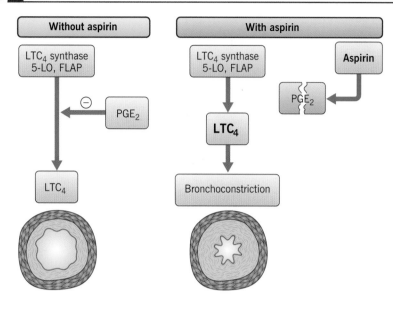

Fig. 7.16 Aspirin-induced asthma is characterized by increased amounts of LTC4 synthase, particularly in eosinophils. The activity of the leukotriene-forming enzyme complex is modulated by prostaglandin E_2. Inhibition of PGE_2 production by aspirin and related NSAIDs results in a marked increase in LTC4 synthesis and a consequential bronchoconstriction. FLAP, 5-lipoxygenase binding protein; 5-LO, 5-lipoxygenase; LT, leukotriene; NSAIDs, non-steroidal anti-inflammatory drugs; PG, prostaglandin.

Uses and administration

As stated above, the use of cyclooxygenase inhibitors in asthma is not usually recommended and is contraindicated to adult patients with AIA. However, they may be of some use in conjunction with H_1-antihistamines in the control of the cutaneous symptoms of systemic mastocytosis where they inhibit the synthesis of mast-cell-derived PGD_2. They may also benefit some patients with delayed pressure urticaria/angioedema. However, some patients with chronic idiopathic urticaria have worsening symptoms with the use of cyclooxygenase inhibitors.

Immunomodulator drugs approved and in development

With the advent of new and better-inhaled corticosteroids, with and without long-acting β-agonists, many individuals with asthma are well controlled. However, as with all treatments, inhaled corticosteroids are not effective for all individuals. Indeed, about 30–35% of both adult and paediatric patients with asthma have a poor or no response to inhaled corticosteroids. Furthermore, inhaled corticosteroids have not been shown to prevent the progression of disease or completely reverse airway remodelling. Thus, there is a need for novel therapies that affect critical immunopathological mechanisms and that induce immune tolerance – that is, change the immune system such that the therapy might actually be able to be discontinued with continued maintenance of disease control in the long term.

Strategies aimed at T cells

Due to the proinflammatory role of activated T cells in asthmatic airways and the observed correlation of increased CD25 expression with asthma severity, attempts have been made to block this arm of allergic disease pathogenesis. Initial attempts included monoclonal antibodies against Th2 cells such as keliximab. Although this treatment showed some modest improvement in patients with severe asthma, because of the potential side effects it has not been extensively studied. Cyclosporin (US ciclosporin) and tacrolimus have similar mechanisms inhibiting T cells and have been used for the treatment of severe asthma. Cyclosporin in early studies was shown to improve pulmonary functions in severe asthmatics, but because of side effects it has not been used extensively. An inhaled form of tacrolimus was used in patients with asthma, but was unsuccessful in meeting primary endpoints.

Daclizumab is a humanized monoclonal IgG1 antibody for the prevention of renal allograft rejection. It is specific for CD25 expressed by activated T cells and inhibits IL-2 induced proliferation by blocking the IL-2 receptor alpha chain. It does not deplete circulating CD25+ cells, however. In a published study, moderate to severe asthma patients placed on intravenous daclizumab showed improved pulmonary functions, reduced asthma symptoms and rescue medication use, increased time to severe exacerbations, and reduced peripheral blood eosinophil and serum eosinophil cationic protein levels.

Another approach to target T and other key cells important in the pathogenesis of allergic respiratory diseases is to use ligands of toll-like receptors. The ligand for the toll-4 receptor is endotoxin/lipid A. A specific form of this, monophosphoryl lipid A (MPL), has been used as monotherapy as well as in combination with allergen immunotherapy for the treatment of allergic diseases. Four preseasonal injections of ultra-short-course vaccines containing MPL can reduce symptoms and medication use, elevate antigen-specific IgG, and blunt seasonal elevations of IgE.

Immunostimulatory DNA molecules, CpG, are toll-9 receptor agonists and have been used as monotherapy and conjugated to antigen in human clinical trials. Initial human experiments showed that immunostimulatory CpG molecules linked to the predominant short ragweed allergen, Amb a 1, stimulated an antigen-specific Th2 to Th1 shift, and improved the safety margin of allergen immunotherapy. Although early studies were promising, large-scale clinical trials have been disappointing.

Another approach using a toll-9 receptor agonist has been shown to be effective in clinical trials. CYT003-QbG10 consists of a virus-like particle, Qb, and a short stretch of DNA from mycrobacteria that activates toll-like receptor 9 present in dendritic and other cells. In a recent publication CYT003-QbG10 plus house dust mite allergen were given for 10 weeks to patients with asthma and allergic rhinitis. Investigators found improvements in symptom scores, quality of life, and skin test responses to house dust mite for up to 48 weeks. This implies that long after discontinuing treatment there is sustained clinical improvement. Interestingly, in an 80 patient seasonal allergic rhinitis study, total rhinoconjunctivitis symptom scores were shown to be improved with QbG10 molecule without allergen.

Another approach targeting T cells and the early phases of allergic inflammation has been to use peroxisome proliferator-activated receptor γ (PPARγ) agonists. PPARγ agonists inhibit gene expression by binding to AP1 and other coactivators inhibiting the production of important inflammatory cytokines. PPARγ agonists have been shown to be effective in murine models of asthma. Human clinical trials are under way and it will be interesting to see whether these agents, already used for Type II diabetes mellitus (glitazones), might also be effective for asthma.

Th-2 cytokine inhibitors

Because of the importance of Th2 cytokines, IL-4, IL-5, IL-9, and IL-13, strategies aimed at inhibiting their production or effects have been tried in numerous clinical trials. Initial attempts to inhibit IL-4 showed some promise, but subsequent large-scale studies with soluble IL-4 receptors and monoclonal antibodies against IL-4 have been unrewarding.

Monospecific anti-IL-13 strategies have been disappointing as well despite IL-13's putative importance in the development of airway hyperresponsiveness, mucus secretion, and IgE and eotaxin production. It is unclear whether this was due to problems with the specific monoclonal antibodies or whether there is too much redundancy in the immune system such that inhibiting either IL-4 or IL-13 is insufficient. Indeed, strategies aimed at both IL-4 and IL-13 may be a better option.

In this regard, there are several strategies aimed at IL-4Rα, the common receptor chain important for both IL-4 and IL-13 signalling. Amgen 317 is a humanized monoclonal antibody to IL-4Rα that has undergone initial human clinical trials. Early trials have been disappointing with some minor biological activity but no clinical effects. None the less, further development of this molecule is warranted since different routes and dosages may be important in showing clinical effectiveness. An inhaled antisense molecule to IL-4Rα, AIR645, has also undergone very early clinical trials, but no positive clinical effects have been reported thus far. A 14 kDa IL-4 mutein that blocks IL-4Rα has been shown to be effective for both atopic dermatitis when given subcutaneously and asthma when given by inhalation. The inhaled form of this molecule, pitrakinra (AEROVANT™) was reported to block early and late phase allergen responses in patients with asthma. Its efficacy in large-scale clinical trials with traditional primary endpoints has yet to be determined.

A monoclonal antibody aimed at IL-9 is in early phase clinical trials. However, no published data are available to ascertain its potential efficacy.

Suplatast tosilate is an oral agent that has been shown to inhibit the synthesis of both IL-4 and IL-5. Suplatast decreases serum IgE and peripheral blood eosinophil counts, improves traditional asthma outcomes and decreases airway inflammation. However, this molecule has to be used in a three times per day regimen – making its utility somewhat problematic since compliance would be an issue.

Anti-eosinophil strategies

Given the prominence of eosinophils in many patients with asthma and their putative role in the pathogenesis of allergic respiratory disorders, several therapeutic strategies have been attempted to block eosinophil-mediated effects. Initial strategies have involved using humanized monoclonal antibodies against IL-5, an important cytokine for both chemotaxis and differentiation of eosinophils. Several older studies have confirmed reductions in blood and sputum eosinophils without significant changes in airway hyperresponsiveness, lung functions, or symptoms in patients treated with anti-Il-5 monoclonal antibodies. In March 2009, two New England Journal of Medicine articles were published using mepolizumab. Unlike previous studies, in order to enroll in these two studies subjects had to have a high sputum eosinophil count, greater than 3%. The investigators once again found a reduction in peripheral blood eosinophil counts. Although clinical effects were modest with either no or little effects on FEV$_1$, airway hyperresponsiveness or symptoms, there were nevertheless significant reductions in asthma exacerbations.

TPIASM8 is an oligonucleotide using RNA silencing. It contains two modified phosphorothiolate antisense oligonucleotides designed to inhibit allergic inflammation by down-regulating human CCR3 and the common beta chain of IL-3, IL-5, and GM CSF. In a recent study, TPIASM8 inhibited sputum eosinophil influx by 46% and blunted the increase in total cells after allergen challenge. TPIASM8 significantly reduced the early asthmatic response, but not the late asthmatic response. The allergen-induced levels of beta-chain mRNA and CCR3 mRNA in sputum-derived cells were inhibited by TPIASM8, but no significant effects on cell surface protein expression of CCR3 and the beta chain were found.

Anti-TNF-α strategies

TNF-α has a number of effects that could be important in asthma. TNF-α can increase airway hyperresponsiveness and the expression of key adhesion molecules important for eosinophil and neutrophil chemotaxis. Moreover, it can stimulate both epithelial and endothelial cells to synthesize and release chemokines and other cytokines. Several small studies in patients with severe asthma have shown TNF-α blockers to improve lung function, quality of life, exacerbation rates, and airway hyperresponsiveness. However, larger multisite studies have been disappointing. Not only has efficacy been difficult to show, but increased adverse events were recorded indicating a relatively poor risk to benefit ratio. Thus, anti-TNF strategies have been placed on hold for further development in the management of asthma and allergic disorders.

Strategies aimed at IgE and mast cells

The mast-cell and mast-cell-mediated events are attractive targets for treating allergic inflammation. Syk kinase is an intracellular protein–tyrosine kinase that is important in mast-cell and basophil activation and mediator release. R112, a Syk kinase inhibitor, demonstrated statistically significant efficacy in ameliorating symptoms of allergic rhinitis including stuffy nose, runny nose, sneezing, itchy nose, itchy throat, postnasal drip, cough, headache, and facial pain in a 2-day seasonal allergic rhinitis park study setting. The onset of action was within 30–90 minutes and the overall clinical improvement over placebo was approximately 25%. An inhaled formulation, R343, is currently being developed for the management of allergic asthma.

Omalizumab, the humanized monoclonal anti-IgE antibody, has been shown to have a number of anti-inflammatory and clinical benefits in patients (Fig. 7.17). Omalizumab decreases free IgE levels rapidly and the expression of the high-affinity IgE receptor expression on key effector cells, including mast cells, basophils, dendritic cells, and monocytes. In addition, lung

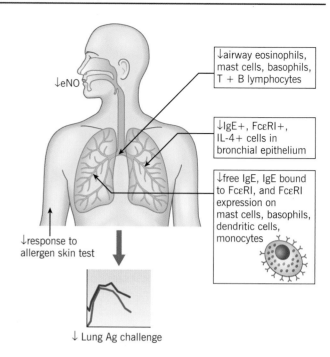

Fig 7.17 Mechanisms of action of omalizumab (anti-IgE).

inflammation has been shown to decrease after only 16 weeks of omalizumab treatment. In patients on inhaled corticosteroids alone or in combination with other agents, the addition of omalizumab has been shown to reduce asthma exacerbations, improve symptom scores, reduce the need for inhaled and oral corticosteroids, and decrease the necessity of rescue medication. Omalizumab has been shown in small studies or case reports to have some benefits in the following disorders: seasonal and perennial allergic rhinitis with and without asthma, atopic dermatitis, food allergies, insect allergy, chronic urticaria with autoantibodies to either the high-affinity IgE receptor or IgE itself, allergic bronchopulmonary aspergillosis, latex allergy, chronic hyperplastic sinusitis, recurrent nasal polyposis, drug allergy, and idiopathic anaphylaxis. However, it has been reported to cause anaphylaxis through unknown mechanisms in first as well as subsequent doses. Recently, concerns about potential adverse cardiovascular events have been raised, and there is still some controversy surrounding earlier associations with malignancies.

Mast cell mediator antagonists

There have been many attempts to develop antagonists to mediators important in asthma. An antagonist to CRTH2 (a G-protein-coupled receptor) has been developed. CRTH2 is present on Th2 cells, eosinophils, and basophils mediating activation and chemotaxis to PGD_2. A recent 28-day phase II study in mild to moderate asthma patients with FEV_1 values between 60 and 80% showed promising trends with ACT-129968, an oral antagonist. Bronchoprovocation to both adenosine monophosphate and methacholine decreased by 1–1.5 doubling doses, FEV_1 increased by 10 to 14%, and there was a decrease in sputum eosinophils and IgE. Moreover, patients had an improved quality of life. Further studies examining the efficacy of CRTH2 antagonists will be necessary to determine their therapeutic potential.

Conclusion

Ultimately, we need better therapeutic options that decrease symptoms, improve quality of life, and prevent or reverse disease. These treatments must also have a favourable risk/benefit ratio and be cost effective, since strategies such as monoclonal antibodies are very expensive to manufacture and to administer.

Summary of important messages

- Allergy comprises a wide spectrum of conditions affecting many organs, each of which requires treatment with different drugs. The primary principles of most pharmacotherapy are the same: symptom relief and reduction of underlying inflammation
- *Adrenaline (US epinephrine)*: potentially lifesaving in anaphylaxis by restoring blood pressure and causing bronchodilatation. Patients at risk should carry a preloaded syringe of adrenaline (EpiPen, Twinject or equivalent) with them at all times and be taught the appropriate use with administration into the lateral thigh
- *Bronchodilators (β_2-agonists)*: increase cyclic AMP to relax bronchial smooth muscle. Short-acting β_2-agonists have an onset of action within 5 minutes and a duration of 4 to 6 hours whereas long-acting β_2-agonists (LABA) work within 30 minutes and last for more than 12 hours. LABA should be used only in combination with inhaled corticosteroids
- *Corticosteroids*: have anti-inflammatory activity in asthma or allergic rhinitis. Should be administered topically whenever possible
- *Leukotriene receptor antagonists*: LTRAs and zileuton improve pulmonary function and symptoms in patients with mild to moderate asthma, have anti-inflammatory effects and complement the anti-inflammatory properties of corticosteroids
- *Methylxanthines*: theophylline is used as a bronchodilator in asthma and may have an additive effect when used in conjunction with small doses of β_2-agonists
- *Anticholinergics*: ipratropium (short acting) and tiotropium (long acting) can be used once daily for the management of COPD, but have not been consistently proven to be of benefit in asthma

- *H_1-antihistamines*: particularly effective in reducing rhinorrhoea and nasal itching in allergic rhinitis; less effective against nasal blockage
- *Intranasal decongestants (α-agonists)*: effective in relieving nasal obstruction, but their use should be limited to no more than 3–5 days because of rebound swelling of the nasal mucosa and drug-induced rhinitis (*rhinitis medicamentosa*)

Further reading

Barnes PJ. Theophylline and phosphodiesterase inhibitors. In: Adkinson NF, Bochner BS, Busse WW et al, eds. Allergy: principles and practice, 7th edn. St Louis: Mosby Elsevier; 2009:1505–1516.

Bousquet J, Khaltaev N, Cruz AA, et al. GA_2LEN; AllerGen. Allergic Rhinitis and its Impact on Asthma (ARIA) 2008 update (in collaboration with the World Health Organization, GA(2)LEN and AllerGen). Allergy. 2008 Apr; 63 suppl 86:8–160.

Camargo CA Jr, Rachelefsky G, Schatz M. Managing asthma exacerbations in the emergency department: summary of the National Asthma Education and Prevention Program Expert Panel Report 3 guidelines for the management of asthma exacerbations. J Emerg Med 2009 Aug; 37(2 suppl):S6–17.

Casale TB, Stokes J. Anti-IgE therapy: clinical utility beyond asthma. J Allergy Clin Immunol 2009 Apr; 123(4):770–771, e1.

Church MK, Maurer M, Simons FER, et al. Should first-generation H_1-antihistamines still be available as over-the-counter medications? A GA_2LEN task force report. Allergy 2010; 65:459–466.

Dimov VV, Stokes JR, Casale TB. Immunomodulators in asthma therapy. Curr Allergy Asthma Rep 2009 Nov; 9(6):475–483.

Edwards AM, Holgate ST. The chromones: cromolyn sodium and nedocromil sodium. In: Adkinson NF, Bochner BS, Busse WW et al, eds. Allergy: principles and practice, 7th edn. St Louis: Mosby Elsevier; 2009:1591–1602.

Spahn JD, Covar R, Szefler SJ. Glucocorticoids: clinical pharmacology. In: Adkinson NF, Bochner BS, Busse WW et al, eds. Allergy: principles and practice, 7th edn. St Louis: Mosby Elsevier; 2009:1575–1590.

Wallace DV, Dykewicz MS, Bernstein DI, et al. Joint Task Force on Practice; American Academy of Allergy; Asthma & Immunology; American College of Allergy; Asthma and Immunology; Joint Council of Allergy, Asthma and Immunology. The diagnosis and management of rhinitis: an updated practice parameter. J Allergy Clin Immunol 2008 Aug; 122(2 suppl):S1–84. Review. Erratum in: J Allergy Clin Immunol 2008 Dec; 122(6):1237.

Zuberbier T, Asero R, Bindslev-Jensen C, et al. EAACI/GA_2LEN/EDF/WAO guideline: management of urticaria. Allergy. 2009 Oct; 64(10):1427–1443.

8

Allergen-specific immunotherapy

Hans-Jørgen Malling, Jonathan Corren and Peter S Creticos

DEFINITION

Allergen-specific immunotherapy (SIT) is the method in which increasing doses of allergen are administered to allergic subjects, thereby modulating the immune system and leading to a reduction in clinical symptoms.

Introduction

The practice of inoculating patients with microorganisms to prevent infectious diseases was first developed in the late 18th century. As hay fever was considered to be caused by an infectious organism, it was logical for Noon and Freeman to prevent hay-fever symptoms by injecting patients with pollen. Although their rationale was later shown to be incorrect, the treatment proved to be effective. During the 1920s and 1930s, at which time therapeutic options for hay fever were limited, desensitizing injections were widely administered to patients and showed varying success rates. During the past 20 to 30 years, the use of immunotherapy in some European countries decreased owing to the introduction of potent and safe antiallergic drugs. Recently, however, standardization of extracts and an increased understanding of immunological mechanisms has led to a renaissance in the use of this treatment. At the same time it has become clear that patient selection and attention to practice guidelines are both vital in achieving successful treatment.

Overall approach to respiratory allergy

The management of allergic airway diseases is based on combining three essential interventions, including allergen avoidance, medications, and allergen-specific immunotherapy, along with education of the patient regarding home management. Initiation of immunotherapy in moderate severe disease is clinically effective. Immunotherapy interferes with the pathophysiological mechanisms of allergic inflammation, with a potential for a prolonged effect compared with symptomatic pharmacological treatment. Although many antiallergic drugs are highly effective with limited side effects, they represent a symptomatic treatment, while immunotherapy represents the only treatment capable of altering the natural course of the disease. Using an appropriately selected allergen extract in patients with allergic rhinitis and asthma, immunotherapy can significantly reduce the severity of symptoms, the need for antiallergic drugs, and improve disease-specific quality of life.

© 2012 Elsevier Ltd
DOI: 10.1016/B978-0-7234-3658-4.00005-6

Mechanisms of immunotherapy
(Fig. 8.1)

Although the precise mechanisms underlying the beneficial effects of SIT are not well understood, a large number of immunological effects have been demonstrated.

Several studies have shown that SIT inhibits both early and late responses to allergen challenge in the nose and lung. Similarly, early and late phase responses following allergen skin tests are reduced during immunotherapy, with greater effects on the late response.

It has long been known that immunotherapy blunts seasonal increases in IgE levels and results in increases in allergen-specific IgG levels (i.e. blocking antibodies), especially of the IgG4 subclass (Fig. 8.2). This results in decreased IgE-mediated histamine release and inhibition of IgE-mediated antigen presentation to T cells. Recent studies have also demonstrated the importance of examining the affinity and specificity of IgG subsequent to

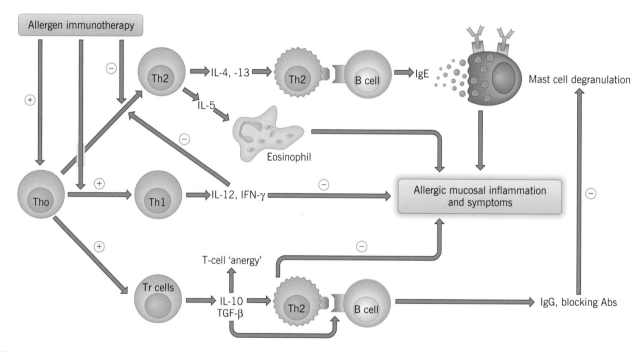

Fig. 8.1 Mechanisms underlying the action of specific immunotherapy (SIT). There is helper T cell type 2 (Th2) predominance in allergic diseases and this is characterized by secretion of interleukin-4 (IL-4), -5, and -13. IL-5 is involved in eosinophil survival, activation, and maturation and IL-4 and -13 are important in class switching of B cells for IgE production. Th1 response induces IL-12 and interferon γ (IFN-γ) production and this dampens the Th2 response. SIT induces Th1 response, dampens Th2 response and induces T-regulatory cells (Tr cells) to secrete IL-10 and transforming growth factor β (TGF-β), and recent studies have shown that IL-10 induces T-cell 'anergy' or 'unresponsiveness' and has other 'anti-allergic properties'. Abs, antibodies.

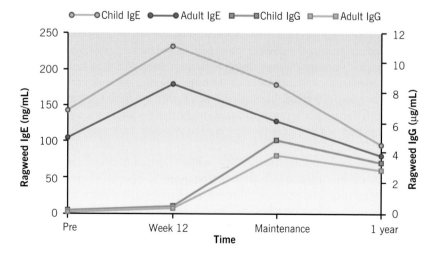

Fig. 8.2 Time course of serological changes during specific immunotherapy. Note the initial rise in allergen-specific IgE and delayed rise in allergen-specific IgG, which follows rather than precedes clinical improvement.

immunotherapy. Following long-term administration of immunotherapy, the binding capacity of IgG4 increases, whereas that for IgE decreases. Although these SIT induced changes in IgG4 concentration may have potential significance pathogenetically, there is no correlation with individual patient IgG4 levels and individual clinical response.

Studies in patients with seasonal allergic rhinitis have shown that immunotherapy affects the influx and function of multiple cell types. These changes include the attenuation of the seasonal influx of eosinophils, basophils, and T cells into the nasal mucosa. In addition to these effects, SIT has been shown to induce a shift in the balance of T-lymphocyte subsets away from the helper T cell type 2 (Th2) phenotype and toward a Th1 phenotype on the basis of preferential production of interferon γ (IFN-γ) and decreased production of interleukin-4 (IL-4) and IL-5. However, these findings have not been shown to be reproducible across all studies.

More recent studies have focused upon T-regulatory (Tr or Treg) cells that are identified by their CD4+CD25+ phenotype. Tr cells are induced by SIT, leading to the production and release of IL-10 and transforming growth factor β (TGF-β), which may have a number of antiallergic effects. Most prominent of these actions is modulation of IL-4-induced B-cell IgE production in favor of IgG4, inhibition of IgE-dependent mast cell activation, and inhibition of human eosinophil cytokine production and survival. IL-10 also suppresses production of 'proallergic' cytokines, such as IL-5, and is able to induce a state of T-cell unresponsiveness or 'anergy', which might occur as a result of IL-10 receptor-dependent blockade of the B7/CD28 costimulatory pathway. The importance of IL-10 and Tr cells cannot be overemphasized. These cells appear to be critical in the therapeutic effects of immunotherapy and further research to define their role is important.

Subcutaneous immunotherapy

Allergen immunotherapy is most commonly administered by subcutaneous infections (SCIT) and requires that an initial very dilute dose of allergen be progressively escalated to higher doses until a maintenance dose is reached. Typically, the incremental (build-up) phase will be given as weekly or biweekly injections over a period of 10–24 weeks (typically 10–13 in Europe, and 12–24 in the United States). In a 'cluster dose' regimen, the maintenance dose is achieved 7–8 weeks after starting and the safety profile of this regimen has been shown to match the conventional, slower dosing schedule.

Maintenance injections are then given at intervals of 4–8 weeks over a total period of 3–5 years. Several variations have been proposed, including 'rush' and 'semi-rush' protocols, in which the incremental phase of the regime is compressed by giving several injections on the same day with 30–60 min intervals. The principal drawback to these protocols is the increased likelihood of side effects, but this must be weighed against the ability to achieve protection within a few days or weeks, which may be particularly useful in patients with Hymenoptera allergy.

Sublingual immunotherapy

A number of alternative routes of administration have been used, the most promising of which is sublingual immunotherapy (SLIT). Many studies have demonstrated that high-dose SLIT is an effective form of immunotherapy for both adults and children. SLIT can be administered by patients at home without supervision by medical personnel, potentially leading to greater compliance. Despite these positive attributes, several issues need to be considered before recommending SLIT as a replacement for subcutaneous immunotherapy. There are very limited data comparing SLIT with SCIT, and those that do exist suggest that the overall efficacy of SLIT is less than of SCIT. We also do not know the long-term effects of SLIT or what immunological changes are evoked by this form of therapy. Finally, although the safety profile appears good with SLIT, long-term studies similar to those done with SCIT are ultimately needed to define the true risk/benefit ratio with SLIT in comparison with SCIT. As more SLIT studies are published, hopefully most of these issues will be resolved and its place as an alternative to SCIT will become more clearly defined. Side effects of SLIT are generally limited to local itching and discomfort in the mouth, throat, and gastrointestinal tract. However, asthmatic reactions following SLIT have infrequently been reported.

Other approaches

Several other non-conventional approaches are in current use. Both oral and local nasal immunotherapy are less effective than SLIT and cannot be considered to be acceptable alternatives. Homeopathic immunotherapy, using extremely dilute doses of pollen, has not been shown to have any convincing activity, and is not recommended.

Efficacy of immunotherapy

Hymenoptera venom allergy

Anaphylactic reactions to Hymenoptera stings are relatively uncommon but can be life threatening; venom immunotherapy to prevent anaphylactic reactions is the treatment of choice. The primary allergen in honey-bee venom is phospholipase A2 (Api m 1) and that of the vespid venoms (yellow jacket, hornet, wasp) is antigen 5 (Ves v 5). Another clinically important insect is the imported fire ant (also a member of the Hymenoptera family). Allergy to the imported fire ant is being reported increasingly often from the USA, Australia, and South East Asia.

Risk assessment is based on the clinical history and measurement of venom-specific IgE. Those who have had systemic symptoms with a previous sting are at much greater risk of anaphylaxis than those who have had only large local reactions. The magnitude of the IgE response is not consistently correlated with the severity or pattern of reaction to a sting, since some patients who experience large local reactions have extremely high venom IgE levels, whereas others who suffer rapid vascular collapse and anaphylactic shock may have barely detectable levels of venom IgE. The frequency of systemic reactions in children and adults with a history of large local reactions and positive venom skin tests is in the range of 5–10%. The reported risk of another systemic reaction occurring in a patient with a previous systemic reaction varies from 30 to 60%, with lower risks in children and patients with milder reactions. The risk of systemic reaction in adults diminishes over 10–20 years towards 15–30%, but does not seem to return to the background 3% prevalence in the general population. Children with a history of cutaneous systemic reactions had less than 5% risk of anaphylaxis during observation for 10–20 years. There is no test that accurately predicts the outcome of the next sting. Live sting challenge is a useful research procedure, but is generally not acceptable for clinical practice – not least because some patients who do not react to a first challenge sting may react to a subsequent sting.

The induction phase of venom SIT may be given weekly for 10 weeks, as a 'semirush' over 2–3 weeks, or as a 'rush induction' in hospital over 2–3 days. Once the maintenance dose is achieved, 95–98% of patients will have no systemic symptoms upon wasp-sting challenge (80–85% for honey-bee venom SIT). Patients not fully protected by the conventional dose of 100 μg may be more effectively treated with a 200 μg maintenance dose. Protection is well maintained during subsequent maintenance therapy; maintenance injections are usually given every 4–6 weeks, but sometimes the interval is up to 8 weeks, especially in long-term maintenance therapy for venom allergy. Maintenance therapy is usually recommended for 3–5 years, with growing evidence that 5 years' treatment provides more lasting benefit, although this has to be balanced against the inconvenience of extended duration of SCIT. More prolonged treatment is offered to those with more severe previous reactions, those who had systemic reactions during venom SCIT, and those allergic to honey bees (as opposed to wasps). The decision to stop therapy may also be based on a

reduction in the skin test response to venom or a reduction in venom-specific IgE. Venom-specific IgG rises in all patients as a result of therapy, and a level of ≥3 μg/mL has been shown to be protective.

A low risk of systemic reaction to stings (10%) appears to remain for many years after discontinuing venom (SCIT). Although post-SCIT systemic reactions to stings have rarely been severe, a few fatalities have been reported, usually in patients with other risk factors (e.g. mastocytosis, severe previous reactions, systemic reactions during venom SCIT, honey-bee allergy). In children who have received venom SCIT, the chance of systemic reaction to a sting is lower, remaining below 5% for up to 20 years after discontinuing therapy. How much of this is due to SCIT and how much to natural resolution of the sensitivity is uncertain, but the clinical message is clear: treatment is effective in the short term and patients are then at relatively low risk of reactions for many years thereafter.

Subcutaneous immunotherapy in allergic rhinitis and asthma

Allergen-specific immunotherapy has been widely used to treat allergic airway diseases. As with any other form of SIT, careful patient selection is crucial. The diagnosis of allergic disease needs to be secure, especially in those with perennial symptoms, and should be based on a careful clinical history supported by documentation of IgE-mediated sensitivity by skin or blood tests.

Published studies indicate that subcutaneous immunotherapy is an effective treatment for allergic airway disease (Fig. 8.3). In meta-analyses reviewing a large number of double-blind, placebo-controlled studies of SCIT in allergic rhinitis or asthma, active treatment (using seasonal pollens, dust mites, animal danders or moulds) was shown to reduce mean symptom-medication scores 45% more than placebo. In this meta-analysis review, a mean improvement of 30% was defined as the minimum level indicative of a clinically relevant difference. In an update of the original meta-analysis review, SCIT resulted in a 40% mean improvement in rhinitis severity and 45% improvement in asthma.

Sublingual immunotherapy in allergic rhinitis and asthma

The majority of clinical trials of SLIT do not comply with modern standards and, based on all studies performed, the efficacy of SLIT seems inferior to SCIT. A small number of recent large-scale studies utilizing grass and birch in allergic rhinitis demonstrated that in separate studies SCIT and SLIT have comparable efficacy. However, currently there are no results available from

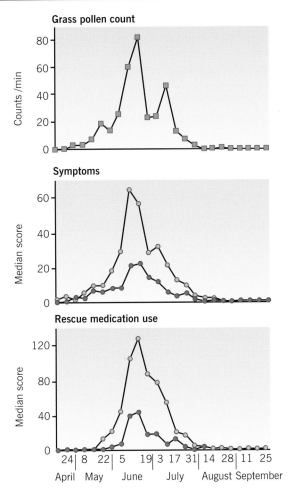

Fig. 8.3 Symptoms and drug scores following immunotherapy with a depot pollen extract or a placebo injection. Note the significant decrease in symptoms and the use of rescue medication after receiving immunotherapy. Green, weekly grass pollen counts for comparison; blue, placebo; red, depot pollen extract. (Data modified from Varney VA, Gaga M, Frew AJ, et al. Usefulness of immunotherapy in patients with severe summer hay fever uncontrolled by anti-allergic drugs. BMJ 1991; 302:265–269.)

adequately powered double-blind studies of SCIT vs SLIT in the same study to determine their comparative efficacy. Some studies of SLIT have shown efficacy in children as well, but experience is limited.

Disease-modifying and preventive capacity of immunotherapy

In a recent study, 205 children aged 6 to 14 years with seasonal rhinitis caused by grass and/or birch pollen (the PAT study) were randomized to receive either active subcutaneous immunotherapy or placebo for 3 years. In children who did not have any symptoms of asthma at the start of the study, actively treated children had

significantly fewer diagnoses of asthma after 3 years (odds ratio, 2.52).

Indications for allergen-specific immunotherapy

Indication for immunotherapy in Hymenoptera venom allergy

Venom immunotherapy is indicated in both children and adults with a history of severe systemic allergic reactions including respiratory and/or cardiovascular symptoms and documented sensitization to the respective insect as determined by skin tests and/or specific serum IgE tests. As for systemic non-life-threatening reactions (urticaria, erythema, pruritus), other factors may influence the decision to initiate venom immunotherapy. These include availability of immediate access to medical care, occupations and/or hobbies where the risk of exposure is high, concomitant cardiovascular disease, the presence of other pathologies such as mastocytosis, and psychological factors arising from anxiety that can seriously impair patient quality of life. Recent guidelines do not recommend immunotherapy in children below the age of 15 with exclusively cutaneous reactions (urticaria). Immunotherapy is not recommended for large local reactions or unusual reactions, like non-IgE-mediated hypersensitivity reactions such as vasculitis, nephrosis or thrombocytopenia.

Indications and contraindications for immunotherapy in respiratory allergy

Allergy immunotherapy is generally indicated in patients with moderate to severe persistent symptoms of allergic rhinitis. Patients with intermittent symptoms easily controlled with oral antihistamines should not be considered as candidates for this therapy. Specific groups of patients who may benefit from immunotherapy include those who: (1) are poorly responsive to available drug treatments, (2) have bothersome side effects with commonly used drugs given at conventional doses, (3) are beginning to develop symptoms of bronchial asthma, and (4) have a secondary complication of rhinitis, such as sinusitis, otitis, or dental malocclusion, despite using conventional medical treatments.

Indications for administering immunotherapy to patients with allergic asthma are less clearly defined. As noted above, SIT may help prevent the progression of allergic rhinitis to asthma, and as such should be considered strongly in patients with new onset allergic asthma. In patients with established allergic asthma, SIT may reduce the intensity of exacerbations caused by exposure to specific allergens. It must be kept in mind that immunotherapy must be administered with great caution to patients with more severe asthma owing to the risk of causing asthma to worsen, particularly in patients with FEV$_1$ <70% of predicted.

In general, children respond to immunotherapy better than adults, which may be most related to the duration of the disease. This suggests that SIT should be started while the natural history of the disease can still be altered prior to the deterioration to a chronic irreversible condition.

As successful immunotherapy in allergic rhinitis and asthma is based on a multitude of elements, it may be advantageous to base the decision to use immunotherapy upon specific patient characteristics that predict a high likelihood of a positive clinical effect and low risk of side effects (Box 8.1).

Absolute contraindications for initiation of subcutaneous allergen-specific immunotherapy with inhalant and Hymenoptera venom allergens include: (1) cardiovascular disease, (2) severe asthma (see above) treatment with β blockers (including topical) (see Hymenoptera below), (3) poor compliance, (4) severe psychological disorder, and (5) pregnancy.

Normally immunotherapy is restricted to patients above 5 years of age. Below this age, inhalation allergens play a less important role. Furthermore, when SCIT is prescribed below 5 years of age it is critical that the physician responsible for the injections has experience in identifying and treating emerging signs of anaphylaxis in this age group.

In contrast to inhalation allergen immunotherapy, immunotherapy for Hymenoptera venom allergy is often indicated in elderly patients with coexisting cardiovascular disease, who are at a special risk to develop severe or even fatal reactions. Such patients are commonly on β blocker treatment. In this situation the risk of stopping the drug must be carefully balanced against the risk of renouncing venom immunotherapy. In coronary heart disease or severe ventricular arrhythmia the risk of stopping the β blocker can be unacceptable. If highly exposed to the relevant insect, venom immunotherapy may be carried out in patients with ongoing β blockade but under careful supervision, including monitoring of blood pressure and electrocardiogram and with expertise and remedies at hand if severe side effects with resistance to treatment due to the β blockade should occur.

Safety of allergen-specific immunotherapy

Injections of allergens into an IgE-sensitized patient (SCIT) always include a risk of inducing anaphylactic reactions. The rate of severe systemic reactions in rhinitics treated with high-potency extract injections, occurs primarily in the induction phase, but can also occur in the maintenance phase. In asthmatics, the risk of systemic reactions is higher, primarily owing to bronchial obstruction. Monitoring the lung function of asthmatic patients before the injections is therefore mandatory and likewise to ensure an optimal antiasthmatic pharmacological treatment.

Data support the view that asthma is a separate risk factor for serious systemic side effects during SCIT. Fatalities have been observed (rate 1 per 2.5 million injections), with an average of 3.4 deaths per year in the USA. This rate of fatalities per immunotherapy injection has not changed much over the last 15 years. The vast majority of fatalities occurred in patients with asthma, most of whom were poorly controlled. Interestingly, some of these reactions occurred more than 30 minutes after the injections (i.e. at a time exceeding the current recommended waiting time for allergen immunotherapy injections). In many of the fatalities, there was either a substantial delay in starting adrenaline (US epinephrine) was not administered at all. Risk factors for systemic side effects are listed in Box 8.2.

Box 8.1 Indication for inhalant allergy immunotherapy based on patient profiling

- Age of patient and duration of disease (in years)
- Organs involved
- Severity and duration of symptoms
- Allergens responsible for clinical symptoms
- Importance of allergen sensitization vs non-specific triggers
- Allergen exposure and effect of allergen avoidance
- Clinical response to pharmacotherapy
- Number and types of drugs needed
- Risk incurred by pharmacotherapy vs immunotherapy
- Impact of disease and treatment on quality of life
- Patients' attitude to and expectations of treatment

Each individual item is evaluated for conditions speaking for or against immunotherapy, and only patients whose overall disease profile favours immunotherapy should be offered the treatment.

Box 8.2 Factors associated with adverse reactions to SCIT

- Induction phase of treatment
- Dosage errors
- Intravenous injection of dose (inadvertent)
- History of previous systemic reaction
- Extreme sensitivity to allergen
- Vigorous exercise after injection
- Change of vial
- Febrile illness
- Uncontrolled asthma
- Environmental exposure to allergen, e.g. during the pollen season
- Administration of β-blocker drugs

Several studies have shown that pretreatment with antihistamines can reduce the frequency and severity of local and systemic reactions during SCIT, but this is not yet standard practice. Efforts to standardize immunotherapy forms and vial labeling will decrease patient and dosing errors. However, clinicians involved in the practice of immunotherapy must constantly assess their patients' current medical status, avoiding the administration of injections to inappropriate candidates, especially patients with poorly controlled asthma. Furthermore, the appropriate and timely administration of adrenaline to treat anaphylaxis is essential.

Sublingual immunotherapy has been introduced predominantly due to the safety. The majority of patients experience some local side effects in the mouth and gastrointestinal tract. Systemic reactions (predominantly asthma reactions) have been infrequently reported. Generally SLIT is a safe treatment that may be given as home treatment.

> **Box 8.3** Rescue equipment essential for subcutaneous immunotherapy
>
> - Adrenaline (1 mg/mL) for injection
> - Antihistamine, corticosteroids, and a vasopressor for injection or oral treatment
> - Syringes, needles, tourniquet, and equipment for infusion
> - Saline for infusion
> - Oxygen and suction equipment
> - Silicone mask and equipment for manual ventilation
> - Equipment for measurement of blood pressure
> - Forms for recording the course and treatment of anaphylaxis
>
> In settings remote from intensive care facilities, equipment for direct laryngoscopy, DC cardioversion, tracheotomy and intracardiac injections may be optional, but the rare situation in which these procedures might be essential does not justify that these procedures are immediately available for subcutaneous immunotherapy.

Practical management of immunotherapy

Patient education

The patient should receive verbal and written information about immunotherapy including a description of: efficacy, possible adverse effects, the need for compliance, the duration of treatment, and the requirement for observation after injections.

Treatment of reactions

Because of the risk of inducing anaphylaxis with SCIT, office personnel should be appropriately trained to treat anaphylaxis and always have an up-to-date emergency cart supplied with all essential drugs (Box 8.3). The physicians should also have a nearby hospital identified in the event that patients need to be transferred for emergency room care or hospitalization for severe anaphylaxis.

Allergen products

The quality of allergen products used for immunotherapy is of essential importance in order to obtain a high clinical efficacy and to minimize side effects. Extracts used for routine immunotherapy should be standardized and be subjected to quality control. In daily clinical practice, only allergen extracts for which clinical efficacy and safety have been documented by controlled studies should be used.

Commercial allergen extracts may be delivered as either aqueous, depot, or modified extracts. Aqueous extracts may be used for administration of multiple injections like rush or cluster immunotherapy. The disadvantages of aqueous extracts are the rapid degradation of allergens and the high frequency of side effects. Depot extracts involve binding of allergens to a carrier in order to diminish the degradation and removal of allergens at the injection site. This may imply a reduction in the frequency of side effects and potentially a better efficacy. The disadvantages are that one (or a few) injection(s) may only be administered in one sequence and that side effects may be observed after 30 minutes. Modified extracts imply either a physical or chemical alteration of allergen structure in order to reduce the allergenicity with retained immunogenicity (and to increase safety). Standardization, however, presents problems for modified extracts, as this could not be based on IgE-binding assays.

A major difference between American and European allergists is the use of allergen mixtures in SCIT. Mixing of unrelated allergens is not recommended in Europe, whereas this is common practice in the United States. Mixing of allergens has not been documented to be effective in clinical studies, but existing data are insufficient to judge whether mixed SCIT is effective. There is no rationale to explain why mixed extracts would not be effective with SCIT other than a mutual degradation or dilution of the dose of each allergen below the optimal dose. Mixtures of cross-reacting allergens like grasses, mites, etc. could be used, but seldom have advantages over single allergens owing to the high sequence of homology for major epitopes. Clinical studies show only a minimal difference in clinical response between single allergens and mixtures of cross-reacting allergens.

Box 8.4 Recommendations to reduce systemic side effects in SCIT

- Postpone injections in patients with airway infections or other significant diseases within the last 3 days.
- Postpone injections in patients with deterioration of allergy symptoms or increased need for antiallergic drugs due to recent allergen exposure within the last 3 days.
- Postpone injections in patients with decreased lung function <80% of personal best value. In asthmatic patients measuring lung function before each injection is mandatory (peak flow is sufficient).
- Reduce the scheduled dose if the interval between injection sessions has been exceeded. The magnitude of reduction depends on the degree of exceeding the time interval.
- Reduce the scheduled allergen dose in case of a systemic reaction at the preceding visit. The magnitude of reduction depends on the severity of the reaction. In case of anaphylactic and other life-threatening reactions the continuation of subcutaneous immunotherapy should be carefully evaluated (except in case of Hymenoptera venom allergy, in which it actually reinforces the indication for immunotherapy).
- Check for any drug intake that may either increase the risk of systemic side effects or render the treatment of anaphylactic reactions more difficult.
- It is recommended not to start induction treatment during allergen seasons. During allergen seasons, injections should not be given if the patient has clinical symptoms.
- Separate allergen injections from other vaccinations for infectious diseases by at least 1 week.

Dose modifications

Detailed guidelines for omission of an injection, repetition of a previous dose, or reduction of a dose exists mostly based on experience and tradition. The recommendations given in Box 8.4 have been documented to be useful. Although a late local reaction at the injection site has been used to adjust the allergen dosing at the next allergen administration, several studies have indicated that the late local reaction at the preceding injection is not related to a risk of developing a systemic reaction at the next injection.

Future directions

Peptide immunotherapy

Peptide immunotherapy is based on the concept that SIT works by altering the function of allergen-specific T cells. To be recognized by T cells, the injected allergen has to be presented to Th cells as short peptide fragments held

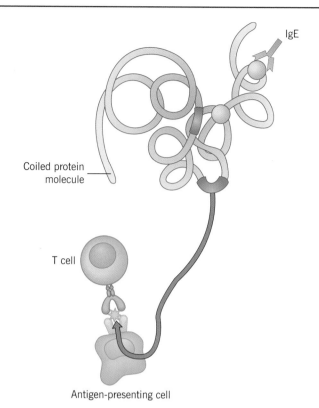

B-cell epitopes on surface of intact molecule, may be formed by ≥ 2 peptide chains or by amino acids that are not contiguous

T-cell epitopes formed by linear fragment of protein, partly digested by APC, and presented in groove of MHC molecule. Can be external on original molecule

Fig. 8.4 Schematic representation of B-cell and T-cell epitopes. Note that T-cell epitopes are linear peptides, derived by partial degradation of the allergen, whereas B-cell epitopes are three-dimensional or 'configurational' and may involve portions from quite separate parts of the primary structure, which are brought together by pleating and folding of the allergenic molecules. APC, antigen-presenting cell; MHC, major histocompatibility complex.

in major histocompatibility complex (MHC) class II molecules on antigen-presenting cells. Since T-cell epitopes are different from the B-cell epitopes recognized by antibodies (Fig. 8.4), it should be possible to give T-cell peptides to target T cells without risking IgE-mediated anaphylaxis. The candidate peptides are identified on the basis of their ability to induce proliferation in lymphocyte lines from a group of patients with specific allergy. Peptide vaccines based on Fel d 1 and Amb a 1 have been tested in patients with cat and ragweed allergy respectively and have shown modest benefit. Up to a third of patients experienced mild systemic reactions between 1 and 3 hours after injection, but these reactions reduced in frequency with continuation of therapy. Occasional immediate reactions were also noted in these studies, suggesting that sensitization to these peptides was possible. At present, peptide immunotherapy remains experimental but there are ongoing studies examining its efficacy and safety.

Anti-immunoglobulin E

Recently, omalizumab has been studied as an add-on therapy to immunotherapy in young patients aged 6–17 years. Individuals allergic to birch and grass pollen were treated by specific immunotherapy and then omalizumab was added after the maintenance phase of allergen immunotherapy was reached. The combination of omalizumab plus immunotherapy showed superior efficacy to immunotherapy alone, with good safety and tolerability. Omalizumab is also being used to try to reduce systemic adverse effects of immunotherapy. Preliminary data indicate that omalizumab has a protective effect against immunotherapy-induced systemic reactions. Cost effectiveness excludes omalizumab as part of standard treatment, however.

Immunostimulatory DNA

Studies in animal models have identified bacterial DNA, and in particular specific palindromic DNA motifs containing unmethylated cytosine residues in the sequence CpG, as potent adjuvants of the Th1 response. CpG DNA exerts its effects via the Toll-like receptor 9 (TLR9) on dendritic cells. When protein antigens are mixed with these immunostimulatory oligodeoxynucleotide sequences (ISS-ODN), a novel type of allergoid for SIT is produced that has several potential advantages. First, this conjugate delivers the ISS-ODN and the allergen to the same antigen-presenting cell; second, no free ISS-ODN reaches bystander cells to produce excess mediators that could cause adverse reactions; third, the conjugate allergoid probably presents fewer B-cell epitopes, reducing the risks of side effects.

This strategy has yielded some encouraging observations in a study of 28 patients with ragweed-induced hay fever. In this study there was no improvement in symptoms during the first postimmunotherapy season, which started 3 weeks after the last injection. A modest symptomatic improvement was noted in the following pollen season, without the subjects receiving any further treatment. These results are encouraging but clearly further studies are required to study the safety and efficacy of these vaccines.

Conclusion

Allergen-specific immunotherapy is the only available treatment with a potential to alter the natural course of allergic disease, provide sustained relief of symptoms, and reduce the risk of progression of rhinitis to asthma. Although there are some risks, these can be minimized when SIT is given in a controlled environment to carefully selected patients following international guidelines for evaluating patients. Combining allergens with CpG-DNA or other adjuvants may also improve the efficacy and safety profile of SIT. SIT is thus a valuable therapy for allergic disease, with the potential for further improvement and wider application in the future.

Summary of important messages

- Allergen-specific immunotherapy represents the only treatment with a capacity to alter the natural course of allergic diseases
- Immunotherapy affects the allergic inflammation by inhibiting the influx and function of a number of inflammatory cells owing to redirection of the T-lymphocyte response into a non-allergic pathway
- Subcutaneous immunotherapy has a well-documented clinical efficacy as well as long-term efficacy (after terminating treatment) in Hymenoptera venom allergy, allergic asthma, and rhinitis
- Sublingual immunotherapy has primarily been documented for pollen rhinitis during ongoing treatment
- The risk of inducing anaphylactic side effects is closely related to subcutaneous immunotherapy, and consequently this treatment has to be reserved for specialists. Sublingual treatment may result in local side effects, but is generally safe and used as home treatment
- Future direction using peptides or immunostimulatory DNA motifs may increase both the clinical efficacy and the safety of immunotherapy

Further reading

Abramson MJ, Puy RM, Weiner JM. Injection allergen immunotherapy for asthma. Cochrane Database Syst Rev 2010; (8):CD001186. Review.

Alvarez-Cuesta E, Bousquet J, Canonica GW, et al. Standards for practical allergen-specific Immunotherapy. Allergy 2006; 61(suppl 82):1–20.

Bousquet J, Khaltaev N, Cruz AA, et al. Allergic rhinitis and its impact on asthma (ARIA) 2008 update. Allergy 2008; 63(suppl 86):8–160.

Bousquet J, Lockey RF, Malling H-J, eds. WHO position paper. Allergen immunotherapy: therapeutic vaccines for allergic diseases. Allergy 1998; 53(suppl 44):1–42.

Calderon MA, Alves B, Jacobson M, et al. Allergen injection immunotherapy for seasonal allergic rhinitis. Cochrane Database of Systemic Reviews 2007, Issue 1. Art. No.: CD001936. DOI: 10.1002/14651858.CD001936.pub2.

Canonica GW. Sub-lingual Immunotherapy: World Allergy Organization Position Paper 2009. Allergy 2009; 64: S1–59.

Cox L, Li JT, Nelson H, Lockey R. Allergen immunotherapy: A practice parameter second update. J Allergy Clin Immunol 2007; 120:S25–85.

Jacobsen L, Niggemann B, Dreborg S, et al. Specific immunotherapy has long-term preventive effects of seasonal and perennial asthma: 10-year follow-up on the PAT-study. Allergy 2007; 62:943–948.

Malling HJ, Weeke B. EAACI Immunotherapy position papers. Allergy 1993; 48(suppl 14):9–35.

Malling HJ. Quality and clinical efficacy of allergen mixtures. Arb Paul Ehrlich Inst Bundesamt Sera Impfstoffe Frankf A M 2006; 95:253–257.

9

Asthma

Thomas AE Platts-Mills, Mitsuru Adachi,
William W Busse and Stephen T Holgate

DEFINITION

Asthma is a chronic
inflammatory disorder in
which the airway smooth
muscle undergoes
exaggerated contraction and
is abnormally responsive to
external stimuli.

Introduction

The symptoms of asthma occur together with variations in the diameter of
medium-sized airways such that it is increasingly difficult to exhale. Narrowing of the airways can occur because of smooth muscle contraction, oedema
or swelling of the wall, or increased mucus in the airways. However, it is
increasingly clear that the pathological event underlying most cases of asthma
is chronic inflammation of the airway walls. The elements of this inflammation are discussed in Chapter 1. The best-defined and most commonly identified cause of this inflammation is inhalation of allergens. Sometimes, the
relationship of these foreign proteins to the symptoms of asthma may be
obvious to the patient (e.g. when wheezing or coughing starts within 10
minutes of entering a house that has a cat in it). On the other hand, many
patients who are allergic to dust mites are not aware of the association
between exposure and their symptoms. In contrast, most patients with
asthma are well aware that their lungs vary in tightness and that many non-
specific stimuli such as exercise, cold air, or passive smoking can trigger
attacks. The fact that the lungs of patients with asthma can react to otherwise
'trivial' stimuli such as cold air is referred to as 'bronchial hyperresponsiveness'. This hyperresponsiveness can be demonstrated in the clinic by using
histamine or methacholine, which narrow the airways directly, or by cold air
or exercise challenge, which are indirect stimuli that narrow the airways following the release of secondary mediators.

The relationship between inflammation in the airways of a patient and
either the symptoms of asthma or bronchial hyperresponsiveness is not
simple. Thus, it is not possible to define the severity of asthma on the basis
of a measurement of inflammation in the lungs. Nevertheless, the production
of mediators by eosinophils, T cells, and mast cells is of central importance
in understanding the pathophysiology of asthma as well as being a target for
treatment. Estimating the prevalence of asthma is dependent on the method
used to define the disease, and in addition the prevalence varies markedly
between countries and between different communities within a country.

The main problem in defining asthma is that the disease varies from occasional episodes of chest tightness or wheezing that will reverse with time or
an inhalation of β2-agonist to a life-threatening condition with severe airway
obstruction that requires high-dose inhaled steroids or oral corticoid steroid
treatment. Although there is a continuum of severity, it is helpful to classify

© 2012 Elsevier Ltd
DOI: 10.1016/B978-0-7234-3658-4.00005-6

the disease in order to discuss aetiology, pathogenesis, and treatment.

The classification of asthma

Classification of bronchial asthma can be based on age, aetiology, associated characteristics, or severity. Classifications based on severity have been primarily designed as an approach to treatment. Thus, management of mild intermittent disease may require only bronchodilator treatment, but frequent attacks with or without persistent mild symptoms require a comprehensive approach to controlling inflammation as well as bronchodilator treatment. Severe asthma can become a major clinical problem that requires specialist care and many different approaches to treatment.

The pattern of disease presenting at different ages is distinct (Table 9.1). In the first 2 years of life, wheezing and bronchiolitis are not distinguishable, and the commonest cause of these episodes is infection with the respiratory syncytial virus (RSV). Infection with RSV is almost universal in the first 2 years of life and in many cases results in no more than a mild upper respiratory infection. An important risk factor for the severity of bronchiolitis or asthma during RSV infection is the size of the lungs at birth. The two major factors that influence the size of the lungs at birth are prematurity and maternal smoking.

In older children and young adults, by far the most commonly identified cause of asthma is sensitization to one of the common inhalant allergens, particularly those encountered indoors. Other important risk factors include a family history of asthma, infection with common cold viruses, especially rhinoviruses, and housing conditions.

Allergen provocation of the lungs of asthmatic patients can induce bronchoconstriction, inflammation in the bronchi, and prolonged increases in bronchial reactivity. In keeping with this, allergen-activated inflammation has become a major target for treatment. This includes reducing exposure to allergens and pharmacological approaches to counteract the inflammatory mediators (e.g. cromolyn sodium, inhaled corticosteroids, and leukotriene-modifying drugs).

People with allergic asthma represent the largest group of asthma patients requiring treatment, and in addition they are also the group on whom most epidemiology studies have been focused. Thus, most of the population-based evidence about the causation for the increased prevalence of asthma has concerned school children or young adults.

Asthma that presents after the age of 20 years provides a complex problem both in management and in investigation. For this age group there is a wider differential diagnosis, and all cases with persistent symptoms require investigation. Major causes include simple allergic asthma in adults, intrinsic asthma associated with chronic hyperplastic sinusitis, allergic bronchopulmonary aspergillosis, wheezing associated with chronic obstructive lung disease, and causes of airway obstruction that are not related to generalized airway reactivity.

Allergic asthma in children

The two strongest risk factors for asthma in childhood are a family history and immediate hypersensitivity to common allergens. This immune response includes both IgE antibodies and helper T cells type 2 (Th2), both of which are thought to contribute to the inflammation in

Table 9.1 Classification of asthma and chronic airway obstruction, based on age of onset and aetiology

Age of onset	Disease	Contributing factors and special features
Infants ≤2 years old	Bronchiolitis/wheezing, single or multiple episodes Bronchopulmonary dysplasia	Respiratory syncytial virus, maternal smoking, and small lungs at birth Prematurity
Children	Allergic asthma	Family history, sensitization to common allergens and intercurrent rhinovirus infection
Adults 20–60 years old	Allergic asthma Allergic bronchopulmonary aspergillosis Late onset/intrinsic asthma Other forms of airway obstruction	Sensitization to indoor allergens and rhinovirus infection High IgE, transient infiltrates, eosinophilia Sinusitis, polyps, aspirin sensitivity Hyperventilation, vocal cord syndrome
>45 years old	Intermittent wheezing complicating chronic obstructive lung disease	Fixed obstruction, $FEV_1 \leq 35\%$ predicted following prolonged smoking

FEV_1, forced expiratory volume in 1 second.

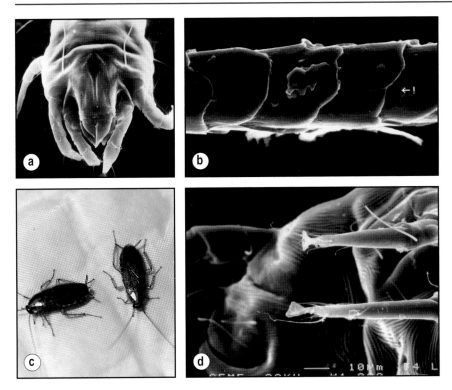

Fig. 9.1 Allergens. (a) Dust mite. (b) Cat hair. (c) Cockroach. (d) Mite legs.

the respiratory tract (see Ch. 1). Children who mount an immune response to inhalant allergens have an increased risk of developing asthma because of this combination of genetics and exposure. However, it is sensitization to indoor allergens (e.g. dust mites, cats, dogs, and cockroaches) that is strongly associated with asthma (Fig. 9.1). By contrast, in some recent studies, immediate hypersensitivity to grass or other pollens has not been found to be significantly associated with asthma. The implication is that a large part of the allergen exposure that contributes to the inflammation in the lungs of patients with perennial asthma occurs inside houses.

The evidence for a causal relationship between exposure to dust mite allergens and asthma has come from many different experiments (Box 9.1). The important features are that:

- there is a very strong association between sensitization to indoor allergens and asthma
- bronchial challenges with the relevant allergens can replicate many features of the disease – acute and delayed airway narrowing, inflammation (which includes an influx of eosinophils), and prolonged increases in non-specific bronchial hyperresponsiveness
- reducing exposure to allergens, whether in the house, hospital room, or sanatorium, can decrease symptoms of asthma.

Thus, the classification of allergic or 'extrinsic' asthma implies not only that the patient has a positive skin test to an allergen but also that exposure to this allergen is contributing to the disease. The main allergens that are

Box 9.1 Evidence that exposure to indoor allergens is causally related to asthma

- There is a very strong association between sensitization to indoor allergens and asthma
- The observations about allergens in houses, sensitization of asthmatics and the association with asthma have been made in many different countries
- The association is only with asthma, and not with any other lung disease
- Bronchial challenge with allergens can reproduce many of the findings of asthma including eosinophil infiltrates and persistent increases in bronchial reactivity
- Reducing exposure to dust mites in a sanatorium or in the home is an effective treatment for asthma
- The mechanism by which allergen exposure causes sensitization and subsequent diseases is biologically plausible

associated with asthma have been purified, cloned, and sequenced (Table 9.2). The immune response to these proteins is very well defined and includes IgE antibodies, IgG4 antibodies, and Th2 lymphocytes. Although this immune response to indoor allergens is well defined as a 'risk factor' for asthma, it is not clear why some allergic people have bronchial hyperreactivity and asthma whereas other apparently equally allergic people do not. In part, this may relate to the many factors that can increase the inflammatory response in allergic people and the many triggers that can induce wheezing. These factors include viral infections, ozone, and passive smoking – all of which

Table 9.2 Allergens associated with asthma

	Species	Allergen	Assays	Size of airborne particles
Indoor				
Arthropods:				
Dust mites	*Dermatophagoides pteronyssinus*	Der p 1	mAb ELISA	10–30 μm
	D. farinae	Der f 1	mAb ELISA	10–30 μm
Cockroach	*Blattella germanica*	Bla g 2	mAb ELISA	>10 μm
Domestic animals:				
Cat	*Felix domesticus*	Fel d 1	mAb ELISA	2–10 μm
Dog	*Canis familiaris*	Can f 1	mAb ELISA	2–10 μm
Rodents:				
Mouse	*Mus muscularis*	Mus m 1	Polyclonal ELISA	2–10 μm
Rat	*Rattus norweigicus*	Rat n 1	mAb	2–10 μm
Outdoors/Indoor				
Molds	*Alternaria alternata*	Alt a 1	mAb/Polyclonal*	10–14 μm
	Aspergillus fumigatus	Asp f 1	mAb	2 μm
Pollens:				
Rye grass	*Lolium perenne*	Lol p 1		
Ragweed	*Ambrosia artemisiifolia*	Amb a 1	Microscopic pollen count	15–30 μm
Oak	*Quercus*			

ELISA, enzyme-linked immunosorbent assay; mAb, monoclonal antibody.
*Also microscopic identification of spores.

are stimuli that induce an epithelial stress response (Fig. 9.2). It is plausible that a fundamental abnormality in asthma is an impaired ability to reconstitute the epithelium in response to environmental stress (Fig. 9.3).

Asthma in adults

Allergic asthma

Asthma in adults is more difficult to classify than asthma in children because there are several overlapping entities and, in addition, a larger number of alternative causes for symptoms of this kind. Among adults with asthma, 30–70% are allergic, depending on the population studied and the severity of the disease. The allergic patients include childhood onset cases, patients who present for the first time, and those allergic patients whose disease goes into remission in their teens but subsequently relapses. The evidence for a direct role of allergens in adults is less complete than it is in children. However, bronchial provocation with allergens can mimic many aspects of the disease, allergen avoidance can reduce both the symptoms and the requirement for medicines, and the epidemiological association between allergen sensitization and asthma in adults has also been found in many countries. In addition, the pattern of sensitization among adults who present to an emergency room with asthma reflects the allergens found in their houses. Patients in this group have positive prick tests to allergens, intermittent wheezing, and significant bronchial hyperreactivity. In addition, their total serum IgE ranges from high normal to high (100 IU/mL up to about 1000 IU/mL), and in general they have moderate eosinophilia (200–500 eosinophils per mL). In most cases of allergic asthma in adults, the chest X-ray is clear and computed tomography (CT) of the sinuses is either normal or shows only mild changes (Fig. 9.4).

Allergic bronchopulmonary aspergillosis

When patients with asthma develop a more severe course (i.e. they require corticosteroids), have persistent symptoms, or start producing sputum, the diagnosis of allergic bronchopulmonary aspergillosis (ABPA) should be considered. In most cases, ABPA is a complication of pre-existing allergic asthma. The diagnostic features are:

- total IgE >400 IU/mL (however total IgE can be suppressed by chronic oral corticosteroid treatment)
- persistent eosinophilia (500/μL)
- productive sputum, which may be brown, orange, or grey in colour and which may grow *Aspergillus fumigatus* or other fungi
- transient infiltrates on chest X-ray
- central bronchiectasis on fine-section CT scan of chest
- immediate hypersensitivity to *A. fumigatus* as judged by skin tests or serum IgE antibodies
- precipitins against the fungus or high-titre specific IgG antibodies.

Colonization of the lungs with *Aspergillus* is very common among patients with cystic fibrosis, and these children often have high total serum IgE and IgE

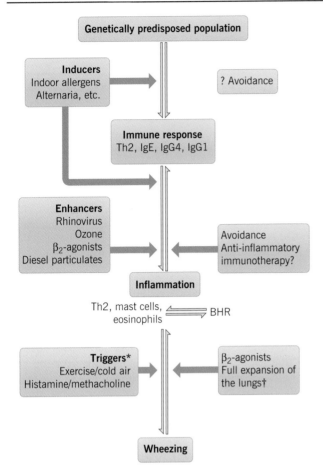

Fig. 9.2 Causes of asthma.

* both inducers and enhancers can act as triggers
† ? exercise

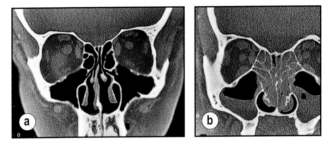

Fig. 9.4 Computed tomography (CT) scans of the sinus. (a) Normal scan. (b) Scan from a patient with severe polypoid changes.

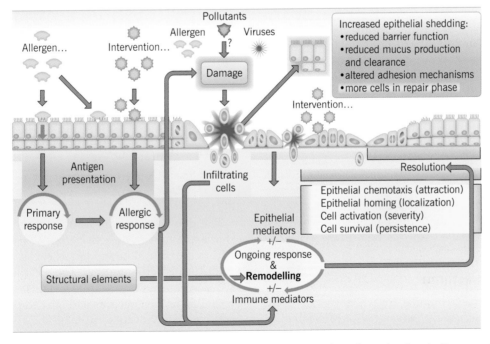

Fig. 9.3 The role of the airway epithelium in disease. The repair cycle in chronic asthma, leading to the secretion of growth factors involved in tissue remodelling.

antibodies to the fungus. Almost all these children have lung damage, including bronchiectasis, but in general they do not have significant eosinophilia. Other fungi can occasionally cause a similar syndrome (e.g. allergic bronchopulmonary curvulariosis or allergic bronchopulmonary candidiasis).

Intrinsic asthma

Intrinsic asthma was defined in 1947 by Rackemann, who drew attention to patients presenting in adult life who showed:

- negative skin tests to common allergens
- no family history of atopic disease
- persistent eosinophilia
- a severe course (often requiring oral corticosteroids and were therefore overrepresented in tertiary care clinics and among hospitalized patients)
- no improvement when admitted to hospital.

In 1956, Samter added the observation that some of these patients had nasal polyps, sinusitis, and aspirin sensitivity. In this form of asthma there is greatly enhanced production of cysteinyl leukotrienes by mast cells and eosinophils with a selective up-regulation of leukotriene C_4 synthase, the terminal enzyme in the generation of these mediators. Although sinusitis is not present in all cases of intrinsic asthma, it is common.

Among adults aged over 40 years who develop severe asthma for the first time, almost 50% may have intrinsic asthma, although these patients do not represent more than 10% of the total population with asthma. In a random sample of adults presenting with asthma to an emergency room, almost 30% have extensive sinusitis on CT. However, this figure includes both those with polypoid sinusitis, typical of intrinsic asthma, and those with acute sinusitis related to intercurrent viral infection (see Fig. 9.4).

Late onset asthma, which is frequently not associated with atopy, may be linked to the workplace. Occupational exposure to sensitizing chemicals (e.g. isocyanates) is an important cause of asthma as the timely removal from exposure can cure the disease or at least prevent progression. In atopic people, exposure to novel foreign proteins (e.g. enzymes in detergents, proteins in rodent urine, etc.) may also lead to occupational asthma. The diagnosis is best established by a careful history, monitoring the peak expiratory flow rate both in and out of work, and occasionally by controlled provocation with the suspected agent or agents.

Virally induced asthma

Viruses are the most common trigger, provoking up to 65% of acute asthma exacerbations. Also, virus infection is associated with particularly severe acute symptoms, with more severe air-flow obstruction and a longer length of stay in hospital. The most common pathogens

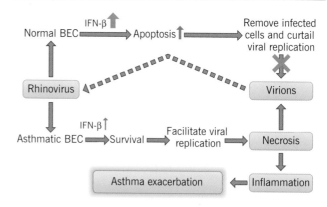

Fig. 9.5 Model of the mechanism of viral asthma. Please see text for explanation. BEC, bronchial epithelial cells; IFN-β, interferon β. (Drawn from Wark PA, Johnston SL, Bucchieri F, et al. Asthmatic bronchial epithelial cells have a deficient innate immune response to infection with rhinovirus. J Exp Med 2005; 201:937–947.)

associated with asthma exacerbations are rhinoviruses, to which allergic asthmatics are particularly susceptible. Infection leads to increased bronchial inflammation and acute exacerbations of existing asthma. The reasons why some asthmatics respond so dramatically to infection are not clear. Some studies suggest that there is an inadequate production of IFN-β (Fig 9.5). On the other hand, rhinovirus challenge consistently shows a positive interaction between allergic inflammation of the lungs and the response to rhinovirus.

Chronic obstructive lung disease

Chronic bronchitis with emphysema, which is also known as chronic obstructive pulmonary disease (COPD), is in most cases a sequel to many years of active smoking. The damage caused by smoking is slow:

- after 5–10 years of smoking, the effect on spirometry may not be detectable
- after 20 years of smoking, the forced expiratory volume in 1 second (FEV_1) and the forced vital capacity (FVC) are usually decreased
- after 30–50 years of smoking, the disease becomes a major clinical problem.

This means that it is unusual for patients to present before the age of 50 years with severe fixed obstruction.

The dominant symptoms of COPD are coughing and shortage of breath on activity, but some patients present with acute breathlessness and wheezing, which is difficult to distinguish from asthma. The treatment of acute episodes in patients with COPD is similar to that of asthma, including bronchodilators and inhaled corticosteroids. In addition, many of these patients show significant reversibility and moderate, non-specific bronchial hyperreactivity to methacholine. The basis for the inflammation in these patients is not clear, but it is usually not related to allergy. In a few patients, colonization of the lungs with fungi may exacerbate the disease; however, even in these cases the patients are usually not 'allergic' to the fungi as judged by skin tests or IgE antibodies.

Establishing that a patient has fixed obstruction is best achieved by spirometry when the patient has been optimally treated. Thus, 2 weeks of full treatment with high-dose inhaled corticosteroids or oral prednisone (about 40 mg/day) is usually sufficient to establish the optimal lung function for that patient. Reversibility of airway obstruction is usually defined in terms of percentage change; however, if obstruction is severe, even a 15% change may represent very little improvement (e.g. a 15% improvement in an FEV_1 of 0.8 L gives an FEV_1 of 0.9 L). Thus, it is necessary to know both the response to bronchodilator and the best FEV_1 and FVC achieved after treatment.

Anatomy and physiology of the bronchi

The pathophysiology of asthma involves the nasal passages, the paranasal sinuses, the mouth, the larynx, the trachea, and the bronchial tree. Each of these may be inflamed and to some degree obstructed, and each can play an important role in symptoms. The anatomy and physiology of the nasal passages and sinuses are considered in Chapter 10. The major focus of asthma is large, medium, and small bronchi, all of which can become inflamed, swollen, and hyperresponsive. The bronchial tree has approximately 16 divisions, or generations, before reaching the terminal, or respiratory, bronchioles. In uncomplicated asthma, the remaining five to seven divisions of the bronchioles and alveolae are normal. The bronchi have cartilage in their walls, which forms complete rings in the trachea; it is present as plates as the bronchi divide but it is absent from the smallest bronchi. All bronchi have smooth muscle in their walls (Fig. 9.6).

The blood supply to the lungs comes from two sources. The pulmonary circulation coming from the pulmonary arteries provides venous (i.e. unoxygenated) blood to the alveoli for gas exchange. The bronchial circulation comes from the aorta and provides blood supply to the bronchial walls. The branches of the bronchial arteries and veins provide a plexus in the submucosa and around the smooth muscles. Changes in the walls of the vessels allow oedema formation and influx of inflammatory cells; in addition, simple changes in the blood vessels may contribute to the thickness of the wall.

The bronchi are lined with a mixture of ciliated and serous cells. For most of the bronchial tree, 60% of the cells are ciliated; however, in the trachea and main bronchi the epithelium is pseudostratified. The proportion of ciliated cells increases as the bronchi divide. The serous cells play a major role in controlling airway lung

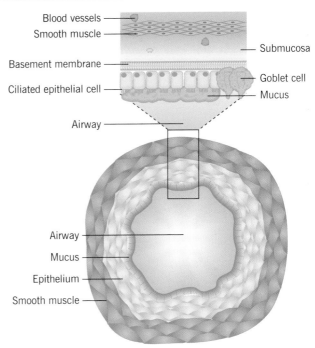

Fig. 9.6 The anatomy of a medium-sized bronchus. The changes in the bronchi that occur in asthma are: (1) increased mucus production; (2) subbasement membrane thickening; (3) epithelial desquamation; (4) submucosal oedema; (5) hypertrophy of smooth muscle; (6) infiltration of submucosa and epithelium with mast cells, eosinophils, T cells, and basophils.

fluid; in addition, there are goblet cells in the epithelium and mucous glands in the bronchial wall and these goblet cells provide the mucous blanket. The best-recognized part of inflammation in asthma is an influx of eosinophils with associated damage, which includes desquamation of the epithelial cell layer (see Fig. 9.3). The response to allergens or other antigens can also include a marked increase in goblet cells and mucus production. The products of this inflammation may be demonstrable in the sputum as mucus, Charcot–Leyden crystals, eosinophil cationic protein, and whorls of desquamated epithelium (Creola bodies), which are indicative of an interaction between infiltrating eosinophils and the epithelium.

Innervation of the bronchi

The bronchi receive nerves from the parasympathetic nervous system, including efferent cholinergic fibres and non-myelinated sensory nerves (C fibres) and from the sympathetic nervous system, primarily from postganglionic adrenergic fibres to the parasympathetic ganglia; the bronchi also receive non-cholinergic, non-adrenergic (NANC) inhibitory fibres, which travel with the cholinergic fibres and provide the only direct neuronal bronchodilator pathway (Fig. 9.7). These nerves provide innervation to smooth muscle, blood vessels, mucous

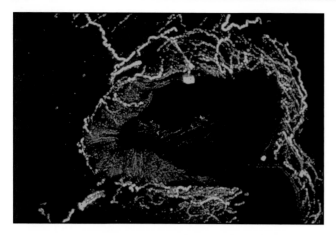

Fig. 9.7 Three-dimensional confocal microscopic reconstruction of sensory nerves surrounding a small asthmatic airway. (Courtesy of J. Polak, RPMS, London.)

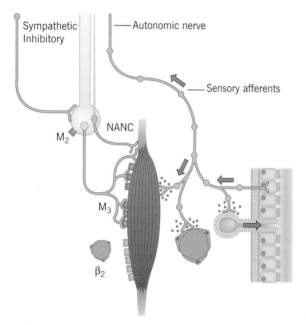

Fig. 9.8 The nerve supply to the airways. The efferent innervation of smooth muscle is cholinergic through M_3 receptors, and sympathetic inhibitory fibres act on adrenergic receptors of the parasympathetic ganglia. Inhibition of smooth muscle is through circulating adrenaline from the adrenal medulla. Activation of sensory non-myelinated fibres with axon reflexes can release neuropeptides [e.g. neurokinin A, substance P, and calcitonin gene-related peptides (CGRP)]. NANC fibres, non-adrenergic non-cholinergic fibres.

glands, the epithelium, and mast cells. Cholinergic fibres from local ganglia stimulate contraction of the smooth muscles and the muscarinic receptor via an M_3 receptor (Fig. 9.8). Adrenergic inhibitory control of the smooth muscle comes from two routes: noradrenaline (norepinephrine) released from postganglionic inhibitory fibres to the vagal ganglia, and adrenaline (epinephrine) released into the circulation from the adrenal medulla. There is

no direct sympathetic innervation to the smooth muscle. In addition, fibres of the NANC system run with the vagus nerve, and their postganglionic fibres innervate smooth muscle. The mediator for the NANC fibres that relaxes smooth muscle is thought to be nitric oxide (NO).

There are two additional elements to the innervation of the bronchi, which may be relevant to the pathophysiology of asthma:

- Sensory fibres that supply the epithelium, blood vessels, and mucous glands contain several mediators, including substance P, neurokinin A, and calcitonin gene-related peptide. Release of these mediators can be triggered by axon reflexes from other sensory endings. The nerve endings can be stimulated by many inflammatory mediators, including bradykinin, mast cell tryptase, and leukotrienes. Damage to the bronchial epithelium exposes sensory nerve endings and can potentially increase reflex stimulation of mucus production, vascular leakage, and smooth muscle contraction.
- Sectioning of mast cells in tissues reveals that most, if not all, have autonomic innervation that can control mediator release. In addition, there are mast cells within the autonomic ganglia. Release of mediators from mast cells in or around the ganglia can dramatically alter the transmission of nerve impulses.

Diagnosis of asthma

Patients may present to clinics or emergency rooms with acute symptoms of breathlessness, wheezing, or coughing. Alternatively, they may present between episodes with normal or near-normal lungs. In the first case, measurement of peak expiratory flow rate or spirometry before and after treatment with bronchodilators will generally establish the diagnosis of reversible airway obstruction. In patients who present without physical signs in the chest or decreased air flow, the diagnosis is dependent on history, serial measurements of air flow over several days using a peak flow meter, or provocation tests to establish bronchial hyperresponsiveness. In children and in young adults, a history of repeated attacks of wheezing combined with waking at night, coughing, or wheezing may be sufficient to recommend a trial of treatment. However, it is always better to establish that there is a decrease in air flow during symptomatic episodes and to establish the best or optimum lung function for each patient.

Further evaluation of patients with asthma involves establishing whether they are allergic (with skin tests for immediate hypersensitivity, measurements of total serum IgE or specific IgE antibodies, and routine blood count focusing on eosinophilia). Evaluation of persistent or severe cases that are not responsive to treatment may also require chest X-ray, sinus CT, and evaluation of the upper airway. Recently several studies have demonstrated the clear correlation between elevated exhaled nitric oxide (eNO) and increased inflammation in the lungs. More importantly, some studies suggest that eNO can be a useful guide to treatment requirements.

History

The cardinal symptoms of asthma are wheezing, coughing, tightness in the chest, and shortness of breath, representing an interaction between inflamed and chronically remodelled airways. In all patients the symptoms fluctuate in intensity, and in the majority of patients the symptoms are intermittent. Thus, most patients have normal or near-normal lung function and no symptoms between episodes. Attacks may occur spontaneously (often at night or first thing in the morning), after exercise, or shortly after exposure to a known trigger factor. In order to define the history, the patient must be questioned about the age at onset of symptoms and about the details of the attacks (Table 9.3). The history should also include details of the response of attacks to treatment. Evidence of severity is based on the occurrence and frequency of acute episodes, emergency room visits, or hospitalizations as well as on treatment requirements, especially the use of bronchodilators and inhaled or oral corticosteroids.

Careful questioning about factors that influence symptoms should distinguish between non-specific triggers (e.g. cold air, passive smoking, emotional events, or strong perfumes) and specific reactions that suggest the patient is allergic (e.g. seasonal hay fever or nasal, eye, or lung symptoms following exposure to known sources of allergens such as domestic animals). Questions about seasonal variations in symptoms are important; however, most patients who are allergic to common indoor allergens do not describe seasonal variation and, conversely, some patients whose attacks are triggered by viral infection report seasonal exacerbations in the autumn. Therefore, the presence or absence of seasonality is not a basis for distinguishing between allergic and non-allergic cases. It is also helpful to ask directed questions about the environment in terms of dampness, mould, domestic animals, pests, and house furnishings. In addition, patients may be aware of reacting specifically to exposures in other houses. Similarly, it is important to know where a child spends his or her time (e.g. other bedrooms, houses of friends or family members, daycare centres).

Attacks of asthma vary from transient wheezing that recovers rapidly, either spontaneously or after treatment with a bronchodilator, to episodes that develop over minutes, hours, or days into severe symptoms that are poorly, if at all, responsive to inhaled medicine. It is essential to know both the severity and the frequency of attacks. In many cases, chest symptoms develop without preceding evidence of an attack; however, in other cases the attack is preceded by or associated with nasal or sinus symptoms or productive cough.

Nasal or sinus symptoms

At least half the patients who are being treated for asthma also have nasal or sinus symptoms of some kind. In a majority of cases, the symptoms are allergic and are

Table 9.3 Classification of asthma based on severity of disease*

Classification	Symptoms	Best FEV$_1$	Investigation
Mild intermittent	Occasional episodes reverse spontaneously or with one dose of bronchodilator	90–100%	History only
Moderate intermittent	Occasional episodes but may require more treatment Attacks after exercise	90–100%	Peak flow meter
Mild persistent	Symptoms several times per week Attacks after exercise Requires regular treatment	>90%	Spirometry, evaluate aetiology, peak flow monitoring, CXR
Moderate persistent	Frequent symptoms, some difficult attacks Difficulty with exercise Requires regular treatment	85–95%	Evaluate causes of increasing severity
Severe persistent	Persistent symptoms requiring continuous treatment, emergency visits and/or hospitalization	60–80%	Spirometry, DLCO, Sinus CT Re-evaluate causes including sinusitis, aspirin sensitivity, fungal infection, etc.

*Occasional patients have rare severe attacks (or even only one severe attack) that requires emergency treatment but have no significant symptoms otherwise.
CT, computed tomography; CXR, chest X-ray; DLCO, diffusion capacity of the lung for carbon monoxide; FEV$_1$, forced expiratory volume in 1 second.

consistent with exposure to allergens and the pattern of positive skin tests. However, many patients report episodes of nasal pressure or pain associated with mucopurulent discharge. Patients may give a history that these symptoms respond to antibiotics. However, the history is a very poor indication of the extent of changes found on sinus CT, and some of these patients will respond to treatment for known allergic sensitization (i.e. allergen avoidance and local anti-inflammatory treatment).

Sinus CT should be reserved for patients who have recurrent episodes that are not responsive to treatment. However, there are many different patterns of sinus disease, and the treatment is not well defined. Extensive sinusitis on CT scan (see Fig. 9.4) is a common feature of intrinsic asthma. In such cases, nasal polyps, eosinophilia, and aspirin sensitivity are also common. Moderate degrees of sinus abnormality are common and may be associated with recurrent episodes of bacterial infection; however, it is not clear to what degree these abnormalities are associated with asthma. Furthermore, very few of these 'infections' are diagnosed bacteriologically. Sinusitis with nasal polyps is very common in cystic fibrosis and the presence of polyps should trigger a sweat test in all patients who are aged less than 25 years. Finally, sinusitis with extensive changes on CT can occur during acute rhinovirus infection. Some adults presenting with acute asthma have extensive sinus abnormalities that resolve over the following few weeks, which strongly suggests that an acute viral infection triggered the asthma attacks (Fig. 9.9).

Evaluation of lung function

Clinical examination of the chest may identify wheezing, prolonged expiration, and poor air entry, but it is an unreliable method of estimating the extent of airway obstruction. The simplest technique for monitoring obstruction is the use of the peak flow meter, which measures the maximum rate of expiratory flow in litres per minute (Fig. 9.10). Peak flow meters are ideal for home monitoring because they are simple to use, inexpensive, and portable. A chart showing repeated measurements over 2 weeks may establish diurnal variation, major changes from day to day, or consistently normal values. However, the results are dependent on effort, require consistent recording by the patient or parents, and do not provide information about the pattern of flow. Spirometry provides a record of the forced expiratory volume (FEV) over time; this is most commonly expressed as:

- the FEV for the first second (FEV_1)
- the midflow FEV (FEV 25–75%)
- the FVC, which is the forced volume over 6 seconds (FVC_6).

In addition, spirometry can provide visual comparison of repeated curves before and after treatment, which can yield clear evidence of reversible airway obstruction. In children or young adults with mild or moderate disease, this is sufficient to establish the diagnosis. In patients with severe disease, spirometry may demonstrate minimal reversibility following bronchodilator therapy (i.e. <15% increase), or may demonstrate reversibility (i.e. >15%

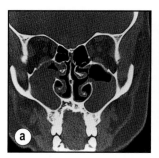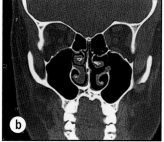

Fig. 9.9 Computed tomography (CT) scans of the sinus. (a) Scan at the time of an acute attack of asthma. (b) Scan 4 months later.

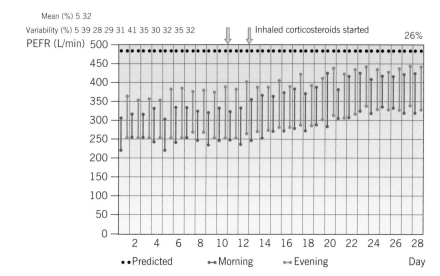

Fig. 9.10 Peak flow measurement. Daily peak flow records taken before and after bronchodilator in the mornings and evenings for 1 month. PEFR, peak expiratory flow rate.

increase) but still show marked obstruction. In such cases, further lung function studies (e.g. diffusion capacity for carbon monoxide and measurements of lung volume, both of which are normal in uncomplicated asthma) may be required to rule out other diagnoses. However, the most useful investigation is to repeat spirometry after 3 weeks' treatment with high-dose inhaled or oral corticosteroids plus bronchodilators. The diagnosis of fixed or irreversible obstruction should be considered only in patients who have obstruction after 2 or 3 weeks of such treatment.

Tests for bronchial hyperreactivity (BHR)

In patients who have normal lung function (i.e. FEV_1 >90% predicted), hyperreactivity or hyperresponsiveness can be demonstrated by several different provocation tests (Table 9.4). Bronchial provocation using specific allergen extract in fine droplets from a nebulizer will produce acute airway obstruction in sensitive patients. However, a similar response, generally requiring a higher dose, occurs in allergic patients who do not have asthma. Furthermore, allergens to which people are exposed naturally are in the form of particles that vary in diameter from 2 μm to 20 μm, not in the form of nebulized droplets (Fig. 9.11). Thus, bronchial challenge with

allergen is not a test for asthma and provides little clinical information that cannot be obtained from skin tests. Non-specific challenge tests to identify bronchial hyperresponsiveness include exercise, inhalation of dry or cold air, histamine, and methacholine.

Exercise challenge

Four minutes of exercise that is sufficiently vigorous to increase the heart rate to 80% of maximum, or random running, will generally be enough to provoke a fall in FEV_1 or peak flow in patients with bronchial hyperreactivity. This test of bronchial hyperresponsiveness is dependent on evaporation from the respiratory tract, and humidification of the inspiratory air will prevent the response. In turn this means that results are very strongly influenced by ambient humidity.

Cold air challenge

Use of cold air (which is by definition dry) for the challenge achieves a very similar effect by inducing evaporation from the lungs, and it is easier to control the conditions of the challenge. Whether exercise or cold air challenge induces mediator release is not entirely clear because it has proved difficult to measure mediators in the lung after challenge. However, these responses can be inhibited by corticosteroids, cromolyn, or leukotriene antagonists, which suggests that mediator release is involved.

Table 9.4 Provocation tests for specific and non-specific bronchial hyperreactivity

	Response				
	Immediate– 15 min	Late 2–8 hours	Depends on BHR	Blocked by	Mechanism
Specific:					
Relevant allergen	++	++	No	Cromolyn, etc.	Triggering of mast cells through specific IgE
Non-specific:					
Exercise or cold air	++	±	Yes	Cromolyn, etc., antileukotrienes, short- and long-acting β₂-agonist	Evaporation of water → hyperosmolar triggering
Histamine*	++	No	Yes	Antihistamine	Direct action on blood vessels, muscles, etc.
Methacholine*	++	No	Yes	Anticholinergics	Direct action on smooth muscles
Others:*					
Water	++	No	Yes	Cromolyn	
Hypertonic saline	++	No	Yes	Theophylline, cromolyn	
Adenosine	++	No	Yes	Steroids	
SO₂	++	No	±	Steroids	

*Given as nebulized drops approximately 2 μm in diameter.

Histamine challenge

Histamine challenge to demonstrate bronchial hyperreactivity was first introduced by Samter in 1935 and adapted by Tifeneau in 1949. There are many different techniques, including tidal breathing over 2 minutes, sequential puffs from a hand-held inhaler, and the use of a dosimeter. The techniques are different in that the response of the lungs to challenge is altered by full inspiratory manoeuvres. The advantage of histamine is that it is a natural substance and has a very short half-life in vivo. The disadvantage is that it can cause unpleasant flushing. As with all challenges, histamine challenge can cause rapid increases in lung resistance; it should therefore be started at a low dose, and it requires medical supervision.

Inhalation of a few (~10–100) mite faecal particles per day

Bronchial provocation with 10^8 droplets in 2 minutes

Local inflammatory responses lead to increased bronchial responsiveness

Diffuse bronchospasm within 20 minutes prolonged effects

(a) (b)

Fig. 9.11 Lung exposure. (a) The natural exposure of the airways to allergen particles – inhalation of a few (10–100) mite faecal particles per day. Local inflammatory responses lead to increased bronchial responsiveness. (b) Exposure to nebulized extract or histamine – bronchial provocation with $\geq 10^8$ droplets in 2 minutes. There is diffuse bronchospasm within 20 minutes, with or without prolonged effects.

Methacholine challenge

Methacholine is an analogue of the cholinergic mediator for smooth muscle contraction in the lung. The assumption is that methacholine challenge works by acting on smooth muscle, although there are other possible pathways and in vitro experiments do not demonstrate very marked hyperresponsiveness of smooth muscle from patients with asthma. A concept that goes some way towards explaining bronchial hyperresponsiveness is thickening of the airway wall. In the submucosa, this thickening will lead to a disproportionate reduction in airway calibre for a given degree of airway smooth muscle shortening; in the adventitia outside the smooth muscle, it will distribute elastic contractile forces over a greater surface area and therefore reduce protection from airway closure. Nevertheless, methacholine provides consistent bronchial challenge results and is widely used for clinical testing (Fig. 9.12). The standard technique uses a dosimeter, but tidal breathing is an alternative. Methacholine challenge is well tolerated and recovery after challenge is rapid.

With all testing of non-specific bronchial hyperresponsiveness, it is assumed that the test does not itself increase bronchial hyperresponsiveness. This is in contrast to allergen challenge, which can produce a late reaction (after 6 hours) and is often followed by prolonged increases in bronchial hyperresponsiveness. With histamine challenge there have been no reports of late reactions or persistent effects on the lung. Most exercise challenges are not followed by late reactions. However, the response to exercise is thought to involve mediator release, and there have been occasional reports of late reactions. Thus it is legitimate to ask whether repeated exercise challenge that results in bronchoconstriction will increase non-specific bronchial hyperresponsiveness. The evidence about methacholine challenge is less clear than about histamine because there have been occasional reports of prolonged effects (particularly coughing) after repeated challenges.

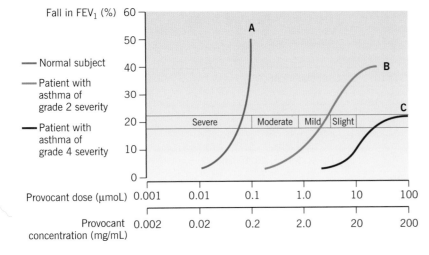

Fig. 9.12 The response of the airways to methacholine challenge. Fall in FEV_1 plotted against amount of provocant (methacholine) that causes that fall.

Other causes of intermittent symptoms that suggest asthma

Asthma is characterized by widespread inflammation of the bronchi, with hyperreactivity that is present in all lobes of the lung. In keeping with this, most diseases that involve localized obstruction, cardiac or other medical causes of shortage of breath, and simple hyperventilation do not present with the typical history of asthma or with typical reversible spirometry. Nevertheless, many patients present in a sufficiently unusual way that they are diagnosed as having asthma and may be erroneously treated for asthma. These alternative diagnoses can be classified as:

- medical conditions involving the lungs that present with symptoms suggestive of asthma
- syndromes characterized by abnormal breathing in which the lungs are structurally normal
- cases of local airway obstruction that present with wheezing audible to the patient or on examination.

On occasion, asthma may present solely as cough without evidence of airway obstruction or bronchial hyperreactivity. In this 'cough variant' form, sputum eosinophilia is invariably present. However, many different medical conditions present with cough or shortage of breath (with or without wheezing) and can easily be confused with asthma. These include:

- cardiac failure with acute pulmonary oedema
- cardiac failure secondary to myocardial infarction
- pulmonary embolism
- pneumonia
- tracheobronchitis.

Chest pain may confuse the situation because anterior chest pain is fairly common in severe cases of asthma. This pain in adults often results in a work-up for myocardial infarction. The distinction from pulmonary oedema is important because narcotics are contraindicated in asthma. Similarly, the recognition of pulmonary embolism as a cause of wheezing and shortage of breath is very important because heparin is life saving in pulmonary embolus. Bronchitis secondary to bacterial or viral infection can produce symptoms very similar to those of the minority of patients with asthma who present primarily with a cough or who have a productive cough.

There are several conditions that present as shortage of breath in which the lungs are not abnormal. The commonest of these is hyperventilation syndrome. If the patient makes severe expiratory noises then these noises are often interpreted as wheezing. However, such patients will have normal spirometry if they can be persuaded to comply. In addition, they have blood gases that are typical of hyperventilation (i.e. normal pO_2 and very low pCO_2). Paradoxical closure of the vocal cords during inspiration or expiration – the so-called 'vocal cord syndrome' – may

present with typical symptoms, but in many cases it is difficult to diagnose. Improvement in symptoms while talking, inconsistent pulmonary function tests, and an absence of markers of atopy or inflammation (i.e. eosinophil count $<0.01\times10^9/L$, or exhaled nitric oxide <25 parts per billion) are all suggestive. The diagnosis should also be considered in patients who rapidly recover fully normal lung function and do not respond consistently to treatment with systemic corticosteroids. Finally, an apparently increasing number of non-asthmatic people present with shortage of breath as a response to exercise exacerbated by poor physical condition or obesity.

Wheezing is a common feature of localized partial obstruction of the bronchi. Local obstruction can be caused by a foreign body, benign tumours such as an adenoma, or malignant tumours. In general, these lesions do not give rise to shortage of breath or variable airway resistance. However, the degree of obstruction may vary with associated inflammation. Malignant tumours are usually visible on the chest X-ray; alternatively, they may present with bleeding. However, even malignant tumours can occasionally present as airway obstruction that is responsive to treatment, including corticosteroids. In doubtful cases, fine-section CT of the chest or bronchoscopy will usually reveal a local obstruction.

Obstruction of the large bronchi or trachea can also be caused by the rare syndrome of bronchomalacia or tracheomalacia, and in some cases the obstruction is intermittent. This diagnosis should also be clear on chest CT. Obstruction of the trachea (e.g. by a tumour) outside the chest can present with symptoms of shortage of breath, but the primary finding is usually inspiratory stridor.

Management of asthma

The fluctuating nature of airway obstruction in asthma means that patients have to play a major role in controlling the symptoms themselves and therefore have to make appropriate decisions. Effective education early in the course of the disease can create a well-informed, confident patient (or parent) who will manage the disease (Box 9.2). This allows less interruption of normal life, a better long-term outcome, and dramatically reduces use of emergency services. The essence of a management plan is that:

- it is simple and effective at controlling symptoms
- it has minimum risk of severe side effects
- it will achieve the best long-term outcome in terms of lung function.

This requires an evaluation of severity (see the History and Diagnosis sections above) based on frequency of attacks, severity of attacks, and previous response to treatment. One of the greatest difficulties is encouraging patients to comply with preventative measures when their symptoms are relatively well controlled. A clear understanding of the nature of asthma and the objectives of treatment is therefore of great value. Effective management of asthma always requires a partnership between the patient and the health professional.

Box 9.2 Role of education in asthma management

1. Education about the nature of the disease and the distinction between causes of inflammation and triggers of acute shortage of breath
2. Techniques for using inhalers, spacers, and nebulizers; distinction between those inhalers that help to control the disease and bronchodilators suitable for short-term use
3. Home monitoring:
   - use of peak flow meter
   - establish normal variability and personal best
   - regular monitoring in a minority of cases only
   - use of meter to help assess attacks and to design response to attacks
4. Side effects of asthma medications:
   - excessive bronchodilator use
   - inhaled steroids
   - oral steroids
   - theophylline
5. Action plan for treating exacerbations
6. Measures to decrease exposure
   - education on relevant avoidance measures: dust mites, domestic animals, cockroaches, fungi, pollens, etc.

Drug treatment

The primary classification of drugs used in asthma (Table 9.5) recognizes:

- bronchodilators, which can relieve symptoms rapidly (relievers)
- anti-inflammatory drugs, which decrease the underlying inflammation in the lungs, and therefore can control symptoms over a longer period of time (controllers).

None of the currently available drugs can be said to offer a cure for the disease. There are several drugs that defy classification but play an important role in some cases. In particular these include:

- theophylline, which may act as an A2b-adenosine antagonist and as a phosphodiesterase inhibitor
- salmeterol and formoterol, which are long-acting β_2-agonists
- the leukotriene-modifying drugs, including both receptor antagonists (montelukast, zafirlukast) and 5-lipoxygenase inhibitors (zileuton), which may have both bronchodilator and controlling effects.

β_2-Adrenergic agonists

β_2-Adrenergic agonists are the primary treatment for bronchospasm both for minor episodes of wheezing during daily life and also in the emergency situation. The inhaled, short-acting β_2-selective agonists generally act within 10 minutes and are very effective at relieving symptoms. Almost all patients with asthma should be

---

Table 9.5 Properties of the commonly used asthma drugs

Steroids	Action				Protects against allergen		
	Route	Control	Bronchodilator	Exercise	Early	Late	Frequency/dosage
Steroids	Inhaled	+ + +	−	+	−	+ +	Daily/b.i.d
	Oral	+ + +	−	−	−	+ +	Daily
Cromolyn	Inhaled	+	−	+ +	+ +	+	q.i.d.
Nedocromil sodium						+ +	
β_2-adrenergic agonist	Inhaled	−	+ + +	+ + +	+ +	−	As needed
	Injected	−	+ + +	nr	nr	nr	
Long-acting β_2-adrenergic agonist (LABA)	Inhaled	+ +	+ +	+ + +	+ +	+ +	b.i.d., nocturnal, or before exercise
Theophylline	Oral	+ +	+	+	+	−	b.i.d., or as needed
Ipratropium bromide	Inhaled	−	+	+ +	−	−	t.i.d.
Leukotriene antagonists	Oral	+ + or ±	±	+ +	−	−	Daily or b.i.d.

nr, not relevant.

taught how to use an inhaler and provided with one. However, these agonists have no controlling effects, and there is some evidence that excessive use of adrenergic agonists without an anti-inflammatory drug can increase bronchial hyperreactivity. In most cases β_2-adrenergic agonists should be prescribed for use in response to increased symptoms or decreased peak flow. In addition, patients should be told that they may need alternative or additional treatment if they require more than two or three doses of bronchodilator per week. Long-acting β_2-agonists (LABAs) are used as a supplement to inhaled corticosteroids in patients who remain symptomatic despite moderate to high doses of corticosteroids. They should be administered in combination with an inhaled corticosteroid in a single inhaler device. LABAs should never be given to patients with asthma in the absence of inhaled corticosteroid.

Inhaled disodium cromoglycate (cromolyn)

In 1970, cromolyn sodium was shown to control the increase in bronchial hyperreactivity that can occur in allergic patients during the pollen season. In addition, it can protect against the effects of exercise challenge and against both the immediate and delayed effects of allergen bronchial challenge. Although the anti-inflammatory or controlling effects of this drug are considered to take 2 weeks for full effect, the protective effect against a challenge is present within 20 minutes. Regular inhaled cromolyn sodium by nebulizer can provide effective long-term control of asthma in children, but it needs to be given frequently for optimal effects.

Inhaled corticosteroids

Corticosteroid inhalers (dry-powder or metered-dose inhalers) have become the primary anti-inflammatory treatment for adults and are very widely used in children. Systemically active corticosteroids (e.g. prednisone or dexamethasone) can be inhaled, but the corticosteroids currently used have been developed specifically for local use in the nose or lungs. These modifications are designed to increase local bioavailability and decrease systemic side effects. The details of local action, absorption, and systemic half-life are different for each preparation.

Local steroids should be used on a regular basis once or twice daily but can also be used as part of an action plan. Regular dosage in children should be kept below 800 µg per day to minimize systemic side effects. In mild exacerbations the dose can be doubled, and in significant attacks the dose should be increased up to 2 mg per day (i.e. 800 µg dose of budesonide or fluticasone three times per day). In the case of metered-dose inhalers, large-volume spacers are advised to reduce oropharyngeal deposition (and therefore the swallowed dose) and to increase the efficiency of intrapulmonary deposition.

Treatment with anti-immunoglobulin E antibody in allergic asthma

Treatment of adult and paediatric allergic moderate-to-severe asthma with humanized monoclonal anti-IgE antibody (omalizumab) results in a decrease in asthma exacerbation rates and reduced usage of inhaled and oral corticosteroids. In addition, improvements in lung function, asthma symptoms, and asthma-related quality of life have been observed in some studies. Treatment with omalizumab leads to decreased IgE levels and partial inhibition of early and late asthmatic responses after allergen bronchoprovocation in allergic asthma. In a range of studies omalizumab also shows reductions in multiple markers of airway inflammation, including eosinophils and high-affinity receptors for IgE. Although omalizumab is more expensive than other controller medications for asthma, it has been demonstrated to save overall treatment costs when used for patients with severe asthma.

Specific immunotherapy (SIT) is effective in patients with allergic rhinitis and allergic asthma if adequate doses of allergens are administered. However, the risks of systemic anaphylactic reactions must be considered. Therefore, treatment with both SIT and omalizumab would provide better clinical efficacy with less adverse events than either treatment given alone. Indeed, a recent clinical study of combined treatment with omalizumab and SIT in polysensitized children and adolescents with seasonal allergic rhinitis showed that combined treatment was more effective than SIT alone, decreasing symptom loads during the pollen season. Therefore, anti-IgE antibody represents a potential therapeutic approach for severe allergic asthma.

Management plans

There is no shortage of guidelines for asthma treatment and all of the national and international guidelines include progressive increases in therapy based on severity. However, many other factors influence the design of treatment plans, including past experience with different drugs, the patient's enthusiasm for, compliance with, and prejudice against corticosteroid inhalers, economics, and the patient's level of anxiety about the symptoms. Effective management of patients with moderate or severe persistent disease includes the use of many different drugs. In addition, it may be necessary to tolerate rather poor control in patients who are opposed to some forms of treatment or unwilling to have close monitoring of their disease.

The introduction of guidelines for the management of asthma has moved the control of airway inflammation with a combination of environmental measures and controller drugs to the centre of management. In order to target therapy effectively, it is important to assess the severity of the asthma. Classifying symptoms as

Table 9.6 Severity-based asthma treatment*

	Treatment plan			
Symptoms	β_2-agonist short acting	Regular	Action plan	Education steps from Box 9.2
Intermittent:				
Occasional symptoms or only after exercise	p.r.n.	Not necessary	No	1 and 2
Symptoms 2–3 times per week	p.r.n.	In some cases	+ or –	1, 2, 3, (6)
Persistent:				
Mild to moderate	p.r.n.	Inhaled steroid/theophylline, LABA, LTRA	Yes	2, 3, 4, (5), 6
Moderate with attacks	p.r.n.	Inhaled steroids and others	Yes	1, 2, 3, 4, 5, 6
Severe	p.r.n.	High-dose inhaled steroids and others	Yes	1, 2, 3, 4, 5, 6

p.r.n., as required.
*Skin tests, or in vitro assays plus specific advice; immunotherapy in seasonal cases related to pollen and other highly allergic cases.

intermittent or persistent and then recognizing attacks as mild, moderate, or severe gives rise to five major groups (Table 9.6). Needless to say, there are many cases that do not fit these groups. However, the key steps involved in management are as follows.

- Does the patient have asthma? If so, establish best lung function, and educate on home monitoring.
- Provide a method of relief of symptoms, plus education about the use of inhalers and how to respond to attacks.
- Does the patient need regular treatment?
  - inhaled, or oral, controlling drugs on a daily basis
  - skin testing combined with education about the role of allergens and methods for avoidance.
- Assess the requirement for additional treatment:
  - management of exercise-induced exacerbations
  - increased treatment in patients with persistent symptoms
  - specific action plans.

Action plans

Patients who have persistent symptoms, with or without exacerbations, should be given an action plan to guide their self-management. In most cases, the plan should be written down (Box 9.3). However, the plans vary a great deal depending on the severity of disease and the level of understanding of the patient. The simplest action plan is for patients to take extra puffs of bronchodilator if they feel 'tight' and to call their doctor if symptoms do not resolve within 3–4 hours. In contrast, for patients who are prone to severe attacks, the action plan will include indications for:

- increasing bronchodilators
- increasing routine treatment (usually in response to increased symptoms or changes in peak expiratory flow rate)
- adding other medications, such as long-acting β_2-agonists, theophylline, or nebulized bronchodilator
- increasing inhaled corticosteroids and starting oral corticosteroids.

Although many clinics have printed action plans, these cannot replace education, including discussion of each step with the patient. Writing the plan down with the patient is more effective than using preprinted forms since a clear understanding of the steps required to control asthma in its different phases is essential for good management. Time spent explaining an asthma plan is time well spent.

Allergen avoidance

The majority of children and young adults with asthma are allergic to one or more of the common inhaled allergens. Evidence that inhalation of these allergens contributes to the disease has come from both the demonstration that allergen challenge can produce the inflammation that is typical of asthma and from studies on allergen avoidance. The avoidance studies in sanatoria, hospital rooms, and patients' houses have shown that decreased exposure to dust mites can improve symptoms and non-specific bronchial hyperreactivity (Box 9.4). In addition, it has been shown that reductions in bronchial hyperresponsiveness are paralleled by decreased numbers of eosinophils in induced sputum. The logical conclusion is that allergen

Box 9.3 Examples of an action plan

Case A. Intermittent symptoms with occasional episodes of prolonged wheezing

I. Take bronchodilator, two puffs, repeated every hour until symptoms improve. (Use peak flow meter if available.)

II. If deteriorating or there is no improvement after 4 hours, consult your physician or call emergency number. (Take action if peak flow is <80% of best.)

Case B. Persistent symptoms with mild to moderate attacks several times per year

I. Increased bronchodilator using either an inhaler or nebulizer. Measure peak flow.

II. If no response (i.e. peak flow ≤80% of best) increase treatment:
   – maintain increased dose of bronchodilator
   – increase or add high-dose inhaled steroids, up to 3000 μg/day BDP or equivalent
   – add delayed-release oral theophylline, 300 mg in the evening or 200–300 mg t.i.d.

III. If there is no response within 2 days or deterioration, consult your physician or call emergency number.

BDP, beclomethasone dipropionate.

Case C. Persistent symptoms with severe attacks requiring emergency treatment or oral steroids

I. Increase inhaled steroids promptly if symptoms are not responsive to bronchodilator; increase dose up to at least 3000 μg/day BDP or equivalent

II. Add oral delayed release theophylline as tolerated to give blood level 2–10 μg/mL

III. If deteriorating or no response within 24 hours and peak flow persistently < 70% of best, start or increase oral steroids. Use standard dosage, i.e. 50 mg/day for 6 days, or 60 mg tailing to 10 mg over 12 days. Consult your physician if starting oral steroids. Seek advice if not responding within 24 hours on steroids

Emergency telephone numbers will depend on the system but all patients with asthma should know how to obtain emergency advice or treatment. Some patients start attacks with increased sinus symptoms and may require antibiotics. However, antibiotics are not part of the normal management of acute attacks of asthma. All patients who receive courses of corticosteroids should be fully educated about the acute and chronic side effects of these drugs.

---

avoidance is a primary form of anti-inflammatory treatment for asthma. Certainly it should be included in the management of all allergic patients with persistent symptoms.

Although many different allergens can contribute to asthma (see Table 9.2), the dominant allergens in most studies have been those found indoors. Furthermore, the measures that can decrease exposure to outdoor pollens and moulds are not well established. The measures for decreasing exposure in houses are allergen specific. The techniques for reducing exposure to dust mites are different from those that are useful in controlling exposure to domestic animals or the allergens derived from the German cockroach. The conclusion is that advice about avoidance is dependent on identifying the specific sensitivity of the patient. Since histories are not a reliable method of defining immediate hypersensitivity, advice on avoidance should reflect the results of skin testing or serum assays for IgE antibodies. Skin testing using prick or lancet techniques is simple, safe, and highly informative for most of the major allergen sources (see Ch. 1). Serum assays using the radioallergosorbent technique or modifications of this test are generally less sensitive. However, in vitro assays provide a reliable test with less discomfort for the patient, can be standardized, and – for some allergens such as moulds – may be more sensitive.

The primary problem in allergen avoidance is encouraging the patient to carry out the recommended steps,

Box 9.4 Measures recommended for allergen avoidance

- Dust mites
  Bedrooms:
  – Impermeable covers for mattress and pillows*
  – Wash all bedding regularly at 130°F/60°C
  – Vacuum clean weekly (wearing a mask)
  – Remove carpets, stuffed animals and clutter
  Rest of house:
  – Minimize carpets and upholstered furniture
  – Reduce humidity
  – Treat carpets with benzyl benzoate or tannic acid
- Cats and dogs:
  – Keep animals outside, or remove
  – Reduce reservoirs and clean weekly
  – Room air filters with HEPA quality
  – Wash animal weekly to reduce allergen going into reservoirs or airborne
- Cockroaches:
  – Obsessional cleaning to remove accumulated allergen and control all food sources
  – Bait stations, bait paste and/or boric acid
  – Close up cracks, etc. to reduce sites for breeding
- These recommendations are only for patients who have been demonstrated to be allergic on the basis of skin tests or in vitro assays for IgE antibodies.

*Impermeable covers are best fine woven with pore size of 10 μm or less. HEPA, high-efficiency particulate air filter.

which by the very nature of the intervention will be beneficial only over the long term. In the case of occupational asthma, when there is clear identification of a sensitizing chemical then removal of the patient from areas of exposure is relatively straightforward. However, with asthma that is activated by major indoor allergens, avoidance becomes more difficult. Without detailed education about both the objectives and the practical steps, patients are unlikely to carry out measures that require effort and expense. Thus, as with so many aspects of asthma management, success is dependent on adequate education as well as full involvement by the patient and the patient's family.

Exercise

The ability of patients to participate in normal exercise is a special concern in management (and sometimes the primary concern). It is one of the best markers of good control and also a primary aspect of the long-term health of the patient. Physical exercise is good for human beings including those who have asthma. In addition, many patients and physicians consider that exercise is specifically good for asthma.

A regimen for controlling exercise-induced bronchospasm is part of the management plan for all patients. Examples of such regimens might be:

- two puffs of a short-acting β_2-agonist 10 minutes before exercise
- 4–20 mg of cromolyn sodium inhaled 20 minutes before exercise plus two puffs of a β_2-agonist immediately before exercise, or
- a long-acting β_2-agonist 1 hour before exercise – both salmeterol and formoterol are long-acting β_2-agonists and are of value in patients with exercise-induced asthma, but should not be taken in the absence of an inhaled corticosteroid.

Recent studies indicate that the leukotriene receptor antagonists (e.g. montelukast, pranlukast) are effective in controlling exercise-induced asthma. However, it is important to recognize that the response to exercise is a reflection of non-specific bronchial hyperresponsiveness; in cases that are not easily controlled, treatment should be directed at the underlying inflammation of the lungs. This can include specific allergen avoidance, regular treatment with leukotriene antagonists, and inhaled cromolyn sodium, theophylline, or inhaled corticosteroids (each of which has been shown to help control the response to exercise).

In addition, all patients should be encouraged to establish a plan for normal exercise. One of the important principles in exercise is that slow warming up, walking or jogging, decreases subsequent responses to more vigorous exercise. Thus, all patients should design a regimen, including pretreatment if necessary, for prolonged (i.e. more than 30 minutes) regular exercise that they can do without developing bronchospasm.

Outcomes of asthma – natural course and the impact of management

In most patients, the long-term outcome of asthma is good. Only a small minority of patients who experience wheezing and require treatment will develop severe disease. In childhood, remission is common, particularly among non-allergic children with virus-induced wheezing or asthma. Although up to 70% of patients have a complete remission, many of these patients will still have bronchial hyperresponsiveness and some will relapse. The factors that influence remission and relapse are poorly understood. However, highly allergic children (especially those with ongoing eczema) and those allergic children who experience symptoms before the age of 3 years are less likely to have a remission. In a birth cohort in Dunedin, New Zealand, the risk factors for persistence of asthma from childhood to adulthood, or for relapse after remission during adolescence were sensitization to house dust mites, airway hyperresponiveness to methacholine, female sex, smoking, and early age at onset. When asthma starts in adult life, it is more likely to become severe and less likely to remit.

Although most physicians believe that good management influences the long-term outcome of asthma, this has not yet been proven. Until recently there was very little evidence that medical management had decreased rates of hospitalization or mortality. It is now clear that the introduction of inhaled corticosteroids has played an important role in decreasing hospitalization for asthma in Scandinavia. Although, in many areas of the world (e.g. the UK, Australia, Japan, and major cities of the USA) asthma remains severe, there is now good evidence for decreases in hospitalization and mortality, which may relate to increased use of inhaled steroids and/or inhaled steroids combined with LABA.

It is commonly implied that the severity of the disease is primarily due to poor medical care and that the full application of the guidelines for the management of asthma would reverse the present situation. The equally plausible view is that the disease has become both more common and more severe.

Another important factor is the influence of Th2-mediated inflammation on the formed airway elements, leading to remodelling. This would explain why drugs such as the long-acting β_2-agonists and leukotriene receptor antagonists, when added to a regimen of inhaled corticosteroids in moderate to severe asthma, are more efficacious than simply doubling the dose of inhaled corticosteroid (Fig. 9.13).

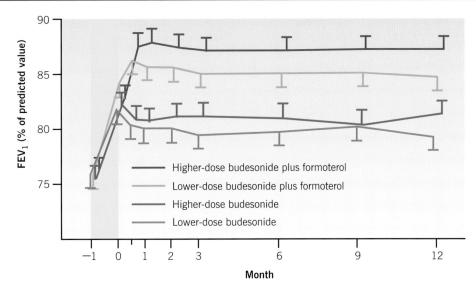

Fig. 9.13 The effect of adding the long-acting inhaled β_2-adrenoceptor agonist formoterol on to high- and low-dose inhaled budesonide on FEV_1. Plotted as an index of airway calibre in a 12-month randomized controlled trial in symptomatic asthma (the FACET study). [Modified from Pauwels RA, Lofdahl CG, Postma DS, et al. Effect of inhaled formoterol and budesonide on exacerbations of asthma. Formoterol and Corticosteroids Establishing Therapy (FACET) International Study Group. N Engl J Med 1997; 337(20):405–411.]

Most patients with intermittent asthma have normal or near-normal lung function between attacks. In contrast, patients with moderate or severe persistent disease often have an FEV_1 of <80% of the predicted value. Follow-up of adults with persistent symptoms of asthma has found that some of them have accelerated decline in lung function, but nevertheless a decline to respiratory failure is rare.

The nature of the long-term damage is not clear. There are changes in the lungs of children and adults with asthma that are more marked in those who have had disease for many years. These include the deposition of repair collagens (types I, III, and V) beneath the basement membrane of the bronchi. These changes, which are sometimes described as 'remodelling', are thought to occur secondary to the release of cytokines, growth factors, and other mediators from mast cells, T cells, eosinophils, and epithelial cells. This has led to the view that aggressive early anti-inflammatory treatment should improve long-term outcome. However, it has not been established that the changes seen in the lung structure are the cause of the decreased lung function, or that early use of inhaled anti-inflammatory drugs will prevent these changes. There is, though, good evidence for proliferative responses of epithelial cells, fibroblasts, smooth muscle cells, and blood vessels. The challenge is to determine the mechanisms and significance of these changes.

Chronic airway inflammation is a major cause of symptoms and abnormal airway physiology in asthma, even in mild disease. Since this inflammation might lead to changes in airway structure (remodelling), causing irreversible air-flow limitation and persistent symptoms, the long-term effect of early intervention with inhaled corticosteroids in patients with mild persistent asthma of recent onset was investigated in the START study (inhaled steroid treatment as regular therapy in early asthma study). Long-term, once-daily treatment with low-dose inhaled corticosteroids decreased the risk of severe exacerbations and improved asthma control in these patients. Although the benefit of inhaled corticosteroids was also noted in lung function measurements, the accelerated decline in lung function over time was only partially prevented by this treatment. It is thus tempting to speculate that, besides chronic airway inflammation, other pathways could be involved in the pathogenesis of airway remodelling.

New approaches to therapy

Pharmaceutical management: agonists and antagonists

Given the evidence that asthma is an inflammatory disease, it is logical to try to manage the disease by blocking the mediators of the inflammatory response. Examples of this approach are the development of cromolyn sodium, delayed-release theophylline, leukotriene antagonists, leukotriene synthesis inhibitors, and locally active corticosteroids. Many different approaches are being developed that range from traditional antagonists to antisense DNA. These approaches include the development of:

- highly active, low-molecular-weight vascular cell adhesion molecule-1 (VCAM-1) antagonists that can prevent eosinophil adhesion
- a soluble interleukin-4 (IL-4) receptor that can block the activity of IL-4 in vivo, which is in clinical trials
- a humanized monoclonal antibody to IL-5 that can effectively reduce blood eosinophil numbers, but fails to improve clinical indices of disease activity in subjects with severe persistent asthma
- antisense DNA, which is designed to block the production of target mediators or their receptors – short sections of DNA that are antisense will block DNA transcription, and, in theory, antisense DNA can be delivered as a pharmaceutical agent directly to the lung and would be active for a period of days
- anti-TNF therapy for severe disease
- humanized monoclonal antibody to IgE, which is specific for the site on human IgE that binds to the high-affinity IgE receptor on mast cells – this molecule has shown significant effects on exacerbations, and is licensed for use in severe allergic asthma in the USA and Europe. Omalizumab is administered subcutaneously as an injection once every month or 2 weeks depending upon the total serum IgE level and body weight. Omalizumab is the first therapy that specifically targets the IgE molecule.

Altering the immune response: immune deviation versus immunotherapy

The best defined target for traditional immunotherapy is the allergen-specific CD4+ T cell. Many different approaches have been proposed to act on these T cells or to deviate the response before initial exposure to allergen (Fig. 9.14).

Recombinant allergens can be modified by random or site-directed mutagenesis in such a way that they have greatly reduced reactivity with specific IgE antibodies but maintain T-cell responses. These molecules would presumably provide a safer version of traditional immunotherapy.

In animal models, DNA plasmids have shown promise both as a method of replacing deficient genes and also as a method of providing transient expression of foreign proteins. Furthermore, the DNA in plasmids includes immunostimulatory signals that can influence the immune response in the direction of either a helper T cell type 1 (Th1) or a Th2 response. Thus DNA plasmids, including the gene for an allergen, can be designed to alter an existing immune response.

High-dose exposure to cats and dogs does not increase the prevalence of sensitization to animal dander. Indeed in some studies, the presence of a cat in the house decreases the risk of sensitization. In some of those patients, high-titre IgG antibodies to cat allergens are found in patients who are clinically tolerant and have no IgE antibodies. This response has been called a 'modified Th2 response'.

Modification of the immune response could be achieved either by immunizing children before they make a natural response or by altering an existing response. Typical approaches are:

- to give nasal or oral immunization to at-risk children, using native protein, in order to try to induce tolerance
- to immunize with antigen linked to IL-12, which will create a Th1 bias
- to use immunostimulatory signal sequences of DNA, such as synthetic oligodeoxynucleotides that contain CpG motifs, linked directly to proteins; the objective is to create a Th1 response that will prevent or replace a Th2 response.

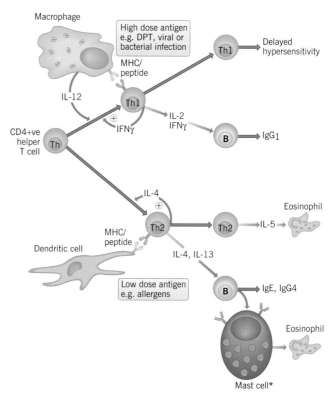

* **activated mast cells produce histamine, tryptase, leukotrienes, and also IL-3, IL-4, IL-5, GM-CSF, TNF-α, RANTES**

Fig. 9.14 Cellular interactions leading to different types of T-lymphocyte responses. DPT, diptherial-pertussis-tetanus.

Approaches designed as a response to the epidemiology of increasing asthma: how to reverse the effects of modern life

The increase in the prevalence of asthma and its morbidity during the second half of the twentieth century is such that at least three-quarters of the cases that present to clinics or to hospitals would not have required treatment in the 1950s. This increase correlates with many different aspects of modern life. We do not want to reverse the conquest of the major infectious diseases; however, there are some aspects of modern life that could be reversed without risk. The changes that have been suggested as causes of the epidemic are summarized below.

Changes in housing

Changes in housing that were designed to make houses more comfortable but that have increased exposure to indoor allergens may have contributed to increasing sensitization and could easily be changed (see Box 9.4).

Decreased rates of infections in early childhood

The incidence of infections in early childhood has decreased as a result of vaccination, decreased family size, and the introduction of antibiotics. The evidence that viral infections have decreased is not clear, however; neither is it obvious how this would have contributed to increasing asthma. In contrast, there is no doubt that bacterial infections in childhood have decreased. Bacterial infections are thought to create a bias towards Th1 responses by stimulating IL-12 production.

Decreased physical exercise

In many Western countries there has been a dramatic decrease in physical exercise such that children typically do several hours of exercise per week rather than the several hours per day that was normal in 1950. The mechanism by which exercise may protect the lungs is not clear, but full inspiration decreases lung resistance and gentle exercise can protect against exercise-induced asthma. In addition, there is now good experimental evidence for an anti-inflammatory effect of exercise.

Changes in diet

Changes in diet have taken many different forms, but there are several aspects that have been common to many countries:

- the pervasive presence of colouring and preservatives in the modern diet
- the increased consumption of animal fat combined with a decreased consumption of vegetables

- excessive protein and caloric intakes, which is the most consistent feature of Western diet – recent data showing a correlation between obesity and asthma suggesting that there has been a change in the phenotype of asthmatics as well as an increase in the prevalence of asthma.

Summary of important messages

- The dramatic rise in asthma cases over the 40 years from 1960 to 2000 triggered intensive studies both to understand the causes and also to develop new approaches to therapy
- Understanding the importance of perennial allergen exposure led to much-improved methods of controlling exposure, particularly for dust mites
- Equally the development of several different inhaled steroids, the long-acting β_2-agonists, and leukotriene antagonists have each contributed to long-term management
- The management of asthma requires extensive education about the causes of the disease, the objectives of different forms of treatment, and the techniques for using inhalers and as well as monitoring the disease. However, the cause of the increase in asthma involves a complex mixture of increased allergic responses, high exposure to the major indoor allergens, and the effects of lifestyle change
- Management in the future will still include avoidance of obvious causes, control of immune responses, and blocking of a wide range of inflammatory mediators. However, it may also be necessary to reverse other aspects of our current lifestyle – including the large number of hours spent in sedentary 'entertainment'

Further reading

Allergy and asthma. Nature 1999; 402 (6760):B1–39.

Barbers R. Asthma. Curr Opin Pulm Med 2000; 6:1–89.

Barnes PJ, Alving K, Kharatonov SA, et al. Exhaled markers in airway disease. Eur Respir Rev 1999; 9:207–253.

Chung KF, Godard P. Difficult therapy-resistant asthma. ERS Task Force Report. Eur Respir Rev 2000; 10:1–101.

Cowan, DC, Cowan JO, Palmay R, et al. Effects of steroid therapy on inflammatory cell subtypes in asthma. Thorax 2010; 65:384–390.

Holgate ST, Chuchalin AG, Hebert J, et al. Efficacy and safety of recombinant anti-immunoglobulin E antibody (omalizumab) in severe allergic asthma. Clin Exp Allergy 2004; 34:632–638.

Klinman DM. Immunotherapeutic uses of CpG oligodeoxynucleotides. Nat Rev Immunol 2004; 4:249–258.

Martinez FD, Holt PG. Role of microbial burden in the aetiology of allergy and asthma. Lancet 1999; 354(suppl II):12–15.

Pauwels RA, Pedersen S, Busse WW, et al on behalf of the START Investigators Group. Early intervention with budesonide in mild persistent asthma: a randomized, double-blind trial. Lancet 2003; 361:1071–1076.

Platts-Mills T, Vaughan J, Squillace S, et al. Sensitisation, asthma, and a modified Th2 response in children exposed to cat allergen: a population-based cross-sectional study. Lancet 2001; 357(9258):752–756.

Platts-Mills TA, Erwin EA, Heymann PW, et al. The evidence for a causal role of dust mites in asthma. Am J Respir Crit Care Med 2009; 180(2):109–113.

Postma DS, Gerritesen J. The link between asthma and COPD: bronchitis VL. Clin Exp Allergy 1999; 29(suppl 2):2–128.

Wark PA, Johnston SL, Bucchieri F, et al. Asthmatic bronchial epithelial cells have a deficient innate immune response to infection with rhinovirus. J Exp Med 2005; 201:937–947.

10

Allergic rhinitis and rhinosinusitis

Glenis K Scadding, Martin K Church and
Larry Borish

DEFINITIONS

Rhinitis: inflammation of the nasal lining, can be defined as two or more of the symptoms of nasal irritation, sneezing, rhinorrhoea, and nasal blockage lasting for at least 1 hour a day on most days.

Rhinosinusitis: inflammation of the nose and sinus linings, is defined by the EPOS guidelines as two of the following symptoms: one of which must be 1 or 2: 1. nasal obstruction, 2. rhinorrhoea, 3. facial pain/pressure, 4. reduction of olfaction, plus evidence of abnormalities at the middle meatus where most sinuses drain – either on nasendoscopy or on CT scans.

Introduction

There are many causes of rhinitis (Fig. 10.1). This chapter concentrates on allergic rhinitis, which is caused by IgE-mediated inflammation, usually to inhalant allergens. There is often an associated allergic conjunctivitis (rhino-conjunctivitis). Rhinosinusitis occurs when both nasal and sinus linings are inflamed (see below). Both rhinitis and rhinosinusitis are common and costly to society because of significant impairment of work/school ability and quality of life. They predispose to and are major exacerbating factors for asthma. Most asthmatics also suffer from rhinitis/rhinosinusitis but this is often ignored, underdiagnosed and/or mistreated.

Functions of the nose and sinuses

The nose is the first line of defence against the inhaled environment and provides 'air conditioning' of inspired air and filtration of potentially harmful particulate matter as well as being the location of the smell receptors – the olfactory mucosa (Fig. 10.2). The nose has a remarkable capacity to humidify inspired air, raising the temperature of room air to 32°C, and humidifying it to 98% relative humidity before it reaches the lungs. This is effected by fluid shift across the highly vascular mucosa and increasing blood flow through the sinusoids. The paranasal sinuses probably lighten the skull, increase vocal resonance, and contribute high levels of nitric oxide, which are toxic to bacteria, viruses, fungi, and tumour cells.

The narrow, irregular shape of the nasal cavity promotes turbulent air flow, and impaction of inhaled particles in the upper airway – a protective function against the inhalation of potentially harmful particles into the bronchial tree. Pollen grains, which are around 10 μm in size, are largely deposited in the nose, whereas turbulent air flow is insufficient to deposit particles less than 2 μm in size, such as mould spores, in the nose. These particles will usually reach the distal airways. Particles trapped in the nose are moved into the pharynx by mucociliary transport within 10–30 minutes of impaction, and subsequently swallowed. Additionally, 99% of water-soluble gases, such as sulphur dioxide, are prevented from reaching the lower airways because of passage over the nasal mucosa.

© 2012 Elsevier Ltd
DOI: 10.1016/B978-0-7234-3658-4.00005-6

Anatomy and physiology of the nose

The nasal cavity commences at the internal ostium, a narrow slit-like orifice about 1.5 cm from the nostrils (Fig. 10.3). This is the narrowest part of the respiratory tract with a cross-sectional area of approximately 0.3 cm². The inferior, middle, and superior turbinates form the lateral wall, and the nasal septum forms the medial wall of the nasal cavity. The turbinates contribute to the irregular outline of the nasal cavity, which is important to its air-conditioning and air-filtering functions. The nasolacrimal duct opens into the inferior meatus, the portion of the nasal cavity lateral to the inferior turbinate. the orifices of the frontal, maxillary, and anterior ethmoidal sinuses open into the middle meatus, lateral to the middle turbinate.

The epithelium changes from stratified squamous in the nasal vestibule to a squamous and transitional epithelium lining the anterior one-third of the cavity. The remaining portion is lined by ciliated pseudostratified columnar epithelium typical of the respiratory tract containing many mucus-secreting goblet cells (Fig. 10.4), except in the

upper part of the cavity where olfactory epithelium is present. The number of goblet cells is highest in the posterior nasal cavity, similar to that in the trachea and main bronchi.

The epithelium rests on the basement membrane – a layer of connective tissue composed of collagen types III, IV, and V, laminin, and fibronectin. The underlying lamina propria is highly vascular. The arterioles have no internal elastic lamina and a porous basement membrane, which increases permeability and allows access for pharmacological agents. There is an extensive capillary network,

Fig. 10.1 Classification of rhinitis.

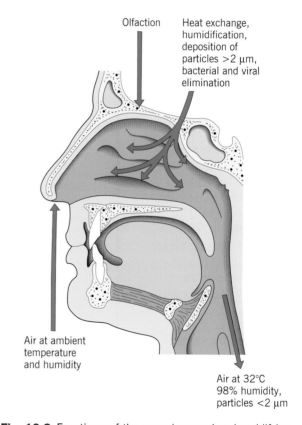

Fig. 10.2 Functions of the nose in warming, humidifying, and filtering inspired air.

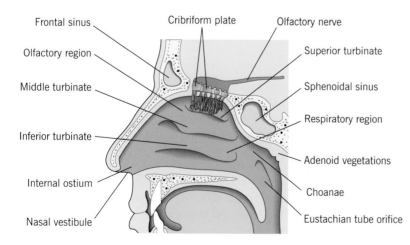

Fig. 10.3 Gross nasal anatomy in sagittal section.

and the capillaries are fenestrated allowing rapid transit of fluid across their walls. Large cavernous vascular sinusoids present in the lamina propria on the turbinates (Fig 10.5) contribute to heating and humidification of inspired air. When chronically or excessively dilated, they are largely responsible for nasal congestion in both allergic and non-allergic rhinitis. Beneath the lamina propria are periosteum and bone.

Innervation (Table 10.1)

Sensory innervation

The trigeminal nerve supplies afferent (sensory) fibres to the nasal mucous membrane. Activation of these produces sensations of irritation or pain, often resulting in sneezing. Olfaction is effected by fibres from the first cranial nerve, which enter the roof of the nose via the cribriform plate.

Vascular innervation

Sympathetic fibres, which mainly follow the blood vessels, predominate. Release of their cotransmitters – noradrenaline and neuropeptide Y – causes vasoconstriction and maintains the sympathetic tone of the sinusoids. This fluctuates throughout the day with an increase in patency in alternate nostrils every 4–6 hours (the nasal cycle).

Parasympathetic fibres that arise in the sphenopalatine ganglion to form the vidian nerve control vasodilatation and glandular secretion. The parasympathetic cotransmitters are acetylcholine and vasoactive intestinal peptide.

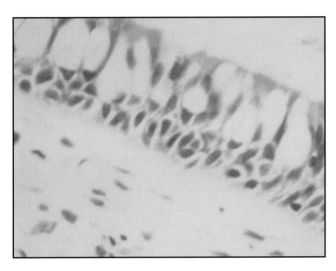

Fig. 10.4 Pseudostratified ciliated columnar epithelium of the nasal mucosa. (Courtesy of Dr M Calderon-Zapata, St Bartholomew's Hospital, London.)

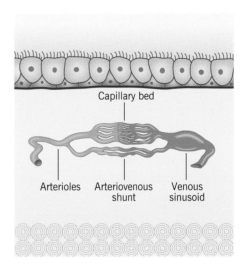

Fig. 10.5 The vasculature of the nose showing the capillary bed, arteriovenous shunt and venous sinusoid. (Courtesy of Professor J-B Watelet, Department of Otorhinolaryngology, Ghent University Hospital, Belgium.)

Table 10.1 Innervation of the nose

	Nerves	Neurotransmitters	Structures	Effects
Smell+other	Cranial nerves 0 and I	Not known	Receptors in olfactory epithelium	Sensory function?
Sensory nerves	Cranial V (Trigeminal: branches V1, V2)	Substance P Neurokinin A CGRP	Blood vessels Mucous glands Epithelium	Sensory reflexes
Parasympathetic nerves	Cranial VII: Vidian nerve to pterygopalatine ganglion	Acetylcholine VIP	Blood vessels Mucous glands	Vasodilatation, congestion, rhinorrhoea
Sympathetic nerves	Thoracic via superior cervical ganglia	Noradrenaline (norepinephrine) Neuropeptide Y	Blood vessels Anastomoses	Vasoconstriction

VIP, vasoactive intestinal polypeptide; CGRP, calcitonin gene-related peptide.

Axon reflexes can be powerful in the nasal mucosa, resulting in vasodilatation and transudation with thickening of the mucosa. These are initiated by irritants and inflammatory mediators at sensory nerve endings and the transmitters include sensory neuropeptides, substance P, neurokinin A, and calcitonin gene-related peptide (CGRP). Additionally, sensory nerve activation can cause vasodilatation via neural connections from the trigeminal to the sphenopalatine ganglia and via central nervous reflexes. There are also nasobronchial reflexes, which may be activated in asthmatics to promote reflex bronchoconstriction in response to nasal obstruction, and naso-ocular reflexes, which result in allergic rhinitis-associated conjunctivitis. Interestingly, cytokines increase neuropeptide production by these sensory nerves, so-called 'neurogenic inflammation', which exacerbates the symptoms of allergic rhinoconjunctivitis.

Control of mucus secretion

Mucus is secreted by goblet and serous cells in the epithelium, by submucosal serous glands, and by deep nasal glands. It is diluted by transudate from the blood vessels. Secretion is controlled by parasympathetic cholinergic nerves, but sympathetic stimulation and axon reflexes also enhance secretion.

Disease mechanisms

Pathophysiology

Allergic rhinitis is a Th2 type inflammatory disorder of the nasal mucosa initiated by an allergic response to inhaled allergens. Dendritic cells, strategically located at nasal mucosal surfaces, capture allergens and present the allergenic peptides to T lymphocytes in the draining lymph nodes. Recent observations suggest that the resulting reponse is driven by the milieu in which the dendritic cell is situated, with molecules such as thymic stromal lymphopoietin (TSLP) promoting a Th2 allergic response. IgE switching occurs locally and locally generated IgE molecules are released and bind to high-affinity receptors on the surface of nasal tissue mast cells and circulating basophils. The activation of mast cells by allergen deposited on the nasal mucosa leads to a rapid release of preformed mediators such as histamine that cause the early symptoms of allergic rhinitis, namely rhinorrhoea, nasal itching, and sneezing. In addition, the influx of inflammatory cells such as eosinophils, CD4+ T lymphocytes, and basophils occurs in response to stimulation of the expression of adhesion molecules on endothelial cells by histamine, the newly generated lipid mediators PGD_2, LTC_4 leukotriene C_4, and cytokines including TNF-α and eotaxin. This response is perpetuated by the generation of CD4+ T lymphocytes cytokines including IL-5, which stimulates eosinopoiesis, eosinophil influx in the mucosa, and prolonged eosinophil survival. The presenting symptoms of this late allergic response are mainly nasal obstruction and nasal hyperreactivity. Allergen-specific IgE and eosinophilic nasal inflammation are typical features of allergic rhinitis that distinguish it from other forms of rhinitis – with the exception of non-allergic rhinitis with eosinophilia (NARES) where nasal eosinophils are found without systemic evidence of allergen-specific IgE, a situation refered to as 'entopy' – localized mucosal allergic disease in the absence of systemic evidence of atopy.

Nasal responsiveness

Nasal hyperresponsiveness, in terms of both symptoms and nasal airway resistance (NAR), can be demonstrated in rhinitics by inhalation of non-specific agents such as histamine and methacholine (Fig. 10.6). Rhinitis alone can cause an increase in bronchial hyperreactivity and probably also up-regulates naso-ocular reflexes. It is likely that the pathogenetic mechanisms of rhinitis and asthma are very similar, with hyperresponsiveness being a cardinal feature in both conditions. Differences such as the lack of correlation between histamine and methacholine responses in the upper airway and poor correlation with rhinitis severity may arise from the absence of smooth muscle in the nose. Histamine reduces upper airway patency by causing hyperemia and oedema of the mucosa, whereas methacholine acts predominantly on glandular secretion, with a less potent effect on vasodilatation because of the dominance of sympathetic vasoconstrictor nerves (Fig. 10.7). The importance of vascular congestion as the mechanism of nasal obstruction is demonstrated by the rapid response to vasoconstrictor sprays, which is not a feature of bronchoconstriction in asthma.

Allergen provocation

Early and late phase responses may be demonstrated in the nose after inhalation of allergen by sensitized individuals. Late phase responses, with associated increases in symptoms and nasal airways resistance, occur in approximately 50% of patients between 2 and 8 hours after allergen provocation. The physiological changes of the late phase can be very subtle compared with the intense blockage and symptoms of the early phase (Fig. 10.8). Small increases in NAR during the late phase may be obscured by the nasal cycle. Recent research suggests that platelet activation factor (PAF) and other mediators can increase the nasal response to bradykinin and histamine.

Priming

During the pollen season, sensitized individuals are exposed to low levels of pollen for a prolonged period. Thus, during the pollen season, a sensitized person may become increasingly responsive to allergen, a process

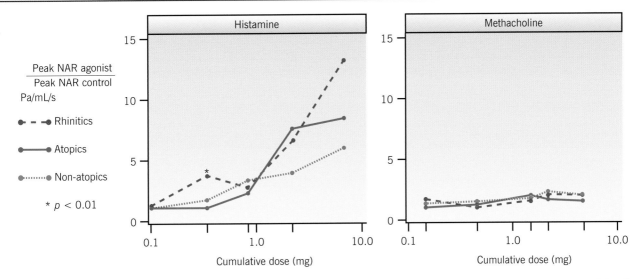

Fig. 10.6 Changes in nasal airway resistance (NAR) following the administration of histamine and methacholine (weighted geometric mean change).

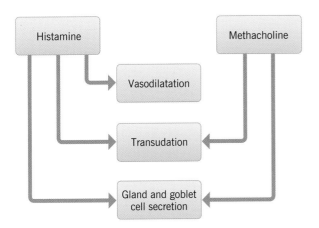

Fig. 10.7 Effects of histamine and methacholine on the nasal mucosa in rhinitis.

known as 'priming'. The mechanisms underlying priming, which are not completely understood, include increased mast cell (Fig. 10.9) and eosinophil numbers and releasability and a cytokine-induced increase in sensory nerve neuropeptides, so-called 'neurogenic inflammation'. This differs markedly from the artificial conditions of allergen challenge in the laboratory where single large doses of allergen are given to evoke a response. Lower-dose challenges repeated over several days are now being employed to better simulate environmental exposure.

Inflammatory cells and mediators

Following allergen inhalation, many diverse inflammatory mediators may be detected in nasal lavage fluid (Table 10.2). Although mast cell mediators, including histamine, prostaglandin D_2 (PGD$_2$), leukotrienes, and tryptase, are responsible for many of the immediate symptoms of nasal

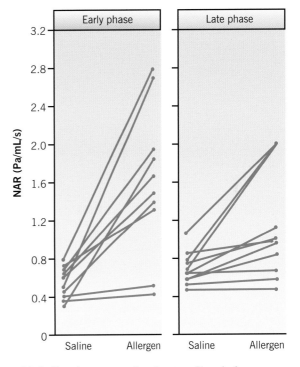

Fig. 10.8 Nasal response to allergen. Nasal airway resistance (NAR) measurements following saline or grass pollen administration to the nasal mucosa. Measurements are taken either 30 minutes after allergen challenge (early response) or 2–7 hours after challenge (late response).

allergy, a large number of other inflammatory mediators have been identified following allergen challenge of the nose. These include sulphidopeptide leukotrienes, primarily from eosinophils; eosinophil cationic protein (ECP), eosinophil peroxidase (EPO), and major basic protein (MBP) from eosinophils; neutrophil peroxidase from neutrophils; PAF from a wide variety of inflammatory

Table 10.2 Inflammatory mediators that act on the nose, their action, and their source

Mediator	Action	Source
Histamine	Vasodilatation, plasma leakage, glandular secretion	Mast cells (early phase), basophils (late phase)
PGD$_2$	Vasodilatation	Mast cells, also platelets, fibroblasts
Tryptase	? activates kallikrein	Mast cells
TAME-esterase	Vasodilatation	Plasma/glandular kallikrein, mast cell tryptase
LTB$_4$	Eosinophil chemotaxis, neutrophil chemotaxis, and activation	Neutrophils in late phase
LTC$_4$ and LTD$_4$	Vasodilatation, Increased blood flow	Mast cells, eosinophils, basophils
Kinins	Vasodilatation, increased capillary flow, pain	Plasma
PAF	Vasoconstriction/vasodilatation, eosinophil, and neutrophil chemotaxis	Macrophages, neutrophils, eosinophils, endothelial cells
ECP, EPO, MBP	Epithelial damage	Eosinophils

ECP, eosinophil cationic protein; EPO, eosinophil peroxidase; LTB$_4$, leukotriene B$_4$; LTC$_4$, leukotriene C$_4$; LTD$_4$, leukotriene D$_4$; MBP, major basic protein; PAF, platelet activation factor; PGD$_2$, prostaglandin D$_2$.

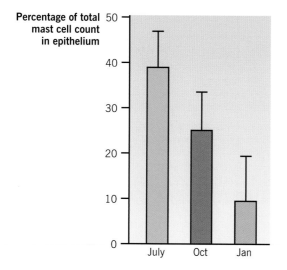

Fig. 10.9 Percentage of total mast cell numbers present in the nasal epithelium in July (in the grass pollen season), compared with October and January, in rhinitics sensitive to grass pollen.

cells; serotonin from platelets; kinins and complement factors from plasma-derived precursors; and substance P, vasoactive intestinal peptide (VIP), and CGRP from nerve endings.

Clinical presentation

Allergic rhinitis

Patients with allergic rhinitis present with symptoms of nasal running, itching, sneezing, and blocking. These may be intermittent or persistent. Intermittent rhinitis is defined by the Allergic Rhinitis and Its Impact on Asthma (ARIA) guidelines as symptoms lasting less than 4 days per week or for less than 4 weeks, and persistent as lasting more than 4 days per week and for more than 4 weeks at a time. This classification is not synonymous with seasonal and perennial; indeed, seasonal rhinitis is often persistent and perennial often intermittent, but it is applicable worldwide and correlates with treatment requirements. ARIA also classifies rhinitis as mild – without effects on quality of life, or moderate to severe – in which the symptoms affect work, school, play or sleep, or are particularly troublesome.

In allergic rhinitis there is usually a clear relationship with exposure to known inhalant allergens, most frequently pollens and house dust mite or household pets. The appreciation of an allergic trigger in the persistent group may be difficult. Some patients with no evidence of allergy (i.e. negative skin prick and absent serum specific IgE tests) present with allergic rhinitis symptoms. Local nasal production of IgE has been shown in the nose of some such patients (entopy).

Epidemiology

A hundred and fifty years ago, allergic rhinitis was a very rare condition but it has increased markedly with civilization so that in some Westernized countries its prevalence is approaching 40%. Furthermore, whereas allergic rhinitis was considered to be a disease primarily of the 15–25-year age group, today the major increases are in younger children (Fig. 10.10). Many environmental reasons have been proposed for this increase: increased pollution, a

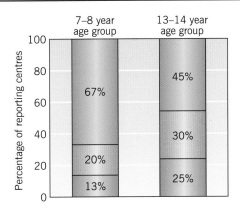

Fig. 10.10 The percentage of centres throughout the world participating in ISAAC studies of childhood allergy who reported increases (red), no change (amber) or a decrease (green) in the prevalence of allergic rhinitis in the 7 years between phases 1 and 3. Reports were received from 66 centres for 7–8 year olds and 106 centres for 13–14 year olds. (Adapted from Asher MI, Montefort S, Björkstén B, et al, Worldwide time trends in the prevalence of symptoms of asthma, allergic rhinoconjunctivitis, and eczema in childhood: ISAAC Phases One and Three repeat multicountry cross-sectional surveys. Lancet 26-8-2006; 368:733–43.)

Table 10.3 Major allergens worldwide

Type of allergen	Examples
Major pollen allergens	**Grasses and weeds**
	Ragweed (USA)
	Bermuda grass (USA)
	Timothy grass (UK and USA)
	Cocksfoot (orchard) grass (UK)
	Trees
	Silver birch (Northern Europe)
	Japanese cedar (sugi tree) (Japan)
	Oak (USA and UK)
	Mesquite tree (South Africa, South America, and Asia)
Domestic and occupational allergens	House dust mite
	Domestic pets
	Flour (bakers)
	Solder (solderers)
	Latex (health workers)

Box 10.1 Factors contributing to the development of allergic rhinitis

Increased by:	Decreased by:
Atopy	Early infection with
Month of birth (May and	hepatitis A
June)	BCG vaccinations
Male gender	Early exposure to domestic
First born	pets (cats and dogs)
Smoking	
Early allergen exposure	
Viral infection	
Environmental pollution	
Family history of allergy	

change to a sedentary, hygienic indoor lifestyle primarily in an urban environment, global warming, lack of vitamin D, exposure to new allergens with globalization, and the increased stress of modern living. Many of these factors are discussed more fully in Chapter 4.

The important allergens in allergic rhinitis vary in different parts of the world: in the UK grass pollinosis is commonest, in some parts of North America ragweed predominates, in Scandinavia birch pollen is common, whereas in Mediterranean areas *Parietaria* species (a nettle-like weed) and olive tree pollen are common allergens (Table 10.3). In tropical climates, allergenic pollens may be present all year round; consequently the symptoms of pollen allergy may be perennial. Conversely, classically perennial allergens, such as the house dust mite, provoke most symptoms during the autumn and winter in temperate climates (see Table 10.3). Moulds are uncommon causes of allergic rhinitis, owing to their small size, as they are more likely to be deposited in the lower airway.

Occupational agents can also cause allergic as well as non-allergic rhinitis (see Table 10.3). Rhinitis is a more common manifestation of sensitization than asthma, the nasal mucosa being more accessible to deposition of dusts and vapours (e.g. baker's flour, isocyanates, wood dusts, and animal allergens), all of which can be associated with an IgE-mediated allergic response. Occupational rhinitis always precedes or accompanies the development of occupational asthma, never the other way round, therefore early diagnosis and removal from the allergen offers an opportunity for asthma prevention. Foods are

sometimes suggested as a cause of allergic rhinitis, particularly in young children, but the rhinitis is usually accompanied by other allergic symptoms (e.g. atopic dermatitis, asthma). This is in contrast to gustatory rhinitis, which is a manifestation of non-allergic rhinitis, triggered by irritant receptors and not associated with IgE sensitization or anaphylaxis.

Much allergic sensitization occurs in very early life when the immune system is immature (Box 10.1). However, allergic rhinitis is occurring de novo in older individuals without a strong history of personal or family atopy, suggesting strong environmental influences. There is evidence that sensitization occurs in the nose with initial local IgE switching and production. Thymic stromal lymphopoietin, described as the 'master switch of allergy'

– up-regulated by cigarette smoke, down-regulated by intranasal corticosteroids, and present on nasal epithelium – may be relevant.

A strong inverse relationship between allergic rhinitis and family size has been noted, with first-born children being at greatest risk. Children with antibodies to hepatitis A and those with positive delayed-type hypersensitivity skin tests to *Mycobacterium tuberculosis* (i.e. those from less clean environments) are less likely to have allergic rhinitis. Early infections may protect against the development of atopy, possibly because of increased production of interferon-γ (IFN-γ).

IgE production is enhanced by cigarette smoking, and the relative risk of rhinitis is doubled for children who live in damp houses and have parents who smoke. Modern energy-efficient 'tight' buildings encourage the growth of house dust mites and moulds, because of higher humidity and warmth, and so increase exposure to potential allergens. However, a reduction in grass pollen exposure caused by production of silage has not decreased the incidence of grass pollen allergy.

Non-nasal symptoms and quality of life

Allergic rhinitis is more than just a runny nose and sneezing: the ramifications are numerous and can have a significant impact on quality of life. It is important not only to detect, investigate, and treat allergic rhinitis but also to identify potential complications.

Over 85% of allergic rhinitis patients have impaired sleep caused mainly by nasal congestion, which is most pronounced during the early hours of the morning and worse when lying down. Partners are often disturbed by snoring; children with allergic rhinitis can experience sleep microarousals and irregular breathing, snoring, and obstructive apnoea. Sleep deprivation leads to physical fatigue, and mental and physical problems (Fig. 10.11).

Allergic rhinitis being common in teenagers, effects on learning and examination performance are of particular concern. Those with symptomatic allergic rhinitis have poorer concentration and impaired learning capacity compared with when asymptomatic (Fig. 10.12); they perform worse compared with when they are symptom free, especially if using sedating first-generation antihistamines. Other complications associated with allergic rhinitis in children are irritability and behavioural problems. Links have been found between allergic rhinitis and attention-deficit/hyperactivity disorder (ADHD), anxiety, and depression.

In adults, allergic rhinitis can result in a reduction in the capacity to work. While few sufferers take time off work, studies have shown up to 35–40% reduced work capacity leading to costs of around 2 billion dollars annually. Questionnaires, such as the SF-36, have shown that

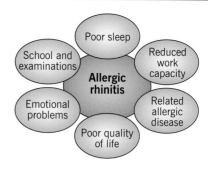

Fig. 10.11 Patients' perception of daily life impairment by allergic rhinitis.

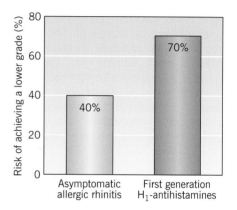

Fig. 10.12 Risk of achieving a lower grade in an examination in students with symptomatic allergic rhinitis and students who have taken a sedating first-generation H₁-antihistamine to control their symptoms. (Drawn from Walker S, Khan-Wasti S, Fletcher M, et al Seasonal allergic rhinitis is associated with a detrimental effect on examination performance in United Kingdom teenagers: case-control study. J Allergy Clin Immunol 2007; 20:381–387.)

more than a third of patients have a significantly reduced quality of life, including poor self-esteem, increased emotional problems, constant fatigue, and reduced sexual function.

Comorbidity of asthma and allergic rhinitis

Almost 90% of patients with allergic asthma have allergic rhinitis and around half of patients with allergic rhinitis have allergic asthma. The relationship between these two conditions may be viewed in two ways. The first is the 'one airway–one disease' concept. Certainly Th2 inflammation is a major common component of both diseases. Also, it is clear that neuronal reflexes stimulated in the nose may affect the bronchi and vice versa. The second is that the nose functions as the 'guardian of the lung' by warming the inspired air to ~35°C, humidifying it to ~95% saturation, and filtering out particles greater than

10 µm in diameter, thus removing most allergenic pollen grains, which are 20–25 µm in diameter. 70% of allergic rhinitis patients with concomitant asthma complain that allergic rhinitis worsens their asthma symptoms. Asthmatics with comorbid allergic rhinitis visit their general practitioner more regularly and are hospitalized more often than those with asthma alone. In fact rhinitis gives an odds ratio around 4 for poor asthma control, similar to that for smoking and twice that of poor concordance with asthma treatment.

Asthma exacerbations usually begin in the upper airway with a rhinoviral 'cold'. Colds are more problematical in rhinitic patients, probably because of pre-existing inflammation (minimal persistent inflammation) and the combination of allergic sensitization; exposure to the relevant allergen and rhinovirus infection leads to an almost 20–fold odds ratio for hospital admission for asthma in asthmatic children. Appropriate treatment of allergic rhinitis can reduce asthma-related events (Fig. 10.13). Thus, physicians treating asthma should be aware of the impact of rhinitis and should ensure their patients are adequately treated.

Comorbidity of oral allergy syndrome and allergic rhinitis

Oral allergy syndrome, sometimes called pollen-food allergy, is caused by primary inhalational sensitization to pollen allergens, primarily birch, mugwort, grasses, and ragweed with cross-reactivity to the same molecules present in food, mainly fruits and vegetables. Symptoms, commonly tingling, erythema, or angioedema of the lips, tongue, and oropharynx and itching or tightness of the throat, result immediately upon eating raw cross-reactive fruit or vegetables. This syndrome was thought to occur only with raw fruit or vegetables and produces mainly oral symptoms because the allergens (profilins) are heat labile and readily destroyed in the gastrointestinal tract. However some cross-reactive allergens are lipid transfer proteins (LTP), are not heat labile and cause more severe symptoms, including anaphylaxis. Details of cross-reactive pollens and foods are shown in Box 6.7 in Chapter 6.

Diagnosis of allergic rhinitis

The diagnosis of allergic rhinitis is based predominantly on the clinical history, a physical examination and appropriately interpreted corroborative testing for allergen-specific IgE – the above definition may exclude a proportion of cases with mild disease or with local nasal IgE only (entopy) who need nasal allergen challenge for diagnosis. Diary recording of symptoms and their circumstances over a 2-week period may be helpful in borderline cases. The additional presence of conjunctivitis makes an allergic cause more likely.

Differential diagnosis

The most common differential diagnosis is non-allergic rhinitis, which encompasses a variety of conditions some of which are amenable to treatment (see Fig. 10.1) – e.g. endocrine disturbances, such as nasal congestion as a complication of pregnancy, oral contraceptives, or hypothyroidism, giving rise to a thickened and oedematous nasal mucosa. Rhinitis medicamentosa with a rebound vasodilatation (the effect of overuse of topical nasal decongestants) often produces an oedematous and red nasal mucosa that should not be confused with true rhinitis. Once these have been discounted there remains

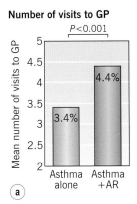

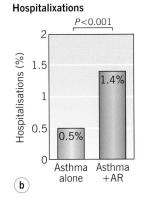

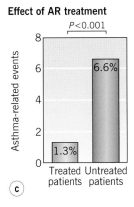

Fig. 10.13 Asthma-related (a) general practitioner (GP) visits and (b) hospitalizations and in asthmatic patients with and without allergic rhinitis (AR). (c) Effect of treatment of allergic rhinitis on asthma-related events. (Data for panels a and b from Thomas M, Kocevar VS, Zhang Q, et al. Asthma-related health care resource use among asthmatic children with and without concomitant allergic rhinitis. Pediatrics 2005 Jan; 115(1):129–134, and data for panel c from Crystal-Peters J, Neslusan C, Crown WH, et al. Treating allergic rhinitis in patients with comorbid asthma: the risk of asthma-related hospitalizations and emergency department visits. J Allergy Clin Immunol 2002 Jan; 109(1):57–62.)

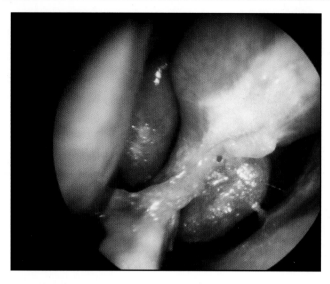

Fig. 10.14 Endoscopic appearances of the nasal mucosa in Wegener's granulomatosis. (Courtesy of Professor VJ Lund.)

either NARES (non-allergic rhinitis with eosinophilia syndrome), which should respond to topical anti-inflammatories, and neurogenic forms of rhinitis, which can be difficult to control.

It is important to be aware of other diseases that may present with nasal symptoms. Uncharacteristic features, such as unilateral nasal blockage, bleeding, or pain, may suggest other pathologies (e.g. malignant tumours or Wegener's granulomatosis; Fig. 10.14). In infants, unilateral nasal blockage and discharge may also be caused by the presence of a foreign body or, rarely, congenital choanal atresia. Chronic rhinorrhoea present from birth plus a wet cough may indicate primary ciliary dyskinesia. Septal deviation, whether congenital or traumatic, may cause nasal blockage, but it is unlikely to be noticed for the first time in adulthood unless there is superadded rhinitis. Chronic infective rhinosinusitis can usually be differentiated by its predominantly greenish secretions and infective exacerbations, although it can occur in association with perennial rhinitis because of impaired drainage from the sinuses.

Further laboratory, radiological, and morphological examinations may also be performed if considered necessary.

History

A detailed history augmented with specific questions, presented in the form of either a structured oral interview or a written questionnaire, is essential to distinguish rhinitis from upper respiratory infections or other nasal complaints. Such a questionnaire should cover the following:

- What is the symptom profile – is there a dominant nasal symptom, such as blockage, sneezes, or nasal secretions?
- How would you describe the symptoms and what is the chronology of their onset?
- Are the nasal problems isolated or are there more extensive symptoms, especially eyes, ears, throat, chest, skin?
- Are there potential allergens in the house environment (e.g. bedding materials, any pets, low quality of housing)?
- Are there any specific precipitating factors (e.g. pollen, animal contact, occupational contact)?
- Is there any relationship to food or drink? Do any fresh fruits or vegetables cause oral itching?
- What are the occupation and leisure activities, particularly those which aggravate symptoms?
- What medications are being taken? Does any drug [e.g. aspirin, non-steroidal anti-inflammatory drugs (NSAIDs)] worsen symptoms?
- What treatments have been tried, How were these used? For how long? Did they help?
- What is the impact of problems on lifestyle?
- Is there a family or past history of atopy?

Symptom presentation

Some patients may present with a comorbidity (e.g. recurrent sinusitis, otitis media with effusion, or poorly controlled asthma) and the underlying contributory rhinitis needs to be teased out by asking about the cardinal symptoms.

Physical examination

Several facial features are associated with the various symptoms of the nasal and ocular disease (Fig. 10.15). These include:

- 'allergic shiners' – infraorbital dark circles, related to venous plexus engorgement
- 'allergic gape' or continuous open-mouth breathing – a result of nasal blockage
- 'transversal nasal crease' – a result of the frequent upward rubbing of the nose 'allergic salute'
- dental malocclusion and overbite resulting from long-standing upper airway problems.

Rhinoscopy

Rhinoscopy is essential in the clinical workup of nasal problems for which there may be several possible explanations. Simple inspection will reveal external nasal deformities, but there may also be inner septal

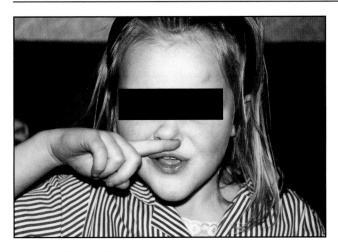

Fig. 10.15 The allergic salute.

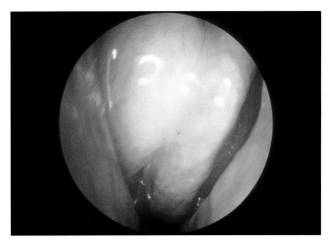

Fig. 10.17 A rigid rhinoscopic examination from a patient with a small nasal polyp in the right nasal cavity, immediately between the middle turbinate and the lateral nasal wall. (Courtesy of Jan Kumlien, MD.)

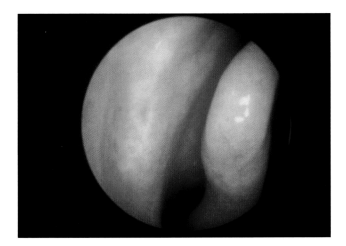

Fig. 10.16 A rigid rhinoscopic examination of a normal nose. The interior of the right nasal cavity is shown with the lateral nasal wall to the right and the middle turbinate on the left. (Courtesy of Jan Kumlien, MD.)

- the presence or absence of polyps should be recorded (Fig. 10.17)
- the amount and the condition of nasal surface liquids (e.g. watery, mucoid, or purulent), which can be useful in differentiating infection from other conditions
- the condition of the mucous membranes and the colour, texture, and signs of scars and lesions should be specifically evaluated – an allergic condition might be indicated by the traditional bluish tint
- unilateral nasal obstruction may also indicate a foreign body.

Since there are several causes for nasal symptoms, these steps are essential.

Examination of extranasal regions

Other regions that should be assessed are the eyes, ears, chest, and skin. The presence or absence of conjunctivitis, or watering with conjunctival injection, and oedema should be noted.

All patients with persistent rhinitis should have a history taken looking for asthma, their chest should be examined and some form of lower respiratory tract functional measurement, such as peak flow or spirometry, should be made.

Since otitis media and middle ear effusions may occur with increased frequency in children with allergic rhinitis, the ears should be examined, looking especially for any middle ear pathology. This is best done using the oto-microscope. Tympanometric examination is also helpful. Atopic skin diseases also may occur with increased frequency, so the physician should check for urticaria or eczematous lesions.

deformities. The rhinoscopic examination can be made using the traditional light-mirror, and a nasal speculum to widen the nasal opening or using an otoscope. Posterior rhinoscopy is performed with a mirror placed below the soft palate to permit the inspection of the epipharyngeal region. When possible this examination should be supplemented with an endoscopic examination of the nasal cavities and epipharyngeal region (Fig. 10.16). This examination is performed using either a short rigid endoscope attached to a good light source – of specific help in the examination of the ostial regions – or a short flexible endoscope, which is also useful for examining the posterior parts of the nasal cavity, as well as permitting examination of the epipharynx and larynx.

The following findings should be noted:

- any structural deformities, such as septal deviations – the site of any deformity should be specified and

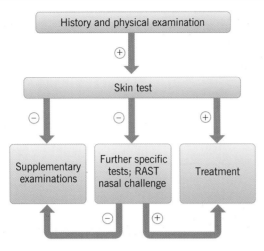

Fig. 10.18 A simplified scheme for evaluating patients with upper airway problems that are suspected of being allergic in origin. If the skin prick test confirms the history, treatment can be instituted. Otherwise, further examinations and tests are indicated. RAST, radioallergosorbent test.

Additional tests

Tests for the presence of allergy

The history and physical examination should be supplemented with an allergen reactivity test.

Skin tests

The routine test for allergy of the upper airways is the skin prick test (SPT). It should be carried out on most rhinitis patients (Fig. 10.18). A clear-cut history of seasonal allergic rhinitis in an adult patient who responds favourably to symptomatic treatment does not necessarily require confirmation by an SPT. Details of skin tests and in vitro tests for specific IgE are contained in Chapter 6.

Nasal challenge

A nasal challenge can be used to test for specific as well as non-specific reactivity. The test for specific reactivity involves the application of the specific allergens to the nasal mucosa. Some of the tests used to monitor the changes in the challenge situation (Table 10.4) may also be used to monitor disease progression.

Nasal allergen challenge can be used to confirm or reject a suspected allergen where the history and skin test are not in agreement since local allergy may be present. Most nasal allergen challenges are performed primarily for research purposes in order to understand nasal pathophysiology and to test potentially beneficial drugs.

There is no generally accepted technique for performing a nasal allergen challenge or for monitoring the clinical response. In the clinical setting, a simple sneeze count and a score for the other symptoms may well be sufficient, but if a graded (quantitative) response is required

Table 10.4 Methods for monitoring nasal symptoms during active disease or after challenge

Symptom	Method
Sneezes	Counting Symptom score
Blockage	Symptom score Nasal peak flow Rhinomanometry Acoustic rhinometry
Secretion	Symptom score Volume measurement Weight measurement Nasal lavage
Itching	Symptom score

for research purposes then more complicated techniques are needed. The risks involved in the nasal challenges are minimal and, even if total nasal blockage occurs, other organs are seldom affected especially if patients hold their breath in inspiration as the allergen is administered.

The allergens used should be well characterized and standardized. An aqueous solution administered by spray allows a widespread distribution of the allergen; conversely, if a biopsy is needed for immunohistology, application of allergen to a small area by impregnated filter paper is preferred.

The reaction to allergen comprises three main symptoms: sneezing, nasal blockage, and nasal secretions. All three are relevant and should be monitored.

Sneezing is the result of a central reflex elicited in the sensory nerve endings in the nasal mucosa. It is easy to grade by counting and is the most reproducible of the nasal symptoms in the challenge procedure.

Nasal blockage is the result of the pooling of blood in the capacitance vessels of the mucosa, and to some degree the result of tissue oedema. Nasal blockage can be assessed subjectively by means of symptom scoring and there are several objective techniques that can be used for assessing the degree of nasal blockage:

- rhinomanometry, which is the determination of nasal air flow and pressure relationships (Fig. 10.19)
- nasal peak flow determination (Fig. 10.20)
- acoustic rhinometry (Fig. 10.21).

Of the rhinomanometric procedures, the active anterior technique is preferred. In this technique, the patient's normal nasal breathing is assessed and the nasal cavities are assessed separately. The presence of a nasal cycle (alternating baseline nasal congestion and decongestion) may give rise to problems in interpretation. There is no uniformly accepted way of determining when a change

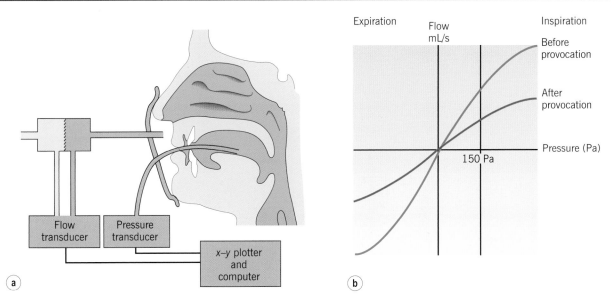

Fig. 10.19 The rhinomanometric examination. (a) The patient breathes through the nose via an anaesthetic mask to which a flow transducer is attached. A further tube is introduced into the mouth and held tightly between the lips. This is attached to a pressure transducer to measure mouth pressure. (b) Pressure and flow are plotted on an *x–y* plotter. Resistance may be calculated by reading flow at constant pressure, usually 150 Pa.

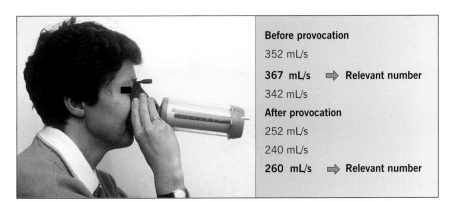

Before provocation

352 mL/s

367 mL/s ➡ **Relevant number**

342 mL/s

After provocation

252 mL/s

240 mL/s

260 mL/s ➡ **Relevant number**

Fig. 10.20 The nasal peak flow determination is usually made on inspiration. A maximum nasal breath is performed with the mask tightly fitted around the nose without influencing the nasal alii. The peak flow is determined at least three times and the highest value is noted. After an allergen challenge, lower values may be obtained.

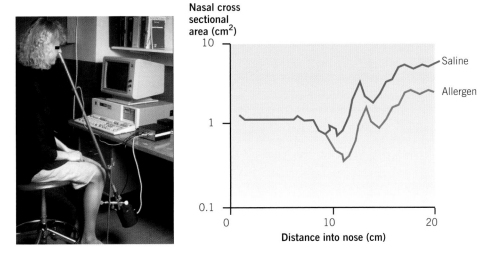

Fig. 10.21 The determination of the nasal geometry using acoustic rhinometry. The spark sound is led to the nasal cavity through the long tube where a microphone is fitted some distance from the nosepiece. The difference in the time and intensity of the sound is monitored and this information is used to compute the nasal geometry with the aid of the computer. Allergen challenge will induce a mucosal thickening, and reduction of the nasal cross-sectional area which can be determined using this method.

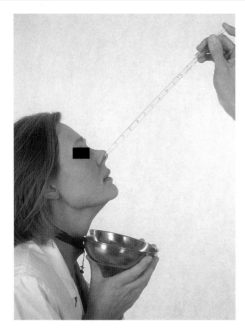
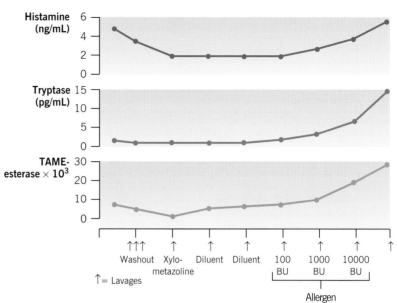

Fig. 10.22 A nasal lavage can be performed by administering normal saline solution (approximately 5 mL/nasal cavity) whilst simultaneously closing the epipharynx. A nasal-allergen challenge can be performed during a series of repeated lavages at a fixed time interval. Increasing doses of allergen in an allergic individual will produce increasing quantities of markers of mast cell activation such as histamine, tryptase, tert amyl methyl ether (TAME)-esterase, and plasma proteins.

in any of these parameters should be considered as positive, and they must still be considered to be mainly research instruments. Acoustic rhinometry uses the reflection of sound to determine the cross-sectional area of the nasal cavity over its entire length. It is more reproducible than rhinomanometry and readings are obtainable even in patients with marked nasal obstruction.

Increase in nasal surface liquid or nasal secretions is the third main symptom. Weighing the blown secretion is a simple way to determine the amount of liquid produced. It may also be of interest to assess any changes in the specific composition of the nasal surface liquid. Lavage of the nasal cavity with saline solution or collection of contents by merocell filters before and after challenge with allergen and the subsequent analysis of various markers of specific cell activation have been performed (Fig. 10.22). Histamine or tryptase may be used as markers of mast cell activation; ECP, MBP, and eosinophil-derived neurotoxin are markers of eosinophil activation, IgA and lysozyme may be used as functional markers for glandular secretion, and albumin and fibrinogen for plasma leakage. Cytokines can also be monitored.

These techniques are primarily useful for research and have contributed to our knowledge of the pathophysiology of upper airway allergic reactions. Their application in the clinical setting remains undefined.

Cytological studies

Cytology of the upper airway mucosa obtained by scrapings or brushings is sometimes used to elucidate whether

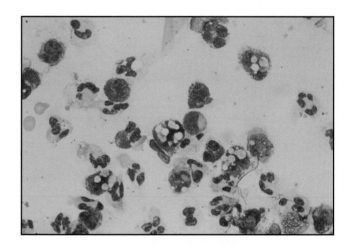

Fig. 10.23 Brush sample from a patient with seasonal allergic rhinitis during natural allergen exposure, showing a few neutrophils, some epithelial cells, and several eosinophils, some with vacuoles indicating ongoing secretory activity. (Giemsa stain, original × original400.) (From Bousquet J, Khaltaev N, Cruz AA, et al. Allergic Rhinitis and its Impact on Asthma (ARIA) 2008 update (in collaboration with the World Health Organization, GA(2)LEN and AllerGen). Allergy 2008; 63 suppl 86:8–160.)

upper airway disease is inflammatory. Eosinophilia over 10% (Fig. 10.23) is a sign of active inflammatory disease, but can be present in some non-allergic rhinitides. The presence and density of mast cells within the epithelium also increases with allergen exposure (see Fig. 10.9).

Ciliary beat frequency can also be analysed from brushings using a polarized light microscope.

Biopsy should be undertaken only by someone familiar with nasal anatomy, and prepared to deal with the sometimes profuse post-biopsy bleeding.

Management of allergic rhinitis

Information

Adequate management of rhinitis can improve symptoms and quality of life and decrease comorbidities. Immunotherapy for rhinitis probably reduces the progression from rhinitis to asthma. As yet there is no generally accepted rhinitis control test, but there are validated quality of life instruments such as the Rhinitis Quality of Life Questionnaire (RQLQ) available to test the outcomes of treatment upon patients' lives.

The most important element is information to the patient and, if the patient is a child, the parent. Successful treatment depends on the patient understanding the nature of the disease: that it may be a life-long ailment in which the treatment response depends on patient cooperation and that treatment is effective, safe, and very worthwhile. Books, videos or pamphlets can be helpful.

Allergen avoidance

Allergen avoidance, when complete, stops symptoms – for example purely seasonal rhinitics are unaffected out of season. This approach should be strictly enforced when there is an allergic reaction to foods, drugs, animals, or latex. Because seasonal pollens and moulds have a widespread airborne distribution. However, complete avoidance of these allergens is difficult if not impossible.

Sometimes a total change of environment might be of value.

Measures designed to reduce the degree of mite exposure in the home have not been proven to be beneficial in double-blind trials – but none such trial has convincingly reduced all mite exposure. In an open small study, improvement occurred in children whose animals were removed and whose homes were superheated steam cleaned with subsequent continuance of avoidance measures. It is also important to try to eliminate other local irritants such as cigarette smoke as much as possible.

Saline douching

Washing the nose with salt water, either isotonic or slightly hypertonic, can reduce nasal symptoms, especially if used after allergen exposure. In children it decreases the need for intranasal steroids.

Drug treatment

Several pharmacological agents are available for the treatment of rhinitis, most of which have different efficacy profiles (Table 10.5). Details of each are contained in Chapter 7. A combination of drugs with different effect profiles can be productive. Allergic conjunctivitis, which is often present and as troublesome as the nasal symptoms, should also be treated. The ARIA guidelines provide a treatment plan based on timing and severity of disease (Fig. 10.24).

Intranasal steroids (INS)

Intranasal steroids have been established by three meta-analyses as the single most effective treatment of allergic

Table 10.5 Efficacy profile of the various drugs used to treat allergic rhinitis*

Drug	Sneezing	Discharge	Blockage	Anosmia	Conjunctivitis
Cromolyn	+ +	+	+	–	++**
Decongestant	–	–	+ + +	–	–
Antihistamine	+ + +	+ +	+/–	–	++***
Ipratropium	–	+ +	–	–	–
Topical steroids	+ + +	+ +	+ +	+	++
Oral steroids	+ +	+ +	+ + +	+ +	??
Antileukotriene	–	+ +	+	+	??

*Some of the drugs inhibit only one nasal symptom (e.g. decongestants only work on nasal blockage), while others have more widespread activity (e.g. topical glucocorticoids).
**Cromolyn is effective against eye symptoms only when given as an ophthalmic preparation.
***The newer, highly potent steroids reduce eye symptoms when administered intranasally.

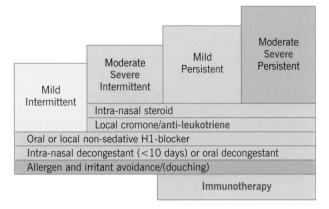

Fig. 10.24 The ARIA guidelines treatment plan based on timing and severity of disease. (Bousquet J, Khaltaev N, Cruz AA, et al. Allergic Rhinitis and its Impact on Asthma (ARIA) 2008 update (in collaboration with the World Health Organization, GA2LEN and AllerGen). Allergy 2008; 63 suppl 86:8–160.)

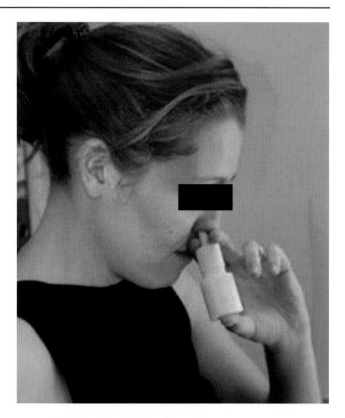

Fig. 10.25 Good technique for administration of an intranasal steroid spray. First gently blow the nose to clear it or douche with saline if secretions are thick. Then, whilst looking slightly downwards as if reading a book, spray towards the lateral wall in two different directions, up and back, using the opposite hand. Do not sniff. This method avoids septal deposition, which can lead to soreness and bleeding and it also wets most of the side wall, allowing the spray to be carried back throughout the nose by mucociliary clearance over about 10–15 minutes. It is during this time that the corticosteroid enters the epithelial cells. Sniffing hard removes the spray too quickly to the posterior nasopharynx from where it is swallowed, not permitting the desired local action. (Adapted from BSACI guidelines for allergic and non-allergic rhinitis. CEA 2008;38:19–42.)

rhinitis. They work on all symptoms, including nasal obstruction, and are more efficacious than antihistamines, leukotrienes, and cromolyn sodium and are the treatment of choice for anything more than mild intermittent rhinitis. INS can be administered conveniently once or twice daily. The correct administration should be explained to the patient (Fig. 10.25). It should, however, be explained clearly to patients that the maximal benefit of glucocorticoids is not immediate but may take several days to be apparent.

The older agents, including beclomethasone dipropionate, budesonide, flunisolone acetonide and triamcinolone acetonide, are less potent than the newer preparations and are metabolized only slowly following systemic absorption. In addition to being more potent, the newer drugs fluticasone propionate, mometasone furoate and fluticasone furoate undergo rapid first-pass metabolism in the liver and thus have negligible systemic effects. Ciclesonide is activated by esterases at sites of inflammation.

If symptoms are already present it may be necessary to open up the nasal cavity with a topical decongestant or a short course of oral glucocorticoids at the same time as starting INS administration.

Some intranasal steroids significantly reduce the ocular symptoms accompanying allergic rhinitis. The mechanism for this is thought to be a reduction in the naso-ocular reflex following the anti-inflammatory actions of the steroids in the nose.

Because of their negligible absorption and rapid metabolism, modern intranasal steroids have limited local and systemic side effects and may be used even for long-term treatment. In this case rhinoscopy is recommended once or twice a year. One should not hesitate to use topical glucocorticoids in children over 4 years old. Long-term treatment should not be instituted without careful

individual evaluation and careful monitoring of growth. The child with asthma, rhinitis, and atopic eczema may be receiving corticosteroids at multiple sites and the potential benefit from adequate rhinitis treatment must be weighed against steroid load. However, the contribution to this from nasal treatment is far less than that from lung and skin, which have much larger absorptive areas, and effective rhinitis treatment may reduce the amount of inhaled steroid needed – therefore a trial period of INS therapy with careful monitoring of growth (which is a sensitive monitor of systemic steroid activity) may be helpful.

Some patients may suffer from local irritation from the spray, with blood spotting. Septal perforation is a very rare side effect, and is probably due to maladministration of spray directly on the septum.

H$_1$-antihistamines

Many drugs with antihistaminic activity are available for use in clinical practice. First-generation antihistamines, including chlorphenamine and diphenhydramine, have a low therapeutic index and can cross the blood–brain barrier. The large doses needed for therapeutic efficacy lead to unwanted effects of sedation, psychomotor retardation, and blockade of cholinergic and α-adrenergic receptors. They should not be used.

The more recent H$_1$-antihistamines, such as cetirizine desloratadine, ebastine, fexofenadine, levocetirizine, loratadine and rupatadine, which have little or no sedative or anticholinergic effect, are useful alone for mild rhinitis, or in combination with a nasal steroid if that is insufficiently effective alone. Their greatest therapeutic benefit is on rhinorrhoea, and they also have a beneficial effect on sneezing and itching, but little effect on nasal blockage. Used on a regular basis, H$_1$-antihistamines may also help to slightly reduce nasal blockage.

The nasal benefits of H$_1$-antihistamines are increased and side effects reduced by administering them as nasal sprays; thus far, azelastine and levacobastine sprays are available. Although the putative sensitizing effect of topically applied antihistamines has been questioned, the risk of such unwanted effects appears to be minimal when it comes to application onto mucous membranes.

H$_1$-antihistamines should be used on a daily basis, rather than on demand, throughout the pollen season for seasonal allergic rhinitis. They may also be taken on a regular basis for persistent rhinitis. There is no evidence of tachyphylaxis or long-term toxicity.

Anticholinergics

An atropine derivative, ipratropium bromide, is poorly absorbed from mucous membranes, and patients with allergic and non-allergic rhinitis whose predominant symptom is that of profuse nasal discharge benefit from this drug. In allergic rhinitis it is usually used in addition to a topical nasal corticosteroid when patients are insufficiently responsive to that drug alone. The spray needs to be used several times daily, with initial application on waking when rhinorrhoea is often most problematical, followed by one or two further doses. The patient should be warned about possible side effects such as urinary retention and glaucoma.

Cromolyn sodium and nedocromil sodium

Cromolyn sodium and nedocromil sodium are traditionally known as mast cell stabilizers, but also down-regulate sensory nerve activation to reduce itching and have some anti-inflammatory properties. These drugs have a similar efficacy to antihistamines but intranasal preparations should be administered at least four times a day. This makes patient compliance difficult. Ophthalmic preparations, being very safe, are especially useful for the treatment of allergic conjunctivitis.

Antileukotrienes

These exist in two forms: drugs that inhibit leukotriene formation (e.g. zileuton), and leukotriene receptor antagonists (LTRAs) (e.g. montelukast, zafirlukast, and pranlukast). These are effective in asthma and in rhinitis, both in allergic rhinitis and in nasal polyposis. In the former, antileukotrienes have an efficacy similar to that of antihistamines; combination with an antihistamine results in very little additional benefit and is not superior to use of a topical corticosteroid alone. In the UK they are licensed for use in patients with combined asthma and hay fever. In nasal polyposis, approximately 60% of patients derive some benefit, with no significant difference between aspirin-tolerant and aspirin-sensitive patients. There is a wide variation in patient responsiveness to the LTRAs, with around 10% of patients deriving marked benefit. Since nasal polyposis is frequently accompanied by asthma, which can be severe, the antileukotrienes are likely to be of most use in such patients, where they may be steroid sparing.

α-Adrenoceptor stimulant drugs (nasal decongestants)

Vasoconstrictors are used by millions of rhinitis sufferers, both as topical preparations and as tablets. All the nasal vasoconstrictors that are available commercially possess α-adrenoceptor stimulant properties to a greater or lesser degree and cause contraction of the smooth muscle of the venous erectile tissues, thereby increasing reactive hyperaemia and rebound congestion. The most popular topical preparations contain xylometazoline or oxymetazoline, which have a long duration of action. Prolonged use can be associated with the risk of rebound congestion, so they can be recommended for occasional limited use for a few days only. The risk of rhinitis medicamentosa, in which nasal obstruction becomes unresponsive to venoconstrictive agents, is lower when the decongestant is administered orally. However, this route is associated with several disturbing and undesirable side effects including bladder dysfunction, restlessness, nausea, vomiting, insomnia, headache, tachycardia, dysrhythmias, hypertension, and angina, and is contraindicated in patients with cardiovascular disease, thyrotoxicosis, glaucoma, and in those taking monoamine oxidase inhibitors. As many of these receptor-blocking drugs are available without prescription, patients at risk should be warned of their possible harmful effects. Patients with hypertension and glaucoma are at particular risk and should avoid oral decongestants.

Intranasal decongestants have a rapid onset of action in improving nasal obstruction, but their use should be limited to no more than 3–5 days because of the concern that prolonged use may lead to rebound swelling of the nasal mucosa and to drug-induced rhinitis (rhinitis medicamentosa).

Systemic corticosteroids

Systemic corticosteroids are highly effective in all inflammatory forms of rhinitis. However, they have systemic side effects, whether given as depot injections or orally, and the benefit/risk ratio should be considered. Depot injections are simple, but have been linked to disfiguring muscle atrophy after repeated injection, and the timing of release does not coincide with maximal effects of seasonal allergen. Severe side effects such as necrosis of the femoral head have been reported after repeated use. In cases of severe seasonal allergic disease, the administration of oral prednisolone or prednisone to cover some peak days may be considered. If, however, more regular treatment fails then specific hyposensitization should be considered.

Immunotherapy

Some 20% of allergic rhinitis patients suffer symptoms that are not controlled adequately by guideline-directed pharmacotherapy combined with avoidance measures. These individuals should be considered for immunotherapy, especially if there is a clear history of symptom causation by one or two allergens with supporting IgE tests and the relevant allergen(s) are available in a standardized form for regular administration.

Subcutaneous immunotherapy (SCIT)

Classic subcutaneous immunotherapy involves repeated injection of the allergen at regular intervals and is effective in allergic rhinoconjunctivitis with clear-cut allergens such as pollens, mites, and animal dander. Before it is started, a careful explanation must be given to the patient, outlining the details and commitment required as it is a long-term programme involving frequent injections of allergenic extracts for at least 3 years. Also, subcutaneous immunotherapy carries the risk of a systemic anaphylactic reaction – thus facilities for resuscitation must be immediately available and the patient has to remain under observation for an hour (30 minutes in USA) after each injection. Because of the possible risks associated with immunotherapy, some countries have introduced guidelines to govern the use of this form of therapy. The mechanism probably involves induction of T-regulatory cells (Fig. 10.26).

Immunotherapy for allergic rhinitis in children has been shown probably to reduce the progression of rhinitis to asthma.

Sublingual immunotherapy (SLIT)

In recent years the efficacy of sublingual immunotherapy has been proved for allergens such as grass pollen and house dust mite. Trials of birch pollen and other allergens are ongoing. This method involves an initial dose under the tongue in a supervised setting followed by self-administration at home. Side effects are common but generally mild – involving itching and sometimes swelling of mouth and throat in around 80% at first – and

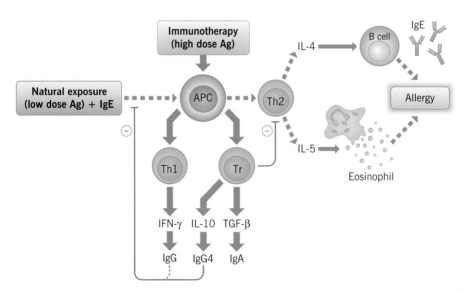

Fig. 10.26 The mechanism of immunotherapy is complex. There is evidence of switching from a Th2 to a Th1 reaction with consequent IgE production. T-regulatory cells may be involved: these produce IL-10, which promotes a switch to IgG4, which is then capable of blocking IgE-facilitated antigen presentation by B cells, and also TGF-β, which switches IgE to IgA production. In contrast, corticosteroids reduce Th2 without augmenting Th1 responses. (Adapted from Robinson DS, Larché ML, Durham SR. Tregs and allergic disease. J Clin Invest 2004; 114:1389–1397.)

disappear in most patients over about 10 days. Systemic anaphylaxis is extremely rare and no death has been reported.

High doses of allergen are needed, but the costs are similar to those of SCIT when all factors such as repeated visits, time off work, professional time, etc. are taken into account.

The mechanisms appear similar to those of SCIT. The efficacy overlaps with that of SCIT when meta-analyses are compared but a large head-to-head trial is needed. There are suggestions that SLIT, like SCIT, can alter the course of disease.

Rhinosinusitis

Structure and function of the sinuses

The paranasal sinuses were thought to lighten the skull and to increase vocal resonance, but have now been found to produce nitric oxide, a colourless, odourless gas capable of killing bacteria, viruses, fungi, and tumour cells. They thus contribute to innate immune defence of the airway.

Despite reaching down as far as the upper jaw, the sinuses drain and ventilate into the upper part of the nose at the level of the nasal bridge, probably as a result of evolutionary changes in posture from moving on all fours to walking upright. Sinus drainage relies on mucociliary clearance moving mucus from the base of the sinus, up and out into the nose via a slit-like orifice. This is easily compromised by swelling of the nasal mucosa, which blocks sinus drainage, leading to stagnation and lack of oxygen in the sinus, reducing mucociliary clearance and nitric oxide production (Fig. 10.27).

Diseases within the sinuses produce one of the most common healthcare problems, affecting ~16% of the population and having significant adverse impact on quality of life and daily functioning. In Europe sinusitis is now termed 'rhinosinusitis' since it nearly always arises secondarily to nasal disease. The exceptions are penetrating injuries, from trauma or dentistry, and diving.

Radiology

A plain radiograph of the sinus regions is rarely useful since a minor degree of mucosal swelling in the maxillary sinuses in conjunction with the allergic ailment is not indicative of sinusitis, but should instead be interpreted as part of the overall allergic condition. Nevertheless, the presence of fluid in one or more of the sinuses, or their complete opacification, needs to be further evaluated by either sinus puncture or sinoscopy. Better visualization of the nasal cavity and the sinus region is obtained using a computed tomography (CT) scan specifically directed towards the ethmoidal and ostial regions where pathology is often present (Fig. 10.28). However, CT scans remain

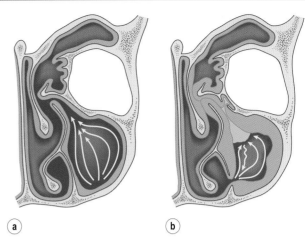

Fig. 10.27 Diagrammatic representation of (a) a normal sinus and (b) a sinus blocked at the normal ostiomeatal complex drainage area to which mucus is still being directed despite a surgically formed inferior meatal antrostomy.

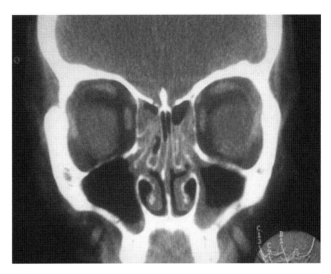

Fig. 10.28 Computed tomography (CT) scan showing ethmoiditis and obstruction of the osteomeatal complex.

abnormal for several weeks following a common cold, therefore they should not be used for diagnosis of sinusitis but to provide a 'road map' for endoscopic surgery, or if malignancy is suspected.

Acute rhinosinusitis (ARS)

This is defined by the European guidelines (EPOS) as lasting under 12 weeks and is a generally self-limited infection of the sinuses produced typically by respiratory viruses, with up to 2% subsequently involving pyogenic bacteria: mainly *Streptococcus pneumoniae*, *Haemophilus influenza*, and *Moraxella catarrhalis*. Treatment with intranasal steroids increases the rate of recovery in mild cases; antibiotics are needed if the symptoms worsen or are initially moderate to severe – that is, fever over 38°C, severe facial pain, and general malaise. In general, only one in eight patients will benefit from antibiotic treatment (i.e. the NNT for antibiotic is 8).

Chronic rhinosinusitis (CRS)

This is a spectrum of inflammatory disorders each with diifferent patterns of infiltrating leukocytes, most of which are characterized by extensive tissue remodelling. In Europe, by definition chronic rhinosinusitis lasts over 12 weeks; like rhinitis it comprises several disorders including presentations distinguished by the absence or prominent expression of eosinophils. Division into mild, moderate, and severe can be simply made by a 10 cm visual analogue scale with divisions at 3 and 7 cm. In the United States the definition is different, being defined as symptoms of nasal irritation, sneezing, rhinorrhoea, and nasal blockage lasting for at least 1 hour a day on most days. The concomitant presence of pressure or pain in a sinus distribution for >6 weeks when corroborated by objective findings defines chronic sinusitis.

The most common etiology of 'sinus' headaches with nasal congestion and rhinorrhea is migraine or mid-facial pain syndrome and the diagnosis of chronic sinusitis categorically requires objective confirmation with either rhinoscopy or radiographic imaging (Fig. 10.29).

Although chronic rhinosinusitis is often associated with the presence of anaerobic bacteria, gram-negative organisms, *Staphylococcus aureus*, and other bacteria, chronic overt infection is rarely a cause in the absence of underlying immune deficiency, human immunodeficiency virus, Kartaganer syndrome, or cystic fibrosis. These patients are identified by prominent neutrophilia and intense bacterial infiltration ($>10^5$–10^6 cfU/mL) within their sinuses.

In contrast, most patients with chronic non-polypoid rhinosinusitis have a predominantly inflammatory disorder. The presence of bacteria in these forms of chronic rhinosinusitis may reflect the loss of the usual mechanisms responsible for maintaining sterility (such as loss of mucociliary clearance) and secondary bacterial colonization, possibly in the form of biofilms. These bacteria may be benign commensal organisms but, alternatively, they probably promote or exacerbate each of the other presentations of chronic rhinosinusitis through their ability to function as sources of antigens, immune adjuvants, and superantigens. The discredited concept that chronic rhinosinusitis is primarily an infectious disorder still leads to an inappropriate focus on antibiotics and surgical drainage as primary modalities of treatment, although these modalities can have a selective role as part of a multi-stranded approach in chronic or recurrent occlusion of the sinus ostia secondary to viral rhinitis, allergic rhinitis, anatomical predisposition, or other causes. These processes lead to recurrent and protracted bacterial infections, possibly in association with barotrauma of the sinus cavities, damage to the respiratory epithelium, ciliary destruction, prominent mucous gland and goblet cell hyperplasia.

Nasal saline irrigation promotes mucus clearance and elimination of bacterial biofilms and often also proves useful.

Eosinophilic rhinosinusitis

This is characterized by the prominent accumulation of eosinophils in the sinuses and associated tissue, and can be diagnosed by histochemical staining of tissue for eosinophils or eosinophil-derived mediators (such as eosinophil cationic protein or major basic protein). The mucosa demonstrates a marked increase in cells that express cytokines, chemokines, and proinflammatory lipid mediators [cysteinyl leukotrienes (CysLTs)] that are responsible for the development of eosinophilia. Eosinophils are a prominent source of many of these cytokines and lipid mediators and, once recruited, they provide the growth factors necessary for their further recruitment, proliferation, activation, and survival. Thus, in contrast to non-eosinophilic sinusitis, this is a self-propagating syndrome and, as such, does not respond well to surgery alone.

The aetiology is poorly understood and does not have a clearly allergic origin despite the predominant

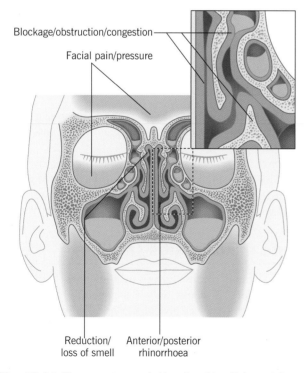

Blockage/obstruction/congestion

Facial pain/pressure

Reduction/ loss of smell

Anterior/posterior rhinorrhoea

Fig. 10.29 The symptoms of rhinosinusitis. (Adapted from Fokkens W, Lund V, Mullol J. European position paper on rhinosinusitis and nasal polyps 2007. Rhinol Suppl. 2007; (20):1–136.)

eosinophilia. Many of these patients display allergic sensitization and allergic mechanisms may be involved in a subset of subjects. Aeroallergens in general do not access healthy sinus cavities and this is likely to be even more true with the occlusion of the sinus ostia that occurs with sinus disease. However, these patients do display worsening of their sinus inflammation after aeroallergen exposures and nasal challenges exacerbate eosinophil influx into the sinuses. In the absence of direct access to the sinuses, these studies suggest a systemic and/or local lymphatic recirculation of inflammatory cells (i.e., eosinophilics, dendritic cells, T-helper lymphocytes) between the nasal epithelium, nasal-associated lymphatic tissue, bone marrow, and the sinuses that could drive this disorder. Alternatively, allergic (IgE) sensitization to commensal fungi and bacteria in the sinuses may be relevant.

These patients often have asthma and this disease shares many histological and immunological features with asthma, suggesting the same disease process attacks the upper and lower airways, respectively. Approaches that are effective in asthma are often effective in eosinophilic rhinosinusitis, including leukotriene modifiers and especially corticosteroids. Surgery is seldom effective alone, but may be essential both to address aggressive hyperplastic disease and to provide access for topically acting agents (i.e. intranasal corticosteroids). As sources of antigens and superantigens, bacteria contribute to disease severity; therefore douching is helpful, and limited use of antibiotics may occasionally be useful. Despite early enthusiasm, current studies do not support the use of topical antifungals, however. The role of allergy-directed therapies (e.g. immunotherapy, anti-IgE, anti-IL5) are under investigation.

Particularly difficult to treat subsets of eosinophilic rhinosinusitis include allergic fungal sinusitis (AFS), aspirin-exacerbated respiratory disease (AERD), and vasculitides such as Churg–Strauss syndrome. Sometimes there is overlap between these conditions, with AFS and AERD appearing together.

Allergic fungal sinusitis

Occasionally mould present as commensals in the sinuses produces a robust Th2-lymphocyte and eosinophilic inflammatory response in individuals with IgE sensitization to the relevant fungus and elevated total IgE concentrations. In contrast to other forms of eosinophilic sinusitis, disease is often limited to one or a few sinuses. The presence of intense eosinophilic infiltration and eosinophil-derived secretory products, along with extensive goblet cell and mucus gland hyperplasia, produces a thick exudate ('allergic mucin') that has a distinct appearance both on CT examination (Fig. 10.30) and during surgical resection. This inflammation often behaves as a space-occupying lesion with expansion into proximate tissue. Treatment of allergic fungal sinusitis requires

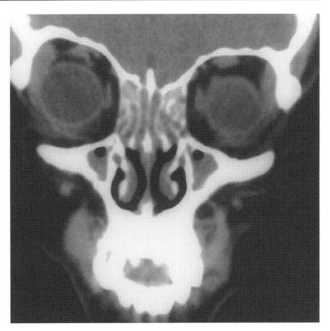

Fig. 10.30 Computed tomography (CT) scan showing calcification in allergic aspergillus sinusitis.

surgical removal with thorough debridement followed by prolonged douching and topical corticosteroid use. No role for topical or systemic antifungals or immunotherapy has been established. This may occur in association with allergic bronchopulmonary aspergillosis (ABPA).

Aspirin-exacerbated respiratory disease

AERD was originally defined by the 'triad' of nasal polyps, aspirin sensitivity, and asthma (Samter's triad) (Table 10.6). The natural history is of a severe 'cold' that does not go away, leaving a non-allergic rhinitis that progresses to nasal polyposis, late onset asthma, and aspirin sensitivity. There is usually a severe and extensive pansinusitis, often with complete opacification of all sinuses. The nasal polyposis of AERD is aggressive with multiple polyps and polypoid changes characterized by rapid growth and – in the absence of medical management – universal recurrence after surgery. Despite the extensive involvement of the sinuses with inflammatory tissue, in contrast to acute or non-eosinophilic chronic sinusitis, patients seldom complain about 'sinus pressure' or headaches. The consistent complaints are anosmia and excessive postnasal mucus and a severe form of asthma that is often difficult to control prior to the use of steroid or LABA combinations. Aggressive remodelling with progressive irreversible decline in lung function is seen in some patients. The lung, sinus, and nasal polyp tissue display robust eosinophilia extending into the circulation. Elevated levels of local IgE, produced polyclonally in response to *Staphylococcus aureus* enterotoxins that engage multiple T cells via the Vb receptor, have been demonstrated. These eventually spill over into the circulation and patients

Table 10.6 Features of aspirin-exacerbated respiratory disease

Onset	3rd or 4th decades of life – later than other forms of asthma
Eosinophilic sinusitis	Extensive pansinusitis often with complete opacification of all sinuses
Nasal polyps	Robust, rapidly growing, and require frequent surgical removal
Anosmia	More frequently associated with complete anosmia than idiopathic eosinophilic sinusitis
Asthma	When present tends to be severe and difficult to control Frequently associated with extensive remodelling and rapidly progressive irreversible decline in lung function
Aspirin sensitivity	Sensitivity to aspirin and other non-selective cyclooxygenase inhibitors Patients generally tolerate selective COX-2 inhibitors
Eosinophilia	Robust eosinophilic infiltration of bronchial airways as well as sinuses and nasal polyps Also significant elevations of circulating absolute eosinophil counts
Cysteinyl leukotrienes	Patients display constitutive overproduction of and overresponsiveness to cysteinyl leukotrienes Aspirin (and other COX inibitor)-induced reactions largely reflect surge in cysteinyl leukotriene production and reactions are mitigated by leukotriene modifiers
Non-atopy	In contrast to other forms of asthma, patients are often non-atopic (do not display IgE sensitivity to aeroallergens or elevated total IgE), although local polyclonal IgE production may occur later in the disease course, probably secondary to stimulation of T cells via Vβ receptors by staphylococcal enterotoxins. This eventually spills into the circulation and patients have multiple positive skin prick tests of uncertain significance When present, allergic rhinitis reflects coincidental presence of this common disorder

develop multiple positive skin prick tests – of uncertain significance.

These patients develop symptoms of nasal congestion, rhinorrhoea, and paroxysmal sneezing, typically with severe exacerbations of their asthma after taking aspirin or other non-steroidal anti-inflammatory drugs that inhibit cyclooxygenase 1 (COX 1). These are not allergic (i.e. IgE-mediated) reactions to these medications but instead directly reflect their pharmacological mechanism. Ingestion of these agents leads to a decline in production of the COX product prostaglandin E_2 (PGE_2) and a surge in secretion of the CysLTs. CysLTs are produced by activated eosinophils and mast cells. PGE_2 inhibits activation of mast cells and eosinophils, and when PgE_2 concentrations are reduced by COX inhibitors these cells become activated. Support for this concept is derived from the observation that exogenously administered PgE_2 prevents this response from developing. The PGE_2 that protects mast cells and eosinophils from activation appears to be derived from COX 1, as selective COX 2 inhibitors are generally well tolerated.

AERD is also explained by the overproduction of and overresponsiveness to the CysLTs. AERD subjects display dramatic up-regulation of enzymes involved in CysLT synthesis. This overexpression drives both the constitutive overproduction of the CysLTs and the life-threatening surge in CysLTs that occurs with ingestion of aspirin. In addition to their overproduction, these patients display greatly enhanced sensitivity to the CysLTs, reflecting overexpression of the CysLT receptors. In addition PGE_2 receptors are down-regulated.

AERD patients are sometimes therapeutically responsive to leukotriene modifiers. These patients also uniquely benefit from aspirin desensitization and subsequent ingestion of daily aspirin. Although the basis for the benefit of aspirin is not known, it is noteworthy that this treatment is associated with both diminished production of the CysLTs and diminished expression of the CysLT receptors. Successful aspirin desensitization produces improved asthma control, fewer requirements for corticosteroid 'bursts', improved (or restored) sense of smell, reduced need for repeat polypectomies, and greatly reduced occurrence of bacterial superinfections of the sinuses.

Churg–Strauss syndrome

A few patients with severe recurrent nasal polyposis and difficult asthma have an eosinophilic vasculitis known as the Churg–Strauss syndrome. Other systemic symptoms include otitis media with effusion, mononeuritis multiplex, rashes, joint pains, and possibly cardiac involvement. Antineutrophil cytoplasmic antibodies are present in 50% of patients. Systemic corticosteroids are helpful but azathioprine or cyclophosphamide may be needed to decrease the steroid requirement and reduce side effects.

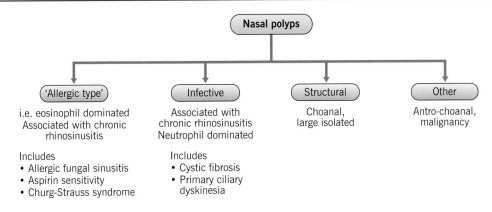

Fig. 10.31 Classification of nasal polyps.

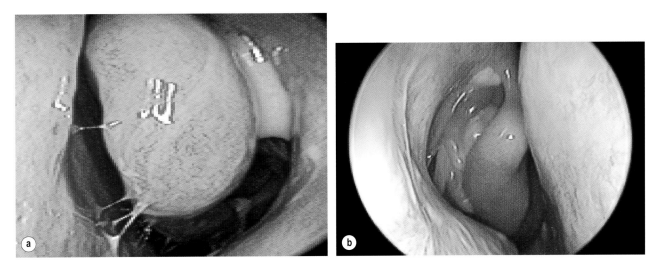

Fig. 10.32 Nasal polyps seen by rhinoscopic examination of the nose. (a) Chronic rhinosinusitis without nasal polyposis. (b) Chronic rhinosinusitis with nasal polyposis.

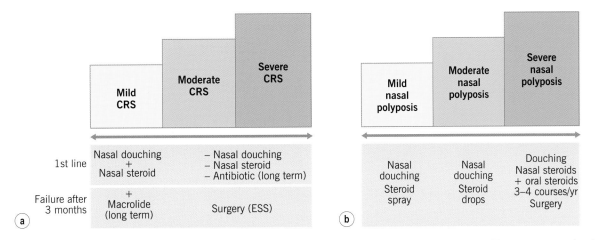

Fig. 10.33 Principles of treatment of chronic rhinosinusitis (a) without and (b) with nasal polyposis. The treatment should be reviewed every 3 to 6 months. (Adapted from Thomas M, Yawn BP, Price D, et al. EPOS Primary Care Guidelines: European Position Paper on the Primary Care Diagnosis and Management of Rhinosinusitis and Nasal Polyps 2. Prim Care Respir J 2008; 17:79–89.)

Nasal polyps (chronic polypoid rhinosinusitis)

These can be classified in the same way as rhinitis (Fig. 10.31). Inflammatory polyps can be predominantly neutrophilic or eosinophilic and probably reflect severe hyperplasia due to many causes. Symptoms are rarely unilateral, although this may occur with choanal polyps or neoplasia and therefore the presence of unilateral 'polyps' requires surgical referral. Occasionally polyps can hide malignancy so new polyps should also be sent to the ENT surgeon. The predominant symptoms of polyposis are nasal blockage and anosmia. Polyps can be seen at rhinoscopy as pale grey-yellow rounded masses (Fig. 10.32).

The principles of treatment of chronic rhinosinusitis with and without polyps are summarized in Figure 10.33.

Summary of important messages

- Rhinitis and rhinosinusitis, although often ignored as trivial, are important conditions warranting careful diagnosis and effective treatment
- Rhinitis and rhinosinusitis adversely affect quality of life, interfere with work/school ability, and have significant comorbidities
- Rhinitis, both allergic and non-allergic, is a risk factor for the subsequent development of asthma. Immunotherapy for rhinitis can probably reduce progression to asthma
- Accurate diagnosis and effective treatment of allergic rhinitis can improve symptoms and quality of life and improve asthma control
- Rhinosinusitis includes a variety of conditions, some of which are serious and can progress to involve other organs (e.g. Wegener's granulomatosis, Churg–Strauss syndrome, and systemic immune deficiency)
- Early diagnosis and therapy of these is vital and can reduce morbidity and mortality

Further reading

Bousquet J, Khaltaev N, Cruz AA, et al. Allergic Rhinitis and its Impact on Asthma (ARIA) 2008 update (in collaboration with the World Health Organization, GA²LEN and AllerGen). Allergy 2008; 63 suppl 86:8–160.

Fokkens W, Lund V, Mullol J, on behalf of the EP3OS group. Rhinology 2007; 45(suppl 20):1. Online at: http://www.rhinologyjournal.com.

Keil T, Bockelbrink A, Reich A, et al. The natural history of allergic rhinitis in childhood. Pediatr Allergy Immunol 2010 Sep; 21(6):962–969; Epub 2010 May 9.

Moscato G, Siracusa A. Rhinitis guidelines and implications for occupational rhinitis. Curr Opin Allergy Clin Immunol 2009; 9(2):110–115.

Portnoy JM, Van Osdol T, Williams PB. Evidence-based strategies for treating allergic rhinitis. Curr Allergy Asthma Rep 2004; 6:439–446.

Powe DG, Jagger C, Kleinjan A, et al. 'Entopy': localized mucosal allergic disease in the absence of systemic responses for atopy. Clin Exp Allergy 2003; 33(10):1374–1379.

Scadding GK, Durham SR, Mirakian R, et al. BSACI guidelines for the management of allergic and non-allergic rhinitis. Clin Exp Allergy 2008; 38:19–42.

Scadding GK, Hellings P, Alobid I, et al. Diagnostic tools in Rhinology EAACI position paper. Clinical and Translational Allergy 2011; 1(2):1–39.

Stelmach R, do Patrocinio TN, Ribeiro M, et al. Effect of treating allergic rhinitis with corticosteroids in patients with mild-to-moderate persistent asthma. Chest 2005;128:3140–3147.

Walker S, Khan-Wasti S, Fletcher M, et al. Seasonal allergic rhinitis is associated with a detrimental effect on examination performance in United Kingdom teenagers: case-control study. J Allergy Clin Immunol 2007; 120(2):381–387.

Wallace DV, Dykewicz MS, Bernstein DI, et al. The diagnosis and management of rhinitis: An updated practice parameter. J. Allergy Clin Immunol 2008; 122(2):S1-S84.

Allergic conjunctivitis

Melanie Hingorani, Virginia L Calder, Leonard Bielory and Susan Lightman

Conjunctivitis is inflammation of the conjunctiva, the mucous membrane lining the anterior sclera and the inner eyelid surfaces, seen in a broad spectrum of conditions, including allergy.

Introduction

Allergic inflammation of the ocular surface (the lid margins, conjunctiva, and cornea; Fig. 11.1) is one of the commonest ocular disorders, affecting 21% of the adult population of the UK. In its mildest form, the conjunctiva becomes inflamed in response to a transient allergen (e.g. pollen in seasonal allergic conjunctivitis), or a persistent allergen (e.g. house dust mite in perennial allergic conjunctivitis), producing unpleasant symptoms but not threatening sight. At the other end of the spectrum are disorders such as vernal keratoconjunctivitis and atopic keratoconjunctivitis that can have blinding complications when the cornea is involved, and for which current therapeutic agents are only partially effective.

Anatomy and physiology

The conjunctiva is a thin, transparent, vascular mucous membrane investing the inner lid surfaces and the anterior sclera (Fig. 11.2). It runs in continuity with the corneal epithelium at the limbus (the transition zone between sclera and cornea) and with the skin at the grey line on the lid margin (Fig. 11.3). There are three major zones of the conjunctiva (Fig. 11.4): the tarsal portion (lining the inner eyelid and firmly adherent to underlying fibrous tissue), the bulbar conjunctiva (lying over the anterior sclera and loosely attached to underlying tissue), and the forniceal conjunctiva (upper and lower), which joins the other two portions and where conjunctiva lies in loose folds.

The normal conjunctiva consists of a non-keratinizing squamous epithelium two to ten cell layers thick, resting on the substantia propria, which is composed of loose vascular connective tissue. The conjunctiva is important in maintaining a suitable environment for the cornea, particularly via its role in the stabilization of the tear film. It is also crucial for defence of the eye against infection and trauma. Many leukocytes are present in the normal human conjunctiva (Fig. 11.5). T cells are the most common cell type, and macrophages the second most common. Eosinophils and basophils are not normally seen. Mast cells (Fig. 11.6) are concentrated around blood and lymphatic vessels and glands, and the vast majority is of the MC_{CT} type (containing both tryptase and chymase in their secretory granules). The conjunctival lymphocytes and plasma cells constitute the

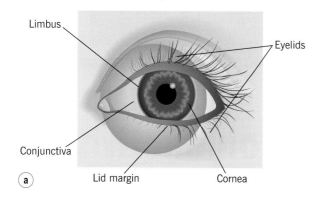

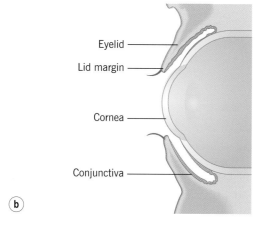

Fig. 11.1 The ocular surface. (a) Anterior view. (b) Cross-sectional view.

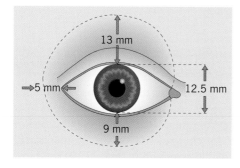

Fig. 11.2 The surface markings of the conjunctiva.

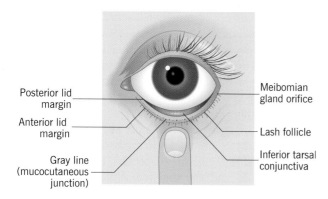

Fig. 11.3 Anatomy of the eyelid margin.

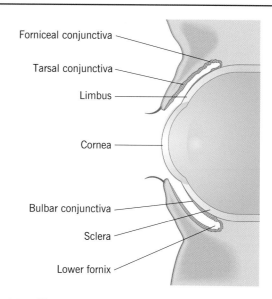

Fig. 11.4 The eyelids and the conjunctiva (forniceal cavities shown are virtual spaces in vivo).

conjunctival-associated lymphoid tissue (CALT), part of the mucosal-associated lymphoid tissue (MALT). The CALT has three components: intraepithelial lymphocytes, scattered substantia propria lymphocytes, and CALT aggregates lying just under specialized, flattened conjunctival epithelium containing M (microfold) cells. IgA plasma cells heavily outnumber other plasma cell types in the substantia propria.

Disease mechanisms

Seasonal allergic conjunctivitis (SAC) is mainly an immediate (type I) hypersensitivity response with conjunctival mast cells and their secreted products orchestrating the inflammatory response. In SAC, conjunctival mast cells become activated as a direct result of allergen cross-linking of surface IgE receptors (FcεR1), resulting in degranulation and release of histamine, leukotrienes, proteases, prostaglandins, cytokines, and chemokines (Fig. 11.7). The rapid secretion of histamine causes the characteristic itching. Upon binding to its receptors (H_1 and H_2), histamine induces vascular leakage, resulting in further cellular infiltration of eosinophils and neutrophils and oedema but little or no T-cell infiltration is observed.

In perennial allergic conjunctivitis (PAC), conjunctival tissue is infiltrated by eosinophils, neutrophils, and a small number of T cells, probably recruited as a result of the release of chemokines that attract these cells to the site of inflammation during the persistent, allergen-driven inflammatory response. These cell types are able to secrete a wide range of proinflammatory cytokines [interleukin (IL)-3, IL-4, IL-5, IL-6, transforming growth factor alpha (TGF-α), tumour necrosis factor alpha

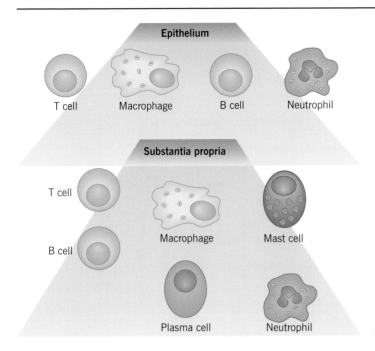

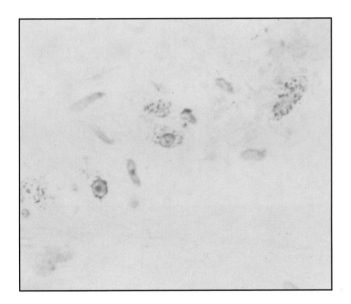

Fig. 11.5 Leukocytes in the normal conjunctiva.

Fig. 11.6 Mast cells demonstrated immunohistochemically in the epithelium and submucosa. (Courtesy of Dr Puman.)

(TNF-α)], chemokines (IL-8, RANTES) and multiple mediators (granule proteins: eosinophil cationic protein, major basic protein, and eosinophil-derived cationic protein, Fig. 11.8) to amplify the inflammatory response. Relative increases in mucosal mast cells (MC$_T$) can be identified in tarsal conjunctival tissue in SAC whereas increased numbers of both MC$_T$ and connective-tissue-type (MC$_{CT}$) mast cell phenotypes have been detected in PAC. The different pattern of mast cell subset activation occurring in PAC probably reflects the more persistent response to allergen.

In the more severe forms of chronic allergic eye disease, other inflammatory cell profiles are detected. During vernal keratoconjunctivitis (VKC), cells of both the innate and adaptive immune responses become activated; T lymphocytes and eosinophils predominate, but mast cells, neutrophils, and other cells also infiltrate the conjunctival epithelium and stroma (Fig. 11.9). In atopic keratoconjunctivitis (AKC) the predominant cell types infiltrating the conjunctival tissues are T cells, eosinophils, and neutrophils. Tarsal conjunctival tissue specimens from VKC patients contain markedly increased numbers of lymphocytes, mainly activated CD4$^+$ T cells, localized to the subepithelial layers of the affected tissue. There is also an increased HLA-DR expression within the epithelium and stroma of the conjunctiva compared with normal subjects and increased numbers of Langerhans' cells and activated macrophages (CD68$^+$). T-cell clones, derived from VKC conjunctival tissues, can be functionally characterized as Th2-type, since in situ hybridization staining demonstrates an increased Th2 cytokine (IL-3, IL-4 and IL-5) mRNA expression. In support of these findings, VKC tear samples contain increased intracellular T-cell expression of IL-4 in more than 60% of specimens and analysis of tear specimens using multiplex bead arrays, demonstrates elevated IL-4, IFN-γ and IL-10 in VKC in comparison with non-atopic controls.

Conjunctival biopsy specimens in AKC contain similarly increased numbers of activated CD4$^+$T cells, HLA-DR expression, and cells of the monocyte/macrophage lineage as well as mRNA expression of the Th2 cytokines (IL-3, IL-4 and IL-5) in the stromal tissues. However, in contrast to VKC, there is also a significant increase in the expression of IL-2 mRNA and IFN-γ-expressing T cells, which suggests a more Th1-type T-cell

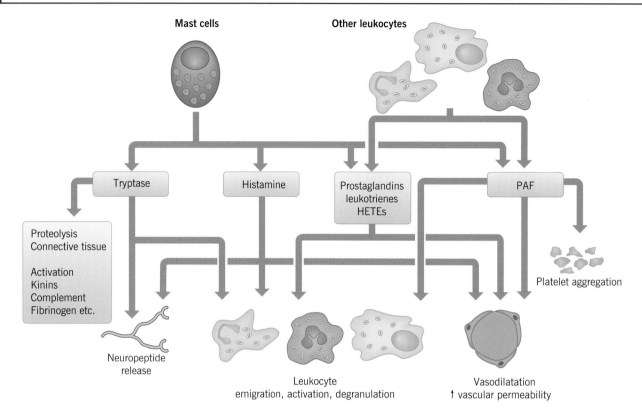

Fig. 11.7 Mediators of allergic conjunctivitis. HETEs, hydroxyeicosatetraenoic acids; PAF, platelet-activating factor.

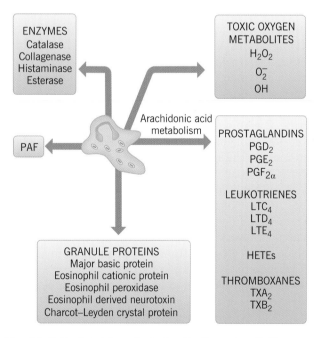

Fig. 11.8 Eosinophil products in allergic conjunctivitis. HETEs, hydroxyeicosatetraenoic acids.

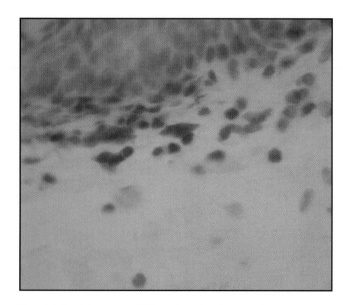

Fig. 11.9 Submucosal T lymphocytes in vernal keratoconjunctivitis demonstrated immunohistochemically.

response in the most severe and chronic of the ocular allergic diseases. In support of this, conjunctival-derived T-cell lines from AKC secrete significantly increased levels of interferon-gamma (IFN-γ). Recent studies have also identified the presence of T_H17 cells in conjunctival tissues and in tear-derived cells in VKC and AKC, but not in SAC, although their role in chronic allergic eye disease remains unclear.

In both VKC and AKC there are also alterations to the epithelium and evidence of tissue remodelling and collagen deposition (Fig. 11.10, Fig. 11.11). It appears that it is the extent of eosinophil activation (expression of ICAM-1 or HLA-DR) that correlates more with disease severity than the overall numbers of eosinophils. There are also differences between VKC and AKC in the patterns of cytokines colocalizing to conjunctival eosinophils; those in VKC mainly express IL-3, IL-5, IL-6, and GM-CSF, whereas in AKC eosinophils express mainly IL-4, IL-8, and GM-CSF.

Although the specific cellular interactions are as still under investigation, these differences in cellular and cytokine profiles point to significantly different disease mechanisms being involved in each form of ocular allergy.

Clinical presentation

General clinical presentation

Although there are a number of allergic conjunctivitis disorders with very different degrees of severity, there are a number of shared features. All present with symptoms of redness, watering, discharge, and discomfort or sometimes pain of the eyes and, most importantly, with ocular itching, which is unusual in non-allergic eye conditions. Visual disturbance is usually minimal except in the more severe disorders. Patients may also complain of swelling of the lids and sometimes of the conjunctival membrane itself, which can give a dramatic gelatinous appearance to the eyes. Many of the conditions are either seasonal or have a seasonal exacerbation during the pollen season. Some have diurnal variations dependent on allergen exposure timing [giant papillary conjunctivitis (GPC), PAC]. Many patients with allergic conjunctivitis will have a history of current or previous non-ocular allergic or atopic conditions (ezcema, asthma, urticaria, rhinitis).

Classic ocular signs of allergic inflammation are lid swelling, diffuse conjunctival redness, and mild swelling, which often combine to give a pink rather than red colour, and a velvety thickening and redness of the tarsal conjunctiva with the presence of fine excrescences called papillae, which may vary from tiny pinprick size (Fig. 11.12) to giant papillae which are >1 mm in diameter and give a cobblestone appearance under the lid (Fig. 11.13). Macroscopic noticeable swelling of the conjunctiva, called 'chemosis', is sometimes seen. Other signs, such as dermatitis of the lid skin (Fig. 11.14), inflammation of the lid margin (blepharitis), conjunctival scarring, and involvement of the cornea occur only in certain of the more severe disorders (Table 11.1).

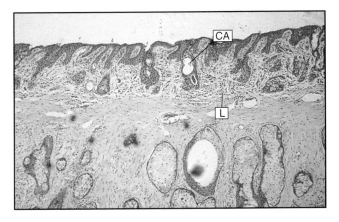

Fig. 11.10 In atopic keratoconjunctivitis, crypt abscesses (CA) are present in the epithelium and there is a band-like lymphocytic infiltrate (L). (Haematoxylin and eosin, ×40.)

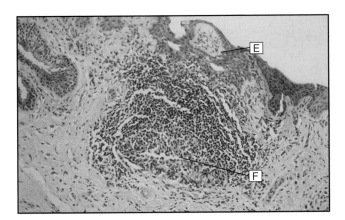

Fig. 11.11 Lymphoid follicle in submucosa in giant papillary conjunctivitis. (Hematoxylin and eosin, ×65.) E, epithelium; F, follicle.

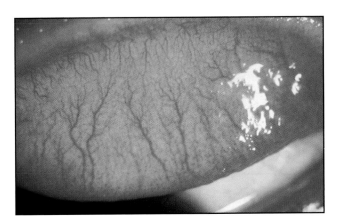

Fig. 11.12 The upper tarsal surface in perennial allergic conjunctivitis.

Table 11.1 Clinical involvement of the ocular tissues in allergic eye disorders

Disorder	Tarsal conjunctiva	Limbus	Cornea	Lid margin
Seasonal allergic conjunctivitis	+	–	–	–
Perennial allergic conjunctivitis	+	–	–	–
Vernal keratoconjunctivitis	+ +	+ +	+ +	+
Atopic keratoconjunctivitis	+ +	+ +	+ +	+ +
Giant papillary conjunctivitis	+ +	–	–	–

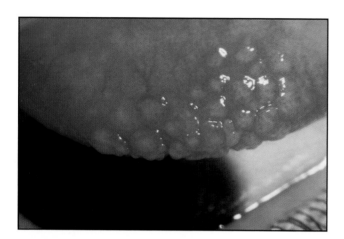

Fig. 11.13 The upper tarsal surface in giant papillary conjunctivitis.

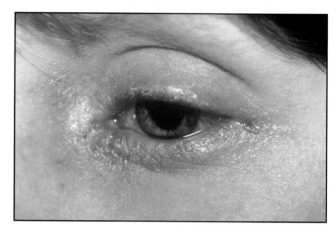

Fig. 11.14 The eyelids in atopic keratoconjunctivitis.

Clinical presentation of disease subtypes

Seasonal and perennial allergic conjunctivitis

These disorders are the commonest forms of allergic conjunctivitis and are similar except in their time course, which is determined purely by the duration of exposure to the causative allergen. In SAC (seasonal allergic conjunctivitis, hay fever), the offending allergens are plant pollens and spores, and clinical manifestations occur only during the seasons in which high atmospheric concentrations of these allergens are reached (Fig. 11.15). In PAC (perennial allergic conjunctivitis), the allergens (most commonly house dust mite, but also animal dander, mould, etc.) and therefore the symptoms and signs, are present all year round (see Fig. 11.12). In both conditions the eyes are itchy, watery, sticky and red but any visual disturbance is mild, caused by excessive tearing and production of mucus. Contact lens wearers may find that their lens tolerance decreases while the condition is active. The clinical appearance is of a mild conjunctival inflammation and clinical signs may be very slight. The bulbar and tarsal conjunctivae show mild to moderate hyperaemia, oedema, and infiltration (loss of transparency and thickening resulting from inflammatory

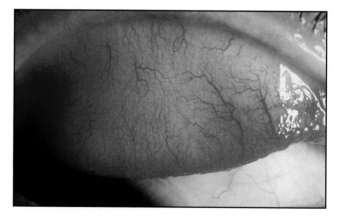

Fig. 11.15 The upper tarsal surface in seasonal allergic conjunctivitis.

infiltration). Small papillae may be seen on the tarsal conjunctiva. There may be chemosis and some swelling of the eyelids after a particularly intense or acute allergen exposure. Differences between the two conditions relate to chronicity, and more infiltration and a greater papillary response are seen in PAC whereas chemosis is more suggestive of SAC. The cornea and limbus are not affected, nor is there any scarring of the conjunctival surface – therefore there is no serious visual threat. There is usually

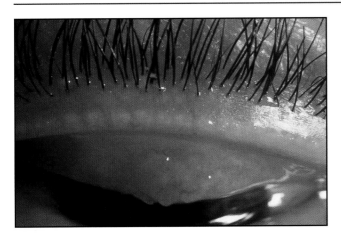

Fig. 11.16 The upper tarsal surface in atopic keratoconjunctivitis.

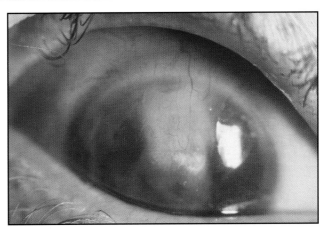

Fig. 11.17 Corneal scarring and neovascularization in atopic keratoconjunctivitis.

a good response to topical therapy using antihistamines and mast cell inhibitors or to systemic antihistamines. Topical steroids are usually not appropriate as their unwanted effects can be far more serious than those of the conditions themselves. These disorders usually affect teenagers and young adults and tend to lessen in severity and eventually resolve with increasing age.

Atopic keratoconjunctivitis (AKC)

AKC is a rare, life-long, sight-threatening condition that affects mainly adults, but occasionally children, who have systemic atopic disease – particularly atopic dermatitis. AKC is a highly symptomatic disorder with severe itching, watering, stickiness, and redness of the eyelids and eye, and sometimes causes ocular pain. There is usually facial eczema involving the eyelids (see Fig. 11.14) and the lid margins show blepharitis (chronic inflammation of the lash follicles and meibomian glands). The lid margins are thickened and hyperemic, posteriorly rounded, sometimes keratinized, and the lid anatomy may be distorted with ectropion (outwardly turning eyelid), entropion (inwardly turning eyelid), trichiasis (in-turning lashes), and notching. The whole conjunctiva is affected and shows intense infiltration, papillae that may be giant, linear and stellate scars, and often shrinkage (Fig. 11.16). Marked limbal inflammation may develop. The cornea is subject to epithelial defects and progressive scarring, and neovascularization (Fig. 11.17), thinning and secondary corneal infections (herpetic, bacterial, and fungal) may occur. Alterations in the volume or quality of the tear film may cause severe dry eye. Corneal plaque similar to that of vernal disease is sometimes seen. Associations between AKC and eye rubbing, keratoconus, atopic cataract, and retinal detachment are recognized.

The management of AKC is difficult and patients cannot be cured. It is crucial to control the facial eczema and lid margin inflammation as much as possible. Topical mast cell inhibitors are used chronically, but the

application of topical steroids is often necessary. A number of these patients require corneal surgery, which, in the presence of AKC, is a high-risk procedure.

Vernal keratoconjunctivitis (VKC)

In the UK, VKC is an unusual, self-limiting, often seasonal ocular allergy that affects children and young adults, males in particular, many of whom have a personal or family history of atopy (Fig. 11.18). The condition is a common and serious cause of ocular morbidity in parts of the Mediterranean basin, the Middle East, the Far East, Africa, and South America, where the disease is perennial and the association with atopy is less consistent.

The symptoms are marked itching, discomfort, photophobia, blepharospasm, stringy inflammatory exudate, blurred vision, and 'morning misery' – an inability to open the eyes in the morning. The superior tarsal conjunctiva and the limbus are the most markedly affected areas and other conjunctival areas show less-specific signs of inflammation. When the disease is active, the conjunctival surfaces are hyperaemic, oedematous and infiltrated, and a tenacious mucus is present (Fig. 11.19). The tarsal conjunctiva is densely infiltrated, with papillae that are often giant (Fig. 11.20). In the later stages, fine subepithelial scarring is also seen but conjunctival shrinkage and distortion does not occur. The limbus may show hyperaemia and infiltration, and discrete swellings may be present. The presence of small white dots, first described by Trantas, is typical of vernal limbitis (Fig. 11.21).

The most serious aspect of the condition is the corneal involvement. At its mildest, there is a punctate disturbance of the epithelium (Fig. 11.22). If not treated the lesions coalesce to form a macroerosion (Fig. 11.23); deposition of mucus, fibrin, and inflammatory debris can then result in the formation of plaque (Fig. 11.24). In VKC the signs can be remarkably different in severity between the two eyes – a phenomenon that has not been satisfactorily explained.

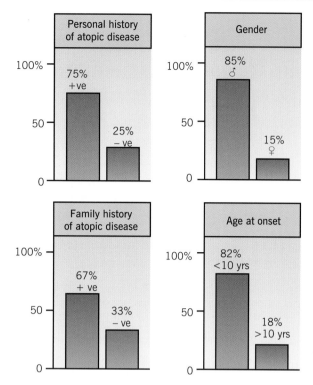

Fig. 11.18 The characteristics of vernal keratoconjunctivitis patients from a series of 100. (Data modified from Buckley RJ. Long-term experience with sodium cromolin in the management of vernal keratoconjunctivitis. In: Pepys J, Edwards AM, eds. The mast cell. London: Pitman Medical; 1980:518–523.)

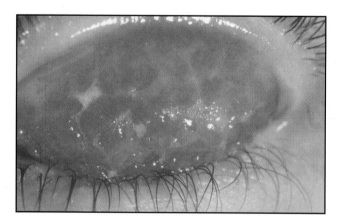

Fig. 11.19 Active vernal conjunctivitis.

Treatment is generally in the hands of the ophthalmologist, because so many cases require topical corticosteroids at some point. For the majority some benefit is obtained from topical mast cell inhibitors and more severe cases benefit from topical ciclosporin A; both these agents act as steroid-sparing agents. Mucolytic drops can provide additional symptomatic relief and may inhibit deposition of plaque material. When the corneal epithelium is breached by a macroerosion or by plaque, topical antibiotic drops are required for antibacterial prophylaxis.

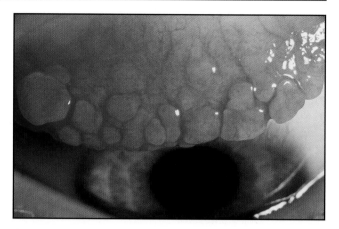

Fig. 11.20 The upper tarsal surface in vernal keratoconjunctivitis showing giant papillae.

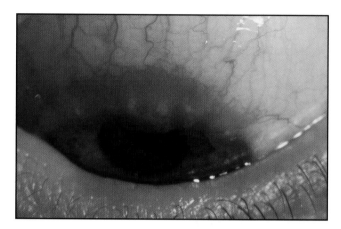

Fig. 11.21 Trantas' dots at the limbus in vernal keratoconjunctivitis.

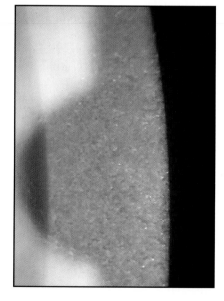

Fig. 11.22 Punctate epithelial keratitis in vernal keratoconjunctivitis.

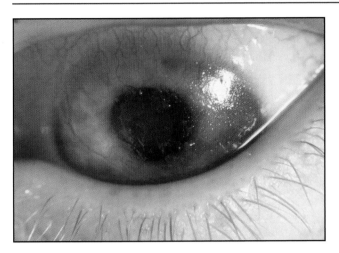

Fig. 11.23 Macroerosion in vernal keratoconjunctivitis.

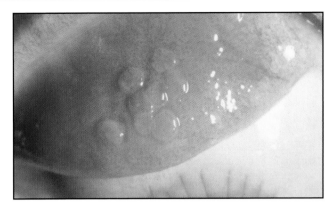

Fig. 11.25 Suture-induced giant papillary conjunctivitis: the offending corneal sutures and the tarsal surface showing giant papillae.

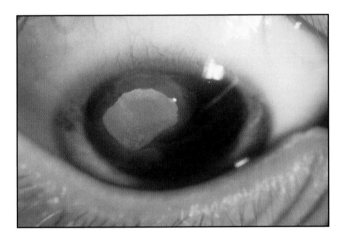

Fig. 11.24 Corneal plaque in vernal keratoconjunctivitis.

When corneal plaque is present, medical therapy is aimed at quietening the conjunctival inflammation as rapidly as possible so that plaque can be surgically removed. This is achieved by lamellar dissection using the operating microscope, usually under general anaesthesia, as most patients are children. Re-epithelialization usually takes place in a few days after this procedure.

VKC usually resolves spontaneously at or after puberty, but it may develop into AKC.

Giant papillary conjunctivitis (GPC)

Foreign body-associated papillary conjunctivitis, as it should properly be called, was first reported in wearers of soft contact lenses in 1974. It is now recognized that it may occur in wearers of all types of lenses and also in association with the use of ocular prostheses and the presence of other foreign bodies and material, such as protruding sutures, extruded scleral buckles, and cyanoacrylate glue, on the ocular surface. Although associations with atopy have been reported, this is not a consistent finding.

The onset of symptoms may occur a few weeks to years after contact lens or prosthesis wear has begun. There is no seasonal variation and GPC occurs in both sexes and at all ages. There is discomfort and accumulation of mucus on the lens. Patients complain of ocular itching when the lens is removed. The tolerance of the lens, as measured by the daily wearing time, is reduced and there is a tendency for the lens to displace upward under the upper eyelid. The patient may notice that the symptoms are alleviated if a brand new lens is worn.

The distribution and nature of conjunctival signs are very similar to those of VKC (see Fig. 11.13) except that the limbus is not commonly involved. Despite the name of the condition, papillae are not always giant. The cornea is not involved.

GPC is managed by careful attention to lens hygiene, by improvement of the fit and surface quality of the lenses or prosthesis, by minimizing the wearing time, and as a last resort by administration of drugs. There is a place for the use of disposable contact lenses. In the case of other foreign bodies (e.g. suture GPC; Fig. 11.25) removal of the offending cause will cure the condition. Mast-cell inhibitors have been shown to be effective in the management of GPC. Topical steroid preparations should not be used as they can be very much more sight threatening than the condition itself, except in the case of ocular prosthesis wearers.

Diagnosis

Each of the clinical entities requires a differential diagnosis that is usually clinical, yet can be substantiated by objective laboratory parameters (Box 11.1).

Differential diagnosis

Although their clinical characteristics allow a relatively convincing diagnosis of most forms of allergic conjunctivitis, in the milder or initial stages of these diseases there can be some diagnostic confusion. Several clinical forms may mimic the clinical pictures of ocular allergy, including tear film dysfunction, subacute and chronic infections, immunological conditions, glaucoma, and toxic and mechanical conjunctivitis (Table 11.2, Fig. 11.26).

History

The history is a vital component of any allergic disorder as the allergic dysfunction rarely targets a single organ, but presents itself as part of the spectrum of an atopic process that includes asthma, atopic dermatitis, urticaria and allergic rhinitis, chronic otitis media, sinusitis, nasal polyposis, and eustachian tube disorders. A family history of various atopic disorders is common. The onset of allergic eye is important as the incidence of seasonal and perennial forms coincide with the development of nasal allergies starting in childhood and with over 80% of individuals developing it before the age of 30. Many patients have specific seasonal exacerbations and it is not uncommon to develop multiseasonal exacerbations during the tree (e.g. birch), grass and weed (e.g. ragweed) seasons.

There are characteristic symptom complexes associated with various forms of conjunctivitis. Tearing, discomfort, and photophobia are common, but not specific. Itching is the primary ocular allergic complaint and leads to eye rubbing. The mucus associated with ocular allergy is profuse, stringy, and sticky. Conjunctival oedema and hyperaemia cause the bulbar surface to take on a 'glassy' appearance that is more pink than red. Blepharospasm is an individual problem associated with AKC and VKC and is particularly troublesome as it takes time to acclimate in the morning.

Box 11.1 Definition and differentiation of allergic conjunctivitis

- Allergic conjunctivitis is characterized by one or more of the following symptoms: itching, redness, tearing (commonly with anterior rhinorrhoea), and swelling (conjunctival and periorbital).
- Conjunctivitis should be classified by aetiology as allergic or non-allergic and differentiated from conditions that mimic symptoms of conjunctivitis.
- Symptoms of allergic conjunctivitis may occur only during specific seasons and be considered intermittent (<4 weeks' duration), may be perennial (or persistent >4 weeks' duration) without seasonal exacerbation, perennial with seasonal exacerbations, or may occur episodically after specific aeroallergen exposures.
- Risk factors for allergic conjunctivitis similar to rhinitis include:
  - family history of atopy
  - serum IgE >100 IU/mL before 6 years of age
  - higher socioeconomic class
  - presence of a positive allergy skin prick test.

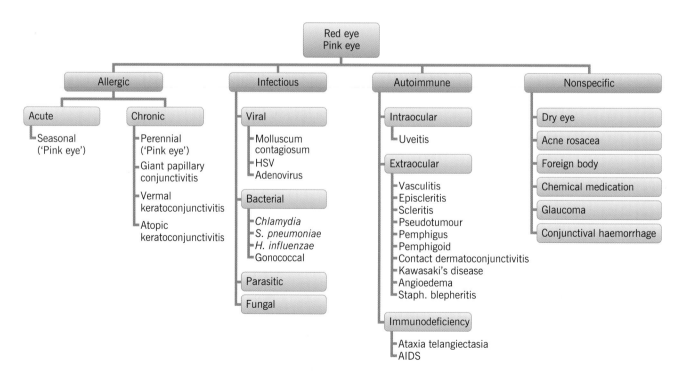

Fig. 11.26 Disorders causing a red eye.

Table 11.2 Differential diagnosis of conjunctivitis

	Predominant cell type	Signs						Symptoms			
		Chemosis	Lymph node	Discharge	Tarsal lid cobblestoning	Limbus	Lid involvement	Pruritus	Gritty sensation	Pain	Seasonal variation
Allergic											
SAC	Mast cell Eos	++	–	Clear mucoid	–	–	+/–	++	+/–	–	+++
PAC	Mast cell Eos	+/–	–	Clear mucoid	–	–	+/–	+	+/–	–	–
VKC	Lymph Eos	+/–	–	Stringy mucoid	++	++	+	+++	+	++*	++
AKC	Lymph Eos	–	–	Stringy mucoid	++	++	+++	++	+	++*	+
GPC	Lymph Eos	–	–	Clear white	++	+/–	–	++	+	–	–
Infectious											
Bacterial	PMN	–	–	Mucopurulent	–	–	–	–	++	+/–	–
Viral	PMN Mono Lymph	–	++	Clear mucoid	Follicles	+/–	–	–	+	+	–
Chlamydial	Mono Lymph	–	+	Clear mucopurulent	Follicles	+/–	–	–	+	+/–	–
Immunological											
Kawasaki's disease	PMN Lymph	+/–	++	Serous mucoid	–	–	–	–	+/–	+/–	–
Uveitis	Lymph	–	–	–	–	–	–	–	–	++	–

Table 11.2 Continued

	Signs							Symptoms			
	Predominant cell type	Chemosis	Lymph node	Discharge	Tarsal lid cobblestoning	Limbus	Lid involvement	Pruritus	Gritty sensation	Pain	Seasonal variation
Sarcoidosis	Lymph	−	−	−	Follicles	+/−	Grey flat papules	−	−	+/−	−
Episcleritis	Lymph	−	−	−	−	−	−	−	+	+/−	−
Contact dermato-conjunctivitis	Lymph	+/−	+	Clear mucoid	−	+/−	++	+	−	+/−	−
Angioedema	Mast cell	++	−	−	−	−	+++	+/−	−	−	−
Staphylococcal blepharitis	Mono Lymph	+/−*	−	++ Mucopurulent	−	−	++	+	++	+/−*	−
Non-specific											
Tear film dysfunction	−	−	−	Serous watery	−	−	−	−	++	+/−*	−
Corneal abrasion/foreign body	−	−	−	Serous watery	−	−	−	−	+/−	+++	−
Chemical	−	−	−	Serous mucoid	−	+/−	++	−	+/−	+++	−
Nasolacrimal obstruction	PMN if secondary infection	−	−	Mucopurulent	−	−	+	−	+/−	−	−

AC, allergic conjunctivitis; Eos, eosinophils; VKC, vernal keratoconjunctivitis; GPC, giant papillary conjunctivitis; PMN, polymorphonuclear leukocytes.
*If cornea involved.

Physical examination

The initial examination begins with the naked eye using a light source such as a penlight or ophthalmoscope for illumination. The ophthalmoscope also offers the advantage of being a source of magnification and illumination with a magnification of approximately 15× and a field of view of 6.5–10°. The slit lamp (biomicroscope) examination used by ophthalmologists offers the widest range of external eye examinations up to a magnification of 16×. The eyelids and lid margins are examined for swelling, discoloration, and drooping of the upper lid (ptosis, Fig. 11.27). The skin of the eyelids may demonstrate induration, scaling, and lichenification. Dennie–Morgan's line in the infraorbital region is a fold or line in the skin below the lower eyelid caused by oedema in atopic dermatitis and is used as a diagnostic marker for allergy. Distortion of the eyelid anatomy may involve entropion (inwardly turning eyelid) or ectropion (outwardly turning eyelid) or inwardly turning lashes (trichiasis). Blepharitis (inflammation of the eyelid) may involve crusting, redness, and swelling of the anterior lid margin. In chronic lid margin disorders, the meibomian gland orifices are unevenly dilated and their secretion is yellow and semisolid, in contrast to the clear fluid that is produced normally; the posterior lid margin may show a rounded margin rather than the normal squared profile.

In allergic disorders of the conjunctiva all areas are involved. The bulbar conjunctiva can be directly examined by asking the patient to gaze in all directions and the lower tarsal surface and forniceal conjunctiva are easily seen when the lower eyelid is drawn downward using a finger. The upper tarsal surface is everted with the assistance of a cotton swab or a similar narrow object while the patient is looking downward (Fig. 11.28). The upper forniceal region requires a special retractor to gain a complete examination of that area of involvement, which is seen in chlamydial and viral disorders (Fig. 11.29). Oedema of the conjunctival surface (chemosis) produces a glassy appearance with a jelly-like consistency. Follicles and papilla are elevations of the tarsal conjunctival surface; follicles are pale, small (1 × 1 mm), and glistening (Fig. 11.30), and papilla are larger and pink with a common central vessel. Scarring of the conjunctival surface appears as pallor in a linear, reticular, or sheet pattern; more marked cicatrization results in shortening of the tarsal surface, loss of the forniceal space, and obliteration of the medial conjunctival anatomy, sometimes with entropion. The cornea should be examined and surface lesions are more easily highlighted with the use of vital stains such as fluorescein and examination with a cobalt blue light. Any surface abnormality should be noted such as a fine dusting indicating punctate epithelial keratitis, and localized epithelial defects such as corneal ulcers; a dry white

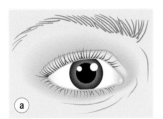
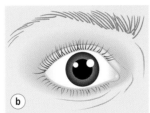
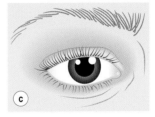

Fig. 11.27 Ptosis. It is important to note the position of the eyelid in respect to the pupil. (a) The normal eye has the lid just touching the iris, but not the pupil. (b) The exophthalmic eye has the eyelid not touching the iris at all, displaying the white of the sclera between the eyelid and the iris. (c) In ptosis, the eyelid covers most of the upper iris and may cover some of the pupil.

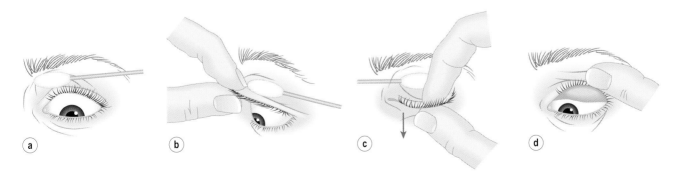

Fig. 11.28 Technique demonstrating the eversion of the upper eyelid. The eversion of the upper lid is performed by the placement of a cotton-tipped swab above the eyelid (a) and then, while the patient is asked to look downward, the upper eyelash is gently grasped (b). The upper eyelid is gently pulled down while placing pressure on the upper portion of the eyelid with the cotton swab (c), and then it is lifted over the surface of the swab (d).

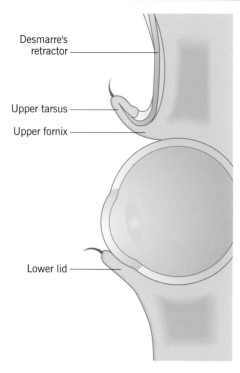

Fig. 11.29 Eversion of the upper eyelid using a Desmarre's retractor.

Labels: Desmarre's retractor, Upper tarsus, Upper fornix, Lower lid

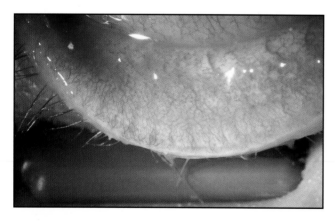

Fig. 11.30 Follicles in the inferior tarsal and forniceal conjunctiva.

Box 11.2 Diagnosis: highlights to the laboratory diagnosis of ocular allergy

- Testing for specific IgE antibody:
  - Preferably by skin testing is indicated
    to provide evidence of an allergic basis for the patient's symptoms
    to confirm or exclude suspected causes of the patient's symptoms
    to assess the sensitivity to a specific allergen for avoidance measures
    to formulate allergen immunotherapy
- In vitro assays for specific IgE:
  - The precise sensitivity of specific IgE immunoassays compared with prick/puncture skin tests is approximately 70–75%

Special diagnostic techniques

- Conjunctival smears for eosinophils:
  - may be a useful adjunct when the diagnosis of allergic conjunctivitis is in question
- Total tear IgE analysis:
  - can be used for the differential diagnosis of IgE-mediated diseases
- Conjunctival allergen challenge:
  - can be used to confirm the diagnosis of systemic allergy
  - to study the clinical features of ocular allergy
  - to study the effects of topical anti-inflammatory medications
- Conjunctival cytology:
  - is an additional useful tool for diagnosis of the chronic forms of allergic conjunctivitis

Investigations and tests

The purpose is to determine that the inflammation is allergic in origin and to identify which of the various forms of ocular allergy is present based on the clinical characteristic observed (Box 11.2).

Skin prick test

Skin prick test is a simple, rapid and inexpensive procedure that is commonly included in the work-up of patients with ocular allergy. It provides evidence of specific sensitivity to environmental and food allergens, and reinforces the concept of allergy to the patient. The test is highly sensitive for systemic allergies, but unfortunately does not always correlate well with the ocular allergic status. Because the conjunctiva can be a uniquely sensitized organ in allergy, the skin test remains a confirmatory test that requires the support of additional local tests such as a conjunctival provocation test.

or yellowish lesion may be indicative of a corneal plaque. Mucus adhering to the corneal surface is considered pathological. The limbus is the zone immediately surrounding the cornea at the interface of conjunctiva. It is normally invisible and becomes visible when inflamed with a pale-pink coloration in an annular pattern. Discrete swellings at this junction may indicate limbal papillae, whereas white dots are characteristic of cellular collections including eosinophils (Trantas' dots, see Fig. 11.21).

Patch test

If there is question of a contact sensitivity, particularly in the presence of eczematous blepharitis or blepharoconjunctivitis, a patch test is necessary. This involves applying to the skin of the back a series of hapten-containing cellulose disks that are removed after 48 hours. Benzalkonium chloride and thimerosal, preservatives present in the ophthalmic and contact lens solutions, should always be tested. If topical agents are suspected, the patch tests can be performed using the exact solution in question. It must be remembered that periorbital skin is quite different from other sites such as that of the back – not only for the depth of epithelial and dermal layers, but also for the limited number of mast cells present and for its limited exposure to the external environment compared with eyelid. It is possible, for example, that sun exposure exacerbates specific and non-specific hyperreactivity reactions only on the eyelid skin.

Haematological assays

The assaying of specific IgE in serum is particularly indicated and preferred over skin tests in certain cases. In children affected by VKC or AKC, the direct determination of serum-specific IgE is recommended for various reasons: the age of patients and their usually insufficient collaboration during skin testing, the frequent presence of cutaneous hyperreactivity and/or eczema, the prolonged use of topical and systemic drugs, the ability to quantify sensitizations to diverse antigens simultaneously, and lastly the ability to compare over time the numerical IgE values obtained. It must be remembered that VKC and AKC are not always associated with specific allergen sensitization. Particularly with VKC, IgE sensitization occurs in only half the population, although the disease is indistinguishable between IgE-positive and IgE-negative patients.

Total serum IgE is no longer considered indispensable for diagnosis since normal values do not exclude an allergic diagnosis and, conversely, high levels of IgE can be observed in numerous pathologies other than atopy.

Eosinophilia, while indicative, is not pathognomonic for allergic disease. Generally, seasonal/intermittent or perennial/persistent allergic conjunctivitis, contact allergy, and GPC are not accompanied by eosinophilia, whereas it is common in AKC and VKC. Conversely, levels of serum eosinophil cationic protein (ECP) do increase significantly in active phases of ocular allergy.

Conjunctival provocation test (CPT) or conjunctival allergen challenge (CAC)

CPT (CAC), also known as 'ocular provocation testing', can be likened to 'skin testing' of the eye. In fact, ocular provocation was the original form of allergy testing in which known quantities of specific allergen are instilled onto the ocular surface and the resulting allergic response is measured. The visible changes in the conjunctiva can be viewed with the naked eye, but for research studies examinations are typically viewed with a slit lamp under high magnification. Mediator release and cellular infiltration are easily measured in tear samples. Although this technique is not routinely used in the clinical setting, it is important in the research laboratory and pharmaceutical industry, especially in the development of new drugs against ocular allergies. Defining the conjunctival allergic response to sensitizing allergens can be extremely helpful in understanding a patient's disease. The CPT may confirm conjunctival reactivity to allergens that were noted to be positive by prick test. It is also particularly useful in patients with a negative prick test or serum IgE and a positive clinical history of allergic ocular disease to evaluate the specific, local conjunctival response. Furthermore, CPT can be used to define the most important allergen(s) in patients with several positive skin tests, to follow the local success of specific systemic immunotherapy, to evaluate the effects of antiallergic drugs, and to study the pathophysiology of the allergic conjunctival reaction.

Standardized allergens are available for the provocation test. At the moment of the test, patients must be asymptomatic and without pharmacological treatment for at least 1 week. The allergen dose is instilled every 15 minutes until a moderate clinical reaction is obtained. The immediate positive response is characterized by the same signs (redness, chemosis, and lid swelling) and symptoms (itching and tearing) that the patients experience after natural exposure to the antigen. The positive reaction usually subsides gradually within 20 minutes. A late phase inflammatory reaction may also occur, depending on allergen dose and patient sensitivity. Systemic side effects (generalized itching, bronchospasm, anaphylaxis) are rare, but possible in particularly sensitized patients.

The use of the test is recommended only in specialized centres, and rapid escape treatment for systemic reactions should always be available. In asthmatic patients, the test should be performed only when necessary.

Non-specific provocation test

Ocular challenge with histamine or hyperosmolar solutions has been used to verify a non-specific hyperresponsiveness of the conjunctiva in allergic patients. VKC patients were shown to respond with lower concentrations of histamine.

Measurement of specific IgE in tears

When an IgE-mediated conjunctival reaction is suspected in the presence of negative systemic tests, tear levels of specific IgE can provide important information. Levels of specific IgE are undetectable in tears of non-allergic subjects. For each assay, at least 50 μL of tears are required, thus it is not always possible to obtain a sufficient quantity of sample. Considering the greater sensitivity of new in vitro diagnostic assay techniques not yet applicable to the tear sample, it is still recommended to perform serum-specific IgE and reserve tear assays for select cases. The assay is identical to that used for serum IgE measurement, even if there are no standardized reference parameters for the eye. The difficulty of tear collection, the potential to induce reflex, and therefore abnormally dilute tears, and all the quantitative limits of sample have led to a preferential use of specific provocation tests in that they better define the level of clinical response of the conjunctiva.

Measurement of total IgE in tears

Normal values of IgE in tears are normally very low, less than 2.5 kUI/L (3 ng/mL), due to the blood-tear barrier. Detectable tear IgE levels indicate local production of antibodies and a diagnosis of allergic conjunctivitis. This test has recently become available for office testing after the commercialization of a simple and rapid diagnostic test for the semiquantitative determination of total IgE in tears – the Lacrytest (Adiatec). The test utilizes paper strips that are applied directly to the lower fornix of the conjunctiva in a manner similar to the Schirmer's test. Inside the strip are anti-IgE antibodies embedded with a colorimetric system, a semiquantitative total IgE result is obtained in a matter of minutes by reading colour intensity.

Conjunctival cytodiagnosis

Evaluation of the number and percentage of leukocytes on the ocular surface in the active phase of conjunctival inflammation can be essential to the decision of how to proceed with further diagnostic tests. The presence of even one eosinophil is highly indicative of an allergic pathology, whereas their absence does not exclude an allergic diagnosis. The presence of mast cells, especially degranulated is also helpful (Table 11.3).

Tear cytology
Tear cytology is rapid and easy to perform: a few microlitres of tears collected from the external canthus with a glass capillary are immediately placed on a precoloured slide.

Conjunctival scrapings
Conjunctival scrapings, performed with a spatula, allow for the collection of more cells than with tear cytology. Samples are placed only on a glass slide, fixed and stained with rapid dyes. This method is also indicated for the differentiation of intracytoplasmic inclusion bodies when there is a suspicion of *Chlamydia*, or in combination with immunofluorescence when looking for viruses.

Table 11.3 Cytological findings in conjunctivitis

Findings	Associated findings
Neutrophils	Bacterial, chemical
Lymphocytes	Viral, allergic, toxic (medicamentosa)
Eosinophils	Allergic, parasitic
Mast cells especially degranulated	Allergic
Mixed neutrophils, lymphocytes, plasma cells, and multinucleated epithelial cells, plus intracytoplasmic inclusion bodies within epithelial cells	Chlamydial

Impression cytology
Impression cytology using nitrocellulose membranes is mostly used for tear film pathology, as it allows for non-traumatic means to evaluate the morphology of the superficial conjunctival epithelium by either light or electron microscopy. It can be performed without topical anaesthetic.

Conjunctival biopsy
Conjunctival biopsy is required for histological and immunohistochemical analyses when a neoplastic pathology is suspected, or for the diagnosis of autoimmune diseases such as pemphigoid.

Brush cytology
Brush cytology is a new investigational technique in contrast to impression cytology, employs a special disposable nylon brush. Brush cytology allows the recovery of a higher number of cells with little trauma to the conjunctival epithelium. The conjunctiva is scraped by several gentle rotations of the brush under direct slit-lamp observation. Collected material is smeared on a slide, fixed, stained, and cover slipped. The specimen is examined by light microscopy. This technique can also be used for flow cytometry to phenotype tear cells. Brush cytology is gaining popularity over impression cytology because it is more efficient at removing surface cells, and is easier and less expensive to perform.

Management

Introduction and goals of management

Allergic conjunctivitis disorders vary considerably in terms of severity and prognosis. Most of the disorders

Table 11.4 Summary of therapy for allergic conjunctivitis

Non-drug	Non-specific drug	Specific drug	Surgical
Allergen avoidance	Lubricants	Antihistamines	Plaque removal
Cold compress	Mucolytics	Vasoconstrictors	Lamellar keratoplasty
Desensitization	Antibiotics	Mast cell inhibitors	Penetrating keratoplasty
	Rx eczema	Ciclosporin	Excimer laser
	Rx lid margins	Non-steroidal anti-inflammatories	Tissue glue lenses
		Steroids	Therapeutic contact

cannot be cured by therapy, but all can be considerably relieved symptomatically with appropriate management, although complete elimination of symptoms may not be safely achievable. The exception to this is GPC, where the disease is usually rapidly reversible if the cause is eliminated; however, most patients wish to continue use of their contact lens or prosthesis, so that elimination of the cause can be impractical or unappealing. In SAC and PAC, symptoms range from mild to severe but there is no risk of damage to the sight or to the anatomical integrity of the ocular surface; a reduction in severity or resolution can also be expected with time in many patients over the years. Therapy therefore aims to reduce symptoms but to avoid drugs such as steroids, which have sight-threatening side effects. In VKC, symptoms are often severe and episodes of high disease activity can cause serious damage to the cornea with a risk of permanent visual reduction, but a spontaneous resolution is probable by puberty or adulthood. The aim in VKC is to get the child through the active disease years, gaining sufficient control over the disease to prevent long-term ocular sequelae, and to allow a good quality of life and regular school attendance without creating iatrogenic problems that may persist once the disease has resolved. This often involves periodic aggressive therapy during disease exacerbations and a rapid reduction of therapy in between. In AKC, however, the disease is often lifelong and slowly progressive with a very high risk of sight damage and compromise to the integrity of the ocular surface. Early recognition of the condition is crucial with management by an experienced specialist and utilization of all other therapies available to reduce dependence on high doses of steroid, and to try and minimize structural damage to the lids, cornea, and conjunctiva.

Patient education

The nature of allergic conjunctivitis and, in particular, the ability to treat but not to cure the disease should be explained to the patient. The likely time course of the condition should also be outlined, as above. Realistic treatment possibilities and aims should be agreed upon early and this depends upon the balance of the risks of therapy with the risks of the disease (Table 11.4); the inadvisability of heavy steroid treatment in milder conditions or during periods of lesser disease activity should be emphasized, even if this means having to accept incomplete symptom resolution at times.

Making information pamphlets and contact addresses available to allergy groups may be helpful.

Management plan

Allergen avoidance

Where an allergen can be identified, reducing exposure often decreases symptoms. In the case of pollen sensitivity, grassy fields, trees, and flowers are to be avoided, car and bedroom windows must remain shut during the pollen season, and patients should ideally attempt to remain indoors on high-pollen-count days. A reduction in exposure to house dust mite may be achieved by:

- zealous household cleaning (regular dusting, use of a special vacuum cleaner on mattresses, carpets, and curtains)
- removal of bedroom carpet and curtains
- laundering bed linen above 60°C
- the use of mite-impermeable mattress and pillow covers
- killing mites with acaricides.

In mould sensitivity, dehumidifying devices may be used and in dander sensitivity elimination of a pet helps. For any allergen, the employment of high-efficiency filters may be useful and, in more serious cases, moving to a new location or even admission to hospital may be necessary to reduce the allergen load.

Immunotherapy, via parenteral and oral routes, has been shown to be effective in SAC and PAC. Its use has been confined to severe cases because of the potential risk and the prolonged duration of treatment. Immunotherapy has not been shown to be effective in the other ocular allergies in which a specific causative allergen is difficult to identify.

In GPC, it may be possible to remove the allergen completely, for example by removal of an exposed suture or by ceasing to wear contact lenses. However, many patients are contact lens or ocular prosthesis wearers who wish to continue use of their device. In this case, a reduction in the wearing time, either temporarily or permanently, is often advisable and provision of a new (non-deposited) lens or device is helpful. The surface quality and edge profile of the lens are optimized, including elimination of any irregularities or scratches, and the fit and lens shape may be changed if necessary, as may the lens material (e.g. from soft to rigid). Lens hygiene must be regular and thorough, with avoidance of preserved solutions where possible and frequent enzymatic protein removal. The use of disposable lenses is helpful in the management of GPC.

Non-specific medical therapy

Cold compresses may be all that is required in mild SAC and PAC and may reduce the need for pharmacotherapy. The use of topical normal saline or lubricants (artificial tears) will reduce symptoms and may help dilute or flush away allergen and inflammatory mediators. They should be used in AKC if there is dry eye. Additional relief is provided by mucolytic drops, which dissolve the abnormal mucus (e.g. acetyl cysteine 5, 10, or 20%) and may speed the resolution of early corneal plaque. Whenever there is a serious breach of the corneal epithelium (macroerosion or plaque), the use of topical antibiotics should be considered.

In AKC, facial and lid eczema are treated – preferably in conjunction with a dermatologist – with emollients, topical steroids, and occasionally systemic therapy. It is important to control the lid margin disease with lid margin hygiene (using cotton buds soaked in weak sodium bicarbonate or baby shampoo solution), application of topical antibiotic (and occasionally steroid) ointment, and systemic antibiotic therapy with a long-term low-dose regimen (e.g. doxycycline 100 mg daily for 3–6 months).

Topical antihistamines

These are commonly prescribed in combination with a sympathomimetic vasoconstrictor (e.g. antazoline–naphazoline) for SAC and PAC, the combination being more effective than either component used alone. They have a rapid onset of action but no preventive effect and prolonged use of these preparations may cause contact blepharoconjunctivitis.

Levocabastine, azelastine, and emedastine are some of the selective and potent topical H_1-receptor antagonists available in eye drop formulations. They have proved effective in decreasing the symptoms and signs of SAC and PAC and have a minor role as adjunctive therapy in the management of the chronic ocular allergic disorders.

Oral antihistamines

These drugs, particularly those with less sedative and anticholinergic side effects (e.g. cetirizine, fexofenadine), are widely used in SAC and PAC. They are occasionally also used in AKC and VKC as an adjunct to break the itch–scratch cycle, particularly at night. They have the added advantage of controlling associated non-ocular atopic manifestations such as rhinitis, but unwanted effects such as drying of the mucous membranes may be uncomfortable.

Topical mast cell inhibitors

These compounds are used topically to reduce mast cell degranulation and also sensory activation, which may be helpful in reducing itch. These drugs are used extensively in all forms of allergic conjunctivitis, are generally well tolerated and have no serious ocular side effects. They offer a preventive action and are most effective if used before the onset of symptoms where possible (e.g. at the beginning of the pollen season), or early in the disease process. As their onset of action is relatively slow (5–7 days) and stinging upon instillation can occur particularly in the presence of active inflammation, patients should be warned that their eyes may initially feel worse. In VKC and AKC, mast cell inhibitors act as steroid-sparing agents.

Cromolyn sodium/chlorphen(ir)amine is the longest established of these drugs and both 2% (UK) and 4% (USA) drops are available for use up to four times daily. Nedocromil sodium is a newer, higher-potency mast cell stabilizer that compares favourably with cromolyn and can be used twice daily in SAC and PAC. Lodoxamide tromethamine is another more recently introduced mast cell stabilizer that may evoke less stinging than other preparations. Both nedocromil and lodoxamide are said to have a more rapid onset of action than cromolyn.

Olopatadine and ketotifen are agents that combine high-potency anti-H_1 receptor effect with inhibition of mast cell degranulation and, particularly for ketotifen, of eosinophil functions. They are useful in SAC and PAC and may also have a role in the treatment of VKC and AKC. They may avoid the initial worsening of symptoms sometimes seen with the use of conventional mast cell inhibitors.

Steroids

Topical steroids are very powerful in controlling allergic conjunctivitis, but have potentially sight-threatening side effects, including glaucoma, cataract, and the potentiation of herpetic, bacterial, and fungal corneal infections. Therefore steroids are generally contraindicated in SAC and PAC, and in GPC (except with an ocular prosthesis where there is no visual potential) as the severity of the side effects outweighs that of the condition. In AKC and VKC, steroids are frequently required, but should be used in as low a concentration and for as short a time as possible to minimize side effects. The use of surface-acting steroids (fluorometholone, rimexolone) may also reduce adverse effects. They are most helpful in periods of increased disease activity or corneal involvement. Other treatment, mast cell inhibitors in particular, should be continued during steroid use. Supratarsal injection of short- or long-acting steroids (e.g. triamcinolone) is occasionally used in refractory cases. In a small number of cases systemic steroids are required in AKC and VKC. As well as considering the serious side effects, the clinician should remember that the reduction in and cessation of use of systemic steroids after the ocular disease has been suppressed can create new difficulties in the management of asthma and eczema by causing rebound activation.

Ciclosporin

Ciclosporin is a potent immunosuppressive agent that acts by inhibiting CD4+ T-cell proliferation and IL-2 production. Topical preparations of 2% ciclosporin have been shown to provide a marked reduction in the symptoms and signs of VKC and AKC, and ciclosporin is particularly helpful as a steroid-sparing agent. An instilled ciclosporin eye drop often causes intense stinging. Also, because of its lipophilic nature, ciclosporin has to be dissolved in oil (e.g. maize) to achieve the therapeutic concentration of 2%, and the oily drops can cause subjective visual blurring for up to 3 hours after instillation. This means that ciclosporin drops, although highly effective, can be very difficult for patients to tolerate. Topical ciclosporin does not produce the serious ocular side effects seen with steroids, but may cause a reversible punctate corneal epitheliopathy and mild lid-skin maceration. Systemic absorption occurs, but serum levels are substantially lower than those required for therapeutic action or systemic side effects, which have not been reported even in prolonged use.

The role for a new, lower concentration (0.05%) but better tolerated ciclosporin ophthalmic emulsion licensed for use in dry eye remains to be established, but early research suggests it may have a beneficial effect in steroid-resistant AKC. The unlicensed use of a veterinary ophthalmic ointment containing 0.2% ciclosporin has, however, proved beneficial and is well tolerated for many patients with VKC and AKC.

Non-steroidal anti-inflammatory agents

Topical non-steroidal anti-inflammatory drugs (NSAIDs) appear to have some beneficial effect in allergic conjunctivitis. Reports of a reduction in symptoms and signs have been published for agents such as suprofen and ketorolac tromethamine in VKC, GPC and SAC. Oral aspirin, as an adjunct to topical therapy, may speed resolution of allergic keratopathy. Topical NSAIDs are not as potent as steroids but have the advantage of a good ocular safety profile and are probably most helpful in treating non-sight-threatening allergic conjunctivitis where antihistamines and mast cell inhibitors are not sufficiently effective.

Surgery

Surgery is usually limited to the treatment of sight-reducing corneal disease in AKC and VKC. For corneal plaque, medical therapy is used to minimize inflammation rapidly and surgical or laser removal of the plaque allows early re-epithelialization. Procedures including lamellar or penetrating keratoplasty, cyanoacrylate glue application or therapeutic contact lens use may be indicated if corneal scarring is reducing visual acuity or if there is extensive thinning or perforation of the cornea; penetrating keratoplasty carries a higher risk of complications in these patients, partly because of the presence of atopy and partly resulting from the compromised ocular environment.

Conjunctival surgical procedures that attempt to influence active inflammation, such as excision of papillae, mucous membrane, or whole tarsus, may provide short-term relief but have long-term adverse effects and are therefore best avoided.

New approaches to therapy

Potential therapeutic agents include leukotriene antagonists, anti-IgE antibodies and platelet-activating factor (PAF) antagonists, antieosinophil granule protein compounds, adhesion molecule antagonists, and drugs that influence cytokine production and action (such as anti-IL-4, -5, -13 or -RANTES monoclonal antibodies) – but none have yet translated to topical ocular preparations of use.

Assessment of effectiveness of disease control

The assessment of disease control involves the severity of symptomatology, the degree of active conjunctival inflammation, and for AKC and VKC the state of the cornea. Frequency of follow-up of patients is determined by these, and can vary considerably over time and during the year. Patients with severe disease known to flare up during the spring and summer months should be seen more often at these times, and the therapy may be increased in anticipation just before the pollen season begins. Those with incipient or active corneal disease may need to be seen weekly or even daily if very severe, especially in young children with VKC.

Conclusions

The vast majority of those suffering from allergic ocular inflammation have a highly symptomatic but not dangerous disorder that can be safely relieved by simple topical medications and allergen control measures and can be managed by the non-specialist. A small proportion of patients, those with severe VKC and AKC, require specialist management and the use of drugs or interventions that can cause ocular damage. In these cases, appropriate therapy by an experienced clinician can minimize the risks of permanent iatrogenic or pathological sight-reducing ocular changes.

Summary of important messages

- Allergic conjunctivitis is frequently associated with systemic allergic diseases
- The cornea may be involved in VKC and AKC, but not in seasonal and perennial allergic conjunctivitis or GPC, and corneal involvement can lead to permanent visual reduction
- Complex subtle pathogenetic differences seem to underlie the different clinical subtypes of allergic conjunctivitis
- The diagnosis of allergic conjunctivitis is mainly clinical, but there are numerous laboratory investigations which may contribute
- Use of topical steroids increases risk of infection, cataract, and glaucoma
- It is crucial to use all modalities of therapy available to minimize the use of steroids

Further reading

Bielory, L. Ocular allergy overview. Immunol Allergy Clin North Am 2008; 28:1–23.

Bonini S, Lambiase A, Sgrulletta R, et al. Allergic chronic inflammation of the ocular surface in vernal keratoconjnctivitis. Curr Opin Allergy Clin Immunol 2003; 3:381–387.

Calder V, Hingorani M, Lightman S. Allergic disorders of the eye: immunopathogenesis. In: Rich RR, Fleischer TA, Shearer WT, et al., eds. Clinical immunology: principles and practice, 3rd edn. London: Elsevier; 2008:Ch 47.

Hingorani M, Calder V, Buckley RJ, et al. The immunomodulatory effect of topical cyclosporin A in atopic keratoconjunctivitis. Invest Ophthalmol Vis Sci 1999; 40:392–399.

Lemp MA, Bielory L. Contact lenses and associated anterior segment disorders: dry eye disease, blepharitis, and allergy. Immunol Allergy Clin North Am 2008; 28:105–117.

Mantelli F, Lambiase A, Bonini S. A simple and rapid diagnostic algorithm for the detection of ocular allergic disease. Curr Opin Allergy Clin Immunol 2009; 9:471–476.

Strauss EC, Foster CS. Atopic ocular disease. Ophthalmol Clin North Am 2002; 15:1–5.

Tabbara KF. Immunopathogenesis of chronic allergic conjunctivitis. Int Ophthalmol Clin 2003; 43:1–7.

12

Urticaria and angioedema without wheals

Marcus Maurer, Clive EH Grattan and Bruce L Zuraw

Urticaria

Introduction

There has been renewed interest in the aetiology, definition, epidemiology, clinical features, health-related quality of life, pharmacoeconomics, pathogenesis, and management of urticaria. Urticaria may affect up to 20% of us over our lifetimes in one form or another. A problem in the past has been the lack of consistency of definition, which in turn has resulted in difficulties with comparing results of studies from different centres and targeting management to specific clinical needs. The advent of new drugs with impressive results in the most severe and difficult patterns of urticaria and angioedema has engaged physicians, patients, and the pharmaceutical industry in looking at new ways of researching and treating this heterogeneous condition.

The fundamental pathological event in urticaria is transient vasopermeability of the cutaneous and submucosal microvasculature resulting in short-lived swellings. The swellings may be superficial, when they are known descriptively as wheals (syn. hives), or deep in the dermis and subcutis, when they are known as angioedema. They may also be somewhere in between if they show properties of both, such as the deep, red swellings that are often seen in delayed pressure urticaria. However, the clinical presentation does not necessarily define the underlying pathogenesis. It is often said that the mast cell is the key effector cell in urticaria and that histamine is the major mediator of itch and wheals. Histamine also causes angioedema, although it should be noted that the clinical pattern of angioedema without wheals may be mediated by bradykinin without mast cell degranulation.

Other illness may also present with urticarial skin reactions as one manifestation of a more generalized systemic disease, such as urticarial vasculitis due to immune complex formation and some hereditary autoinflammatory syndromes mediated by interleukin-1β rather than histamine release or bradykinin formation.

Recent guidelines on urticaria have highlighted the preferred use of 'urticaria' to describe a disease characterized by wheals, angioedema or both, rather than an eruption of wheals. The clinical pattern of angioedema without wheals is important for clinicians since it includes patients with mast-cell-dependent histaminergic angioedema and bradykinin-mediated mast cell-independent angioedema, which has a different clinical course and management. Non-mast-cell-mediated angioedema is discussed in the second part of this chapter.

Because there are many types and subtypes of urticaria, the main elements of diagnosis have been included within the sections on the individual types rather than as a separate section.

Pathophysiology and disease mechanisms of mast-cell-mediated urticaria

Urticaria symptoms are brought about by activation of cutaneous mast cells. Mast cells are resident skin cells with characteristic metachromatic cytoplasmic granules that contain preformed mediators including histamine and proteases. In the skin, mast cells are colocalized with sensory nerves and small blood vessels. Their main physiological role is to provide a first line of defence against pathogens and other environmental threats. Mast cell activation and the subsequent release of preformed and de novo synthesized mediators induce sensory nerve stimulation (pruritus, burning sensation, pain), vasodilatation (erythema), increased plasma extravasation (oedema) and the recruitment of neutrophils, and other immune cells (infiltrates). Mast cell activation is a complex process that can be initiated by a large array of signals, many of which act via specific mast cell surface receptors.

Clinical presentation

Wheals are short-lived superficial skin swellings of variable size that are associated with itching or burning (Fig. 12.1). They are associated with flare reactions (reflex erythema) of the surrounding skin. They resolve spontaneously, usually within several hours. Angioedema swellings are sudden, deeper, pronounced, and sometimes painful swellings of the lower dermis and subcutis of longer duration and slower resolution (usually within several days) (see Fig. 12.1). They frequently affect mucous membranes. Urticaria symptoms can develop spontaneously, or they can be induced by a specific trigger or eliciting factor, depending on the type of urticaria. In chronic spontaneous urticaria (see Table 12.1), wheals develop most often during the evening hours and on the arms and legs, whereas angioedema is most commonly located in the head region (e.g. eyelids, lips, tongue) as well as the hands and feet. In contrast, lesion development in inducible urticaria occurs at those skin sites exposed to the eliciting trigger. The appearance of urticaria skin lesions in all types of urticaria can be accompanied or preceded by extracutaneous symptoms such as feverishness, headaches, joint pain, or gastrointestinal symptoms including indigestion and diarrhoea.

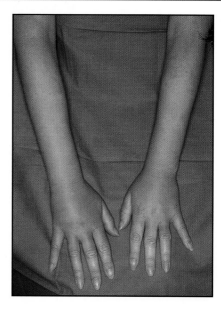

Fig. 12.1 Urticarial wheals of chronic spontaneous urticaria by the elbows occurring simultaneously with angioedema of the hands.

Disease activity in spontaneous urticaria is measured by using the urticaria activity score, which combines the daily score values for numbers of wheals and intensity of pruritus. In chronic spontaneous urticaria disease activity can also be measured by the disease-specific quality of life (QoL) instrument CU-Q$_2$oL and other QoL questionnaires. Disease activity in inducible urticarias is highly dependent on the presence of and exposure to the eliciting stimulus. In some inducible urticarias such as cold contact urticaria and solar urticaria, disease activity can be assessed by measuring exposure time or trigger thresholds.

Classification

Urticarias are classified by their duration as acute (<6 weeks) or chronic (≥6 weeks) and by their clinical presentation as spontaneous or inducible (Table 12.1). In spontaneous urticaria (also sometimes called ordinary urticaria), wheals/angioedema arise spontaneously – that is, they can usually not be induced by a specific trigger or eliciting factor. Inducible urticarias, in contrast, are characterized by wheals/angioedema that develop in response to specific triggers, which can be exogenous physical triggers (physical urticarias) or other stimuli (other types of urticaria). Triggers of physical urticaria include skin contact with cold and heat, electromagnetic radiation (solar radiation), and mechanical triggers (friction, pressure, vibration). Triggers of symptoms in the other types of inducible urticaria are contact with urticariogenic substances (contact urticaria), water (aquagenic urticaria), physical exercise (exercise-induced urticaria), and increased body core temperature (cholinergic urticaria).

Differential diagnoses of mast-cell-mediated urticaria include cutaneous mastocytosis (urticaria pigmentosa), urticarial vasculitis, and non-histaminergic angioedema (e.g. hereditary or acquired C1 esterase inhibitor deficiency) (Box 12.1). Wheals and angioedema may also be features of several syndromes (Box 12.2).

Forms of urticaria

Spontaneous urticaria

Most cases of acute spontaneous urticaria resolve within several days or weeks, and the risk for acute urticaria

Table 12.1 Classification of urticaria

Type	Classification
Spontaneous urticarias	
	Acute spontaneous urticaria
	Chronic spontaneous urticaria
Inducible urticarias	
Physical urticarias	Symptomatic dermographism
	Delayed pressure urticaria
	Vibratory urticaria
	Cold contact urticaria
	Heat contact urticaria
	Solar urticaria
Other forms of urticaria	Cholinergic urticaria
	Exercise-induced urticaria
	Contact urticaria
	Aquagenic urticaria

Urticaria of all types can present with an immediate wheal and flare and/or angioedema, except for delayed pressure urticaria, which is characterized by deep swellings arising with a ½ – 12 h latency and symptomatic dermographism, which does not present with angioedema. (Adapted from Zuberbier T, Asero R, Bindslev-Jensen C, et al. EAACI/GA²LEN/EDF/WAO Guideline: Definition, classification and diagnosis of urticaria. Allergy 2009; 64:1417–1426.)

Box 12.1 Differential diagnoses of urticaria

- Cutaneous mastocytosis (urticaria pigmentosa)
- Urticarial vasculitis
- Non-histaminergic angioedema (e.g. HAE)

Box 12.2 Syndromes that include wheals/angioedema

- Cryopyrin-associated periodic syndrome (CAPS), including Muckle–Wells syndrome
- Schnitzler's syndrome
- Gleich's syndrome
- Well's syndrome

patients of developing chronic disease is considered to be low. The most common causes of acute spontaneous urticaria are viral infections of the upper airways and drugs, especially non-steroidal anti-inflammatories.

The mean duration of chronic spontaneous urticaria is 4 years, with 50% of patients showing spontaneous remission within the first 10 years of disease in a recent series. Most chronic spontaneous urticaria patients exhibit both wheals and angioedema, whereas about 1 in 3 patients show only wheals and 1 in 10 patients develop only angioedema. In 10% of chronic spontaneous urticaria patients, symptoms occur every day (or almost every day). In the majority of cases, however, the disease is characterized by periods of time in which no symptoms occur for several days to several months. In some classifications, this intermittent course is called 'episodic' or 'recurrent' urticaria.

Chronic spontaneous urticaria can result from many different causes, the most common ones being autoreactivity, infection, and intolerance to food components. Autoreactivity (i.e. the presence of circulating mast-cell-activating factors), which is readily detectable by the autologous serum skin test (ASST), is found in about 40% of patients. Some of these patients exhibit autoantibodies to IgE or the high-affinity IgE receptor.

Infections that can cause chronic spontaneous urticaria include viral infections (e.g. hepatitis A and B), bacterial infections of the nasopharynx or gastrointestinal tract (e.g. *Helicobacter pylori*), and parasitic infections (e.g. *Blastocystis hominis*, *Strongyloides*). Generally, chronic spontaneous urticaria patients do not exhibit an increased prevalence of infections and they should be held responsible only in patients who show remission of their urticaria upon successful eradication of the infectious pathogen. The most common infections known to cause chronic spontaneous urticaria are *H. pylori* gastritis, infections of the upper respiratory tract (e.g. by group A streptococci), and dental infections.

Chronic spontaneous urticaria may be aggravated or caused by intolerance – that is, non-allergic, dose-dependent and delayed (4–12 h) onset hypersensitivity – to food components such as colourants, preservatives, taste intensifiers, and naturally occurring substances (e.g. aromatic compounds, biogenic amines, and natural salicylates). Chronic spontaneous urticaria related to intolerance is diagnosed in patients who show decreased disease activity following a 3–4-week diet low in pseudoallergens or increased disease activity following challenge tests with pseudoallergens. Responder rates vary and range from 30% to 90% depending on the study following elimination, and from 20% to 60% following challenge testing with pseudoallergen-rich foods.

Other less frequent causes of chronic spontaneous urticaria include type I allergies (less than 1%) and non-infectious chronic inflammatory processes such as gastritis, reflux oesophagitis, inflammation of the bile duct or bile gland, and autoimmune disorders, for example systemic lupus erythematosus (SLE).

Independent of the underlying cause, chronic spontaneous urticaria symptoms may be induced or worsened by non-specific triggers. For example, approximately 50% of all chronic spontaneous urticaria patients report that symptoms are increased in frequency or intensity after physical exertion or stressful events. Strategies aimed at avoiding or reducing relevant non-specific triggers have been demonstrated to result in less disease activity and a better quality of life.

In all patients with chronic spontaneous urticaria, a thorough history (Box 12.3) should be obtained to confirm the diagnosis, to identify the relevance of common eliciting factors, and to assess the impact of disease. The daily documentation of symptoms by the patient (diary or calendar) can help to determine disease activity and response to therapy. Major internal conditions should be excluded by a physical examination and basic blood work-up. Provocation tests for skin responses to physical triggers and exercise are useful to verify or rule out inducible urticaria when suggested by the history. Chronic spontaneous urticaria patients who exhibit frequently recurring symptoms for more than 1 year and high disease activity should be checked for underlying causes (Table 12.2) – especially autoreactivity with the autologous serum skin test (ASST), infections (e.g. tests for *H. pylori* and ENT/dental infections), and intolerance to dietary pseudoallergens (elimination diet, oral provocation tests).

Inducible urticaria

In contrast to spontaneous urticaria, symptoms in all inducible urticarias occur only in response to specific triggers and the underlying causes of inducible urticarias are largely unknown. Therefore, the diagnostic work-up in inducible urticaria patients is aimed at the identification of the relevant trigger, by means of a suggestive medical history and positive provocation testing. Since patients may present with more than one inducible urticaria, all triggers that appear to be relevant from the medical history should be tested. Inducible and spontaneous urticaria may occur in the same patient. Patients exhibit individual trigger thresholds, and threshold testing in most inducible urticarias allows for an estimation of the activity of the disease at that time point. Since provocation tests in patients with a severe inducible urticaria may result in systemic symptoms including shock, care must be taken and emergency treatment should be available. Inducible urticarias frequently have important occupational and employment implications.

Physical urticaria

Physical urticaria is a heterogeneous group of inducible conditions in which symptoms are induced by exogenous physical triggers acting on the skin such as mechanical stimuli (symptomatic dermographism/urticaria factitia, delayed pressure urticaria, vibratory urticaria/angioedema), cold and heat (cold contact urticaria, heat contact urticaria), and electromagnetic radiation (solar urticaria).

Symptomatic dermographism (syn. urticaria factitia, dermographic urticaria) is the most common subtype of physical urticaria. It is characterized by rapidly occurring pruritic whealing after moderate scratching, stroking, or rubbing of the skin (Fig. 12.2). Provocation testing should be performed by stroking the skin of the upper back or volar forearm lightly with a smooth blunt object (e.g. the tip of a closed ballpoint pen or a wooden spatula) or a calibrated dermographometer, where one is available. The test response should be read 10 minutes after testing

---

Box 12.3 Relevant questions to ask patients with chronic spontaneous urticaria

1. When did your urticaria first present? (Life events?)
2. How often do you have wheals and how long do they last?
3. What time of day are the wheals and itchiness worst?
4. What is the usual shape and size of wheals and what skin areas are affected?
5. Do you get angioedema? How often? Where? For how long?
6. What problems do the wheals/angioedema cause? (e.g. itch/pain/burning?)
7. Does or did anyone in your family also suffer from urticaria (or allergies)?
8. Do you have allergies/other diseases? What do you think is the cause?
9. Can you induce the onset of wheals/angioedema (e.g. by rubbing the skin)?
10. What drugs do you use (e.g. analgesics or anti-inflammatories, hormones, laxatives, alternative medicines)?
11. Do you see a relationship between the onset of wheals or angioedema and the food you eat?
12. Do you smoke/drink alcohol? Do you see a relationship with urticaria?
13. What type of work do you do? Do you see a relationship with urticaria?
14. What do you do for fun? Do you see a relationship with urticaria?
15. Does your urticaria change on the weekend/during holidays or vacation?
16. Do you have surgical implants?
17. Do you react normally to insect stings/bites (e.g. bees, yellow jackets)?
18. What therapies have you tried and what were the results?
19. Does stress trigger wheals?
20. Is your quality of life affected by the urticaria? How?
21. In female patients: do you see a relationship with your menstrual cycle?

Table 12.2 Basic and advanced diagnostics in chronic spontaneous urticaria

Step	Diagnostic measure	Goal
Basic	• History • Calendar/diary • Physical examination and differential blood count, ESR/CRP • Discontinue suspected drugs • Provocation tests (e.g. dermographism, pressure, cold, UV, heat, exercise)	• Confirm diagnosis, assess QoL • Assess activity and response to therapy • Exclude major internal condition • Rule out drug intolerance • Verify/rule out inducible urticarias (e.g. physical urticaria)
Advanced	• Test for autoreactivity (e.g. autologous serum skin test, thyroid: hormones and autoantibodies, ANAs, MCAAs) • Test for infectious diseases (e.g. stool for *H. pylori* and parasites, ENT and dental examination) • Test for intolerance to food (e.g. elimination diet for pseudoallergens, provocation with pseudoallergens) • Test for chronic inflammatory conditions, type I allergy (e.g. skin prick test, total, and specific IgE)	• Verify/rule out chronic spontaneous urticaria due to autoreactivity • Verify/rule out chronic spontaneous urticaria due to infection • Verify/rule out chronic spontaneous urticaria due to intolerance • Verify/rule out chronic spontaneous urticaria due to other causes

ENT, ear, nose, and throat; ESR, erythrocyte sedimentation rate; CRP, c-reactive protein; ANA, antinuclear antibodies; MCAAs, mast-cell-activating antibodies; UV, ultraviolet; QoL, quality of life.

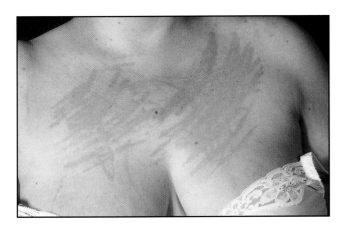

Fig. 12.2 Linear wheals of symptomatic dermographism (urticaria factitia) induced by scratching.

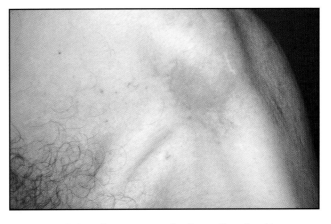

Fig. 12.3 Delayed pressure urticaria on the shoulder induced by carrying a heavy pipe 6 hours earlier.

and is considered positive in patients who show a wheal response and report pruritus at the site of provocation.

Delayed pressure urticaria is defined by skin-swelling responses after sustained perpendicular pressure (Fig. 12.3). Responses usually occur 6–8 hours (between 30 minutes and 12 hours) after exposure and may last up to 3 days. The reaction is not usually itchy, but may be associated with a burning/painful sensation. Testing for delayed pressure urticaria can be done by suspending weights over the shoulder (7 kg on a 3 cm shoulder strap), or by applying weighted rods supported in a frame to the patient's back, thighs, or forearm, and by using a dermographometer. Test responses should be assessed after 6 hours and are considered positive if the site of provocation shows a deep-red palpable swelling.

Vibratory urticaria, a rare subtype of physical urticaria, is defined by the rapid onset of itching and swelling within minutes at skin sites exposed to vibration. For diagnostic purposes, the patient's forearm is placed on a laboratory vortex mixer and the response is assessed for swelling 10 minutes after testing.

Cold contact urticaria (syn. acquired cold urticaria) is characterized by the rapid appearance of whealing or angioedema after contact cooling of the skin. This reaction will in most cases be itchy and/or associated with a burning sensation. Cold provocation is done on the volar forearm using the traditional ice cube test or by testing with cool packs, cold-water baths, or TempTest®. If an ice cube is used for testing, it should be melting and contained in a see-through plastic bag to avoid cold damage of the skin. The use of cool packs and localized immersion in cold water requires special care, because these methods carry the risk of inducing systemic reactions. A palpable and clearly visible wheal and flare-type skin reaction at 10 minutes after the end of provocation testing is indicative of a positive response.

Heat contact urticaria is a rare condition defined by the quick appearance of whealing responses, which in most cases are itchy and/or associated with a burning sensation, after contact heating of the skin within minutes of exposure. Provocation tests are done using metal/glass cylinders filled with hot water, localized hot water exposure, or TempTest®, usually at temperatures of up to 45°C. The test should be considered positive if the test site shows a palpable and clearly visible wheal and flare-type skin reaction 10 minutes after provocation.

Solar urticaria is defined by the appearance of a whealing response, which in most cases is itchy and/or associated with a burning sensation, within minutes of exposure to sunlight. Provocation testing should be done on the buttocks separately in the UV-A, UV-B and visible light range. Positive provocation leads to a rapid palpable and clearly visible wheal and flare-type skin response at the site of exposure within 10 minutes.

Other forms of inducible urticaria

This group of urticarias that are not characterized by exogenous physical triggers of skin lesions comprises cholinergic urticaria, exercise-induced urticaria, aquagenic urticaria, and contact urticaria (see Table 12.1).

Cholinergic urticaria is defined by itching and whealing induced by an increase in the body core temperature – for example, because of exercising or passive heating (sauna, warm bath, stress, or spicy foods). It typically presents on the trunk and limbs with small short-lived wheals with a pronounced flare reaction, and must be distinguished from exercise-induced urticaria/anaphylaxis. The latter is induced by exercise but not passive warming. In exercise-induced urticaria/anaphylaxis, symptoms are also induced by physical exercise, but not passive heating, and it is more often associated with systemic symptoms than cholinergic urticaria. Food- or drug-dependent exercise-induced anaphylaxis should be considered in the differential diagnosis. Aquagenic urticaria and contact urticaria symptoms are brought about by skin contact with water and other urticariagenic substances, respectively.

Management of urticaria

Management is primarily directed towards symptom control because an avoidable or treatable cause of urticaria is usually not found, in the expectation of eventual natural resolution without long-term damage. Disease-modifying drugs are increasingly being used, which may lead to a shorter duration of disease, although the evidence for this is lacking. An understanding of the mediators involved in the different clinical patterns of urticaria should logically help with the choice of treatment.

Removal of the cause

Acute urticaria

Upper respiratory tract viral infections appear to be the commonest cause where one can be identified. There is some evidence that streptococcal and staphylococcal infections may be causative. Immediate hypersensitivity reactions to foods are frequently suspected by patients as a cause of their acute urticaria, but are probably rarely responsible for acute spontaneous urticaria and more relevant in atopic children than in adults. Anisaki infection, or eating infected fish in patients who are already sensitized, may be a cause of acute urticaria in Mediterranean countries. The importance of endoparasitic infection as a cause of acute urticaria in endemic countries is unknown.

Chronic urticaria

The evidence linking chronic bacterial infection as a cause of spontaneous urticaria is based mainly on reports and small series dating from the last century of patients with dental abscesses. Although the strength of evidence is low, it is still good practice to identify and treat chronic abscesses if they can be identified. Of possible greater relevance is *Helicobacter pylori* infection of the stomach. A meta-analysis concluded that more patients with chronic spontaneous urticaria treated successfully for *H. pylori* infection responded than those in whom eradication was unsuccessful. Anecdotal reports of infection causing cold contact urticaria responding to 'curative' antibiotic therapy have not been substantiated by clinical trials. Avoidance of dietary pseudoallergens in chronic spontaneous urticaria will be reviewed in the section below on targeted non-pharmacological interventions. Minimizing exposure to physical triggers of inducible urticarias may reduce or prevent symptoms.

Acute urticaria

The majority of patients can be managed with non-sedating H_1 antihistamines. Oral corticosteroids given for a few days at the onset of the disease can lessen the severity of acute urticaria and reduce its duration. Parenteral adrenaline (epinephrine) may be necessary in addition for patients who also present with symptoms of anaphylaxis.

Chronic urticaria

Non-pharmacological interventions

It is often possible to identify aggravating factors from the history that worsen spontaneous urticaria but do not cause it. These may occur singly or in combination. They include overheating, localized pressure or friction, stress, viral infections, and non-steroidal anti-inflammatory drug intake. Dietary pseudoallergens such as artificial food additives, natural salicylates and amines, alcohol, and spices may also aggravate spontaneous urticaria.

Targeted non-pharmacological interventions include a low-pseudoallergen diet, which is taken for 3 weeks. Foods are re-introduced at intervals of 3 days for responders to identify those foods that were previously making the condition worse. These need to be avoided for at least 6 months after disease remission.

Phototherapy has been used for spontaneous and physical urticarias. A recent open pilot study of narrow-band ultraviolet B phototherapy for patients with symptomatic dermographism not responding to a licensed dose of fexofenadine reduced whealing and pruritus in nearly all patients, but the benefit was lost between 6 and 12 weeks after stopping. Successful desensitization has been described in primary cold contact urticaria and solar urticaria by repeated cold and UV light exposures respectively, but is unrealistic for most patients.

Partial desensitization can be achieved by a few patients with cholinergic urticaria by exercising to the point of bringing out symptoms, but the benefit is short lived.

Pharmacological treatments

Non-sedating H_1 antihistamines are the first-line treatment for all patients with urticaria. They are the only treatment for which there is high-quality evidence when used at licensed doses. There is increasing evidence to support their use at above licensed doses for spontaneous urticaria and cold urticaria. The addition of an H_2 antihistamine may provide additional benefit, although the evidence for this is of low quality. Classical sedating antihistamines are effective but carry important risks of unwanted anticholinergic and sedating side effects. Even though tolerance to sedation may develop with chronic usage, impairment of performance is maintained. Recent consensus guidelines (see Zuberbier et al 2009 in Further reading) recommend against the use of sedating antihistamines as first-line agents for urticaria.

A wide range of unlicensed drugs has been proposed as targeted therapies for chronic urticaria, but with low-quality evidence to support them (Table 12.3). There are,

nevertheless, some agents that are used for specific clinical indications that appear to be selectively helpful and should be considered. More work is needed to identify clinical and biochemical biomarkers that might identify individuals likely to respond.

Oral corticosteroids

The quality of evidence for using oral corticosteroids in urticaria is low. However, clinical experience shows that they are effective and safe in short courses (days) for all patterns of urticaria and may have to be given for longer courses in severe delayed pressure urticaria and urticarial vasculitis if safer treatments have failed. Long-term treatment should be avoided if possible.

Antileukotrienes

The most widely used antileukotriene is montelukast. It is generally taken with a non-sedating antihistamine. It may be more effective than H_1 antihistamines alone for delayed pressure urticaria.

Danazol

This may raise the exercise threshold for patients with cholinergic urticaria, but androgenic side effects are often dose limiting in women.

Dapsone

Use of this drug has been reported for chronic spontaneous urticaria, but anecdotal experience suggests that it may be more targeted usefully for patients with delayed pressure urticaria in aspirin-sensitive patients or urticarial vasculitis. Dapsone hypersensitivity syndrome is a potential concern and patients need to be monitored for anaemia.

Sulfasalazine

This may be very effective for delayed pressure urticaria, but there is a risk of associated spontaneous urticaria being aggravated by its aminosalicylate moiety.

Disease-modifying treatments

Immunomodulatory and immunsuppressive treatments were first trialled after the description of functional histamine-releasing autoantibodies in a subset of patients

Table 12.3 Targeted therapies for mast-cell-mediated urticaria to be taken in conjunction with non-sedating H_1 antihistamines

Generic name	Drug class	Dose	Clinical indication
Prednisolone	Corticosteroid	½ mg/kg/day	Short term for severe urticaria
Montelukast	Antileukotriene	10 mg/day	Delayed pressure urticaria
Danazol	Anabolic steroid	200–400 mg/day	Severe cholinergic urticaria
Dapsone	Sulfone	50–150 mg/day	Aspirin-sensitive delayed pressure urticaria
Sulfasalazine	Aminosalicylate	1–4 g/day	Delayed pressure urticaria

with severe chronic spontaneous urticaria in the 1990s. A small series of patients treated with plasma exchange as a proof of concept treatment supported the use of other immunomodulatory treatments. Intravenous immunoglobulins also appeared to be effective in open studies, but are generally no longer used because of a relative shortage of supply and concerns about the use of pooled plasma products. Ciclosporin has the best evidence base and appears to be effective in about two-thirds of patients, especially those with a positive basophil histamine release assay as a marker of autoimmune urticaria. It is usually given at 4 mg/kg/d at a reducing schedule over 3–4 months. Other immunosuppressive agents include mycophenolate mofetil and methotrexate. Azathioprine, tacrolimus, and cyclophosphamide have also been reported to be beneficial. The advent of biologicals has provided a new and potentially important advance in the management of patients with severe disabling urticaria. Omalizumab (anti-IgE) has been reported to be successful for most patients with chronic spontaneous urticaria and inducible urticarias in four controlled trials and small open series and case reports respectively. Further studies are needed to identify potential responders, dosing regimens and why it works.

Non-mast-cell-mediated angioedema

Angioedema can be regarded as a disease as well as a physical sign when it presents without wheals. It is most commonly recognized on the mouth, eyelids, and genitalia but may occur anywhere on the skin and may also affect the oropharynx and bowel. Angioedema may be hereditary, acquired, or drug induced.

Angioedema is characterized by an asymmetric non-dependent swelling that is generally not pruritic (Fig. 12.4). The pathophysiologies of mast-cell-mediated wheals and angioedema are similar and have already been discussed. This section will address the non-mast-cell-mediated forms of angioedema, specifically hereditary angioedema (HAE), acquired C1 inhibitor deficiency, angiotensin-converting enzyme inhibitor (ACE-I)-associated angioedema, and non-histaminergic idiopathic angioedema. In general, these diseases present as recurrent angioedema in the absence of wheals and are generally thought to represent bradykinin-mediated swelling.

Pathophysiology of non-mast-cell-mediated angioedema

Hereditary angioedema with C1 inhibitor deficiency

HAE results from a functional deficiency of the plasma protein C1 inhibitor, which is the primary inactivator of the contact system, proteases, plasma kallikrein, and Hageman factor (coagulation factor XIIa) as well as the complement proteases C1r and C1s. Two major types of HAE have been described (Table 12.4). Both type I and type II HAE are caused by mutations in the C1 INH gene. The discrepancy between antigenic and functional C1 INH levels in type II HAE results from the secretion of a dysfunctional protein. Over 280 different mutations of the C1 INH gene have been reported in HAE patients (website http://hae.enzim.hu/), and the prevalence of HAE is estimated to be between 1 : 30 000 to 1 : 80 000 in the general population, without evidence of any gender, ethnic, or racial differences. Compelling laboratory and clinical data have now demonstrated that bradykinin generated through activation of the plasma contact system is the primary mediator of swelling in HAE.

Hereditary angioedema with normal C1 inhibitor

An additional form of inherited angioedema has been described in which multiple generations are involved in a pattern consistent with an autosomal dominant inheritance; however, the C1 inhibitor gene and protein are completely normal. This has been called 'type III HAE with normal C1 inhibitor'. The original descriptions of type III HAE with normal C1 inhibitor described families

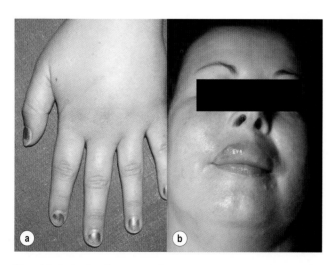

Fig. 12.4 Angioedema (a) of the hand, (b) of the face.

Table 12.4 Types of hereditary angioedema

	C1INH antigenic level	C1INH functional activity	Percent of all HAE
Type I	Low	Low	85
Type II	Normal	Low	15
Type III	Normal	Normal	??

in which all the affected subjects were women. Furthermore, attacks of angioedema were felt to mirror states of high endogenous oestrogen (i.e. pregnancy) or administration of exogenous oestrogen. Subsequently, however, a number of families have been described with affected male subjects and with affected female subjects whose angioedema does not depend on high oestrogen levels (Fig. 12.5). Mutations in Hageman factor (coagulation factor XII) have been found in a minority of type III HAE kindreds, which may result in enhanced generation of bradykinin. The underlying cause of type III HAE in patients without this Hageman factor mutation remains unclear; however, it is likely to involve bradykinin as the final mediator.

Acquired C1INH deficiency

Angioedema due to C1INH deficiency also occurs on an acquired rather than hereditary basis. The syndrome of acquired C1 inhibitor deficiency is not associated with a mutation of the C1 inhibitor gene, or impaired synthesis of functional C1 inhibitor. Rather, it occurs because of increased catabolism of C1 inhibitor that outstrips the capacity of the host to synthesize new C1 inhibitor. Patients with acquired C1 inhibitor deficiency often have an underlying disease leading to continuous activation of the classic complement pathway with consequent depletion of C1 inhibitor, especially lymphoproliferative disorders including malignancies and monoclonal gammopathies. Some patients with acquired C1 inhibitor deficiency also

have autoantibodies that specifically recognize normal C1 inhibitor, promoting an ineffective interaction between C1 inhibitor and its target proteases wherein the C1 inhibitor is cleaved into an inactive form by the protease without inactivating the protease. Like HAE, attacks of angioedema in patients with acquired C1INH deficiency are accompanied by elevated bradykinin levels.

ACE-I associated angioedema

Angiotensin-converting enzyme (ACE) is a protease that cleaves the carboxyl amino acid from certain peptides, including bradykinin and substance P (Fig. 12.6). When ACE is inhibited, bradykinin degradation is expected to be prolonged and thus may contribute to the resultant angioedema. Patients experiencing ACE-I associated angioedema have been reported to have increased plasma bradykinin levels. It has been speculated that the susceptibility to ACE-I-induced angioedema may be determined by the level or activity of other bradykinin degrading enzymes. Indeed, clinical studies with a combined ACE and neutral endopeptidase inhibitor resulted in a higher incidence of angioedema than seen from an ACE inhibitor alone.

Non-histaminergic idiopathic angioedema

A subpopulation of patients with idiopathic angioedema and normal C1INH do not respond to treatment with high-dose antihistamines. Increased plasma bradykinin

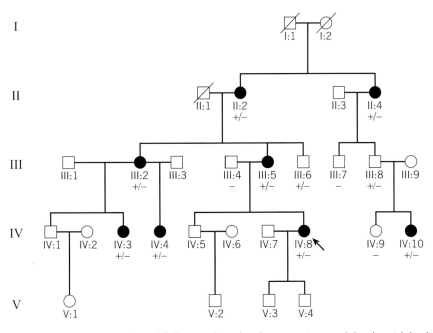

Fig. 12.5 Pedigree of a family with type III HAE and fXII mutation showing an autosomal-dominant inheritance. Filled symbols, individuals affected by recurrent angioedema; +/−, heterozygous presence of the p.Thr309Lys mutation; −, absence of the mutation. Individual IV:8 (arrow) is the index patient. Individual III:8 is an unaffected male transmitting the disease. (From Bork K, Wulff K, Hardt J, et al. Hereditary angioedema caused by missense mutations in the factor XII gene: Clinical features, trigger factors and therapy. J Allergy Clin Immunol 2009; 124:129–134.)

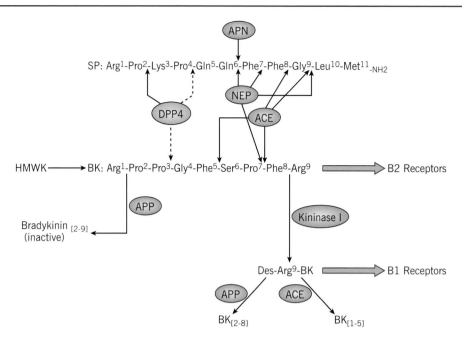

Fig. 12.6 Degradation of bradykinin, des-Arg9-bradykinin, and substance P. APN, aminopeptidase N or M; APP, aminopeptidase P; BK, bradykinin; DPP4, depeptidyl peptidase IV; HMWK, high-molecular-weight kininogen; NEP, neutral endopeptidase; SP, substance P. (From Byrd JB, Adam A, Brown NJ. Angiotensin-converting enzyme inhibitor-associated angioedema. Immunol Allergy Clin N Am 2006; 26:725–737.)

levels have been measured in these patients during attacks of angioedema. Whether these patients have abnormalities in the bradykinin-generating or bradykinin-catabolizing pathways has not been determined.

Clinical presentation of non-mast-cell-mediated angioedema

Hereditary angioedema with C1 inhibitor deficiency

Patients with HAE typically present with a history of discrete episodes of non-pruritic, non-pitting angioedema involving the extremities, genitourinary tract, abdomen, face, oropharynx, or a combination of the above. HAE attacks are usually distinguished from allergic or idiopathic angioedema by their longer duration. Patients with HAE may also experience prodromal manifestations (such as an erythematous non-urticarial rash called 'erythema marginatum', localized tingling, or a sense of skin tightness) for several hours or up to a day prior to the onset of an attack. The swelling in HAE is always episodic and is not continuous daily swelling. The typical HAE attack tends to worsen progressively for 24 hours and then slowly remit over the following 48–72 hours; however, attacks can occasionally last longer particularly if the swelling moves from site to site.

Attacks involving the extremities and abdomen are the most common, each representing almost 50% of all attacks. Over a lifetime, almost 100% of HAE patients experience both extremity and abdominal attacks. The latter can result in severe abdominal pain with intractable nausea and vomiting, and third spacing of fluid can induce significant hypotension. Because of the severe presentation of some abdominal attacks, many HAE patients undergo unnecessary and inappropriate surgical interventions. The most dangerous attacks occur in the oropharynx and threaten laryngeal patency, with a significant risk of mortality. Although these types of attacks occur much less frequently than the extremity or abdominal attacks, more than 50% of HAE patients experience at least one oropharyngeal attack during their lifetime. All HAE patients must be considered at risk for a potential oropharyngeal attack irrespective of their disease severity or whether they have ever had a facial or oropharyngeal attack in the past.

Patients with HAE typically experience their first attack during childhood (Fig. 12.7); 50% of HAE patients begin swelling under the age of 10 years, with some patients manifesting angioedema by 1 year of age. Most patients then experience a worsening of symptoms around puberty. Disease severity in HAE is highly variable. Some patients experience attacks one or more times per week, whereas rare patients with HAE have been reported who never experience angioedema. Several stressors have been associated with precipitating HAE attacks, especially trauma (even relatively minor trauma such as sitting on a hard surface for a prolonged time) and emotional stress. Of particular concern are iatrogenic trauma stimuli such as dental work, medical procedures, and surgery.

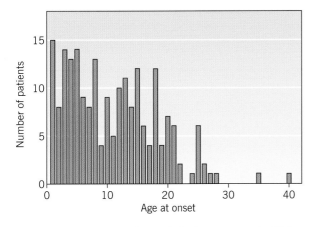

Fig. 12.7 Age at onset of the clinical symptoms in 209 patients with hereditary angioedema due to C1 inhibitor deficiency. (From Bork K, Meng G, Staubach P, Hardt J. Hereditary angioedema: new findings concerning symptoms, affected organs, and course. Am J Med 2006; 119(3):267–274.)

Hormonal changes can affect disease severity. Birth control pills containing oestrogen and oestrogen replacement therapy both appear to increase frequency of swelling. The impact of pregnancy on HAE disease severity is variable; however, women appear to be relatively protected against swelling at the time of parturition. Because angiotensin-converting enzyme (ACE) inhibitors decrease the catabolism of bradykinin, ACE inhibitors can precipitate attacks of angioedema and should be avoided in HAE patients.

A potential role for *Helicobacter pylori* infection in triggering abdominal attacks has been reported, although not all investigators have observed this relationship. No clear precipitating cause can be determined for many if not most HAE attacks.

Hereditary angioedema with normal C1 inhibitor

Although the clinical presentation of type III HAE resembles that of HAE with reduced C1INH function, a number of important differences have been observed. Compared with types I and II HAE, type III HAE is characterized by: more likely to be female, less likely to present prior to puberty, fewer attacks and more attack-free intervals, significantly more facial and tongue episodes, and fewer abdominal attacks and multiorgan attacks. Triggers of attacks are similar to types I and II HAE, and include trauma, stress, and states of increased oestrogen levels.

Acquired C1INH deficiency

The most striking clinical differences in acquired C1INH deficiency compared with HAE are its relatively late age of onset and lack of family history. Attacks of angioedema in patients with acquired C1INH deficiency are otherwise similar to those in patients with HAE.

ACE-I-associated angioedema

Angioedema associated with the use of ACE-I typically involves the lips, tongue, and face. Abdominal attacks are far less commonly seen than in patients with HAE. The ability of ACE-I to cause angioedema is a class effect based on their pharmacological activity, thus any of the ACE-Is can cause angioedema. Whereas the overall incidence of ACE-I-associated angioedema is less than 1% of exposed patients, the incidence is strikingly increased (2.8–6%) in black Americans. Other factors that increase the risk of ACE-I-induced angioedema are a history of smoking, increasing age, and female gender. Diabetics appear to be at a reduced risk. The interval between starting an ACE-I and developing angioedema is usually less than 1 month; frequently it begins within the first week, but is greater than 6 months in over 25% of cases and can be as long as 10 years.

Non-histaminergic idiopathic angioedema

The attacks of angioedema in these patients resemble HAE attacks; however, these patients have normal C1INH function and no family history of angioedema. Because of the difficulty in diagnosing these patients, little is currently known about this disorder.

Diagnosis

Patients with recurrent angioedema in the absence of typical wheals should be evaluated for the possibility of a bradykinin-mediated angioedema. The diagnosis may be suggested by clinical features (Table 12.5); however, laboratory confirmation is frequently necessary.

A diagnosis of C1INH deficiency requires laboratory confirmation. In general, testing for C4, C1INH antigen, and C1INH function will reliably identify these patients, although complement values must be interpreted with care in patients under the age of 1 year. All C1INH-deficient patients should have a low C4 during attacks, and almost all will have a low C4 even between attacks. Type I and II HAE are primarily distinguished by the C1INH antigenic level. Acquired C1INH deficiency is frequently associated with a decreased C1q level and presence of high levels of C1INH autoantibody. Figure 12.8 shows a standard algorithm for interpreting these tests, and Table 12.6 summarizes the values expected in each of these diseases. In cases where there is a low index of suspicion for C1INH deficiency, measuring the C4 alone is typically sufficient, particularly if the sample is drawn during an acute episode of swelling.

At the current time, there is no diagnostic test for type III HAE. A subset of these patients has a mutation in codon 309 of coagulation factor XII; however, the absence

Table 12.5 Clinical characteristics of different types of angioedema

	HAE type I and II	HAE type III	ACID	ACE-I	AE in csU
Typical age of onset	6–20 yrs	2nd decade	>50 yrs	Any	Any
Usual sites of swelling	Extrem., GI, genital, facial, oral-laryngeal	Facial, tongue	Extrem., GI, genital, facial, oral-laryngeal	Facial, tongue, laryngeal	Extrem., facial, tongue
Duration of attacks (h)	48–96	48–96	48–96	Prolonged	2–48
Response to corticosteroids or antihistamines	No	No	No	Unproven	Yes
Family history of angioedema	Usually	Yes	No	No	No
Underlying disease	No	No	Malignancy or gammopathy	Hypertension	No
Worsened by exogenous estrogens	Yes	Yes	Yes	No	No

ACID, acquired C1INH deficiency (acquired angioedema); csU, chronic spontaneous urticaria.

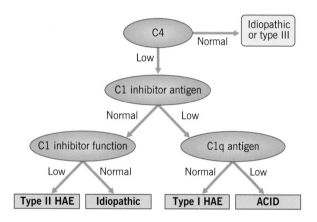

Fig. 12.8 Algorithm for interpretation of complement testing in HAE. C4 is almost always low in HAE types I and II, but is normal in type III or idiopathic angioedema. In patients with low C4 and normal C1INH levels, the C1INH function distinguishes type II HAE from idiopathic angioedema with complement activation. In patients with low C4 and low C1INH levels, the C1q level helps distinguish type I HAE from acquired C1INH deficiency. ACID, acquired C1INH deficiency.

of this mutation does not exclude the diagnosis and the mutation itself has not yet been unequivocally demonstrated to cause the disease. Angioedema occurring in patients taking an ACE-I is assumed to be due to the ACE-I until proven otherwise. The diagnosis of non-histaminergic idiopathic angioedema is largely a diagnosis of exclusion with normal C1INH, a lack of family history, and a lack of efficacy of high-dose antihistamines.

Management

The standard angioedema treatment modalities used for histamine-mediated angioedema such as adrenaline, corticosteroids, or antihistamines do not have a significant impact on the swelling in bradykinin-mediated angioedema. There is no evidence that corticosteroids or antihistamines have any beneficial impact on HAE attacks. Adrenaline probably has a temporary effect on the permeability defect and may provide transient benefit; however, there is no evidence that it changes the overall course of the attack.

Hereditary angioedema with C1 inhibitor deficiency

The management of HAE involves both treatment of acute attacks and prophylaxis. Acute attacks involving the abdomen or larynx are associated with significant risk of morbidity and mortality. Even extremity swelling can lead to prolonged and frequent absence from school or work. Plasma-derived C1INH (pdC1INH) given by intravenous injection has been the standard of care for acute attacks in parts of Europe and elsewhere for more than 20 years, but was not available in the United States until recently. Fortunately, randomized placebo-controlled studies of five drugs have been performed over the past several years and have led to the emergence of improved options for treating angioedema attacks.

Three different C1INHs (two pdC1INHs and one recombinant human C1INH) are currently approved for use in the treatment of attacks in patients with HAE

Table 12.6 Laboratory profile of different types of angioedema

	C1-INH level	C1-INH function	C4 level	C3 level	C1q level
HAE type I	Low	Low	Low	Normal	Normal
HAE type II	Normal or increased	Low	Low	Normal	Normal
HAE type III	Normal	Normal	Normal	Normal	Normal
Acquired C1INH deficiency	Low	Low	Low	Normal/low	Low
ACE inhibitor	Normal	Normal	Normal	Normal	Normal
Idiopathic angioedema	Normal	Normal	Normal	Normal	Normal

Table 12.7 Drugs effective for treatment of acute angioedema attacks in HAE patients

Drug	Mechanism	Dose	Route	Potential side effects
Plasma-derived C1INH	Inhibits plasma kallikrein and activated factor XII	500–1000 units based on clinical anecdotal experience; 20 U/kg per clinical trial	Intravenous	Anaphylaxis (rare); infection (theoretical)
Recombinant human C1INH	Inhibits plasma kallikrein and activated factor XII	50–100 U/kg	Intravenous	Anaphylaxis (uncommon)
Ecallantide	Inhibits plasma kallikrein	30 mg	Subcutaneous	Prolonged PP; anaphylaxis (uncommon)
Icatibant	Antagonizes bradykinin at the bradykinin B_2 receptor	30 mg	Subcutaneous	Discomfort at injection site (common)

(Table 12.7). In addition, each of these drugs appears to be highly effective. Although extensive open-label experience suggested that 500–1500 U of pdC1INH was highly effective, a recent randomized study of pdC1INH demonstrated that 20 U/kg was required to see significant benefit. Uncontrolled studies have shown that home administration of pdC1INH early in an attack (on-demand), results in better and faster relief of symptoms. Ecallantide is a potent inhibitor of plasma kallikrein – the protease that cleaves kininogen and releases bradykinin. Subcutaneous injection of ecallantide 30 mg is approved for treatment of acute attacks in the United States. Because of a potential risk of allergic reactions, ecallantide must be given in a medical facility. Icatibant is a selective bradykinin B_2 receptor antagonist that is also administered subcutaneously. Injection of icatibant 30 mg is approved for treatment of acute HAE attacks in Europe. Hypotension due to decreased intravascular volume may require aggressive intravenous fluid replacement, and laryngeal angioedema with impending airway compromise may require emergent intubation or tracheotomy.

HAE patients may also require prophylactic treatment (Table 12.8). Short-term prophylactic therapy is meant to protect patients against the likelihood of experiencing acute attacks during a defined temporal window following a stimulus known to precipitate HAE attacks (such as extensive dental work, invasive medical procedures, or surgery). Long-term prophylactic treatment of HAE is meant to decrease the frequency or severity of HAE attacks.

All HAE patients are candidates for short-term prophylaxis for times when they are exposed to situations or procedures that are likely to trigger attacks of angioedema. When undergoing a relatively minor procedure (such as dental cleaning), the ready availability of one of the acute treatment drugs described above is sufficient. Alternatively, exposure to a major procedure or lack of availability of acute treatment requires that the patient be pretreated with pdC1INH, FFP/SDP, or high-dose anabolic androgen.

Not all HAE patients require long-term prophylaxis, and the decision regarding who should receive it must be individualized based on attack frequency, attack severity, access to acute care or on-demand treatment, and comorbid conditions. Several modalities of prophylaxis are available. Prophylactic treatment with pdC1INH (1000 U twice per week) provides effective prophylaxis for patients with severe HAE. Anabolic androgens are

Table 12.8 Drugs effective for prophylactic treatment of HAE patients

Drug	Mechanism	Dose	Route	Potential side effects
Plasma-derived C1INH	Inhibits plasma kallikrein and activated factor XII	1000 units every 3–4 days	Intravenous	Anaphylaxis (rare); infection (theoretical)
17α-Alkylated androgens				
Danazol	Increase C1INH levels modestly; may also increase kininase levels	Long-term: 100 mg every 3 days to 200 mg/day; short-term: 400–600 mg/day	Oral	Common: weight gain, virilization, acne, altered libido, headaches, irritability, increases in liver enzymes, depression, hypertension, alternations in lipid profile.
Stanozolol		Long-term: 1 mg every 3 days to 2 mg/day; short-term: 4—6 mg/day		Uncommon: decreased growth rate in children, masculinization of female fetus, cholestatic jaundice, peliosis hepatis, hepatocellular carcinoma. Best avoided in children.
Oxandrolone		Long-term: 2.5 mg every 3 days to 10 mg/day; short-term: 20 mg/day		
Antifibrinolytics				
Tranexamic acid	Inhibits plasminogen activation	20–50 mg/kg/day divided into twice or thrice per day	Oral	Common: nausea, vertigo, diarrhoea, postural hypotension, fatigue, muscle cramps with increased muscle enzymes.
ε-aminocaproic acid		1 g twice daily to 1.5 g thrice daily		Uncommon: thrombosis

also very effective, but may cause bothersome or serious side effects. Both the efficacy and adverse effects of anabolic androgens are dose related. Antifibrinolytics such as tranexamic acid (available in Europe) and ε-aminocaproic acid (available in the United States) are less effective than anabolic androgens, but can be useful particularly in children in whom anabolic androgens are relatively contraindicated.

Hereditary angioedema with normal C1 inhibitor

Somewhat surprisingly, most patients with type III HAE who were treated with pdC1INH for acute attacks have reported benefit. Anecdotal reports suggest that icatibant may also be useful in treating acute attacks in type III patients. Both progesterone and anabolic androgens have been reported to be helpful for long-term prophylaxis in type III HAE.

Acquired C1INH deficiency

There are several important differences in the treatment of acquired C1INH deficiency compared with HAE. First, treatment of the underlying disorder (such as a lymphoreticular malignancy) has been reported to result in the resolution of the acquired C1INH deficiency. Secondly, rituximab has been reported to induce a sustained remission in a small group of patients with acquired C1INH deficiency and severe frequent attacks. Successful treatment of acute attacks of angioedema in these patients with pdC1INH has been reported; however, some patients require a higher dose of pdC1INH or are even resistant to pdC1INH treatment. Icatibant or ecallantide may be potentially useful in these patients. Finally, treatment with antifibrinolytics appears to be more effective than anabolic androgens for long-term prophylaxis in many patients with acquired C1INH deficiency.

ACE-I associated angioedema

The key step in managing these patients is to discontinue the ACE-I. It appears that these patients can be safely switched to an alternative class of antihypertensive. Preliminary anecdotal experience suggests that icatibant may be useful in treating acute angioedema in these patients.

Non-histaminergic idiopathic angioedema

No specific treatment has yet been demonstrated to be effective in these patients.

Summary of important messages

- Urticaria is a group of diseases characterized by wheals and/or angioedema
- Urticarias are classified by their duration as acute or chronic and by their clinical presentation as spontaneous or inducible
- Chronic spontaneous urticaria can result from many different causes, which should be looked for in patients with high activity and long duration of disease
- The underlying causes of chronic inducible urticarias are largely unknown. Provocation tests are performed to verify the relevance of triggers and to assess their thresholds
- Non-sedating antihistamines are the first-line treatment for all patients with urticaria and should be increased in dose if standard doses do not work
- Treatment options for chronic urticaria patients who do not respond to non-sedating antihistamines include add-on antileukotrienes and/or H_2 blockers, ciclosporin, omlizumab and other immunomodulatory and immunosuppressive treatments
- Angioedema can be mast cell-mediated (e.g. in urticaria patients) or bradykinin-mediated (e.g. in hereditary or acquired C1 inhibitor deficiency)
- Hereditary angioedema with C1 inhibitor deficiency is characterized by swelling attacks involving the extremities, the abdomen and, most dangerously, the upper airway
- The diagnostic work-up in patients with recurrent angioedema in the absence of wheals should include testing for C4 and C1 inhibitor antigen and function
- Patients with hereditary angioedema with C1 inhibitor deficiency must be provided with effective on-demand treatment and should be considered for prophylactic treatment
- Plasma-derived or recombinant C1 inhibitor, the plasma kallikrein inhibitor ecallantide and the bradykinin B2 receptor antagonist icatibant are highly effective on-demand treatments for hereditary angioedema with C1 inhibitor deficiency
- Non-mast-cell-mediated angioedema may also be hereditary with normal C1 inhibitor (called HAE type III), acquired angioedema with C1 inhibitor deficiency, ACE-inhibitor-induced, or idiopathic

Further reading

Bork K, Wulff K, Hardt J, et al. Hereditary angioedema caused by missense mutations in the factor XII gene: Clinical features, trigger factors and therapy. J Allergy Clin Immunol 2009; 124:129–134.

Grattan CEH, Humphreys F. Guidelines for evaluation and management of urticaria in adults and children. Br J Dermatol 2007; 157:1116–1123.

Konstantinou GN, Asero R, Maurer M, et al. EAACI/GA²LEN task force consensus report: the autologous serum skin test in urticaria. Allergy 2009; 64:1256–1268.

Magerl M, Borzova E, Giménez-Arnau A, et al. The definition and diagnostic testing of physical and cholinergic urticarias – EAACI/GA²LEN/EDF/UNEV consensus panel recommendations. Allergy 2009; 64:1715–1721.

Magerl M, Pisarevskaja D, Scheufele R, et al. Effects of a pseudoallergen-free diet on chronic spontaneous urticaria: a prospective trial. Allergy 2010; 65:78–83.

Metz M, Gimenez-Arnau A, Borzova E, et al. Frequency and clinical implications of skin autoreactivity to serum versus plasma in patients with chronic urticaria. J Allergy Clin Immunol 2009; 123:705–706.

Młynek A, Zalewska-Janowska A, Martus P, et al. How to assess disease activity in patients with chronic urticaria? Allergy 2008; 63:777–780.

Zuberbier T, Asero R, Bindslev-Jensen C, et al. EAACI/GA²LEN/EDF/WAO Guideline: Definition, classification and diagnosis of urticaria. Allergy 2009; 64:1417–1426.

Zuberbier T, Asero R, Bindslev-Jensen C, et al. EAACI/GA²LEN/EDF/WAO Guideline: Management of urticaria. Allergy 2009; 64:1427–1443.

Zuraw BL. Hereditary angioedema. New Engl J Med 2008; 359:1027–1036.

Atopic dermatitis and allergic contact dermatitis

Thomas Werfel and Alexander Kapp

Atopic dermatitis is a common inflammatory skin disorder, characterized by severe pruritus, chronically relapsing course, a distinctive distribution of eczematous skin lesions, and often a personal or family history of atopic diseases.

Allergic contact dermatitis, which is not linked to atopy, is the prototype of a delayed-type hypersensitivity reaction (so-called type IV reaction), which is mediated largely by lymphocytes preciously sensitized to low-molecular-weight allergens causing inflammation and oedema in the skin.

Introduction

Eczema is a pattern of inflammatory responses of the skin that can be defined either clinically or histologically. Clinically, acute eczema is associated with marked erythema, superficial papulae, and vesiculae that easily excoriate and lead to crusts. Chronic eczema is composed of rather faint erythema, infiltration, and scaling (Fig. 13.1). Histologically, eczema is characterized by oedema and spongiosis of the epidermis, oedema of the papillary dermis, and a mononuclear infiltrate in the dermis that extends into the epidermis (Fig. 13.2).

Eczema accounts for a large proportion of all skin diseases and is the most common cause for consultation with a dermatologist. The condition may be induced by a range of external and internal factors acting singly or in combination. The individual classification of the clinical form may be difficult because multiple causative factors may be implicated and more than one form of eczema may be present in the same patient simultaneously. Table 13.1 gives a classification of the most common forms of eczematous skin diseases. Since allergic mechanisms play a major role in only the atopic and allergic contact forms of dermatitis, this chapter will concentrate on these diseases. The reader is referred to dermatological textbooks to learn more about the other forms of eczematous skin diseases. Generally, the terms 'eczema' and 'dermatitis' are synonymous but the term dermatitis will be used preferentially in this chapter to describe all forms of diseases that involve the eczematous process.

Both atopic dermatitis and allergic contact dermatitis belong to the group of eczematous skin diseases. In both diseases, a mononuclear infiltate, dominated by CD4+ T-helper cells, is found in the dermis; in acute phases of the disease epidermal involvent is often clearly visible. Although both diseases have many features in common, their causes and clinical presentations are so different that the diseases are presented here separately.

© 2012 Elsevier Ltd
DOI: 10.1016/B978-0-7234-3658-4.00005-6

Table 13.1 Classification of eczematous skin diseases

Disease	Feature
Allergic contact dermatitis	Provoked by local contact with allergen Haematogenous/drug induction possibly with allergen
Photoallergic dermatitis	Provoked by local contact plus UV radiation Haematogenous/drug induction possibly
Atopic dermatitis/neurodermatitis	Extrinsic type (i.e. atopic dermatitis) Intrinsic type (i.e. neurodermatitis)
Irritant contact dermatitis	Provoked by local contact
Phototoxic dermatitis	Provoked by local contact plus UV radiation
Seborrhoeic dermatitis	Provoked by *Malassezia sympodialis* plus endocrine factors
Nummular dermatitis/discoid eczema	Provoked by inflammatory focus
Varicosis dermatitis/stasis eczema	Provoked by a state of chronic venous insufficiency

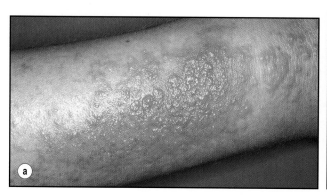
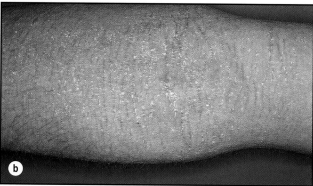

Fig. 13.1 Morphology of acute versus chronic eczema. (a) Acute eczema characterized by marked erythema, superficial papulae, and vesiculae. (b) Chronic eczema characterized by faint erythema, infiltration, and scaling (chronic atopic dermatitis).

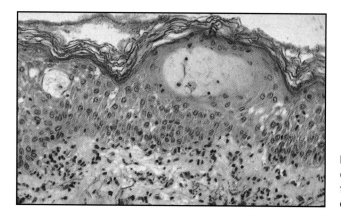

Fig. 13.2 Histological appearance of allergic contact dermatitis. The epidermis is oedematous with microvesicle formation; mononuclear cells have infiltrated the dermis and epidermis (×130).

PART I Atopic dermatitis

Atopic dermatitis (AD) is a common inflammatory skin disorder, characterized by pruritus, a chronically relapsing course, a distinctive distribution of eczematous skin lesions, and often a personal or family history of atopic diseases.

Anatomy and physiology

Histological examination of the skin in acute dermatitis/eczema reveals a picture in atopic dermatitis similar to that of allergic contact dermatitis, with microvesiculation in the epidermis and a lymphohistiocytic infiltrate in the dermis.

Disease mechanisms

It appears that different disease mechanisms are important for different subgroups of patients suffering from atopic dermatitis. This is reflected by the fact that a multifactorial trait involving numerous gene loci on different chromosomes (3, 5, and 11) has been observed. Described genetic polymorphisms in AD involve mediators of atopic inflammation on different chromosomes; some of these may also play a role in respiratory atopy.

More recently, strong associations have been shown with mutations in the filaggrin gene also associated with ichthyosis vulgaris, highlighting the predisposing barrier defect in AD patients. That means that, for a substantial percentage of patients, abnormal skin barrier function ('dry' skin) due to abnormal lipid metabolism and/or epidermal structural protein formation (e.g. filaggrin loss-of-function mutations, protease inhibitor deficiency) may be relevant for the initiation of the disease.

These may be combined with pathological factors of innate immunity leading to abnormal microbial colonization with pathogenic organisms such as *Staphylococcus aureus* or *Malassezia furfur* (compared with *Staphylococcus epidermidis* in normal individuals) and subsequent increased susceptibility to skin infection. Some of the innate immune defects observed in atopic dermatitis are primary defects such as defects in signalling or expression of innate receptors (e.g. TLR2, NOD2). Others may be secondary to the effects of the adaptive immune response. For example, deficiencies in antimicrobial peptides may be due to the overexpression of Th2 cytokines such as IL-4 and IL-13 in acute eczema.

A number of immune deviations in the adaptive immune system have also been described. Like in other atopic diseases, there is a general overexpression of Th2 cytokines in many patients with atopic dermatitis. This is closely linked to the regulation of IgE, which is higher than normal in 80% of all patients. Specific IgE is commonly associated with food or environmental allergens. More recent studies point to the fact that specific immune responses including T lymphocytes and specific IgE are directed against autoantigens, and microbial antigens as well. Those T lymphocytes and specific IgE antibodies may be directly involved in the eczematous skin reaction.

Eczematous patch-test reactions to house dust mites, pollen, animal dander, or foods are frequently observed in sensitized patients (Fig. 13.3). These tests have helped to understand the pathophysiological role of different haematopoietic cell populations in the early eczematous reaction. In the acute phase of eczema, the majority of T cells express Th2 cytokines (IL-4, IL-13, IL-31); during

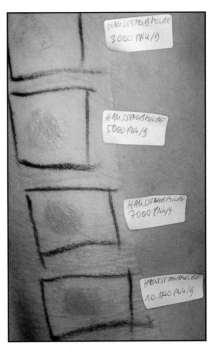

Fig. 13.3 Patch-test reactions to house dust mite allergens provoked on the back of a highly sensitized patient with atopic dermatitis. Note the dose-dependent strength of the reactions.

chronification the Th1 cytokine IFN-γ is increased in the skin. More recently it became clear that IL-17 and IL-22, two T-cell cytokines acting on constitutive epithelial cells, are also secreted into the skin in atopic dermatitis (Fig. 13.4).

Antigen-bearing dendritic cells, binding IgE mainly via the high-affinity Fc receptor FcεRI, are present in the epidermis and mainly in the dermis in atopic dermatitis. Binding of allergens to Fc receptors of those cells is thought to facilitate antigen presentation to specific T cells (Fig. 13.5). Those cells, many of them expressing the skin-homing molecule cutaneous lymphocyte antigen (CLA) have been identified in the circulation and in the skin in atopic dermatitis. At present, epidermal and dermal milieu factors such as TSLP are being investigated that may directly or indirectly influence the different cytokine pattern of infiltrating T cells.

Many activated eosinophils are seen early in spongiotic epidermal lesions. Later, secretory proteins, such as major basic protein or eosinophil cationic protein, from the eosinophils can be detected but no intact cells can be found in the lesional dermis. A major clinical symptom of AD is itch. It is a matter of current research how strong is a psychosomatic influence with an imbalance in the autonomic nervous system, with subsequent increased production of mediators from various inflammatory cells (e.g. eosinophilic leukocytes) in AD.

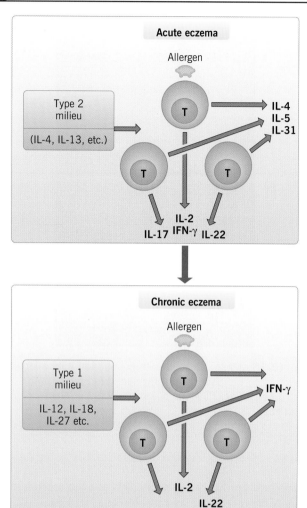

Fig. 13.4 Switch of cytokine pattern in acute versus chronic dermatitis.

Suggestions on causes and disease mechanism from epidemiological studies

During the last decades a marked increase in the frequency of atopic dermatitis has been observed and it is now the most frequent inflammatory skin disease, with a prevalence of more than 10% in children in Northern Europe and in the USA. A number of possible expression factors are currently being considered (Fig. 13.6). Some studies point to a higher prevalence of atopic dermatitis in children who live in areas with a greater degree of air pollution. The comparison of genetically similar populations who have been exposed to different types of air pollution (i.e. of children from former East and West Germany shortly after reunification) did not, however, reveal marked differences in the prevalence of atopic dermatitis.

The manifestation of atopic dermatitis in childhood appears to be greater in families with a higher income and a more privileged lifestyle. The reduced incidence of infection observed in early childhood and reduced contact with agents that elicit cellular immune responses associated with a type 1 cytokine pattern of T lymphocytes (i.e. vaccination responses) are currently felt to be associated with manifestations of atopic diseases. However, differences of prevalence of respiratory allergic diseases often do not parallel prevalences of atopic dermatitis in larger epidemiological studies, which points to independent risk and manifestation factors being critical for the atopic skin disease. Changes in the quality and quantity of food and environmental antigens that have contact with the immune system may also be involved in the increased prevalence.

Clinical presentation

Classification of atopic dermatitis

Atopic dermatitis is characterized by severe pruritus, a chronically relapsing course, a distinctive distribution of eczematous skin lesions, and a personal or family history of atopic diseases. It often begins in early infancy and follows a course of remissions and exacerbations. The role of exogenous and endogenous factors in the pathophysiology of atopic dermatitis has been intensively discussed in recent years. There is increasing evidence that T-cell responses to environmental or food allergens are important for the pathogenesis of atopic dermatitis. In patients with atopic dermatitis, the skin disease is most often associated with the existence of environmental or food allergen-specific IgE. This variant of the disease, which is also associated with environmental allergen-specific IgE, is usually called the 'extrinsic' form of atopic dermatitis. The 'intrinsic' variant is found in 20% of diseases with the typical clinical appearance of atopic dermatitis but without specific IgE. In this respect, atopic dermatitis resembles bronchial asthma, which also has an extrinsic and an intrinsic variant (Fig. 13.7). Perhaps the old term 'neurodermatitis' might be reintroduced to differentiate the intrinsic form from atopic dermatitis associated with specific IgE to food or inhalant allergens.

Provocation factors in atopic dermatitis

A number of different trigger factors of atopic dermatitis are well established (Fig. 13.8). Although there is still no consensus about the relative importance of these factors, the points given below should be considered in the management of individual patients.

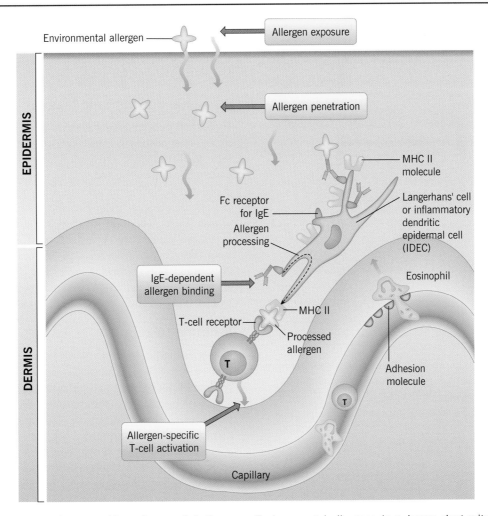

Fig. 13.5 Scenario in patch tests with environmental allergens. Environmental allergens (e.g. house dust mite extracts, cat epithelia, or grass pollen extracts) are applied onto uninvolved skin of the back for at least 24 hours. This allows allergens to penetrate into the skin and bind to the epidermal Langerhans' cells. These cells can present allergens either via molecules of the major histocompatibility complex (MHC II) or via IgE bound to Fc receptors for IgE for skin-infiltrating T lymphocytes.

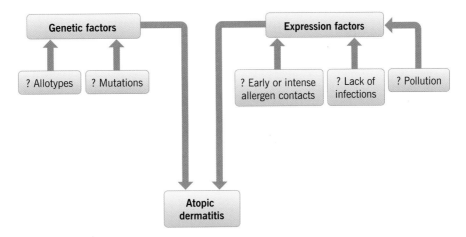

Fig. 13.6 Genetic and expression factors in atopic dermatitis.

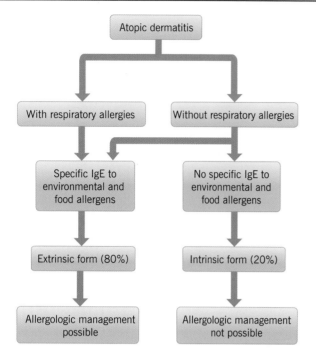

Fig. 13.7 Classification of atopic dermatitis. (Modified from Wüthrich B. Atopic dermatitis flare provoked by inhalant allergens. Dermatologica 1989; 178(1):51–53.)

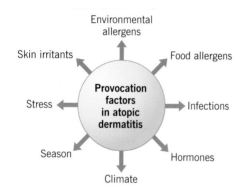

Fig. 13.8 Common provocation factors in atopic dermatitis.

Hormonal and emotional factors

Intraindividual fluctuations in the severity of atopic dermatitis are frequently observed in women. This points to hormonal influences with menstruation, pregnancy, birth, and menopause as possible trigger factors. However, more recent data suggest that hormonal factors may also play a role in male patients. Many studies emphasize the importance of psychological factors, such as personality traits or psychosocial stress, in the exacerbation and maintenance of skin symptoms. Stressful life events may be associated with an increase in itching, which leads to scratching and, by this mechanism, to a deterioration of the skin condition. The action of neuropeptides, an increasing number of nerve fibres that have close contact with mast cells and interactions of inflammatory mediators from inflammatory cells (e.g. histamine acting via the H_3 or H_4 receptor, IL-31 from Th2 lymphocytes) may be possible links between the nervous system and the skin condition in atopic dermatitis.

Seasonal and climatic factors

Individual patients show a seasonal variation in the severity of their problems: most patients tend to experience a flare in the autumn and winter months whereas few are affected in the spring and summer. Those who experience problems in the spring and summer may be sensitized to pollen allergens, or belong to the small group of patients whose skin deteriorates upon exposure to ultraviolet (UV) radiation. Large temperature fluctuations and continental climates also lead to a worsening of the skin condition. This is one reason why those patients not sensitive to UV radiation are encouraged to spend some weeks every year at the seaside if possible.

Irritating factors

The most consistent perturbators of atopic skin conditions are irritants. The skin response to sodium lauryl sulphate is increased in atopic individuals with or without apparent dermatitis. Occupational substances have particular clinical and social relevance and it appears that a history of atopic dermatitis, rather than of respiratory allergies, is a better prognostic factor of future work-related dermatitis. Intolerance to wool is based on its irritating effect on atopic skin, and cigarette smoke may elicit irritating eczema on the eyelids in atopic dermatitis. It is speculated that an altered composition of the epidermal lipids, an enhanced release of histamine, or a latent subclinical inflammatory reaction in the skin may play a role in the enhanced vulnerability of the atopic skin.

Infections

Both systemic and local infections can trigger the eczematous response in atopic dermatitis. *Staphylococcus aureus* has been studied extensively as a possible trigger factor. It is detected on the skin in more than 90% of all atopic dermatitis patients, which may at least in part be due to the decreased expression of antimicrobial peptides in the acute phase of eczema in atopic skin. Cell wall components from *S. aureus* may directly stimulate inflammatory cells via Toll-like receptors. In addition, exotoxins are detectable in more than 50% of all cultures containing *S. aureus* that have been generated from skin swabs in atopic dermatitis. They may function as superantigens that can bind to major histocompatibility complex class II (MHC II) molecules of monocytes and dendritic cells and release a number of proinflammatory molecules such as IL-1 and tumor necrosis factor α (TNF-α). Moreover, T cells that express reactive T-cell receptor Vβ chains can be stimulated to proliferate and secrete cytokines (e.g.

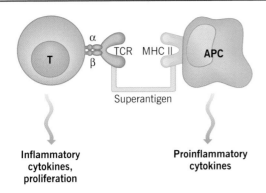

Fig. 13.9 The action of superantigens in atopic dermatitis. T, T lymphocyte; APC, antigen-presenting cell; TCR, T-cell receptor; MHC II, major histocompatibility complex class II (i.e. HLA-DR, HLA-DQ, HLA-DP).

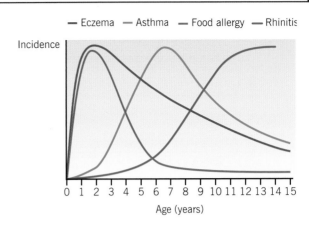

Fig. 13.10 Age-related incidences of atopic diseases. Atopic dermatitis usually presents during the first year of life, and is often outgrown by the age of 14 years. Food allergy also usually presents in the first year of life, and is often outgrown by the age of 5 years. Asthma develops later, usually between the ages of 3 and 7 years, and is often outgrown by the age of 14 years. Allergic rhinitis presents later still, around the age of 7 years, and continues into adulthood.

IL-22, IL-31) in response to superantigens, which may maintain the eczematous skin response (Fig. 13.9).

In addition to *S. aureus*, the saprophyte *Malassezia sympodiales* is thought to elicit a specific immune response and thus provoke eczema on the face and neck of atopic dermatitis patients – a substantial number of clinical and laboratory data support this hypothesis. *Candida albicans* is also considered to be a possible trigger factor of eczema; however, there are no immunological data that point directly to a pathogenetic role for an infestation of the gastrointestinal tract or the skin with *Candida* species in atopic dermatitis.

Environmental and contact allergens

The identification of sensitizers with a subsequent reduction of individual allergens is particularly important in the clinical management of atopic dermatitis, although allergens are certainly not the only trigger factors in this condition.

Hypersensitivity to house dust mite antigens is found in 5% of all people in Western nations, whereas it is found in up to 90% of adolescents or adults suffering from atopic dermatitis. Exacerbations of atopic dermatitis caused by house dust mites are presumed to be related to both inhalation and skin contact. Several clinical studies have reported improvement of the skin condition after a reduction in the level of house dust mites.

In addition to mites, sensitization to pollen or animal dander may be associated with eczematous skin reactions. Sensitization to cat, dog, or horse dander is frequently detected in patients with atopic dermatitis. Repeated contact with such animals should be avoided in case of chronic or severe atopic dermatitis and individual sensitizations – even if the patients do not suffer from respiratory symptoms.

Of note, the frequency of 'classic' allergic contact dermatitis to haptens is generally not reduced in patients with atopic dermatitis. The risk of contact allergy to ingredients of commonly applied topical preparations

(e.g. vehicles, preservatives, fragrances, antibiotics, steroids) appears to be even higher in this group. Thus, classic patch testing should not be neglected in adolescents or adults with atopic dermatitis because it may reveal important cofactors in the development of eczematous skin lesions in these patients.

Food

The role of food antigens as trigger factors of atopic dermatitis has been discussed for more than 60 years. Early studies on passively sensitized individuals have demonstrated that immunologically active food proteins can enter the circulation and are distributed throughout the body, including skin sites. It is possible that intestinal permeability is enhanced in atopic individuals and this may facilitate the resorption of food proteins. The incidence of atopic dermatitis and IgE-mediated food allergies peaks in early childhood (Fig. 13.10), which suggests that these two clinical entities may be associated.

Most young patients with atopic dermatitis (or their parents) suspect that certain foods trigger their skin abnormalities. The tendency to try restrictive diets that have uncertain benefits may lead to a risk of malnutrition or additional psychological stress. Placebo-controlled oral food challenges represent the 'gold standard' for the diagnosis of food allergy. Many food-inducible symptoms are immediate, occurring within 15 minutes of food ingestion, but a subpopulation of patients suffers from late symptoms, such as pruritus and worsening of their eczema, 8–24 hours later. In some patients the late symptoms follow directly on from the immediate manifestations (e.g. erythematous flush of the face leading to

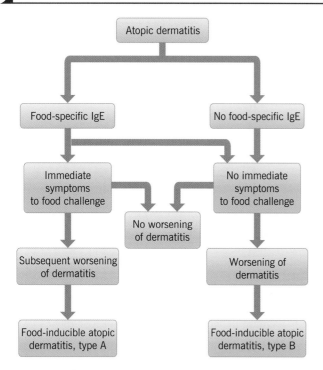

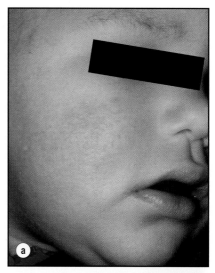

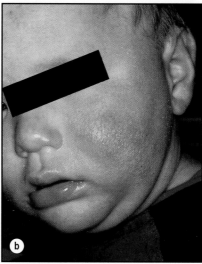

Fig. 13.11 Association between food allergy and atopic dermatitis.

Fig. 13.12 Clinical presentation of an 18-month-old boy with atopic dermatitis sensitized to cow's milk casein: 1 day before (a) and 30 minutes after (b) provocation with 30 mL cow's milk. The erythematous flush led to a late phase dermatitis during the following days.

eczema of the face) – a situation analogous to the dual reaction in asthma (Fig. 13.11). Immediate reactions are easily related to the suspected foodstuff in most cases (Fig. 13.12). The causes of isolated late eczematous reactions – which are also observable to pollen-associated foods in adolescent and adult patients with atopic dermatitis – are difficult to identify, and evaluation of the skin condition at least 24 hours after food challenges is proposed as an aid to identification.

A high proportion of children with food intolerance – particularly cow's milk allergy – will outgrow the problem and the controlled reintroduction of the previously offending foodstuffs 12 months after the first problem occurred will not be associated with further deterioration. However, IgE-mediated food allergy is not the whole story so far as food intolerance is concerned. A lack of correlation between specific IgE and the clinical response to food has been reported for food-responsive atopic dermatitis in several studies and this may point to the relative importance of allergen-specific T lymphocytes in these reactions. Moreover, many patients assert that consumption of citrus fruits exacerbates their eczema; also, adult patients observe that alcoholic beverages (particularly in excess!) cause worsening of their eczema on the day following alcohol consumption. It seems, therefore, that both food allergy and food intolerance due to non-immunological mechanisms are complicating factors in atopic dermatitis.

Diagnosis of atopic dermatitis

Differential diagnosis

Table 13.1 summarizes the most common eczematous skin diseases. Allergic contact dermatitis is reviewed in the second part of this chapter. A number of rare immune deficiency syndromes should be considered if eczema occurs in combination with other symptoms. In children, atopic dermatitis may be generally overdiagnosed. It is always important to remember that, besides skin eczema, a number of other red skin conditions with superficial (epidermal) involvement of the skin may occur in childhood (and of course in adults as well). Important and more common examples are infections and infestations of the skin (e.g. mycosis, scabies), other inflammatory skin diseases of unknown origin (e.g. psoriasis), and neoplasia (e.g. Langerhans cells histiocytosis, cutaneous lymphoma).

Investigations and tests

History

The highest incidence of atopic dermatitis is found within the first 2 years of life, although the disease can begin virtually at any age (see Fig. 13.10). A small proportion of patients present with atopic dermatitis before the age of 6 months and, in this situation, it is important to exclude the common dermatological problem of infantile seborrhoeic dermatitis. In the young infant the trunk, cheeks, and the extensor sites of the extremities are frequently involved and, as the infant develops, the limbs also become affected.

Symptom presentation

Many infants with atopic dermatitis have erythematous oozing lesions, predominantly on the cheeks. As the child grows, the affected sites tend to be the hands, the neck area, and the feet, particularly under the straps of footwear. The older child has predominant involvement behind the knees (Fig. 13.13), in the elbow folds, and frequently also on the face. The adult patient has a more generalized distribution, commonly with diffuse involvement on the trunk and upper thigh area.

With continual rubbing and excoriation, the skin becomes lichenified and develops a thickened, coarse appearance. A clinical variant found in adolescents and adults is the pruriginous form of atopic dermatitis, which is probably caused by repeated localized scratching.

The facial appearance of a patient with chronic atopic dermatitis is characteristic, with premature small wrinkles underneath both eyes – Dennie– Morgan folds – and frequently the loss of the outer third of the eyebrow through rubbing the face on the pillow while sleeping. This is referred to as 'Hertoghe's sign' (Fig. 13.14). The characteristic white dermographism (Fig. 13.15) of the atopic patient gives rise to an unhealthy pallor. Although most patients with atopic dermatitis are encouraged to keep their nails cut very short to avoid excoriation of the skin by scratching, many patients buff or rub at their skin using the flat surface of the nail, which gives the nails a highly polished appearance.

Young women with atopic dermatitis may develop persistent and, at times, severe dermatitis around the nipple and periareolar area (Fig. 13.16). In a proportion of patients with hand dermatitis their condition is associated with atopy. This should be considered particularly with regard to hairdressers, nurses, and others whose work involves persistent exposure of the skin to detergents, soaps, and other degreasing materials.

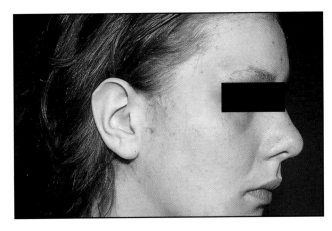

Fig. 13.14 Hertoghe's sign.

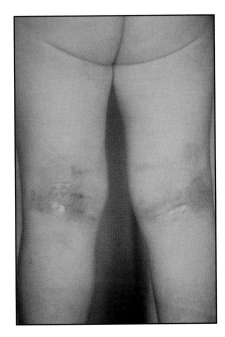

Fig. 13.13 Child with flexural (mild) atopic dermatitis.

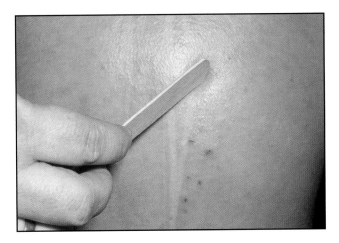

Fig. 13.15 White dermographism.

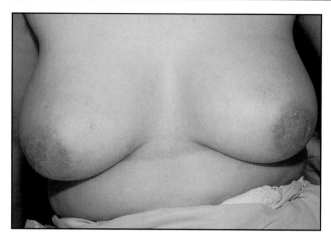

Fig. 13.16 Nipple dermatitis.

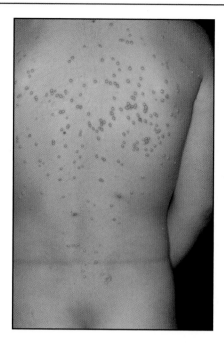

Fig. 13.18 Infection with molluscum contagiosum virus as a stigma for atopic children.

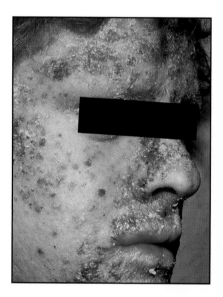

Fig. 13.17 Atopic dermatitis with obvious secondary infection and impetiginization on the face.

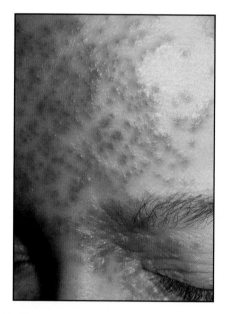

Fig. 13.19 Eczema herpeticum.

A large proportion of patients with chronic atopic dermatitis have an associated dry skin that is frequently hypersensitive and mildly pruritic; its control may help to alleviate the pruritus of atopic dermatitis.

Some patients with atopic dermatitis do not develop their first lesions until later childhood, adolescence, or even adulthood. There are individual case reports of patients who develop atopic dermatitis for the first time after acute intercurrent infection (e.g. infectious mononucleosis) or after successful marrow transplantation for leukaemia.

Patients with atopic dermatitis are unusually susceptible to certain cutaneous viral and bacterial infections and, of these, *S. aureus* infection is the commonest (Fig. 13.17). There is evidence of a causative relationship between *S. aureus* colonization and the severity of the disease.

Furthermore, these patients have a higher than expected incidence of warts caused by human papilloma virus or infections by molluscum contagiosum virus (Fig. 13.18). They are also susceptible to severe infection when exposed to the herpes simplex virus type I, which may spread and cause eczema herpeticum (Fig. 13.19). In a patient with severe excoriations caused by pre-existing dermatitis, it may be difficult to identify these new vesicles. Herpes simplex infection is an important, and at times severe, complication of atopic dermatitis and if it

Box 13.1 Diagnostic criteria of atopic dermatitis according to Hanifin and Rajka

Major features (at least three must be fulfilled):

- Pruritus
- Typical morphology and distribution:
  - flexural lichenification or linearity in adults
  - facial and extensor involvement in infants and children
- Chronic or chronically relapsing dermatitis
- Personal or family history of atopy (asthma, allergic rhinitis, atopic dermatitis)

Minor features (at least three must be fulfilled):

- Xerosis
- Ichthyosis/palmar hyperlinearity/keratosis pilaris
- Immediate (type 1) skin-test reactivity
- Elevated serum IgE
- Early age of onset
- Tendency towards cutaneous infections (esp. *Staphylococcus aureus* and *Herpes simplex*) or impaired cell-mediated immunity
- Tendency towards non-specific hand or foot dermatitis
- Nipple eczema
- Cheilitis
- Recurrent conjunctivitis
- Dennie–Morgan infraorbital fold
- Keratoconus
- Anterior subcapsular cataracts
- Orbital darkening
- Facial pallor/facial erythema
- Pityriasis alba
- Anterior neck folds
- Itch when sweating
- Intolerance to wool and lipid solvents
- Perifollicular accentuation
- Food intolerance
- Course influenced by environment/emotional factors
- White dermographism/delayed blanch

From Hanifin JM, Rajka G. Diagnostic features of atopic dermatitis. Acta Derm Venereol 1980; 92:44.

Box 13.2 Simplified diagnostic criteria of atopic dermatitis according to the UK Working Party's diagnostic criteria for atopic dermatitis

- Itchy skin condition (obligatory)
- Plus three of more of the following:
  - history of flexural involvement
  - history of asthma/hay fever
  - history of generalized dry skin
  - onset of rash under the age of 2 years
  - visible flexural dermatitis

According to Williams HC, Burney PG, Pembroke AC, et al. Validation of the UK diagnostic criteria for atopic dermatitis in a population setting. UK Diagnostic Criteria for Atopic Dermatitis Working Party. Br J Dermatol 1996; 135(1):12–17. © Blackwell Science Ltd.

frequently have eosinophilia and approximately 80% of patients have abnormally high serum levels of IgE, the highest levels being recorded in those patients with additional respiratory symptoms and in those with apparently associated food allergy. However, up to 15% of the normal population has serum IgE levels above the normal range, and a number of other diseases (e.g. helminthic infestations, cutaneous T-cell lymphoma) are also associated with high serum IgE levels. Thus, total serum IgE levels are not specific markers of the atopic dermatitis patient.

In vitro or skin prick tests to identify IgE levels specific to allergens have a higher specificity than total serum IgE in the diagnosis of atopy. In the young child, the bulk of IgE is directed against ingested foodstuffs; however, later in life, a large proportion of IgE appears to be directed against inhalant allergens. It is important to note that these tests show a sensitization, but often do not prove that the patient has a clinically relevant allergy.

Management of atopic dermatitis

Management of exacerbated atopic dermatitis is a therapeutic challenge as it requires efficient short-term control of acute symptoms, but without compromising the overall management plan that is aimed at long-term stabilization, flare prevention, and avoidance of side effects. Exacerbation may sometimes uncover relevant provocation factors – for example contact allergy or infection. Consequently, the initial work-up must include a detailed enquiry about the circumstances of the flare, and a careful dermatological examination including lymph nodes, orifices, and all skin folds. Professional attitude in face of exacerbated disease is setting the stage for future compliance. Patient fears regarding side effects of treatment must be taken seriously, and with a constructive attitude. Instruction of patients or parents about the necessary know-how regarding basic skin care is of primary importance.

Figure 13.20 summarizes approaches to the management of atopic dermatitis according to allergy and severity; Figure 13.21 assigns single treatment modalities to the severity of the disease.

is not identified and treated appropriately it can prove lethal.

Additional tests

The diagnosis of atopic dermatitis is usually made by evaluation of anamnestic data and clinical presentation. According to Hanifin and Rajka, three of their major and three of their minor criteria (Box 13.1) must be fulfilled to classify a skin disease as atopic dermatitis. Since this list is too long to be evaluated in daily practice, easier diagnostic criteria have been subsequently defined. Box 13.2 displays a simplified proposal, which was evaluated by a multicentre study group from the UK.

Laboratory data may sometimes be helpful in the diagnosis of atopic dermatitis. Patients with atopic dermatitis

Basic therapy

Basic therapy of atopic patients usually begins with control of the commonly associated dry skin. If this is treated then the need for topical steroid therapy will be greatly reduced. Most patients benefit from an emollient added to a bath, used after a bath, or applied continuously to the skin. The use of soap should be restricted in favour of a syndet, and an emollient substituted. Most patients will learn by trial and error which specific emollient preparations best suit their skin. A structured patient education programme, performed with groups of approximately 10 patients or with 10 parents of young patients suffering from atopic dermatitis, has recently been evaluated in a German controlled multicentre trial. It proved to be effective in the management of atopic dermatitis with respect to sustained improvement of the skin condition and of quality of life.

Avoidance of skin irritants

Patients with atopic dermatitis should avoid materials that irritate the skin. These frequently include both natural products, such as wool, and synthetic fibres. The majority of patients find that pure cotton is the most comfortable clothing. Rapid movement from one environmental extreme to another should also be avoided because large changes in ambient temperature, particularly from cold to heat, and in humidity are associated with deterioration of the skin condition.

Allergen avoidance

Reasonable steps to reduce the environmental exposure to allergens should be taken. This can be difficult with some allergens, but with others the precautions are obvious (e.g. households with a severely atopic child should not keep a cat). Although the house dust mite is ubiquitous and difficult to control, every effort should be made to reduce the prevalence of the mite in the environment, particularly in the sleeping area. The established and recommended avoidance procedures include removal of the carpet and curtains from the bedroom, encasing

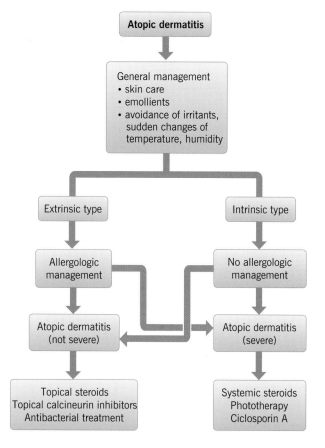

Fig. 13.20 Management of atopic dermatitis.

Severe: objective SCORAD >40/ persistent eczema	Hospitalization, systemic immunosuppression: oral glucocorticosteroids, cyclosporin A, PUVA, azathioprin, oral tacrolimus, mycophenolate mofetil
Moderate: objective SCORAD 15–40/ recurrent eczema	Sedating antihistamines (doxepin, hydroxyzine), UV therapy (UVB 311 nm, UVA 1), psychosomatic counseling, climate therapy
Mild: objective SCORAD >15/ transient eczema	Topical glucocorticosteroids or depending on local cofactors: topical calcineurin inhibitors, antiseptics incl. silver/AEGIS underwear, non-sedating antihistamines (controversial)
Baseline basic therapy	Educational programmes, emollients, bath oils, elimination diet in food-allergic patients, allergen avoidance (encasings, if diagnosed by allergy tests)

Fig. 13.21 General treatment of atopic dermatitis according to the position paper of ETFAD/EADV Eczema Task Force. Most international guidelines follow this four-step scheme of managing atopic dermatitis. For every phase, additional therapeutic options are given. In cases of visible superinfections, antiseptics/antibiotics should be added. Compliance (adherence) and diagnosis must be considered if therapy has no effect. (Adapted from Darsow U, Wollenberg A, Simon D, et al. ETFAD/EADV Eczema Task Force 2009 position paper on diagnosis and treatment of atopic dermatitis. J Eur Acad Dermatol Venereol 2010; 24(3):317–328.)

mattresses, pillows, and blankets in impermeable synthetic material, and hot washing of all bedding once a week.

Dietary measures

Two differing approaches, preventive and curative, can be adopted. The preventive approach involves the exclusive breastfeeding of infants known to be at high risk. A lower incidence of atopic dermatitis has been found in children who have been breastfed, or fed with extensively hydrolysed milk formula for at least 4 months. After 4 years, however, there are no differences in the prevalence of atopic diseases between the diet and control groups. Supplementation of the maternal diet during the last trimester of pregnancy and into lactation probably has no further protective effect on the manifestation of atopic dermatitis. Recent epidemiological data do point, however, to a preventive effect of fish consumption of the mother during pregnancy and lactation and of the infant with regard to manifestation of childhood eczema. Although elimination diets during early childhood are not sufficient to prevent the manifestation of atopic dermatitis generally, breastfeeding or the feeding of a hypoallergenic formula during the first 4 months of life should be recommended for high-risk infants.

The curative approach concerns dietary control of the established disease. This may be either by exclusion of an item of food that the patient or parent has noticed specifically exacerbates the disease or by non-specific exclusion of foods (e.g. dairy foods and other protein sources). The first approach is logical, but identification of provoking foods can be difficult – particularly if there is a long interval between ingestion and the onset of symptoms.

Exclusion of dairy products is a very popular move with parents of affected children. However, this should be recommended only for a prolonged period, and after a positive oral provocation test, because there is a very real danger of malnutrition and only about 10% of patients notice a benefit. A very small number of patients with severe and intractable disease derive benefit from an elemental diet.

Treatment with topical drugs

Anti-inflammatory and antimicrobial agents

The mainstay of control in atopic dermatitis is the appropriate use of topical corticosteroid creams or topical anti-inflammatory calcineurin inhibitors. Topical steroids must be handled with care and under regular supervision because they may be absorbed through the skin and the inappropriate use of potent steroids may lead to unwanted topical and systemic effects. In Europe, topical steroids are divided into four classes, with increasing potency

Table 13.2 European classification of the external corticosteroids

Group	Substance (examples)	Concentration (%)
I (low)	Hydrocortisone	0.500; 1.000
	Hydrocortisone acetate	0.250; 1.000
	Prednisolone	0.400
II (medium)	Hydrocortisone butyrate	0.100
	Triamcinolone acetonide	0.100
	Prednicarbate	0.250
III (strong)	Betamethasone (betametasone) valerate	0.100
	Fluocinolone acetonide	0.025
	Mometasone furoate	0.100
IV (very strong)	Clobetasol	0.050

ranging from grade I, containing hydrocortisone, to grade IV (Table 13.2). It is important to note that this classification differs from the one used in the USA (which has seven classes) and that there is no direct link between these classes and prednisone-equivalent doses calculated for systemic applications of steroids. It is normal dermatological practice to use a topical steroid no more potent than grade I on the face, and then only for a short time, and only moderately potent steroids (grade II) on other body sites. Preparations vary widely throughout the world, so current national formularies should be consulted.

Topical calcineurin inhibitors such as tacrolimus or pimecrolimus are also effective in atopic dermatitis. Because they do not have the same local side effects as topical steroids, such as the induction of skin atrophy, their use may be particularly favourable at sensitive skin regions such as the face or intertriginous areas. The use of intermittent topical anti-inflammatory therapy, with corticosteroids or calcineurin inhibitors applied twice a week over a period of some months upon healing of lesional skin, has been proved to lead to a better permanent skin condition and a reduced need of symptomatic therapy. This concept is now sometimes designated as 'proactive' therapy.

Treatment with systemic drugs

Systemic histamine H_1-receptor antagonists are frequently prescribed for patients with atopic dermatitis, but their value is disputed. It is found that these antihistamines are initially of some benefit to individual patients, particularly with regard to pruritus at night and loss of sleep. Newer non-sedating histamine H_1 antagonists are suitable for daytime use, but many patients with chronic severe atopic dermatitis will find the older antihistamines of more value – possibly because of the sedative effect rather than the specific antihistaminic actions of the drugs. Antihistamines binding to alternative receptors (H_4 receptors) are currently under study in atopic dermatitis and other inflamatory skin diseases.

Severe chronic atopic dermatitis will benefit from the use of systemic corticosteroids; however, long-term treatment must be reserved for exceptionally stubborn cases because of the side effects.

Ciclosporin, a polypeptide of fungal origin, is a potent inhibitor of T-lymphocyte-dependent immune responses and was originally introduced as an immunosuppressive agent to facilitate allogenic organ transplantation; it is also very effective in patients with atopic dermatitis in doses from 2.5 to 5 mg/kg per day. It is approved for the treatment of atopic dermatitis in most Western countries. Acute eczematous skin lesions usually clear after 4–6 weeks of therapy but, as with steroids, improvement is only temporary and flare-ups frequently occur after discontinuation of the drug therapy. Other immunosuppressive substances (azathioprine, mycofenolate mofetil, methotrexate) and newer biologicals (anti-CD20, anti-IgE) have been described to work in some patients with severe atopic dermatitis as well; however, these substances have to be used 'off label' (i.e. without formal appraisement).

Many dermatologists find that the addition of a topical antibacterial agent (such as triclosan) to the steroid preparation will apparently improve atopic dermatitis, and for many this is routine practice. Topical antibiotics should, however, not be applied in the long term because these may induce resistances and sensitizations. Intermittent short courses of systemic antibiotics with antistaphylococcal action (e.g. clindamycin, cephalosporin derivates, or flucloxacillin) should be used only if there is clinical sign of baterial superinfections of the skin in addition to the eczema.

Management of eczema herpeticum requires systemic aciclovir or related derivates, which are given either orally or intravenously depending on the severity of the exacerbation and on the need to obtain a rapid response.

Phototherapy

Phototherapy – including UVB (290–320 nm), UVA (320–400 nm), and combinations of UVA and UVB – and photochemotherapy (PUVA) have long been used to treat atopic dermatitis. The recent development of specific emission spectra has resulted in a re-evaluation of the efficacy of phototherapy for atopic dermatitis. Compared with conventional UVB, narrow-band UVB (311 nm) radiation is less erythemogenic and causes fewer side effects and, according to recent studies, atopic dermatitis appears to respond well to the therapy. Long-waved UVA (UVA1, 340–400 nm) is used successfully for the treatment of atopic dermatitis as well; it is less erythemogenic than conventional UVA.

Specific immunotherapy

Specific immunotherapy with extracts of airborne allergens that attenuate the cutaneous late phase response to aeroallergens appears to be a promising treatment. Allergen desensitization has been shown to be effective in some therapeutic trials in patients who have a history of exacerbation after exposure to the suspected allergens. These data appear to be sufficient to recommend specific immunotherapy in those patients who suffer from respiratory symptoms and atopic dermatitis. It has to be proved in ongoing or future prospective studies whether atopic dermatitis alone may be the indication for specific immunotherapy.

New approaches to therapy

New drugs that are discussed for the therapy of atopic dermatitis include inhibitors of signal transduction pathways such as p38 MAPK, inhibitors of angiogenesis such as VEGF inhibitors, and cytokine and/or T-cell activation inhibitors such as WBI-1001. More experimental approaches include topical siRNA applications or kinase inhibitors from oncology, but these need far more investigation before developments are possible.

PART II Allergic contact dermatitis

Allergic contact dermatitis of a delayed-type hypersensitivity reaction (so-called type IV reaction), mediated largely by previously sensitized lymphocytes, that causes inflammation and oedema in the skin. It is not linked to atopy.

Anatomy and physiology

The main histological findings of contact dermatitis have been summarized earlier; Figure 13.2 shows some of these. The earliest histological change, which is seen about 4 hours after epicutaneous challenge with an antigen, is a periappendageal and perivascular mononuclear cell infiltrate. By 8 hours, mononuclear cells begin to infiltrate the epidermis. The infiltrates increase to a maximum at 48–72 hours — by which time there is oedema of the epidermis — after which the reaction subsides. The majority of infiltrating cells are CD4+, although the quantity of CD8+ T cells can be as high as 50%. Basophils are also observed in the early infiltrate of allergic contact dermatitis. The numbers of Langerhans' cells increase in the epidermis at 24–48 hours, and CD1a+ cells are found in the dermal infiltrate as well. Macrophages invade the dermis at 48 hours.

Disease mechanisms

Most allergens in allergic contact dermatitis are of low molecular weight (less than 1 kDa) and, though many of them have a complicated structure, they are often called 'simple chemicals'. Contact allergens are haptens and need to link with proteins (so-called carriers) in the skin before they become antigenic. Haptens may be readily absorbed transcutaneously. Of clinical interest, humidity and warmer ambient temperature increase allergen penetration. An intact skin surface decreases penetrability, whereas maceration by sweating, occlusion, water immersion, or genetically inherited barrier defects (such as filaggrin loss-of-function mutations) increases the accessibility of antigens and irritants. Generally, a dry or inflamed skin presents a broken barrier and a greater vulnerability.

Once in the extravascular spaces, most haptens bind in a covalent fashion to their carrier proteins – usually serum proteins – or to the cell membranes of antigen-presenting cells. For example, nickel binds, through its interaction with the amino acid histidine, to peptides present in the specialized peptide-binding groove of MHC class II molecules.

The most potent cells that are able to present antigens to T lymphocytes are epidermal Langerhans' cells and dermal dendritic cells. Langerhans' cells form an extensive network in the epidermis to trap and process epicutaneously applied antigens (Fig. 13.22). These cells are dendritic cells derived from bone marrow and are characterized by the membrane expression of Langerin (CD207), CD1a, and MHC class II antigens; also, they contain a unique organelle, the Birbeck granule, which is seen on electromicroscopic examination. In the corium, dermal dendritic cells – composed of at least three subpopulations – and certain types of macrophages are available for antigen presentation, which is the key event in delayed hypersensitivity.

The development of contact hypersensitivity usually occurs in only a minority of individuals exposed to potential allergens, although certain substances have a greater likelihood of inducing sensitivity. For example,

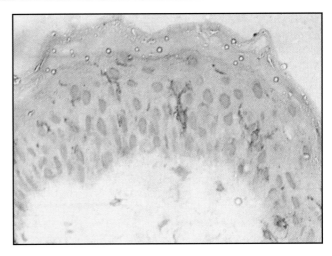

Fig. 13.22 Langerhans' cells in a skin section stained using a monoclonal antibody to CD1a. These dendritic cells comprise 3% of epidermal cells (×312).

dinitrochlorobenzene will sensitize over 90% of normal individuals upon repeated skin contact. Some studies suggest that the allergeneity of a molecule may be associated with its potential to induce intracellular activation steps with the subsequent release of proinflammatory cytokines – such as IL-1β – from antigen-presenting cells. Sensitization takes 10–14 days to develop. If examined prospectively, it is characterized clinically on about the 10th day by an eczematous flare reaction at the site of the sensitizing application. Most epicutaneously applied allergens that attach to the cell membrane of cutaneous dendritic cells are internalized. Activated dendritic cells up-regulate certain chemokine receptors (particularly CCR7) and follow a gradient of the respective receptor ligands in the dermis and draining lymphatics after they have moved out of the epidermis until they reach the regional lymph nodes. There they may congregate in the paracortical areas of the regional lymph nodes and have the opportunity to present the processed antigen (associated with MHC class II molecules) to a large number of T lymphocytes (Fig. 13.23). If sensitization develops, a population of antigen-specific sensitized CD4+ T lymphocytes is produced.

Inflammatory cells and mediators

Figure 13.24 illustrates that an antigen applied epicutaneously to the skin of a sensitized individual is again processed by Langerhans' cells and expressed on the cell surfaces in association with MHC class II molecules. Langerhans' cells then present antigens not only in the lymph nodes but also in the skin to specific memory T lymphocytes. T cells become activated both by the direct contact of antigen receptors to the antigen–MHC complex and by cytokines secreted from antigen-presenting cells, from other cells of the skin (e.g. keratinocytes), and from

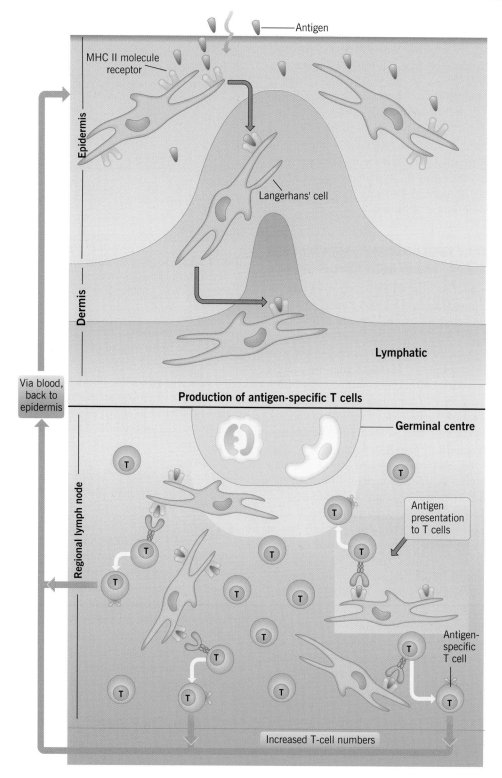

Fig. 13.23 Antigen-bearing Langerhans' cells migrate, via the lymphatics, to the regional lymph nodes. In the paracortical area they interdigitate with CD4+ T lymphocytes, resulting in the generation of antigen-specific memory T cells.

other skin-infiltrating T cells. The latter produce a mixed cytokine pattern – including IL-4 and IFN-γ – in acute allergic contact dermatitis and a more pronounced type 1 cytokine pattern in the chronic phase of dermatitis. The production of cytokines and chemokines results, through a variety of mechanisms, in the accumulation of antigen-specific and non-antigen-specific effector T cells and in the expression of adhesion molecules and MHC class II molecules on the cell membranes in the skin (Fig. 13.25). Less than 10% of T cells in allergic contact dermatitis are

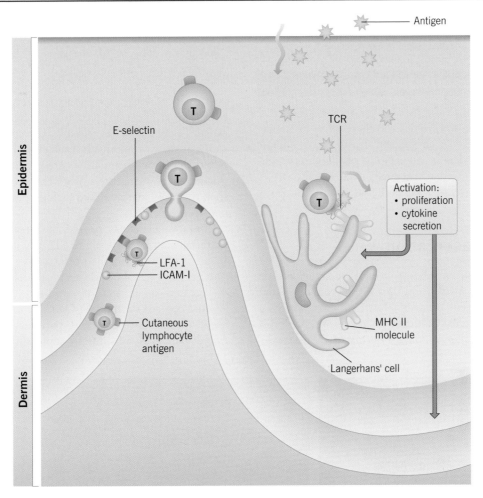

Fig. 13.24 The presentation by Langerhans' cells of processed antigen to T cells results in a cascade of events leading to the influx of mononuclear cells into the dermis and epidermis and the development of dermatitis. For the purpose of clarity, most constitutional cutaneous cells are deleted from the scheme. LFA-1, leukocyte-function-associated antigen 1; ICAM-1, intercellular adhesion molecule 1; T, T lymphocyte; MHC II, major histocompatibility complex class II; TCR, T-cell receptor.

allergen specific. Endothelial cells are stimulated early by cytokines to express molecules involved in lymphocyte adhesion such as the intercellular adhesion molecule (ICAM-1) or E-selectin. Circulating T lymphocytes, through their expression of corresponding ligands such as leukocyte function antigens (LFA) or CLA, recognize adhesion molecules on the surface membranes of endothelial cells and can bind to these cells. This further increases the transport of mononuclear cells through the skin.

Spontaneous resolution occurs after the antigen is removed and the T-cell mediators disappear. A number of mechanisms are involved in the down-regulation of the inflammatory response. Macrophages and keratinocytes produce prostaglandins of the E series, which inhibit the production of (proinflammatory) cytokines. Other mediators, such as leukotriene B$_4$, transforming growth factor, or IL-10, may be involved in down-regulation of the eczematous reaction as well. In addition, T-regulatory cells inhibit T-cell proliferation by cell-to-cell contacts. The role of skin-infiltrating CD8+ T cells is not clear yet,

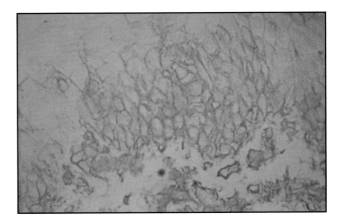

Fig. 13.25 MHC class II antigen expression by keratinocytes in allergic contact dermatitis (×400).

but a subpopulation of these cells may function as suppressor cells that dampen down the reaction.

Clinical presentation

Women present more commonly than men with allergic contact dermatitis, and there is an increase in incidence with advancing age. The clinical features of allergic contact dermatitis depend on the type of allergen responsible (Fig. 13.26). Dermatitis usually occurs at the site of allergen application, but a spreading of the dermatitis is also possible.

Symptom presentation

A number of common allergens have been defined in several parts of the world, and they differ from continent to continent. In some areas of North America, plants – particularly poison oak and poison ivy – are the most common cause of allergic contact dermatitis. Worldwide,

however, nickel sulphate is now the leading cause of allergic contact dermatitis.

Common sources of allergens in Europe and North America are shown in Table 13.3. Many patients find it difficult to understand that material handled for many years can suddenly give rise to an allergic contact dermatitis; similarly, allergy to a regular cosmetic or washing powder may not be regarded by the patient as a possible cause of their problems. In such cases it must be remembered that new formulations are continually being introduced and also that it is often the preservative – rather than the main ingredient of such preparations – that gives rise to problems.

Contact dermatitis caused by an allergy to airborne material may be difficult to identify, but this can occur (e.g. with plants, volatile preservatives in wall colours, or fine particles of rubber dust in cars). If a contact allergen is ingested or inhaled it can lead to haematogenous allergic contact dermatitis. Due to the common involvement of the buttocks, this particular characteristic is called 'baboon syndrome' by some authors (Fig. 13.27).

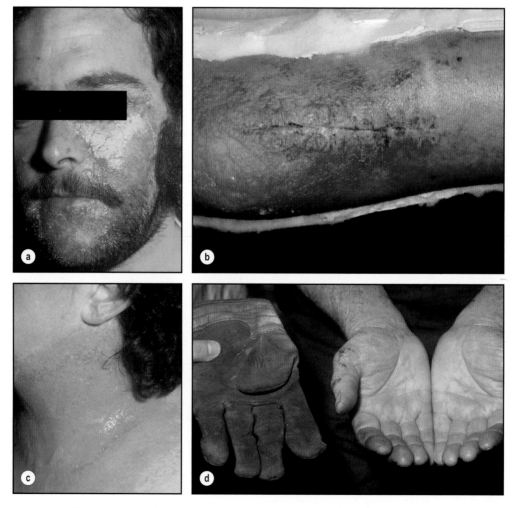

Fig. 13.26 Contact dermatitis: (a) caused by eyedrops containing neomycin; (b) caused by mercury (applied as disinfectant); (c) caused by perfume spray; (d) caused by industrial gloves.

Table 13.3 Common agents causing allergic contact dermatitis and their sources

Agent	Found in
Nickel	Clothing clasps, earrings, spectacle frames, jewellery, coins, household utensils
Chromate	Leather, bleaches, matches, cement
Formaldehyde	Preservatives, cosmetics, cigarettes, newsprint, fabric softeners, wrinkle-resistant clothes
Chloroisothiazolinone	Preservatives in creams and technical fluids
Dibromocyanobutane	Preservatives in creams and cosmetics
Mercaptobenzothiazole	Rubber products (especially boots and gloves), catheters
Thiurams, paraphenylenediamine	Rubber products, fungicide in paint and soap, hair dye, clothing dye, stockings and tights
Plants	*Primula obconica* (Europe), *Rhus*, (poison ivy – North America), Compositae, tulips

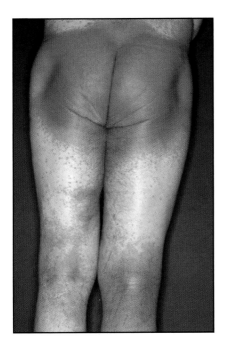

Fig. 13.27 Haematogenous contact dermatitis ('baboon syndrome').

Diagnosis of allergic contact dermatitis

History

Important clinical information comes from the patient's history. Points that should be considered in particular are any recent and continous direct contacts of lesional skin with substances from the private and professional individual environment. Since airborne and haematogenous allergens may rarely also be relevant, these points have to be addressed in the history.

The important points in the clinical identification of allergic contact dermatitis are shown in Figure 13.28. In taking the patient's history, it is important for the clinician to consider occupational, household, and recreational exposure to possible allergens.

Patch testing

Once there is a suspicion of allergic contact dermatitis, patch testing is warranted. The selection of test batteries for patch tests is highly dependent on the clinical presentation of the disease and on anamnestic data. It has been estimated that 2800 of the more than 6 million chemicals that are in the environment have contact-sensitizing properties, which underlines the need for a rational selection of substances for individual tests. It is crucial, however, to realize that many patients are unaware of any relevant exposures, despite a careful history. Done appropriately, patch tests always provide useful information – whether the results are positive or negative.

False positive reactions may be due to patch testing too soon after treatment of acute dermatitis, and false negatives may be due to prior UV radiation, or the use of steroids or other immunosuppressant drugs. Systemic antihistamines have no effect on eczematous patch-test results. The technique of patch testing is deceptively simple. The European standard battery of allergens, shown in Table 13.4, is a collection of the allergens that most often lead to epicutaneous sensitization; a similar battery is available for North America. In addition to the European standard battery, additional batteries are available for certain body sites and for certain occupations.

The allergens are prepared in appropriate concentrations in an appropriate diluent – usually white soft paraffin – and are applied to the skin on inert metal disks such as Finn chambers (Fig. 13.29). After 24–48 hours, the battery of chambers is removed and areas of erythema or induration are noted (Fig. 13.30 and Table 13.5). A

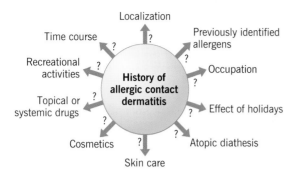

Fig. 13.28 Important points of the patient's history of allergic contact dermatitis.

similar reading is taken 24 hours after removal of the chambers (i.e. 48–72 hours after application of the prepared allergens).

Antigen selection and patch-test interpretation can be difficult; a well-demarcated, red, raised area is in most cases due not to an allergic contact dermatitis but to an irritant reaction. Adverse reactions during patch testing include a severe irritant reaction, which may cause blistering, sensitization to material that previously produced no response, the development of a Koebner reaction if the patient has a tendency to psoriasis or lichen planus, and a flare of pre-existing dermatitis.

The sensitivity of patch tests depends on individual contact allergens and, on the whole, is about 60–80% in different studies. However, around 10% of healthy people

Table 13.4 The European standard contact dermatitis testing battery

Compound	Concentration % (w/w) in petrolatum	Compound	Concentration % (w/w) in petrolatum
Potassium dichromate	0.5	Epoxy resin	1.0
4-phenylenediamine base	1.0	Myroxylon pereirae resin	25.0
Thiuram mix	1.0	4-tert-Butylphenol formaldehyde resin	1.0
Tetramethylthiuram monosulfide (TMTM)	0.25	Mereaptobenzothiazole (MBT)	2.0
Tetramethylthiuram disulfide (TMTD)	0.25	Formaldehyde	1.0†
Tetraethylthiuram disulfide (TETD)	0.25	Fragrance mix	8.0‡
Dipentamethylenethiuram disulfide (PTD)	0.25	Cinnamic alcohol	1.0
Neomycin sulfate	20.0	Cinnamic aldehyde	1.0
Cobalt chloride	1.0	Hydroxycitronellal	1.0
Benzocaine	5.0	α-Amylcinnamic aldehyde	1.0
Nickel sulfate	5.0	Geraniol	1.0
Clioquinol (Chinotorm and Violorm)	5.0	Eugenol	1.0
Colophonium	20.0	Isoeugenol	1.0
Parabens	16.0	Oakmoss absolute	1.0
Methyl-4-hydroxybenzoate	4.0	Sesquiterpene lactone mix	0.1
Ethyl-4-hydroxybenzoate	4.0	Alantolaetone	0.033
Propyl-4-hydroxybenzoate	4.0	Dehydrocostus lactone + Costunolide	0.067
Butyl-4-hydroxybenzoate	4.0	Quaternium-15 (Dowicil 200)	1.0
N-Isopropyl-N-phenyl-4-phenylenediamine	0.1	Primin	0.01
Lanolin alcohol	30.0	Cl + Me-isothiazolinone (Kathon CG, 100 p.p.m.)	0.01†
Mercapto mix	2.0	Budesonide	0.01
N-Cyclohexylbenzothiazyl sulfenamide	0.5	Tixocortol pivalate	0.1
Mereaptobenzothiazole	0.5	Methyldibromo glutaronitrile	0.5
Dibenzothiazyl disulfide	0.5		
Morpholinylmercaptobenzothiazole	0.5		

Modified from http://www.escd.org/aims/standard_series/European_Standard.pdf.

† in water.

‡ with emulsifier sorbitansesquiloleat 5%.

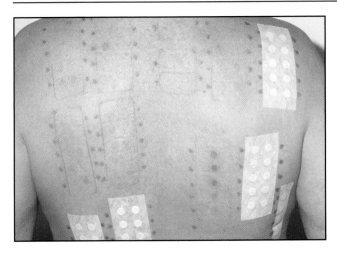

Fig. 13.29 Patch testing. General view showing the number of allergens that can be tested for at any one time.

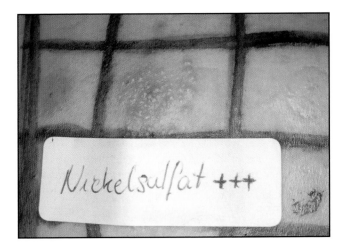

Fig. 13.30 Patch testing showing 48 hours' positive reaction to nickel sulphate.

Table 13.5 Interpretation of patch-test reactions

?	Doubtful reaction, faint macular erythema only
+	Weak (non-vesicular) positive reaction: erythema, infiltration, possibly papules
+ +	Strong (vesicular) positive reaction: erythema, infiltration, papules, vesicles
+ + +	Extreme positive reaction: bullous reaction
–	Negative reaction
IR	Irritant reaction of different types
NT	Not tested

in populations who have no skin disease will have unexpected, apparently irrelevant, positive results. In the case of some potential allergens, the classic 48-hour closed patch test is inappropriate because it does not give a true reflection of the individual's contact with the allergen in normal daily life. Consequently, some alternatives have been introduced – the most important being the open patch test, which is recommended for the investigation of irritating substances.

The identification of a photosensitizer is performed with the photopatch test. Each substance has to be applied at two symmetric sites on the back, as in classic patch-test procedures. One set of the duplicate patches will be irradiated with UVA light, whereas the non-irradiated set serves as a control.

For many years there have been efforts to develop in vitro tests that are more sensitive. Lymphocyte proliferation has been found, in published studies, to be elevated in patients with positive patch tests to some allergens. However, as the risk of false positive reactions is high in

routine diagnosis, it is not recommend in current guidelines of allergic contact dermatitis.

The basic battery of standard antigens is helpful in the great majority (80%) of cases. Substances that commonly cause allergic contact dermatitis include rubber, cosmetics, preservatives, fragrances, dyes, chemicals, topical medicaments, and metal salts.

Common allergen sources and special clinical features of allergic contact dermatitis

Metal allergies

Nickel dermatitis is extremely common in women, and in Northern Europe more than 10% of the female population is affected. A high proportion of patients with allergic contact dermatitis first develop their problem after skin piercing. The frequency of nickel dermatitis has increased in the male population during the last decade, which may be due to an increased popularity of piercing in this group. In the European Union, it is now illegal to sell earrings and other items of jewellery that release a high concentration of nickel. Obvious areas of involvement are beneath rings, watches, bracelets, spectacle frames, coins in pockets, jeans studs, and other sites of direct contact with metal (Figs 13.31, 13.32). Less-obvious areas are the eyelids and the nape of the neck. A serious problem in occupational dermatology is the well-known induction of hand dermatitis in individuals sensitized to nickel who have to work in a wet environment. This may be due to additional effects of continuing skin irritation and contact with low concentrations of nickel ions in fluids.

To determine whether a metal contains nickel, a spot test can be carried out using dimethylglyoxime – a pink colour develops if nickel is present in the material tested. There is continuing controversy over whether the nickel content of a normal diet can provoke or aggravate pre-existing nickel dermatitis. Such a diet may be beneficial in those patients who clearly respond to oral

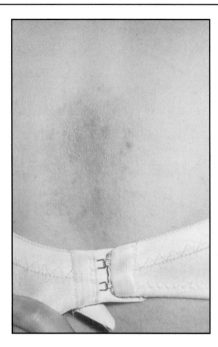

Fig. 13.31 Nickel sensitivity to metal clips in underwear.

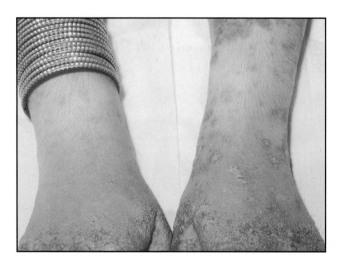

Fig. 13.32 Nickel sensitivity to bracelets.

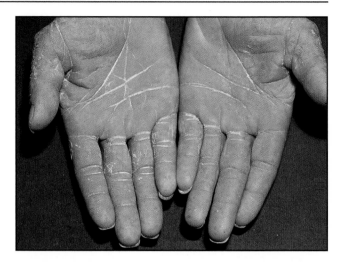

Fig. 13.33 Hand dermatitis caused by chromates.

provocation with nickel sulphate within 24–48 hours with a dyshidrosiform eruption on the hands and feet, but the rate of nickel-allergic patients who respond to nickel upon oral provocation is less than 3%.

Dry, lichenified hand or foot dermatitis is frequently caused by chromates (Fig. 13.33). Hexavalent metal salts of chromate are among the most important causes of contact reactions. They are found in cement, detergents, bleaches, and match heads and are used in tanning leather. In some countries the chromate is removed from cement because of its association with contact dermatitis.

Preservatives

These are ubiquitous antibacterials used in the industry to prevent contamination. Cosmetic products with a high water content (e.g. lotions, gels – also in hair cosmetics) require more preservatives than do pure ointments (e.g. petroleum jelly), which can be preservative free. Formaldehyde, bronopol, quaternium-15, imidazolidinyl urea, dimethyloldimethyl hydantoin, dibromocyanobutane, methylchloroisothiazolinone, and parabens are common sensitizers. Quaternium-15, imidazolidinyl urea, and dimethyloldimethyl hydantoin are potential formaldehyde releasers and may therefore cause problems with formaldehyde-sensitive patients. Each preservative can be identified by a vast number of synonyms and the clinician must be familiar with these when reading product labelling.

Rubber ingredients and ingredients in dark colours

Patients with hand, foot, waistband, and chest rashes should be suspected of being allergic to rubber ingredients in gloves, shoes, elasticated skirts/trousers, and bra straps respectively. Knee braces, elbow braces, and other prostheses are also common culprits. Shoes present a particular challenge in these patients as virtually every commercially available shoe contains some rubber.

Rubber allergies are common among those involved in rubber manufacturing and the possible allergens include the thiurams, mercaptobenzothiazole, and p-phenylenediamine (PPD). Mercaptobenzothiazole and thiurams are accelerators used in the manufacture of both natural and synthetic rubber, and PPD derivates are found in dark rubber. Sensitizations to PPD can also occur upon application of dark colourants (e.g. in temporary tattoos) on the skin. These substances are also major components of most hair dyes, and of dyes for some stockings and tights.

Plant dermatitis

Although common, plant dermatitis is not evaluated by standard patch testing. The most common plant

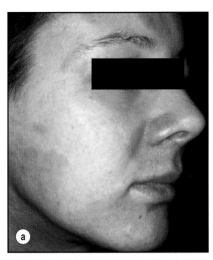

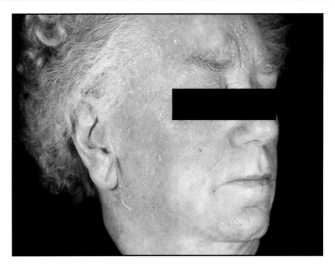

Fig. 13.35 Photoallergic contact dermatitis.

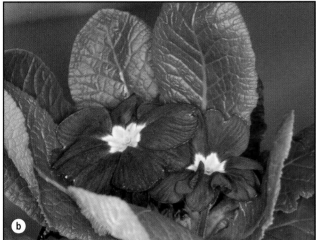

Fig. 13.34 Plant dermatitis. (a) Facial dermatitis eruption (with the characteristic patchy distribution), caused by *Primula* (b).

dermatitis in the USA is caused by poison ivy and/or poison oak; their allergenicity is due to the antigen urushiol. There is also cross-reactivity with other related plants such as cashew, mango (skin), and ginkgo (leaves). Patients with acute perioral dermatitis due to these foods are usually unaware of the cross-relationship. Sesquiterpene lactones are found in members of the Compositae family (chrysanthemum, ragweed, artichoke, chamomile, daisy, dandelion, etc.), but also in unrelated plants; in Northern Europe, *Primula obconica* is a common cause of such problems (Fig. 13.34). The allergen involved is primin, which is airborne and can cause an acute reaction. Tulip bulb handlers may also develop a problem with a dry cracked dermatitis on the fingertips, which is caused by handling the bulbs.

Photosensitizers

The most frequent sites of allergic photocontact dermatitis are exposed areas (e.g. face, neck, back of the hands, etc.), but any skin area receiving sufficient light and a photosensitizing chemical may manifest a reaction (Fig. 13.35). The most important differential diagnoses are airborne or phototoxic contact dermatitis – the latter being based on a non-immunological mechanism and often manifested clinically as exaggerated sunburn reactions. The most common phototoxins and photoallergens are activated by UVA radiation (320–400 nm). Paradoxically, sunscreen agents have become the most common causative substances of photoallergic contact dermatitis; p-aminobenzoic acid (PABA) – and its esters – and oxybenzone are the most frequent sensitizers. Other frequent photoallergens are fragrances, chlorpromazine, and phenothiazine and its derivatives. The last two substances are used as sedatives in veterinary medicine, as insecticides, and as antipsychotic agents.

Some individuals who develop a photoallergic contact dermatitis will retain a persistent reactivity to light long after the exposure to photosensitizing compounds. The mechanism of this reaction remains obscure. A plausible theory may be that the patient has become autophotosensitized to a carrier protein that absorbs photons in the UV range, thereby producing an eczematous response.

Management of allergic contact dermatitis

General principles

The initial management of all types of suspected allergic contact dermatitis consists of reduction or, if possible, elimination of all suspected allergens and the use of a topical steroid of appropriate potency or – particularly in the face – a topical calcineurin inhibitor to return the skin to a normal state. The use of a systemic steroid, such as prednisone in doses of 30 mg or greater daily, will be necessary in the treatment of allergic contact dermatitis that involves more than 30% of the body surface. Once the likely causes of the patient's dermatological problems have been determined by patch testing, it is very important for the clinician to communicate this information to the patient in a way that is easy to understand. This involves careful explanation of the material or materials that contain the offending allergen. In some countries the patient is given an 'allergy passport', which usually contains both the designation and information about identified allergens. This information should also be given to other physicians involved as their support will be needed.

Allergen avoidance

Allergen avoidance can be rather simple at times (e.g. topical antibiotics), whereas at other times it can be virtually impossible (e.g. chromate or nickel). A visit to a patient's place of employment may be necessary to identify an occupational causative substance. Skin protection from chemicals known to cause allergic contact dermatitis is sometimes difficult and barrier creams or gloves should be used whenever possible. The prognosis of allergic contact dermatitis varies, depending on the individual's sensitization pattern. Unfortunately, 70% of patients sensitized to ubiquitous allergens will still have some degree of dermatitis after some years, in spite of avoiding substances containing high concentrations of such allergens.

Conclusions

All allergists must be familiar with atopic dermatitis and allergic contact dermatis, the most common inflammatory skin diseases related to allergy.

Summary of important messages

- Atopic dermatitis and allergic contact dermatitis belong to the group of eczematous skin diseases with an involvement of the most upper layer of the skin: the epidermis
- Atopic dermatitis consists of subgroups; however, allergic trigger factors may be relevant for a significant group of the patients
- Management of atopic dermatitis consists of basic treatment modalities, symptomatic anti-inflammatory approaches, and allergological procedures
- Allergic contact dermatitis is not related to atopy; however, atopic individuals including those suffering from atopic dermatitis may develop allergic contact dermatitis as well
- A good history and patch testing form the mainstay in the diagnosis of allergic contact dermatitis
- The management of allergic contact dermatitis consists of allergen avoidance and symptomatic anti-inflammatory therapy

Identification of relevant allergens can be difficult since there is usually a delay of onset of clinical symptoms after contact with allergens. That implicates that there is still a great need for the development of better diagnostic in vitro tests for both diseases. Due to a continous increase in the knowledge base, it can be anticipated that more-specific symptomatic treatment modalities will be developed both for acute exacerbations and for the chronic forms of both diseases.

Further reading

Akdis CA, Akdis M, Bieber T, et al. AAAAI/EAACI/ PRACTALL consenus report. Diagnosis and treatment of atopic dermatitis in children and adults. J Allergy Clin Immunol 2006; 118:152–169.

Ale IS, Maibacht HA. Diagnostic approach in allergic and irritant contact dermatitis. Expert Rev Clin Immunol 2010; 6:291–310.

Bieber T. Atopic dermatitis. N Engl J Med 2008; 358:1483–1494.

Boguniewicz M, Leung DY. Recent insights into atopic dermatitis and implications for management of infectious complications. J Allergy Clin Immunol 2010; 125:4–13.

Breuer K, Werfel T, Kapp A. Safety and efficacy of topical immunomodulators in the treatment of childhood eczema. Am J Clin Dermatol 2005; 6:65–70.

Darsow U, Wollenberg A, Simon D, et al. ETFAD/EADV eczema task force 2009 position paper on diagnosis and treatment of atopic dermatitis. J Eur Acad Dermatol Venereol 2010; 24:317–328.

Fonacier LS, Dreskin SC, Leung DY. Allergic skin diseases. J Allergy Clin Immunol 2010; 125(2 suppl 2):S138–149.

Kerr A, Ferguson J. Photoallergic contact dermatitis. Photodermatol Photoimmunol Photomed 2010; 26:56–65.

Lee PW, Elsaie ML, Jacob SE. Allergic contact dermatitis in children: common allergens and treatment: a review. Curr Opin Pediatr 2009; 21:491–498.

Mortz CG, Andersen KE. New aspects in allergic contact dermatitis. Curr Opin Allergy Clin Immunol 2008; 8:428–432.

Niebuhr M, Werfel T. Innate immunity, allergy and atopic dermatitis. Curr Opin Allergy Clin Immunol 2010; 10:463–468.

Nosbaum A, Vocanson M, Rozieres A, et al. Allergic and irritant contact dermatitis. Eur J Dermatol 2009; 19:325–332.

Ong PY. Emerging drugs for atopic dermatitis. Expert Opin Emerging Drugs 2009; 14:165–179.

Valenta R, Mittermann I, Werfel T, et al. Linking allergy to autoimmune disease. Trends Immunol 2009; 30:109–116.

Werfel T. The role of leukocytes, keratinocytes and allergen-specific IgE in the development of atopic dermatitis. J Invest Dermatol 2009; 129:1878–1891.

Food allergy and gastrointestinal syndromes

Stephan C Bischoff and Hugh A Sampson

DEFINITION

Gastrointestinal allergy is an immune-mediated adverse reaction of the gastrointestinal tract in response to ingested food. It may result in variable gastrointestinal symptoms such as pharyngeal pruritus, dysphagia, vomiting, abdominal pain, diarrhoea and malabsorption.

Introduction

Food allergy is a common and often underdiagnosed disorder, which frequently has been neglected even by allergologists. A major reason for this disregard is an uncertainty on the part of many physicians about the appropriate diagnostic means to confirm the disease, which is mandatory because only a small portion of patients with adverse reactions to food suffer from true food allergy. In industrialized countries approximately 20–30% of the population claims adverse reactions to food; however only approximately one-quarter of these cases in children and one-tenth of the cases in adults are caused by immune-mediated food allergies. In young children, the major manifestations of food allergy concern the skin or the gastrointestinal (GI) tract, whereas in adults the spectrum of afflicted organs is much broader and less specific. However, also in adults, the skin, GI tract, and mouth/throat area are most common sites of manifestations, followed by the respiratory tract, and less specific manifestations involving the vascular and nervous systems.

In about one-third to one-half of the cases with food allergy, depending on age and other unknown factors, the major symptoms involve the GI tract. These food allergies that manifest in the GI tract are often referred to as 'GI allergy'. The remaining adverse reactions to food are defined as clinically abnormal reactions to ingested food or food additives based on non-immune reactions (food intolerances). Food intolerances include carbohydrate intolerances (lactose, fructose, sorbit, etc.), amine intolerances (histamine, serotonin, etc.), and other forms of intolerances. They have to be considered in the differential diagnosis of GI allergy. Although diagnosis of food allergy remains a particular challenge, therapy is clear and well established. An individual elimination diet, and if required emergency treatment with drugs, is the therapy of choice – as stated in several guidelines around the world. A number of therapeutic trials investigating various means of treating IgE-mediated food allergies (e.g. oral immunotherapy, sublingual immunotherapy, recombinant protein vaccines, etc.) are showing promise, but these are all considered experimental at this time.

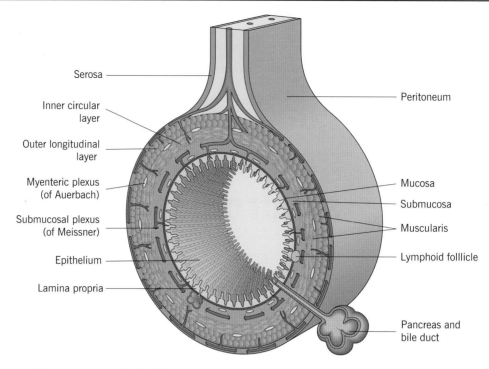

Fig. 14.1 Anatomy of the intestinal wall. The histological anatomy of the small intestine is shown. A similar architecture of the bowel layers is found at other sites of the gastrointestinal tract.

Anatomy and physiology of the intestinal tract

The gastrointestinal tract comprises the largest surface area of the body – approximately equivalent to the size of one tennis court. It must prevent the entrance of harmful pathogens whilst readily absorbing various nutrients.

Anatomy

In general, the GI tract is comprised of four concentric layers; from the lumen outward, they are the mucosa, submucosa, muscularis propria, and serosa (Fig. 14.1). The mucosa comprises the epithelium, the lamina propria – a loose connective tissue rich in immune-competent cells – and the circular muscularis mucosae. The epithelium may invaginate to form glands or ducts that extend to organs outside the GI tract, such as the pancreas or liver. The mucosa (and submucosa) may also project into the GI lumen as folds (plicae) or villi. The submucosa is a more densely collagenous, less cellular structure than the mucosa, and contains major blood vessels, lymphatics, nerves, ganglia, and occasionally lymphoid collections. The tunica muscularis comprises at least two muscular layers: the inner circular layer and the outer longitudinal layer. The tunica serosa consists of loose, connective tissue with fat, collagen, and elastic fibres.

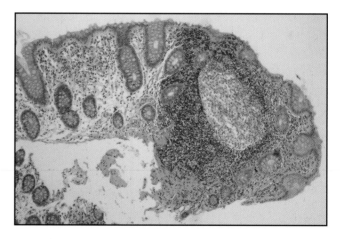

Fig. 14.2 Gut-associated lymphoid tissue. A large lymphoid follicle can be seen in the mucosa of the caecum (haematoxylin and eosin stain, original magnification ×100).

Lymphoid tissue

The gut-associated lymphoid tissue (GALT) is primarily located in the lamina propria (Fig. 14.2). It may be present diffusely or as solitary or aggregated nodules, known as Peyer's patches, in the small intestine. Lymphoid follicles surrounded by a plexus of blood vessels and lymphatic capillaries are found in all sections of the GI tract, and contain both B and T lymphocytes. The lymphoid cells form part of the mucosal immune system and secrete IgA as well as other immunoglobulins and cytokines. Lymphocytes are found in the lamina propria [mostly CD4+ helper T cells (Th cells)] and between the epithelial cells (mostly CD8+ T cells). It is believed that both T and B lymphocytes migrate out of the epithelium to the lymphoid follicles where Th cells aid in the differentiation of B cells to antibody-producing plasma cells. T cells also migrate to mesenteric lymph nodes where they proliferate and enter the systemic circulation, returning back to the mucosa as memory T cells. Antigen-presenting cells (APC) are predominantly found in Peyer's patches or as scattered cells in the lamina propria. The most efficient antigen sampling occurs in the flattened epithelial cells overlying lymphoid aggregates.

The M cell, which is an epithelial cell with microfolds, endocytoses macromolecules and transports them to the basolaterally located intraepithelial lymphocytes. Mucosal plasma cells produce predominantly IgA and IgM antibodies. The Ig monomers are linked by J chains to dimeric secretory IgA or pentameric IgM, which bind to the secretory component – a receptor on glandular epithelial cells that mediates the transport of IgA and IgM to the lumen. IgG and IgE are secreted into the lumen as monomers and the majority diffuse directly into the lymphatics. Apart from lymphocytes, other haematopoietic cells found in the GI tissue, particularly in the small and large bowel, are eosinophil granulocytes (4–6% of the lamina propria cells), neutrophil granulocytes (rare in non-inflamed GI tissue), monocytes, mast cells (2–3% of lamina propria cells), and various types of endocrine cells producing hormones and neurotransmitters such as somatostatin, vasoactive intestinal polypeptide, serotonin, motilin, and substance P (Fig. 14.3).

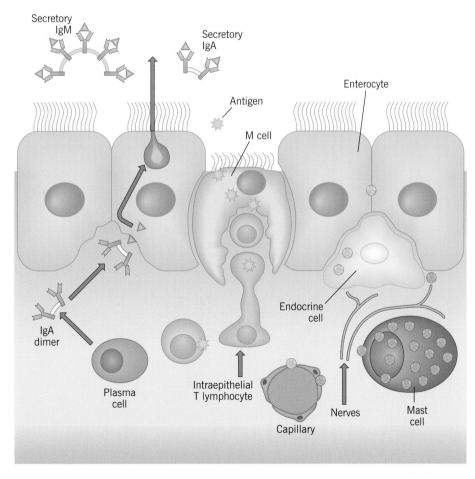

Fig. 14.3 Immune regulation of the intestinal barrier. Lamina propria plasma cells synthesize IgA dimers (linked by J chains), which bind to secretory components expressed on the basal surface of epithelial cells. They are secreted together into the gut lumen. Pentameric IgM is similarly transported. M cells take up and process luminal antigens for presentation to intraepithelial T lymphocytes. Endocrine cells exert a local modulatory activity on neighbouring exocrine and endocrine cells of the gut by direct cell-to-cell contact, or by secretory products diffusing into the interepithelial spaces or across the basal membrane into the lamina propria, where they affect nerve endings, blood vessels, and smooth muscles. Mediators of mast cell release, such as histamine, cause contraction of the muscularis mucosae and blood vessels, modulation of lymphocyte function, and increases in mucus secretion and permeability.

Innervation

The enteric nervous system (ENS) is the most complex portion of the peripheral nervous system. It differs from the sympathetic and parasympathetic division of the autonomous nervous system because most of its component neurons do not receive direct input from the brain or the spinal cord. Therefore, it can mediate reflex activity independently of the central nervous system (Fig. 14.4). The ENS contains integrative circuiting, consisting of interneurons within the ganglia that process information from intramural and mucosal sensory receptors (e.g. fluidity, volume, chemical composition, and temperature of luminal contents) and, via the motoneurons, programmes the appropriate behaviour of the effector system. The majority of the neurons from the submucosal ganglia project into the mucosa.

Neurons of the parasympathetic ganglia are located in the submucosal plexus (Meissner's plexus) and in the myenteric plexus (Auerbach's plexus) lying between the circular and longitudinal layers of the tunica muscularis propria. The myenteric plexus generates the basic electrical rhythm of the gut, but it is not necessary for propagation of the interdigestive myoelectric complex. However, Meissner's and Auerbach's plexuses are interconnected into a single functional system. Stimulation of the parasympathetic neurons usually increases circulation, secretion, and muscular activity, whereas stimulation of the sympathetic system has the reverse effects.

Disease mechanisms

Pathophysiology of food allergy manifesting in the GI tract

As noted above, the GI mucosa has to meet the challenge of protecting the host against possibly harmful nutrients, microbes, and toxins while assuring the uptake of nutrients and antigens indispensable for life. To achieve this, the GI barrier is equipped with an innate immune system and other non-specific defence systems including gastric acid, mucus, and bicarbonate secretion as well as an intact epithelial layer forming tight junctions, peristaltic movement, digestive enzymes, phagocytes, alternative complement pathways, and antimicrobial peptides like defensins and cathelicidins. Macrophages and neutrophils, as well as mast cells and eosinophils, are important effector cells involved in such innate immune responses. Conserved bacterial structures are recognized by these cells through 'pattern recognition receptors', including the Toll-like receptor family. Upon recognition of 'danger signals', these effector cells trigger and/or support adaptive immune responses required for effective host defence

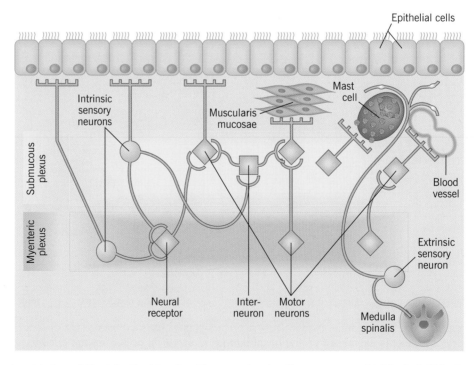

Fig. 14.4 Neuronal regulation of the intestinal barrier. Diagram showing the presence of intrinsic (within the gut wall) and extrinsic (paravertebral neuronal cell bodies) sensory neurons and motor neurons regulating the function of epithelial cells, smooth muscles, blood vessels, and mast cells. Motor neurons are interconnected by interneurons forming a largely autonomous enteric nervous system.

and protection. On the other hand, the GI immune system has the unique capacity to develop 'oral tolerance', a state of acceptance of foreign antigens such as food or particular bacterial antigens, which is achieved by down-regulation of normal immune responses and is necessary for normal gut function.

In some cases, this immunological tolerance is impaired and food proteins are inappropriately recognized by the immune system as harmful antigens, resulting in an abnormal immune response and a subsequent inflammatory reaction of variable extent and duration. The best-defined immune reaction against food involves IgE-mediated hypersensitivity to food. Such reactions lead to an increased release of inflammatory mediators in mast cells, basophils, and eosinophils, and play a central role in the pathogenesis of many cases of asthma, rhinitis, atopic skin diseases, and GI food allergy. Apart from type I reactions, type IV reactions are thought to be involved that are characterized by the activation of food antigen-specific T cells. The type IV reactions are difficult to distinguish from the 'late phase type I reactions' that are observed in about 25% of afflicted individuals. Both forms of delayed reactions have in common the fact that they consist primarily of a so-called 'Th2 immune response', defined not by the antigen-recognizing molecule but by the set of cytokines released during such immune reactions. The most relevant Th2 cytokines are IL-4, IL-5, IL-9, and IL-13. In patients with food allergy, priming of naive lymphocytes of the GALT leads to cytokine-producing Th2 effector cells or IgE-producing plasma cells (Fig. 14.5).

The cause of allergic inflammation that occurs only in selected individuals is still unclear. Apart from a hyper-responsive mucosal immune system, a sufficient amount of allergen is required for an intestinal allergic inflammation. Reasons for the increased antigen exposure could be genetically determined alterations of key molecules of the GI barrier, immaturity of the GI barrier, acquired disturbances of the GI defence system such as enteric infection, or a combination thereof. An impaired mucosal barrier caused by reduced mucus production, decreased defensin expression, challenge to particular toxins, or bacterial/viral infection might be an initial step for the development of immunological hypersensitivity. In addition, a genetic predisposition favouring Th2 responses is required.

Eosinophils (see Ch. 19) have been proposed as major contributors to allergic inflammation because they are typically found in increased numbers at sites of allergic inflammation and are activated for mediator release in the course of IgE-mediated allergic reactions. The responsible factors for eosinophil recruitment identified include interleukins (IL-5, to a lesser extent also IL-3 and GM-CSF) and chemokines [CCL-5 (formerly named RANTES), CCL-11 (formerly named eotaxin), and

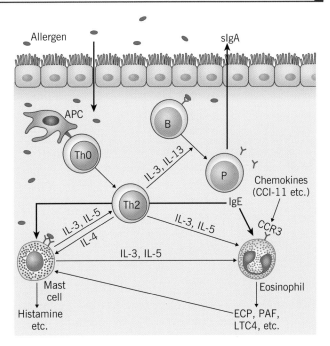

Fig. 14.5 Mechanisms leading to immunological hypersensitivity in the GI tract. APC, antigen-presenting cell; B, B cell; EO, eosinophil; MC, mast cell; P, plasma cell; T, T cell; Th, T-helper cell; IgA, immunoglobulin A; IL, interleukin; ECP, eosinophil cationic protein; PAF, platelet-activating factor; CCR, chemokine. (Modified from Bischoff SC, Crowe SE. Gastrointestinal food allergy: new insights into pathophysiology and clinical perspectives. Gastroenterology 2005; 128:1089–1113.)

others]. The mechanisms of eosinophil activation during allergic reactions are less clear. Eosinophils produce and release highly bioactive inflammatory mediators such as eosinophil cationic protein (ECP), eosinophil-derived neurotoxin (EDN), eosinophil peroxidase (EPO), and major basic protein (MBP). Furthermore, they are a rich source of cytokines and reactive oxygen species, thus participating in cytotoxic and immunoregulatory processes within the allergic reaction (see Fig. 14.5). The clinical symptoms and the organ dysfunction following allergic reactions can be attributed to a large extent to such products. The association between eosinophils and allergy is particularly striking in the GI tract. In contrast to other mucosal sites, the small and large intestine, but not the oesophagus, constitutively contain eosinophils – most probably for defence against parasites and other infections. About 80% of individuals with eosinophilic gastrointestinal disorders (EGIDs) are atopic, and dietary exclusion of the allergen can sometimes reverse disease severity. Furthermore, about 50% of patients with GI allergy show mucosal eosinophilia, further arguing for a major function of eosinophils in GI allergic disorders. Peripheral eosinophilia, which is defined as more than

Table 14.1 Common symptoms of gastrointestinal allergy

Oropharynx	Lip and oral pruritus; lip and tongue swelling
	Pharyngeal pruritus and oedema (oral allergy syndrome)
Stomach	Reflux disease
	Nausea
	Vomiting
Small intestine	Crampy abdominal pain
	Malabsorption
	Vitamin deficiency
Large intestine	Diarrhoea
	Constipation
	Faecal blood loss

Box 14.1 Clinical presentation of food allergy

Immediate food allergy (IgE-mediated in most cases)

- Skin: urticaria, angioedema, flushing, maculopapular rash, pruritus, aggravation of atopic dermatitis
- GI: oral allergy syndrome (OAS), angioedema of the lips, tongue and/or palate, nausea, vomiting, diarrhoea, colic, abdominal pain
- Respiratory: repetitive 'dry' cough, hoarseness, rhinoconjunctivitis, wheezing, dyspnoea
- Cardiovascular: tachycardia, occasionally bradycardia, dysrhythmia, hypotension
- Systemic: anaphylaxis
- Other: uterine contractions, feeling of 'pending doom'

Possible (unproven) food allergy (IgE-Independent reactions? Eosinophilic reactions? Non-immune-mediated reactions?)

- Joints: arthritis
- Nervous system: migraine, headache, fatigue, hyperkinetic syndrome (children)
- GI: bloating, IBS-like symptoms
- Systemic: oedema

400 eosinophils per microlitre, can be seen in approximately 50% of patients with GI eosinophilia.

Pathophysiology of food allergy manifesting outside the GI tract

Over 60 years ago, Walzer and colleagues unequivocally demonstrated the ability of food antigens to traverse the GI barrier and disseminate rapidly throughout the body, even in normal individuals. More recently Husby and coworkers found that about 2% of ingested food protein can reach the circulation in an immunologically intact form. Consequently, the ingestion of food results in potential allergens circulating throughout the body where they can come into contact with IgE bound to mast cells in various tissues (e.g. skin, respiratory tract, and cardiovascular system, as reviewed in Ch. 1). With activation of sufficient mast cells and perhaps other cell types (basophils, antigen-presenting cells), mediators are released that lead to vascular leakage, smooth muscle contraction, mucus secretion, and inflammation in target organs, which result in the classic allergic symptoms depicted in Table 14.1.

Clinical presentation

General clinical presentation

The first scientific report on the ability to transfer allergy with a serum factor involved the use of a food allergen. A small amount of serum was transferred from a Dr C Küstner, a fish-allergic individual, to the non-allergic Dr H Prausnitz. Subsequent challenge of Dr Prausnitz resulted in a wheal-and-flare reaction at the site of serum injection. This study, the Prausnitz–Küstner or PK-reaction, was published in 1921. During the next three decades, increasing numbers of cases of allergic reactions to foods

were described and the spectrum of clinical abnormalities in these cases was broadened to include reactions that were often slower in onset and involved the GI tract, skin, and respiratory and cardiovascular systems. Nowadays, we distinguish between IgE-mediated reactions, presenting in most cases with classical symptoms, and IgE-independent reactions, which often present with more non-specific symptoms involving many organs (Box 14.1).

Clinical presentation of disease subtypes

In children with food allergy either skin symptoms or GI symptoms tend to dominate, whereas in adults the oral allergy syndrome (OAS) is the most frequent manifestation of food allergy. This difference is related to the spectrum of most relevant allergens, which varies according to both the age of the patients and the countries in which they are living (Box 14.2). In children, milk and milk products as well as eggs and peanuts are the most relevant food allergens. In adults, pollen-associated food allergens are of major importance – a phenomenon that is based on the cross-reactivity between food and pollen allergen components such as Bet v1 and Bet v2. Allergens such as fish, shellfish, tree nuts, and peanuts are the most common causes of systemic allergy in adults.

Food allergy manifesting in the GI tract

The symptoms of food allergy manifesting in the GI tract are variable and, to a large extent, non-specific.

Box 14.2 Most frequent food allergens in children and adults

Children	Adults
Milk and milk products	Pollen-associated food allergens (e.g. apple, nuts, celery, carrots, paprika, spices)
Egg	
Wheat	Tree nuts and seeds
Soy, peanuts	Peanuts, soy
Nuts	Fish and shellfish
Fish	Milk and milk products, egg
	Latex-associated food allergens (e.g. banana, avocado, kiwi)

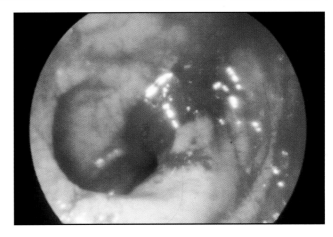

Fig. 14.7 Eosinophilic enterocolitis: macroscopic findings. Endoscopic view of the mucosa of the small intestine (ileum). Note the severe mucosal inflammation with mucosal thickening, loss of normal mucosal surface, and spontaneous bleeding of the mucosa. The photograph was taken from a patient with eosinophilic enterocolitis due to intestinal hypersensitivity reactions toward multiple food allergens.

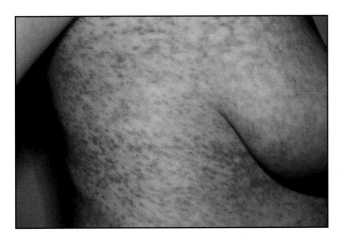

Fig. 14.6 Mastocytosis. Cutaneous manifestation of systemic mastocytosis (urticaria pigmentosa). The patient also suffered from gastrointestinal mastocytosis and hypersensitivity reactions against multiple food allergens.

Depending on the site of mucosal reaction and the type of allergic reaction, the patient may suffer from swelling of the lips, pharyngeal itching, and laryngeal oedema (OAS); reflux, nausea, and vomiting (gastric reactions); abdominal pain, malabsorption, and vitamin deficiency (small intestine); and diarrhoea, constipation, and faecal blood loss (colon and rectum). Macroscopic or histological evidence for inflammatory infiltration and tissue destruction is facultative and may be related to late phase or delayed-type hypersensitivity reactions. In some cases, intestinal food allergy is accompanied by histological findings typical for intestinal mastocytosis (Fig. 14.6), eosinophilic enterocolitis (Figs 14.7–14.9), or coeliac disease (Fig. 14.10). Typically, in patients with active GI allergy the lamina propria is infiltrated with high numbers of eosinophils (see Fig. 14.8). In rare cases, GI allergy may cause a total loss of intact intestinal mucosa, and therefore severe malabsorption, thus making oral nutrition almost impossible (see Fig. 14.9).

The time interval between food challenge and onset of clinical symptoms may vary from a few minutes to many hours. In general, early reactions – occurring within minutes – involve the upper part of the GI tract (e.g. lips, pharynx, stomach, duodenum), whereas late reactions starting after several hours (or days) are often related to the small or large intestine. Early reactions are more frequently IgE-mediated (type I hypersensitivity reactions) and can be readily diagnosed by skin tests or measurements of serum allergen-specific IgE. In contrast, delayed reactions are often based on other mechanisms and are much more difficult to confirm on an objective basis. IgE-mediated reactions, but not delayed reactions, are frequently associated with atopy (atopic dermatitis, allergic rhinoconjunctivitis, extrinsic asthma, atopic relatives, etc.). The relationship between GI allergy and other chronic idiopathic diseases of the gut, such as eosinophilic enterocolitis, coeliac disease, IBD, and irritable bowel syndrome (IBS), is unclear at present. Evidence comes from clinical and pathophysiological observations that such a relationship may exist, at least in subsets of afflicted individuals, and therefore GI allergy should be considered in the differential diagnosis of chronic inflammatory or functional GI diseases of unclear origin.

The prevalence of food allergy is largely unknown. It has been estimated that, depending on the methods used for diagnosis, 1–4% of the general population suffer from food allergy. A population study of food intolerance in adults, published by Young et al in 1994, reported a prevalence of 1.4% based on a questionnaire involving 20 000 individuals who had undergone oral food challenges. Of

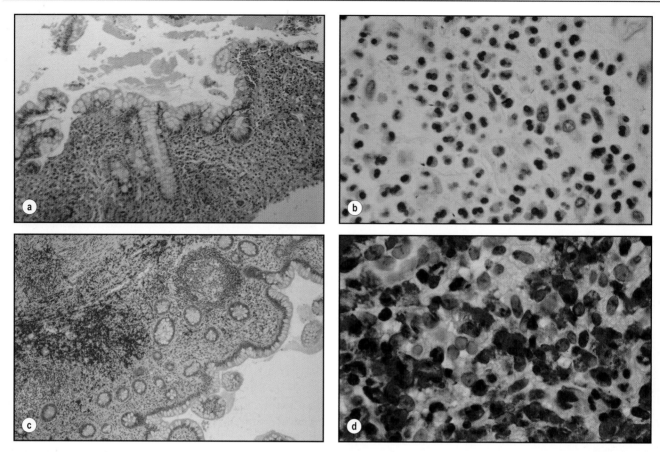

Fig. 14.8 Eosinophilic enterocolitis: histological findings. Large-bowel sections (same patient as in Fig. 14.7). (a) Mucosal destruction and cell infiltration (haematoxylin and eosin stain, ×100). (b) Eosinophilia in the submucosa (haematoxylin and eosin stain, ×500). (c) Immunohistochemical staining using an antibody directed against eosinophil cationic protein stored in the granules of eosinophils (EG2 monoclonal antibody stain, ×100). (d) Same as (c) (×1000).

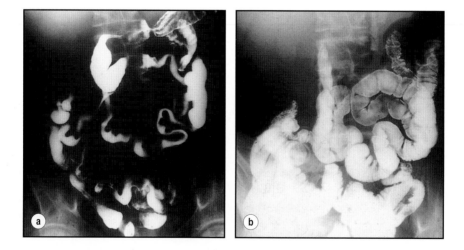

Fig. 14.9 Eosinophilic enterocolitis: radiological findings. X-ray photographs of the small intestine after barium contrast filling (same patient as in Fig. 8.9). (a) Complete loss of normal intestinal mucosa. At that time, the patient suffered from malabsorption syndrome, excessive weight loss, and anaemia. (b) Almost normal mucosa after 8 months of total food allergen avoidance (home-parenteral nutrition). At that time, the patient started to eat following an individual elimination diet without recurrence of the initial symptoms.

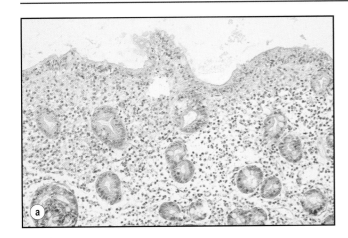

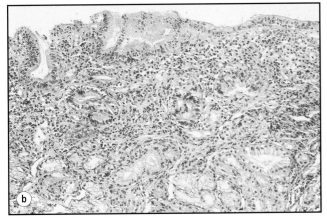

Fig. 14.10 Coeliac disease. (a) Two examples of duodenal tissue sections derived from patients with active coeliac disease. (b) See the complete loss of mucosal villi and dense infiltration of the lamina propria with mononuclear cells and eosinophils. (Courtesy of Rolf Rüdiger Meliβ, Institute of Pathology, Medical School of Hanover, Germany.)

the individuals testing positive in the food challenge, 28% had intestinal symptoms. Two recent meta-analyses suggested that about 1.5%–4.5% of the general population is affected by food allergy. In children during their first 3 years of life, the prevalence of GI food allergy may be somewhat higher (4%–6%). On the other hand, it has been repeatedly reported that 20–45% of the general population believe that they suffer from adverse reactions to food, indicating the necessity of objective diagnostic means.

Food allergy manifesting in the skin

One of the most common food-induced symptoms in the skin is acute urticaria, which may develop within minutes to a few hours of food ingestion. In a subset of patients, an adjuvant factor such as exercise, alcohol, or NSAIDs is necessary in combination with the ingestion of a food in order to induce urticaria (i.e. adjuvant-associated, food-induced urticaria). In contrast, chronic urticaria is

rarely due to food allergy. Other common cutaneous manifestations on the skin include a markedly pruritic, erythematous maculopapular rash, especially in children with atopic dermatitis, flushing, and angioedema. Cutaneous symptoms will often persist for 1–4 hours following an isolated ingestion. In some children with atopic dermatitis, symptom onset is not immediate and only apparent after several hours.

Food allergy induces flares of eczema in about one-third of children with atopic dermatitis. In general, the younger the child and the more severe the atopic dermatitis, the more likely the child is to be affected by food allergy. Egg allergy is the most common trigger, but milk, peanut, soy, wheat, and other cereal grains may also be involved. Elimination of the responsible food allergen often leads to significant clearing of the eczema in affected patients, but food allergy is only one factor involved in the pathogenesis of this disorder. The role of food allergy in adults is less clear, but there is evidence that ingestion of *Bet v 1*-related foods in birch-pollen-allergic individuals may lead to worsening of skin symptoms.

Food allergy manifesting at other body sites

In children, food-induced symptoms of the upper airway alone are uncommon, but are frequently seen in combination with symptoms manifesting in other target organs. Nasal congestion, rhinorrhoea, and sneezing, as well as periocular pruritus, conjunctival erythema, and tearing, are frequently seen with IgE-mediated cutaneous and gastrointestinal symptoms during oral food challenges. Lower respiratory symptoms (e.g. chest tightness, dyspnoea and wheezing) are less common, but typically indicate a more severe reaction. Pulmonary failure is the predominant cause of life-threatening and fatal food-allergic reactions in children.

In severe, life-threatening reactions to foods, the cardiovascular system may be involved manifesting as hypotension (e.g. light-headedness and syncope) and changes in cardiac function (e.g. dysrhythmia, tachycardia, and less often bradycardia). Cardiac failure is the major cause of life-threatening and fatal food-allergic reactions in adults, and occasionally may be the sole manifestation of anaphylaxis.

Anaphylaxis is a generalized allergic reaction that is rapid in onset and may lead to death. Cutaneous symptoms are most frequently involved in combination with gastrointestinal, respiratory, and cardiovascular symptoms, but occasionally are absent – especially in life-threatening or fatal cases. In a subset of patients, adjuvant factors, such as exercise, alcohol, NSAIDs, and menstrual cycle in women, in combination with ingestion of the food allergen are necessary to induce an anaphylactic reaction. Food allergy is the leading cause of anaphylaxis treated in emergency departments in the USA, and accounts for more than 125 000 visits per year.

Table 14.2 Diagnosis of gastrointestinal allergy

History	Symptoms
	Atopy
	Other disease
Gastroenterological examination	Endoscopy (gastroduodenoscopy, colonoscopy)
	Sonograph of the abdomen
	X-ray examinations of the GI tract
	Malabsorption tests
	Histology of biopsy specimens
Laboratory studies	Routine laboratory parameters
	Microbiological examinations (serum, titres, faeces)
	Total IgE and specific IgE (UniCAP®, Immunlite®,) in serum
	Eosinophil-derived cationic proteins in serum and faeces (EPX)
	Basophil histamine release test (BHR)
	Cellular allergen stimulation test (CAST)
Provocation tests	Skin prick tests
	Elimination diet and stepwise rechallenge
	Double-blind placebo-controlled food challenges (DBPCFC)
	Colonoscopic allergen provocation test (COLAP)
Diagnostic trial	Disodium cromoglycate
	Swallowed fluticosone or budesonide spray (metered-dose inhaler)
	Enteral nutrition (tube feeding with elemental diet)
	Total parenteral nutrition

Abbreviations: EPX, eosinophil protein X.

Diagnosis

The diagnosis of food allergy is based primarily on a comprehensive history, which attempts to identify potential relevant food allergens and guide further evaluation, exclude disorders other than allergies, and guide the selective use of established allergy tests (Table 14.2).

Differential diagnosis

The differential diagnosis of food allergy is dependent on the affected organs and the type of symptoms. Most relevant and extensive is the differential diagnosis in cases of GI allergy triggered by food, since so many individuals claim to suffer from adverse reactions to food, but only a minority suffer from true food allergy (Box 14.3).

Investigations and tests

History

A comprehensive history is essential in order to optimize the evaluation and make the diagnosis of food allergy. The following questions should be addressed:

1. What symptoms are associated with the reaction?
2. What food precipitated the symptoms and has it occurred more than once?

Box 14.3 Differential diagnosis of GI allergy

Food intolerances

- Carbohydrate intolerances (lactose, fructose, sorbit malabsorption)
- Histamine intolerance

Inflammatory bowel disease

- Crohn's disease/ulcerative colitis
- Microscopic colitis
- Coeliac disease
- Chronic infectious GI disease (e.g. *Campylobacter jejuni*, *Clostridium difficile*, etc.)
- Other chronic inflammatory bowel diseases
- Extraintestinal inflammation (pancreatitis, acute appendicitis, etc.)

Malignant disease

- Colon carcinoma
- Small intestinal tumour disease (lymphoma, stroma tumours, endocrine tumours)
- Mastocytosis

Irritable bowel syndrome, functional dyspepsia, gastroesophageal reflux disease

3. How much food was ingested when the symptoms occurred?

4. Was the food in a baked (extensively heated) or native (raw) form?

5. How long after ingesting the food did the symptoms occur?

6. Has the food been eaten on other occasions without these symptoms occurring?

7. Have the symptoms been present at times other than following exposure to a given food?

8. Were other factors involved such as exercise, alcohol, or use of aspirin or NSAIDs?

9. What treatment was given, and for how long did the symptoms last?

With this information in hand, the food and type of allergy involved often become evident, which enables the physician to undertake the appropriate confirmatory allergy testing. The practice of obtaining large batteries of skin tests or allergen-specific IgE levels to screen for immediate-type food allergies is rarely appropriate. The history is particularly important in diagnosing GI allergy because of the lack of specific clinical symptoms and laboratory tests specific for GI allergy; therefore the diagnosis of GI allergy to foods or other antigens is largely based on the exclusion of other diseases.

Physical examination

The physical examination includes a general examination of major body functions as well as specific examinations, such as inspection of the skin, the oral cavity and the pharynx, the palpation and percussion of the abdomen, and the digital examination of the rectum. Unless the patient is seen shortly after developing an allergic reaction, the physical exam is likely to be normal. However, normal findings on physical examination do not exclude food allergy.

Exclusion diagnosis tests

In order to exclude other disorders, especially in the GI tract, additional diagnostic means are often required, such as endoscopy of the upper and lower GI tract, histological examinations of GI biopsies, radiological examinations, laboratory tests, microbiological examinations, and stool analyses for parameters of malabsorption. The classic gastroenterological studies for the exclusion of non-allergic GI diseases have to be combined with in vitro and in vivo allergy tests to confirm GI-related food allergy on an objective basis.

Tests for the presence of IgE-mediated food allergy

Definitive laboratory tests for the diagnosis of food allergy are basically lacking. Skin prick tests are useful for excluding IgE-mediated food allergies and suggesting or supporting the diagnosis, but alone they are known to be of limited value in establishing the diagnosis. The measurement of total IgE in serum may predict atopy, but has limited value for the confirmation of food allergic disease. Similarly, the absence of specific serum IgE against food proteins (negative UniCAP®, Immunlite®, or similar test systems) may largely exclude IgE-mediated reactions, but the positive predictive accuracy of these tests is low. In general, the larger the prick skin test wheal size or the greater the level of food-specific IgE in the serum, the more likely it is that the individual will experience an allergic reaction if the food is ingested. However the magnitude of the wheal size or quantity of food-specific IgE does not correlate with the severity of the allergic reaction. The clinical value of these tests is limited in the evaluation of OAS (pollen-food syndrome) because of the instability of the reactive allergens. In addition, studies have shown that patients with food allergy, as confirmed by oral challenges, have intestinal mast cells that release histamine when challenged with food antigen in vitro or in vivo, but skin tests and tests for allergen-specific IgE are positive in only about 50% of these patients. This implies that local IgE production may explain some GI hypersensitivities not generally considered to be IgE mediated. Nevertheless, skin tests and allergen-specific IgE tests should be performed in patients with suspected GI food allergy for two purposes: they may raise evidence for atopy or atopic diseases within or outside the GI tract, and they may be useful in patients suffering from IgE-mediated, immediate-type GI allergy. In patients testing positive for particular food allergens, the skin test and tests for allergen-specific IgE may aid selection of relevant allergens for further testing (e.g. by provocation tests).

Laboratory tests other than skin tests and tests for food-specific IgE have been developed, although most of them have not been thoroughly validated for clinical sensitivity and specificity. For example, IgE, IgA, and IgG4 have been quantified in serum and faeces, but a diagnostic role for these antibodies has not been conclusively demonstrated. Tests such as the basophil histamine release (BHR) assay and the cellular allergen stimulation test (CAST) may be used. In both assays, peripheral blood leukocytes containing basophils are challenged with allergen extracts and subsequently histamine (BHR) or leukotrienes (CAST) are quantified in the cell supernatants. The sensitivity and specificity of both tests evaluated are possibly better than that of prick skin tests and tests for allergen-specific IgE, based on controlled food challenges, but nevertheless await further validation. A major advantage of BHR and CAST is that freshly prepared extracts of labile foods can be used. However, 5–10% of the population have circulating basophils unresponsive to in vitro challenges and therefore such tests will not be useful in such individuals. Intestinal mast cell histamine release (IMCHR), performed by adding food antigen to dispersed mast cells, was shown to correlate most closely with oral food challenge results in patients experiencing only GI symptoms compared with skin prick tests, tests for allergen-specific IgE, and BHR test.

Another approach to diagnose or monitor GI allergy independently of IgE is measurement of eosinophil-derived cationic proteins, such as eosinophil cationic protein (ECP) and eosinophil protein X (EPX). Increased serum ECP levels were found in children with food hypersensitivity. Even more interesting could be the quantification of ECP and EPX in stool samples, because it reflects eosinophil activation in the GI tract more accurately than do serum measurements, as shown by Bischoff and colleagues.

Provocation studies

The double-blind placebo-controlled oral food challenge (DBPCFC) and the utilization of exclusion diets and rechallenge have been proposed as gold standards for the confirmation of food allergy.

The diagnostic dietary regimens include allergen avoidance (e.g. water–rice diet, hydrolysed proteins, elemental diet, or total parenteral nutrition) and allergen investigational diets in which the patient is placed first on an allergen-free diet (e.g. water–rice diet) and then challenged stepwise (in 8–12 steps, each for 2–3 days) with different groups of food proteins. An example is shown in Table 14.3. Together with the diet, patients record their symptoms in a diary. The allergen investigational diet has several potential disadvantages, such as risk of anaphylaxis (therefore the patient must be hospitalized in case of suspected anaphylaxis in history), the time requirements (16–36 days), and the lack of controlled studies indicating the sensitivity and specificity of the test procedure.

The DBPCFC has been used successfully by a number of investigators, in both children and adults, to examine a variety of food-related complaints. However, the test is limited because:

- only one or a few allergens can be tested at one time
- the test has the risk of systemic anaphylactic reactions
- certain delayed symptoms, such as those occurring in GI allergy, may be difficult to interpret
- underlying pathogenic mechanisms cannot be studied by this test – for example, milk allergy and lactose intolerance could provoke similar symptoms (although other tests should differentiate the mechanisms involved).

In particular for GI manifestations of food allergy, the interpretation of the DBPCFC is difficult because the read-out system is poorly defined and it is often dependent on patients' subjectivity with regards their symptoms following oral challenge. To overcome the limitations of the DBPCFC, Bischoff and coworkers developed a diagnostic approach for intestinal food allergy: the colonoscopic allergen provocation test (COLAP test). Local provocation tests have been established for the nasal, conjunctival, and bronchial mucosa, but so far not for the GI mucosa. In the COLAP test, the caecal mucosa is challenged endoscopically with three food antigen extracts selected according to patient history, skin tests, and tests for allergen-specific IgE (Fig. 14.11). The mucosal wheal-and-flare reaction is registered semiquantitatively 20 minutes after challenge. The COLAP test has been performed in adult patients with abdominal symptoms suspected to be related to food allergy and in

Table 14.3 Diagnostic dietary regimen

Step	Principle	Examples
1	Hypoallergenic diet	Rice, potatoes, sunflower oil, salt, white sugar, water
2	Milk and milk products	Milk, butter, cheese, cottage cheese, yoghurt
3	Cereals	Wheat (bread, rolls, noodles), oats, maize, honey, yeast
4	Vegetables and legumes	Tomatoes, carrots, broccoli, celery, peanuts, soya, garlic
5	Eggs and poultry	Eggs, omelette, chicken, turkey
6	Meat	Pork, beef, lamb
7	Fruit and nuts	Apple, strawberry, peach, cherry, kiwi fruit, hazelnut, walnut
8	Fish and shellfish	Codfish, shrimps
9	Spices and herbs	Pepper, paprika, oregano, curry, caraway, mustard
10	Additives, preservatives	Ready-to-serve meals, frozen foods, wine, beer, coffee

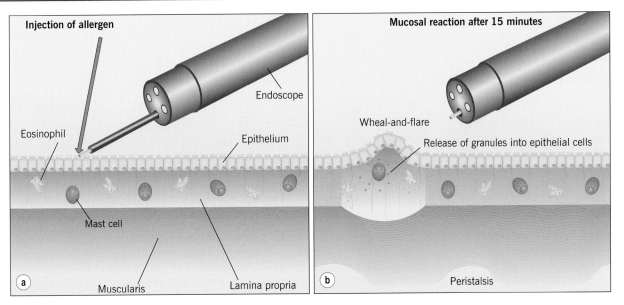

Fig. 14.11 Technique of colonoscopic allergen provocation. (a) Allergen extracts are injected into the intestinal mucosa by a fine needle during colonoscopy. (b) After 15 minutes, a mucosal wheal-and-flare reaction, accompanied by mast cell and eosinophil degranulation and increased peristalsis, can be observed in cases reacting positively toward the administered allergen.

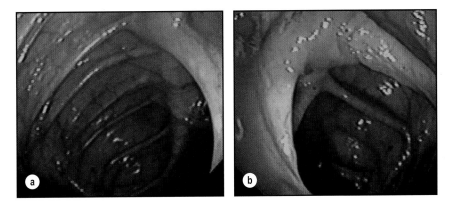

Fig. 14.12 Mucosal reaction after colonoscopic allergen provocation. (a) Normal mucosa before challenge. (b) Mucosal reaction 15 minutes after administration of milk allergen extract.

healthy volunteers. Half of the selected antigens cause a significant wheal-and-flare reaction of the mucosa in patients, whereas no reaction in response to antigen is observed in healthy volunteers (Fig. 14.12). Antigen-induced wheal-and-flare reactions could be related to the patient's history of adverse reactions to food, but not to serum levels of specific IgE or skin test results. No severe systemic anaphylactic reactions have been observed in response to intestinal challenge. It has been found that antigen-induced wheal-and-flare reactions are closely correlated with intestinal mast cell and eosinophil activation (Fig. 14.13). The studies suggest that the COLAP test may be a useful diagnostic means in patients with suspected intestinal food allergy and an interesting tool for the study of the mechanisms of GI allergy and oral tolerance.

Final diagnosis

The final diagnosis of food allergy is based on a patient's history, personal and family history of atopy, on exclusion of other disorders, specific allergy tests and – in cases of doubt – controlled provocation tests. For the final diagnosis of food allergy, a particular flow chart is proposed that has been proved of value in clinical practice (Fig. 14.14).

Management

Introduction

The diagnosis and treatment of food allergy is often difficult, time consuming, and sometimes even hazardous

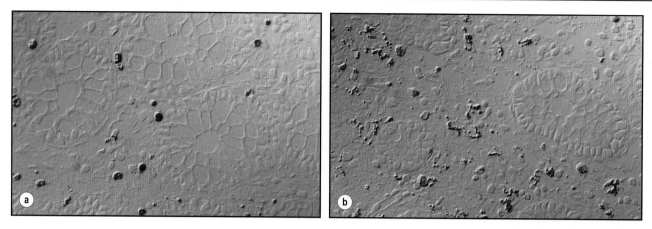

Fig. 14.13 Mast cell activation after colonoscopic allergen provocation. Immunohistochemical staining of histamine in tissue sections of caecal mucosa. Biopsies were taken: (a) 20 minutes after challenge of a patient suffering from pork allergy with wheat antigen extract, which induced no macroscopic reaction, and (b) after challenge with pork antigen extract, which induced a significant wheal-and-flare reaction of the mucosa. Note the more widespread distribution of histamine, which is black (×400).

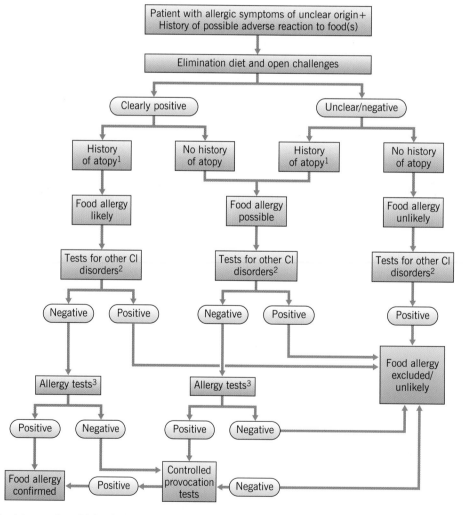

Fig. 14.14 Flow chart to confirm GI food allergy. For details see text. (Adapted from Bischoff SC, Crowe SE. Gastrointestinal food allergy: new insights into pathophysiology and clinical perspectives. Gastroenterology 2005; 128:1089–1113.)

for the patient. Therefore, affected patients need intimate care by a competent specialist with a sympathetic understanding of the symptoms and effect on quality of life issues, the diagnostic procedures, and the treatment options. Even in cases of confirmed food allergy, the treatment remains difficult because allergen avoidance requires a high degree of vigilance and discipline by the patient, and drug treatment options are limited. Moreover, immunotherapy and prevention of GI allergy are not yet established. Only breastfeeding of newborns who are at an increased risk of developing atopic disease has been shown to have a significant effect in preventing allergy. Apart from the physician, experienced dietitians are required to advise afflicted patients how to perform exclusion diets, to identify potential risky ingredients in food, and to avoid malnutrition and vitamin deficiencies.

Goals of management

The major goals of treatment are symptom relief, enhancement of quality of life, and avoidance of life-threatening anaphylactic reactions.

Patient education

Patients with confirmed food allergy need education in:

- reading food labels and understanding the content of food
- learning to recognize unsafe situations, e.g. buffets; Asian restaurants for peanut and nut allergic patients
- learning about cross-reactivities in cases of pollen-associated food allergy
- knowing about the risk of anaphylaxis and how to combat it.

Their families should be advised about allergy prevention by breastfeeding newborns for 4–6 month, stepwise introduction of solid food to the baby, and possibly by the administration of probiotic lactobacilli strains to the mother in the perinatal phase.

Management plan (Table 14.4)

Allergen avoidance

The only proven therapy in the management of confirmed food allergy is avoidance of the triggering allergen or allergens. However, this approach requires that the allergen(s) responsible has been clearly identified, and that it is possible to exclude the allergen(s) completely from the diet without risk of malnutrition. The success of allergen avoidance depends on the patient's compliance, the quality of advice, the number of allergens to be avoided, and the kind of allergens responsible for the

Table 14.4 Treatment of food allergy

Allergen avoidance	Hypoallergenic diet Elimination diet according to history and test results (Total parental nutritional)
Drug treatment	Cromolyn sodium (GI symptoms) Corticosteroids (local or systemic administration) Swallowed fluticosone or budesonide spray Anti-IgE antibodies H_1 blockers? Leukotriene antagonists?
Future concepts	Immunotherapy (induction of oral tolerance) Cytokine treatment (e.g. IL-10; anti-IL-5)

reactions. The ten foods most commonly implicated in GI food allergy are milk, egg, hazelnut, peanut, wheat, soy, apple, fish, shellfish, and pork. Some allergens, such as nuts and apple, are relatively easy to avoid; others, such as milk, egg, and wheat, require enormous efforts to eliminate them completely from the diet. Patients have to be selected for their capacity to follow sophisticated dietary regimens and to be advised by experienced personnel. They should be cautioned to read the ingredient labels on all foods they consume, and they need education on how to read food labels, to understand the technical names and abbreviations, and to appreciate that some ingredients are not always indicated. They need instructions about the effects of cooking on the allergenicity of food proteins, and about eating away from home. They must be informed about the cross-reactivities within different food allergens and between some food allergens and pollens. Finally, patients who follow an extensive exclusion diet need monitoring of body weight, body composition, vitamin status, electrolytes and bone density.

Drug treatment

Controlled studies on the medical management of GI allergy are not available. Therefore, the recommendations for drug therapy of food allergy in general should be followed (see Ch. 7). One must distinguish between treatment of acute reactions (see 'Treatment of emergencies' that follows) and of chronic or recurrent symptoms.

Long-term drug therapy of GI allergy is required in patients who cannot, for whatever reason, achieve a complete avoidance of food allergens. Drug treatment and dietetic regimens are not mutually exclusive, since partial exclusion of relevant allergens may help to reduce the doses of drugs required to become free of symptoms. In our experience, H_1 blockers are in most cases not effective for the treatment of chronic GI symptoms – except for pruritus in patients suffering from OAS. Cromolyn administered orally (200 mg four times a day) may be useful in some cases with mild reactions of GI allergy. The advantages of this drug are that it is well tolerated by most individuals and that no relevant side effects have been reported. In moderate to severe cases, additional treatment with oral corticosteroids (e.g. prednisolone 5–40 mg per day, or, in cases of GI allergy, budesonide 3–12 mg per day) may be useful. In eosinophilic oesophagitis, swallowed fluticosone or budesonide spray has been shown to be successful in ameliorating symptoms in the majority of patients. Only anecdotal reports of successful use of other long-term treatments, such as non-steroidal immunosuppressants and cytokine antagonists, exist at present. In extremely severe cases, treatment with higher doses of corticosteroids and total parenteral nutrition may be indicated for a limited time period. If such cases are accompanied by symptoms of systemic anaphylaxis, the general recommendations for management of anaphylaxis should be followed. In particular cases of severe food allergy (e.g. triggered by highly potent food allergens such as peanuts or lipid transfer proteins), not only should emergency drugs be prescribed, but systemic anti-IgE treatment may be considered on an experimental basis.

Evidence to support the use of classical allergen immunotherapy by parenteral administration of food allergen extracts in any form of food allergy is lacking. Other treatment options (e.g. leukotriene antagonists, or cytokines such as IL-10) still have to be evaluated in patients with GI allergy.

Treatment of emergencies

Patients with food allergy and a history of systemic anaphylaxis, or sensitization against dangerous allergens such as peanuts, tree nuts, or lipid transfer proteins found in peaches and other fruits should be equipped with emergency medications including adrenaline [automatic syringe for intramuscular or subcutaneous injection (0.3 mg for patients >25–30 kg; 0.15 mg for patients >10–25 kg)], H_1 blockers, such as clemastine (2 mg), cetirizine (10 mg) or diphenhydramine (1.25 mg/kg up to 50–75 mg), and prednisolone (1–2 mg/kg up to 100 mg). In children, half the adult doses indicated here should be used. These drugs must be prescribed every year and usage of the drugs must be carefully explained to the patient and his relatives.

Assessment of effectiveness of disease control

Patients with food allergies who are started on allergen elimination diets should be followed-up in about 3 months to verify the effectiveness of the individual diet with regard to the treatment goals (see above) and to exclude malnutrition related to the elimination diet. Subsequent visits depend on the complexity of the diet and the effectiveness of the therapy.

Summary of important messages

- Food allergy is still the 'black box' in the field of allergy, because the mechanisms have not been unravelled, the diagnostic means are sophisticated, time consuming and non-specific, and the success of dietetic treatment is dependent on accuracy of the diagnosis
- About 20–30% of the general population believes that they suffer from adverse reactions to food, but only one-quarter of children and one-tenth of adults suffer from true food allergy
- The diagnosis of food allergy needs objective confirmation and must be distinguished from malabsorption syndromes, food intolerances, and other diseases
- The diagnosis of food allergy can be confirmed accurately in most patients, by employing a comprehensive diagnostic strategy including a comprehensive patient and family history, an accurate use of allergy tests, and exclusion of non-allergic disorders
- Once the diagnosis is confirmed, the therapy of choice is strict avoidance of the responsible food allergy; additionally, antiallergic drug treatment can be employed in some cases
- In cases with suspected anaphylactic reactions, patients must be equipped with an emergency set of drugs consisting of self-injectable adrenaline, antihistamines, and corticosteroids

Further reading

Bischoff SC, Mayer J, Wedemeyer J, et al. Colonoscopic allergen provocation (COLAP): a new diagnostic approach for gastro-intestinal food allergy. Gut 1997; 40:745–753.

Bischoff SC. Role of mast cells in allergic and non-allergic immune responses: comparison of human and murine data. Nat Rev Immunol 2007; 7:93–104.

Bock SA, Sampson HA, Atkins FM, et al. Double-blind placebo-controlled food challenge (DBPCFC) as an office procedure: a manual. J Allergy Clin Immunol 1988; 82:986–997.

Liacouras CA. Pharmacologic treatment of eosinophilic esophagitis. Gastrointest Endosc Clin N Am 2008; 18(1):169–178.

Mehr S, Kakakios A, Frith K, et al. Food protein-induced enterocolitis syndrome: 16-year experience. Pediatrics 2009; 123:e459–464.

Monsbakken KW, Vandvik PO, Farup PG. Perceived food intolerance in subjects with irritable bowel syndrome

– etiology, prevalence and consequences. Eur J Clin Nutr 2006; 60:667–672.

Nowak-Wegrzyn A, Muraro A. Food protein-induced enterocolitis syndrome. Curr Opin Allergy Clin Immunol 2009; 9:371–377.

Sicherer SH, Sampson HA. Food allergy. J Allergy Clin Immunol 2010; 125(suppl. 2):S116–125.

Turner JR. Intestinal mucosal barrier function in health and disease. Nat Rev Immunol 2009; 9:799–809.

Zuidmeer L, Goldhahn K, Rona RJ, et al. The prevalence of plant food allergies: a systematic review. J Allergy Clin Immunol 2008; 121(5):1210–1218.

Occupational allergy

Piero Maestrelli, Piera Boschetto and
Mark S Dykewicz

DEFINITION

Occupational allergy is defined as allergy caused by exposure to a product that is present in the workplace. Both elements of this definition are important, as the agent should be specific to the workplace and be causally related to the disease.

Introduction

The recognition of occupational allergy goes back to Olaus Magnus who, in 1555, wrote:

When sifting the chaff from the wheat, one must carefully consider the time when a suitable wind is available that sweeps away the harmful dust. This fine-grained material readily makes its way into the mouth, congests in the throat, and threatens the life organs of the threshing men. If one does not seek instant remedy by drinking one's beer, one may never more, or only for a short time, be able to enjoy what one has threshed.

Since then, many agents encountered at the workplace have been associated with allergic reactions in various organs. These include, for example, high-molecular-weight agents in flour, castor beans or vegetable gums, and low-molecular-weight agents such as platinum salts, diisocyanates or those in wood dust.

Reactions can lead to permanent impairment and disability. Due to its significant medical, social, and possibly legal consequences, a definitive diagnosis of occupational allergy, including identification of the causative agent, is imperative. Whenever possible, prevention programmes should be set up in high-risk workplaces.

Occupational allergy can affect many target organs, including the lungs, nose, eyes, and skin. This chapter focuses on occupational allergy affecting upper and lower airways – that is, occupational asthma and occupational rhinitis.

Disease mechanisms

Understanding the pathogenesis of occupational allergy is critical for optimal prevention and management of the disease. The several hundred causes of occupational allergy can be classified conveniently into high-molecular-weight (HMW) and low-molecular-weight (LMW) compounds. By convention, HMW sensitizers are >10 kd, common examples being inhaled protein agents, whereas LMW agents are often reactive chemicals. A list of aetiological agents according to industries, jobs, or work processes where the exposure can be found has recently been prepared (see Malo & Chang-Yeung in

Further reading) or available on the websites: (http://www.remcomp.fr/asmanet/asmapro/index.htm; http://www.asthme.csst.qc.ca).

Box 15.1 summarizes the most important causes of occupational asthma and rhinitis.

Occupational asthma (OA) and rhinitis are probably the result of multiple genetic, environmental, and behavioural influences. A dose–response relationship between the level of exposure and the development of OA is well established for several sensitizing agents. Recent evidence indicates that chemical respiratory allergens may induce respiratory tract sensitization by routes different from inhalation, mainly dermal exposure. Genetic susceptibility, probably in combination with occupational and environmental exposures, can affect the development of occupational allergy by modifying the impact of a given gene on complex phenotypes. In this respect, interactions between genes and environment, in part through epigenetic mechanisms (see Ch. 2), seem to be more important in causing disease than the influence of either genetics or environment considered separately.

HMW compounds, which are often from biological sources, generally induce occupational allergy through an immunoglobulin (Ig)E-dependent mechanism, comparable to that operating in non-occupational atopic asthma. In contrast, most LMW agents induce occupational allergy through non-IgE-dependent mechanisms. The pathogenesis of OA caused by LMW agents remains largely uncertain. The mechanisms of 'induction' or sensitization, by which many LMW agents induce asthma and rhinitis, are believed to be mainly related to immunological sensitization. However, relevant immunological mechanisms involve IgE-mediated immunity in only

some cases, and probably involve novel cell-mediated and mixed immune reactions. It is well recognized that diisocyanates and plicatic acid cause OA that has the clinical and pathological features of immunological asthma, but do not consistently induce specific IgE antibodies.

The immune response may be initiated by recognition of the agent bound to protein by antigen-presenting cells (Fig. 15.1). Subsequent production of sHLA-G (a non-classical HLA class I molecule with tolerogenic and anti-inflammatory functions), up-regulation of immune pattern-recognition receptors (chitinase-1) by macrophages and release of damage-associated molecular patterns from injured epithelium (danger signals) may represent an immunological cascade by which isocyanates stimulate innate immune responses and contribute to the activation of immunocompetent cells. In isocyanate-induced OA, a mixed CD4–CD8 type 2/type 1 lymphocyte response or induction of γ/δ specific CD8 cells may play a role. Th2 (IL-5) and Th1 [interferon γ (IFN-γ)] cytokines, and other proinflammatory chemokines produced by macrophages [migration inhibitory factor (MIF), monocyte chemoattractant protein 1 (MCP-1), tumor necrosis factor α (TNF-α)] induce recruitment and activation of inflammatory cells. These cells, mainly eosinophils and mast cells, characterize airway inflammation, which contributes to the functional alterations of

---

Box 15.1 Classification and major causes of occupational asthma

High-molecular-weight compounds

- Plant products
- Animal products
- Enzymes
- Seafood proteins

Low-molecular-weight compounds

- IgE-dependent causes:
  - acid anhydrides
  - metals
- Non-IgE-dependent causes:
  - diisocyanates
  - wood dust
  - amines
  - colophony
  - pharmaceutical products
  - glutaraldehyde
  - formaldehyde
  - pot-room aluminium-induced asthma

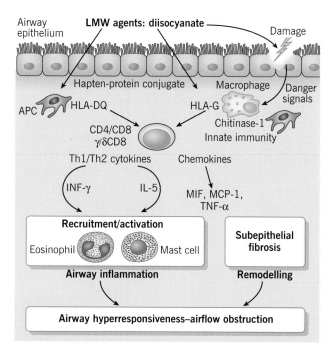

Fig. 15.1 Schematic diagram of mechanisms in OA induced by low molecular weight (LMW) chemicals, in particular diisocyanates. APC, antigen-presenting cell; eos, eosinophil; mast, mast cell; Th, T-helper cell; IL, interleukin; HLA, human leukocyte antigen; INF, interferon; TNF, tumour necrosis factor; MIF, migration inhibitory factor; MCP, monocyte chemoattractant protein.

OA – that is, bronchial hyperresponsiveness and air-flow limitation. Subepithelial fibrosis due to thickening of the reticular basement membrane is considered a histopathological feature of OA. However, the role of this remodelling of the airways on lung function remains undetermined (see Fig. 15.1).

In occupational rhinitis (OR), there is some evidence that non-allergic neural mechanisms may play an important role in pathogenesis by promoting neurogenic inflammation that can cause vasodilation and oedema leading to nasal obstruction. It is thought that neurotrophins such as the nerve growth factor up-regulate the synthesis and release of sensory neuropeptides such as substance P, neurokinin A and neurokinin B, and calcitonin gene-related peptide. Neuropeptides have been recovered after airway challenge with isocyanates, ozone, and allergens. Various occupational exposures to irritant agents such as chlorine, formaldehyde, and volatile organic compounds have been demonstrated to cause nasal inflammation, usually with a neutrophil predominance.

Clinical presentation

Occupational asthma

General

Occupational asthma is defined as the new onset of asthma due to exposure to a product present in the workplace. In contrast, and much more common, is the occurrence of work-exacerbated asthma – that is, asthma that was present before the work exposure, but then is aggravated or exacerbated by conditions at work (this can be chemical exposures, but could also include physical conditions such as changes in the temperature or exertion). Together, occupational asthma and work-exacerbated asthma comprise the spectrum of work-related asthma (Fig. 15.2).

Occupational asthma can be subdivided into two types depending on whether it is induced by sensitization to a specific HMW substance (e.g. an inhaled protein) or a LMW chemical at work, termed 'sensitizer-induced OA', or by exposure to an inhaled irritant at work, which is termed 'irritant-induced OA' (see Fig. 15.2). OA due to a sensitizer appears after a latency period of exposure necessary for the worker to acquire immunologically mediated sensitization to the causal agent. It encompasses OA that is induced by an IgE mechanism (proteins and some chemicals), and OA caused by agents (usually reactive chemicals) for which an immunological mechanism is strongly suspected, yet an antigen-specific immune response cannot easily be identified in most affected workers.

OA caused by a high level of irritant exposure has no apparent latency period and its most definitive form is reactive airway dysfunction syndrome (RADS), which describes an acute onset of asthma after a single, very

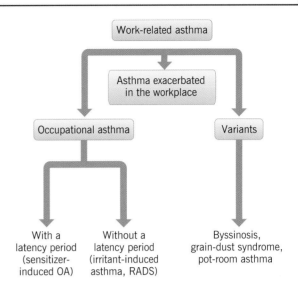

Fig. 15.2 Occupational asthma and asthma-like occupational variants. RADS, reactive airway dysfunction syndrome.

high irritant exposure. Although its functional characteristics resemble those of OA, symptoms of RADS cannot be reproduced by re-exposure of the affected patients to lower, non-irritant levels of the offending agent. Also, the airway pathology of RADS is different. The bronchial epithelial damage and subepithelial fibrosis are more pronounced, whereas inflammatory cell infiltration in the bronchial wall is generally less evident than in asthma, and the presence of eosinophils is inconsistent.

These definitions are interpreted with the understanding that work-exacerbated asthma and OA are not mutually exclusive and may coexist in the same worker. Of different types of work-exacerbated asthma, OA from specific sensitizers is the most common type studied in most case surveillance series. A history of childhood or pre-existing adult onset asthma does not exclude the possibility that OA may develop after an appropriate workplace exposure.

Epidemiology

The reported prevalance of OA has been increasing (and is more frequent than pneumoconioses such as asbestosis and silicosis), based upon the number of cases referred or accepted for medicolegal compensation and on the number of cases reported by sentinel physicians. The causes of this increase are incompletely understood, but may reflect heightened recognition of the problem as well as a broader range of environmental exposure. Besides medicolegal and sentinel-based programme statistics, the frequency of OA can be assessed in general populations and in specific at-risk workplaces. It has been estimated that 23.4% of the US total workforce (7.8 million out of 33.4 million) is exposed to at least one of the 367 potentially asthmogenic products in the workplace. An important prospective study in a general population, the European Community Respiratory Health Survey (ECRHS), which started around 1990, showed a very high attributable risk fraction for asthma due to occupation: 10–25%.

Recently, focus has been put on exposure differences that may explain variation in frequency between different countries. Analysis of the geographical distribution of asthma identified a greater prevalence among English-speaking countries. Comparison of prevalance between countries is important; there are similarities in the frequency of work-attributable asthma for some jobs, such as cleaners. Data from South Africa and Brazil taken from sentinel-based studies have shown relatively low risks for OA, with an incidence of less than 2 per 100 000, in contrast to almost 12 per 100 000 incidence in Finland. A geographical pattern occurring within different areas of the same country is also likely to be present for OA. Data from the ECRHS showed large variations in prevalence of sensitization to ubiquitous allergens in Spanish and French cities as well as variations in the attributable risk of asthma due to sensitization.

Gender seems to play a role in OA, but the direction depends on agents and occupations; for example, in Finland examination of the risk of occupation on the incidence of asthma has been performed from data of three national registers that showed different risks for men and women. Unfortunately, most surveillance data are not stratified by gender. Some gender differences have been reported, although many apparent differences could relate to different exposures. Education also plays a significant role; work-related asthma being commoner in workers with only a primary education.

Table 15.1 describes longitudinal general population cohort studies of asthma published June 1999–2007 in which the population attributable risk (PAR) for occupational exposure and asthma was either published or can be derived. Most epidemiological surveys of OA in specific workplaces have been cross-sectional and have, therefore, assessed the prevalence of the condition. The main pitfall of this approach is that it is likely to be influenced by the 'healthy worker effect', which can result in an underestimate of the rate of disease. Asthma symptoms can be very troublesome and even life threatening, so it is likely that many subjects will leave the workplace before a survey can be conducted. It is suspected that this bias is more pronounced in the case of OA than for slowly progressing conditions such as pneumoconiosis. Another difficulty lies in the diagnostic tools available for assessing the prevalence. Surveys rely on questionnaires, immunological testing, assessment of airway calibre and bronchial responsiveness, and peak expiratory flow (PEF) monitoring, used alone and in combination. Only rarely are surveys performed in a stepwise fashion leading to the identification of cases that are then confirmed either by PEF monitoring or by specific inhalation challenge. Other possible problems of epidemiological studies include: misclassification due to the overlap between asthma and other chronic obstructive lung diseases, attribution bias in responses to questions on symptoms after starting exposure, and varying symptoms, as workers may experience chest or nasal symptoms without wheezing.

Occupational rhinitis

According to a 2008 consensus statement of the European Academy of Allergy and Clinical Immunology

Table 15.1 Frequency of occupational asthma: synthesis of population attributable fraction (PAR) for occupational exposure and asthma obtained by Toren and Blanc (current review) and previous review studies

Type of study	Studies included	Range (%)	Mean (%)	Median (%)
Current review				
Longitudinal	6	8.6–44	19.3	16.3
Case-control	3	9.5–21.4	14.8	13.5
Cross-sectional	7	7.0–31.3	16.1	13.6
Current and earlier review				
Longitudinal	6	8.6–44.0	19.3	16.3
Case-control	6	9.5–36.0	20.7	12.2
Cross-sectional	14	7–51	21.1	17.6
All	26	7–51	20.7	17.6
All, adult onset asthma only	17	8.6–44.0	18.5	16.9

(From Torén K, Blanc PD. Asthma caused by occupational exposures is common – a systematic analysis of estimates of the population-attributable fraction. BMC Pulmonary Medicine 2009; 9:7.)

(EAACI), occupational rhinitis (OR) has been defined as an inflammatory disease of the nose, characterized by intermittent or persistent nasal symptoms (i.e. nasal congestion, sneezing, rhinorrhoea, itching) and/or variable nasal air-flow limitation and/or hypersecretion attributable to a particular work environment and not to stimuli encountered outside the workplace. However, as some forms of non-occupational rhinitis are well recognized to have nasal symptoms in the absence of consistent findings of nasal inflammation, it is plausible that some clinical presentations of OR actually may not be accurately characterized as an inflammatory process.

Analogous to consensus definitions of work-related asthma, 'work-related rhinitis' may be distinguished into: (1) OR that is due to causes and conditions attributable to a particular work environment, and (2) 'work-exacerbated rhinitis' that is pre-existing or concurrent rhinitis exacerbated by workplace exposures. Similar to OA, OR can be subdivided into 'allergic OR' and 'non-allergic OR'. In allergic OR, work-related rhinitis symptoms develop because of immunologically mediated hypersensitivity responses that occur via antibody- or cell-mediated mechanisms, with development of nasal symptoms upon exposure to a specific occupational agent after a latent period of sensitization. Allergic OR can be further subdivided into 'IgE-mediated OR', generally caused by HMW agents, and 'non-IgE-mediated OR', induced by LMW agents such as isocyanates.

Non-allergic OR includes several subtypes of rhinitis caused by work exposures that elicit irritant, non-immunological mechanisms. Single or multiple exposures to very high concentrations of irritant agents can lead to acute onset of 'irritant-induced OR', which is analogous to RADS, so use of the term 'reactive upper airways dysfunction' or RUDS has been proposed. In chlorine-induced RUDS, histological findings include epithelial desquamation, lymphocytic inflammation of the lamina propia, and increased numbers of nerve fibres. Irritant-induced OR may also refer to rhinitis symptoms that develop in subjects who have repeated work exposures to irritants (dusts, vapours, fumes) but without known acute exposures at high concentrations. In a more severe form of irritant-induced OR, 'corrosive OR', exposures to high concentrations of chemicals result in permanent nasal mucosal inflammation, sometimes with mucosal ulcerations and nasal septal perforations.

Generally, the same work environments cause OA and OR. Rhinoconjunctival symptoms may occur from HMW occupational sensitizers such as protein allergens, including laboratory animals (e.g. mice, rats, guinea pigs), natural rubber latex, enzymes and storage mites, and LMW sensitizers including anhydrides, diisocyanates, platinum salts, and drugs. Irritant workplace exposures that have been reported to cause OR include grain dust constituents (e.g. endotoxin), flour dust, fuel oil ash, and ozone.

Epidemiology

Based upon cross-sectional studies, prevalence rates of OR are two to four times more prevalent than OA, and range from 2 to 87% in work environments having exposure to HMW sensitizers, and from 3 to 48% with exposures to LMW agents. The development of specific IgE to a HMW occupational sensitizer is a strong predictor for the development of rhinitis or asthma symptoms. Atopy is associated with OR from HMW agents, but not clearly to OR from LMW agents. A relationship between smoking and OR is uncertain. There is some evidence from cohort studies that non-specific bronchial hyperresponsiveness is associated with increased risk for future development of work-related nasal symptoms.

Rhinitis symptoms are typically present in the vast majority of patients with OA, whether from HMW or from LMW agents, although the intensity of nasal symptoms is more pronounced with exposure to HMW agents. It has been reported that symptoms of nasal and ocular itching and nasal secretions in relation to work exposure are good predictors of OA from HMW agents as confirmed by specific inhalation challenges. OR may occur as the only manifestation of occupational respiratory disease, precede the onset symptoms of OA in many individuals, have concurrent onset with OA, or occasionally develop after the onset of OA. Symptoms of OR have been reported to precede the development of OA in 20–78% of affected subjects, with higher rates more often reported with HMW agents (Fig. 15.3). These data support the concept of 'the united airway' in occupational respiratory disease, in which the respiratory mucosa forms a continuum from the nose to the lower airways that is vulnerable and responsive to similar environmental exposures.

Diagnosis

Work-related asthma

The recently published consensus statement on work-related asthma from the American College of Chest Physicians (ACCP 2008) is an updated and authoritative guideline addressing most of the relevant aspects of diagnosis of occupational asthma.

Studies have shown that both early diagnosis of OA and early removal from exposure to the causative agent in the workplace improve the chance of recovery. However, the diagnosis of OA still remains complicated and controversial. Suspecting work exposure as a cause of asthma in all individuals with new onset or worsening asthma, and asking key questions about work exposures while history taking, is crucial in the work-up of OA. Information on exposures in various jobs can be accessed from several websites (see below).

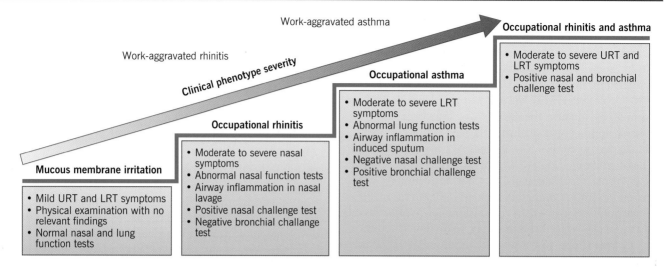

Fig. 15.3 The clinical spectrum of work-related rhinitis and asthma indicating the relative clinical severity of symptoms and main clinical features. Although the temporal progression from occupational rhinitis to occupational asthma occurs in many patients, occupational rhinitis does not necessarily precede or accompany occupational asthma. Work-aggravated rhinitis and asthma occur in the context of pre-existing airway disease. LRT, lower respiratory tract; URT, upper respiratory tract. (From: Castano R, Malo JL. Occupational rhinitis and asthma: Where do we stand, Where do we go? Curr Allergy Asthma Rep 2010; 10:135–142.)

The confirmation of the disease by demonstration of reversible bronchoconstriction and/or airway hyperresponsiveness requires criteria similar to those applied in non-OA. This is justified by the findings that OA and non-OA have similar functional features. These similarities are also found in types of asthma in which an IgE-mediated mechanism is not demonstrated – that is, between intrinsic asthma and OA induced by many LMW chemicals.

A scheme summarizing a proposed approach in the investigation of OA is shown in Figure 15.4. All patients with asthma should be questioned about their current and past workplaces as persistent asthma can be attributed to past exposure. This holds for OA with a latency period as well as for RADS. Two clues in a patient's history should point to the possibility of OA: the symptoms, and the job and products at work. Worsening from work exposures may occur with every work shift, or may be intermittent. Symptoms may be worse almost immediately at work or only after several hours – even after leaving work at the end of a shift or during the night. Sometimes, the job and product at work can suggest the diagnosis. For example, if the medical history reveals that an asthmatic patient is a nurse, possible exposure to a sensitizing product such as latex should be considered. Being an asthmatic and being exposed to polyurethane at work should suggest the possibility of OA caused by isocyanates.

Databases of high-risk jobs and products can be obtained from national agencies, for example the National Institute for Occupational Safety and Health (NIOSH) in the USA and the Health and Safety Executive (HSE) in the UK. Interesting databases have been developed in France

(asmanet.com) and in Québec (asthme.csst.qc.ca). The clinician should obtain information on the nature of all products present in the workplace, not only those handled by the subject, by requesting safety data sheets. There could be products present that have not been listed as known causes of OA (but this does not preclude the possibility of their being so).

Objective confirmation of asthma as a generic diagnosis should be sought in all patients by various means whenever feasible. A compatible history of OA, such as improvement of symptoms when away from work and worsening on returning to work, is very suggestive, but not specific. A key practical aspect for the investigator is to perform the tests for diagnosis of asthma (bronchodilator response manifested by spirometric assessment or a test of airway hyperresponsiveness by methacholine or histamine challenge) preferably during the working week or at least when the asthmatic has had recent symptoms. In fact, these tests may be normal and yet not exclude work-related asthma, if performed after removal of the relevant exposure and at a time when the patient has not had recent symptoms.

After establishing the diagnosis of asthma, the next diagnostic step is to establish its relationship to work. This can lead to one of the following diagnoses of work related asthma:

- occupational asthma from an irritant exposure
- occupational asthma due to a sensitizer
- work-exacerbated asthma.

For irritant-induced asthma, a work relationship is best obtained by history (i.e. for RADS, the occurrence of one or more high-level irritant exposures, with the new onset

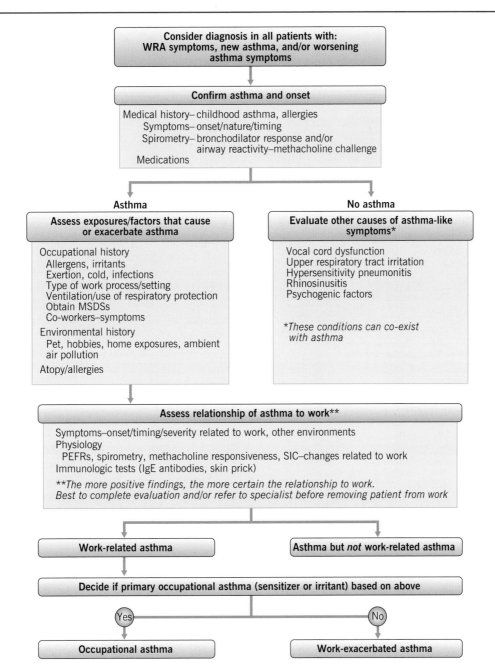

Consider diagnosis in all patients with:
WRA symptoms, new asthma, and/or worsening
asthma symptoms

Confirm asthma and onset

Medical history– childhood asthma, allergies
Symptoms– onset/nature/timing
Spirometry– bronchodilator response and/or
airway reactivity–methacholine challenge
Medications

Asthma

Assess exposures/factors that cause or exacerbate asthma

Occupational history
  Allergens, irritants
  Exertion, cold, infections
  Type of work process/setting
  Ventilation/use of respiratory protection
  Obtain MSDSs
  Co-workers–symptoms
Environmental history
  Pet, hobbies, home exposures, ambient
  air pollution
Atopy/allergies

No asthma

Evaluate other causes of asthma-like symptoms*

Vocal cord dysfunction
Upper respiratory tract irritation
Hypersensitivity pneumonitis
Rhinosinusitis
Psychogenic factors

*These conditions can co-exist
with asthma*

Assess relationship of asthma to work**

Symptoms–onset/timing/severity related to work, other environments
Physiology
  PEFRs, spirometry, methacholine responsiveness, SIC–changes related to work
Immunologic tests (IgE antibodies, skin prick)

***The more positive findings, the more certain the relationship to work.*
Best to complete evaluation and/or refer to specialist before removing patient from work

Work-related asthma

Asthma but *not* work-related asthma

Decide if primary occupational asthma (sensitizer or irritant) based on above

Yes

No

Occupational asthma

Work-exacerbated asthma

Fig. 15.4 Diagnosis of work-related asthma. (From Tarlo SM, Balmes J, Balkissoon R, et al. Diagnosis and management of work-related asthma: American College of Chest Physicians Consensus Statement. Chest 2008; 134(3 suppl):S1–41.)

of asthma symptoms within 24 h of the exposure, usually leading to an emergency department visit or unscheduled outpatient physician visit). Asthma symptoms must continue for at least 3 months after the exposure, and pulmonary function testing must confirm reversible airway obstruction or airway hyperresponsiveness.

Occupational asthma due to a sensitizer is further investigated by objective tests providing evidence of specific sensitization whenever possible (see below).

Work-exacerbated asthma can range from a single short-term worsening of asthma at work up to daily worsening at work on a consistent basis. A single short-term

exacerbation may be documented by history alone and further investigations are probably not necessary, unless similar episodes recur frequently enough to be documented by means of a symptom and peak flow diary. Work-exacerbated asthma with symptom worsening on a daily or near-daily basis can be investigated in a similar manner to that for sensitizer-induced occupational asthma.

Eosinophilic bronchitis, presenting as a non-productive cough without evidence of airway obstruction or airway hyperresponsiveness, but associated with increased sputum eosinophils, has been reported from exposure to

Box 15.2 Differential diagnosis of asthma

- Obstructive sleep apnoea
- Bronchiectasis
- Bronchiolitis
- Laryngeal dyskinesia
- Chronic respiratory disease of prematurity
- Cystic fibrosis
- Tracheoesophageal fistula
- Deglutition disorders
- Viral and bacterial infections
- Heart failure
- Hypopharyngeal masses
- Mediastinal masses
- Chronic obstructive pulmonary disease
- Gastroesophageal reflux
- Eosinophilic bronchitis
- Loeffer's syndrome
- Hyperventilation syndrome

Box 15.3 Causes of asthma-like symptoms*

- Vocal cord dysfunction
- Upper respiratory tract irritation
- Hypersensitivity pneumonitis
- Rhinosinusitis
- Psychogenic factors

*These conditions can coexist with asthma.

some occupational agents. These include acrylates, latex, lysozyme and mushroom spores.

Box 15.2 indicates the principal diseases that should be differentiated from asthma. Other conditions that may coexist with asthma are listed in Box 15.3.

Besides chest symptoms, those related to ocular and nasal involvement should be evaluated. These symptoms are more common in cases of OA due to HMW rather than LMW agents and, as mentioned earlier, they may precede those of asthma, particularly in the case of HMW agents. Work-related dysphonia (suggestive of vocal cord dysfunction) is negatively associated with OA.

Work-related rhinitis

By itself, the clinical history has low specificity for the diagnosis of OR. Nevertheless, the diagnosis of OR is supported by a history of nasal symptoms (congestion, pruritus, sneezing, rhinorrhoea) and associated eye symptoms that increase when the person is at work and resolve when away from work. Currently, the diagnosis of OR to HMW sensitizers or a limited number of LMW sensitizers (e.g. platinum salts, reactive dyes, acid anhydrides) is often made by a history of work-related rhinitis that correlates with demonstrated sensitization to a specific agent encountered in the work environment. However,

immunological sensitization is not specific for OR. Because of this and other limitations in the diagnosis of OR, recent guidelines have encouraged the greater use of objective physiological measurements of nasal airway responses. Consistent with this, an algorithm for a diagnostic approach to work related rhinitis is indicated in Figure 15.5.

Environmental assessment

Although air sampling can be undertaken at the workplace, the most important information is whether or not a product is actually present. In many instances, a causal agent can be released into the air in minute amounts, which makes its detection difficult even with sophisticated instruments. Product information is often difficult to obtain, so a good relationship should be established with the employer and the manufacturers of suspect products, as well as with local, regional, and national health and safety agencies. Generally, it is not mandatory for safety data sheets to give information on products present at concentrations below 1%, despite such concentrations being sufficient to cause OA.

Intensity of exposure to a respiratory sensitizer is an important determinant of OA. Many studies have shown dose–response relationships for several agents such as flour, laboratory animal protein, Western red cedar, colophony, and acid anhydrides. However, there is still a lack of information regarding the existence of 'no effect' levels and whether peak or mean exposures to LMW agents are the more important in causing sensitization and OA. The level that provokes symptoms in already sensitized workers is lower than that which would cause sensitization.

The possibility that a proportion of non-RADS work-related asthma is due to low-level irritant exposure (1) alone, or (2) in the presence of atopy, or (3) combined with allergen exposure has also been raised. Previous studies have examined the interaction of irritants and allergens. A report of 'not so sudden' irritant-induced asthma noted the significant contribution of underlying atopy and/or asthma; conversely, irritant exposure may increase the allergic exposure, possibly via disruption of epithelial structure and an easier crossing of allergen through the epithelium. General air sampling of a workplace does not usually provide an accurate reflection of what workers are exposed to, particularly if they are at any distance from the sampling apparatus. Personal samplers have been developed to overcome this problem, allowing sampling of aerosols, mists, and dusts close to the worker.

The respiratory tract is believed to be the main route of exposure and site of initiation of the immune response toward occupational–chemical allergens. There is, however, growing evidence that chemical exposure can induce sensitization of the respiratory tract by routes

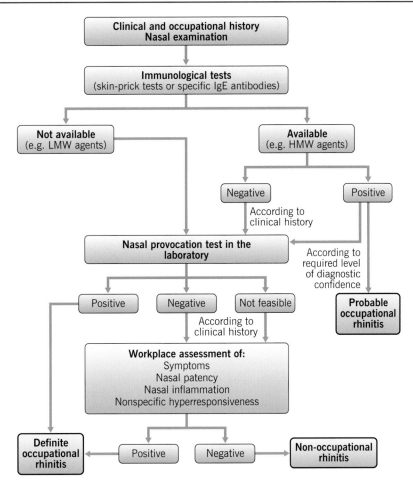

Fig. 15.5 Diagnostic algorithm for diagnosing occupational rhinitis. (From Moscato G, Vandenplas O, Gerth Van Wijk R, et al. EAACI Task Force on Occupational Rhinitis. Occupational rhinitis. Allergy 2008; 63:969–80.)

other than inhalation – mainly dermal exposure. Indeed, isocyanate skin exposure in various animal models induces systemic Th2-like sensitization that leads to asthmatic-like responses of the lung on subsequent specific inhalation challenge.

Immunological assessment

Specific IgE or IgG antibodies against an occupational sensitizer have been detected mainly for HMW agents. The value of in vivo or in vitro tests in establishing a sensitization to LMW chemicals has proved to be limited. In addition, the presence of immediate skin reactivity or increased specific IgE or IgG may reflect exposure or sensitization, but it does not imply that the target organ is involved. This has been shown for common allergens and occupational sensitizers. With HMW allergens, negative skin tests to such allergens almost completely exclude the possibility of OA. The worker may still be sensitized to another agent found in the workplace, or to another component of the offending agent. With LMW allergens, such as isocyanates and red cedar, negative skin tests or

specific IgE or IgG neither refute nor confirm the diagnosis of OA or OR; skin tests are also usually unavailable. Immunological testing is not helpful in identifying worked-exacerbated asthma or rhinitis due to non-allergic work triggers and is not indicated for the detection of irritant-induced asthma and rhinitis.

Skin tests

If the offending agent has been identified and is known to induce asthma or rhinitis through an IgE-mediated mechanism, and the appropriate antigen is available, an immediate-type percutaneous diagnostic skin test can be used to confirm sensitization. Suitable preparations of antigens (extracts, complete allergens, or, in the case of limited number of reactive LMW agents, protein conjugates) are necessary that contain the biologically active substance and give a positive skin reaction in sensitized subjects, whereas the same preparations should give negative results in non-exposed subjects. Since commercial preparations of occupational agents are not usually available, the quality control of 'home-made' antigens is particularly important. Assessment of the relative sensitivity and specificity of prick tests is recommended for each preparation of antigen. Skin prick tests are quick, inexpensive, simple to perform, and safe. Allergy skin testing with common inhalants should be performed in order to define the atopic status of the patients and to check for non-occupational aetiological factors. Skin prick tests can also be carried out in patients with impairment of lung function. There are limitations to immediate-type skin testing: they are not applicable for most LMW agents, when the mechanism of asthma or rhinitis is not IgE mediated, and when the offending agent is unknown.

In vitro tests

Specific antibodies to allergens may be demonstrated in biological fluids using a variety of tests. They confirm a sensitization demonstrated by skin test, but are often less sensitive. They represent an alternative to the skin test when the preparations of antigens have irritant, toxic, or mutagenic effects, and in patients under pharmacological treatment that blunts normal skin reactivity. Control for specificity is required, especially when protein conjugates are used. Different factors, such as total IgE level, characteristics of the conjugate, carrier specificity, and cross-reactivity with other antigens, may affect the results. The test sensitivity of in vitro specific IgE antibody assays, as well as that of skin tests, may decrease after the cessation of exposure. Assessment of the chemokine MCP-1 produced in vitro by diisocyanate-stimulated blood

mononuclear cells exhibited higher test efficiency than specific antibodies for identification of isocyanate asthma. However, like other in vitro tests such as histamine release from basophils, the assays are less standardized.

Physiological assessment in suspected asthma

The presence of airway obstruction with demonstrable reversibility after inhaling a bronchodilator is a well-recognized confirmatory step for asthma, whether or not it is occupational. If there is no significant airway obstruction, the demonstration of increased bronchial responsiveness is suggestive of asthma, but not necessarily of OA.

Simple pre- and post-workshift comparisons of forced expiratory volume in 1 second (FEV_1) are not sensitive or specific enough to be useful in the investigation of OA. Serial PEF monitoring has been proposed for both the investigation and the assessment of OA. The sensitivity and specificity of PEF monitoring, as compared with the 'gold standard' specific inhalation challenges, varies from 72 to 89% depending on the study. PEF graphs can be generated by plotting individual values or maximum, mean, and minimum values (Fig. 15.6). Serial measurements of PEF are best performed in triplicate a minimum four times a day for at least 2 weeks at work and 1–2 weeks off work.

There are several problems associated with PEF monitoring:

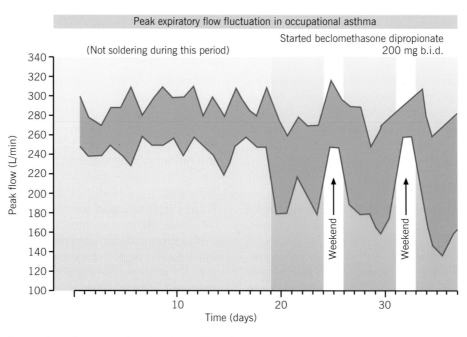

Fig. 15.6 Peak expiratory flows in occupational asthma. Plot of daily maximum (top line) and minimum (bottom line) peak flow in an asthmatic electronics worker who was exposed to colophony fumes. The days at work have a blue background, and the days away from work a pale yellow background. There is definite occupational asthma with deterioration on return to work, and improvement each weekend. (Data modified from Burge PS, Moscato G, Johnson A, et al. Physiological assessment. In: Bernstein IL, Chang-Yeung M, Malo J-L, et al, eds. Asthma in the workplace, 3rd edn. New York: Taylor & Francis; 2006:199–226.)

- it requires good collaboration and honesty on the part of the subject
- re-exposure of the subject to the same environment may be not feasible if the patient left work, or it may be dangerous
- the interpretation requires specific expertise
- the interpretation is generally based on a visual reading (although automated reading programmes have been recently proposed).

At times it is difficult to distinguish between PEF responses from a non-specific irritant exacerbation of asthma at work and OA. It has been found that compliance with PEF self-monitoring is often unsatisfactory and that a substantial number of data are falsified, which may limit interpretation. To prevent fabrication of PEF readings, guidelines recommend consideration of a device data logger to record measurements. Additional helpful information is obtained by concurrent recording by the patient of the frequency of symptoms, medication use, and specific tasks at work.

Another functional asthma test is the measure of airway responsiveness (such as methacholine challenge), which should be conducted serially at more than one time point – for example towards the end of a working period and near the end of a period away from the suspected work factor(s), preferably after at least 10 days away (e.g. the end of a holiday period without exposure).

Specific inhalation challenge (SIC) is intended to demonstrate a direct relationship between exposure to a test agent and an asthmatic response. SIC involves exposing workers who are suspected of sensitizer-induced OA to suspected agents in a safe and controlled fashion. The SIC has often been referred to as the 'gold standard' for the diagnosis of sensitizer-induced OA. However, SICs are performed in only a few centres and patients who undergo these tests are not necessarily representative of all patients with suspected OA. The clinical indication for SIC when available (which can take ≥4 days to perform) is likely to be in cases where other tests were not performed or were inconclusive. Patients in whom the index of suspicion is high because of occupation (e.g. painter, baker, red cedar lumber worker), who have a positive skin test response to a relevant work allergen, and/or increased peak flow variability, and/or increased methacoline responsiveness while working compared with off-work, have a strong case for the diagnosis of work-related asthma and are unlikely to undergo SIC. Finally, SIC with suspected sensitizers is not without risk; it needs to be undertaken only in a laboratory properly equipped and by trained staff.

The use of non-invasive tools to assess airway inflammation (induced sputum, exhaled nitric oxide, breath condensate) is promising. Induced-sputum cell counts may add useful information to the diagnostic process. Indeed, preliminary reports support the diagnosis of sensitizer-induced OA in workers who have a greater proportion of sputum eosinophils during a working period, as compared with the end of a period away from exposure. Conversely, there is limited evidence for the use of exhaled nitric oxide levels as an additional tool in the investigation of sensitizer-induced OA. Further research needs to be conducted to establish the usefulness of these tests in the diagnosis and management of OA.

Physiological assessment in suspected rhinitis

Physiological assessments to make the diagnosis of OR are not well validated, but are used to provide objective information in support of the diagnosis. Nasal physiology can be measured by several techniques including rhinomanometry, acoustic rhinometry, and peak nasal inspiratory flow. There is conflicting data about the degree of correlation between different techniques and with subjective symptoms. Physiological techniques can measure interval changes that occur with workplace exposure or with nasal allergen challenge (see Fig. 15.5). Laboratory nasal allergen challenges may be performed at some specialized centres to confirm sensitization and clinical response to some occupational HMW allergens, and some LMW sensitizers. Anterior or posterior rhinomanometry is used to measure functional obstruction to air flow in the upper airway. Acoustic rhinometry produces an image of cross-sectional dimensions of the nasal cavity. Peak nasal inspiratory flow (PNIF) has been proposed as a simple, inexpensive tool for evaluating nasal airway patency.

Only a few studies suggest that measurement of nasal nitric oxide (nNO), as a marker of nasal inflammation, might be useful in the diagnosis of OR.

Management

The natural history of OA is illustrated in Figure 15.7.

Among host markers of susceptibility, atopy is a well-known predisposing factor to asthma and OA due to HMW agents. Genetic polymorphisms of HLA class II, glutathione S-transferase, N-acetyltranferase may modify the susceptibility to OA induced by LMW agents (isocyanates, western red cedar, acid anhydrides, platinum salts). Smoking increases the risk of sensitization in subjects exposed to platinum salts, snow crab, and acid anhydrides. However, the high prevalence of smoking, atopy, and certain genetic markers among the general population, compared with their low predictive value toward the risk of occupational sensitization, precludes use of such parameters as useful screening strategies. It is unlikely that pre-existent asthma is a predisposing factor in the development of OA due to LMW agents. Although

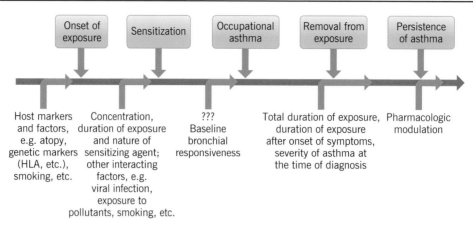

Fig. 15.7 The natural history of occupational asthma.

this conclusion is based almost entirely upon retrospective studies, most subjects who develop OA do not have a history of asthma before exposure began.

The outcome of OA after diagnosis is often poor. Several factors associated with an adverse outcome have been identified. These include a longer symptomatic exposure, lower lung volumes, higher bronchial hyper-responsiveness (BHR), or greater bronchospastic response to specific inhalation challenge at diagnosis, and older age. Moreover, HMW agents seems to cause longer duration of BHR compared with LMW allergens. In contrast, there is no relationship between atopy or smoking at the time of diagnosis and outcome of occupational asthma. More research is needed in order to assess the effects on the outcome of OA of gender and the type of asthmatic response to specific bronchial challenge.

Management plan

Primary prevention

Since all cases of occupational allergy are avoidable, policies related to primary prevention must be encouraged. Elimination of the sensitizing agent(s) is the most effective way of primary prevention, although this is often not practicable. Other options may include isolating or enclosing the process using the causative agent, reducing exposure by improving workplace ventilation or using respiratory protective devices (respirators), and education of workers about avoidance manoeuvres.

Once the diagnosis of OA is made, it is important to remove the subject from exposure as soon as possible. If this is done, it is less likely that the subject will be left with the permanent sequelae of asthma and bronchial responsiveness requiring medication. However, OA is associated with substantial long-term morbidity, as complete avoidance of exposure to the causal agent results in symptom recovery and resolution of BHR in less than one-third of affected workers. Moreover, complete

avoidance of exposure is associated with a substantial socioeconomic impact in terms of employment, income, healthcare resource utilization, and quality of life.

Persistence of exposure to the causal agent is less likely to result in the resolution of asthma symptoms and BHR, and more likely to be associated with an accelerated decline in FEV_1 compared with complete avoidance of exposure. Relocation to jobs with less exposure may be successful in some workplaces, but available evidence is insufficient to recommend this approach as a first-line therapeutic strategy. A beneficial effect was observed in workers with OA due to platinum salts transferred to low-exposure areas. Reduction of exposure to natural rubber latex was associated with clinical improvement and fewer negative socioeconomic consequences than cessation of exposure. However, placing workers with diisocyanate-induced OA in low-level exposure workplaces has not been as successful.

Respiratory personal equipment can result in an improvement, but not a complete suppression, of respiratory symptoms and airway obstruction in the short term in a few selected cases of OA. Note that, in western red cedar asthma, wearing a conventional face-mask while continuing to work does not reduce the risk. In some subjects, it may be worthwhile to consider wearing a helmet respirator whenever short periods of exposure to a sensitizer occur.

Secondary prevention

The early detection of workers with established disease, and their subsequent removal from exposure, is the most effective way to prevent progression to moderate or severe disease with its associated morbidity and disability. An individual diagnosis of OA represents a potential sentinel event for a careful evaluation of the workplace to identify and prevent other cases of OA. In addition, screening programmes may provide a means to measure the impact of primary prevention measures. Therefore, adequate worker medical surveillance has to be ensured. This can be done by routine skin testing with HMW occupational agents; it is feasible and can identify subjects who have become immunologically sensitized and who should be followed more closely in terms of the development of bronchial hyperresponsiveness and asthma symptoms. In subjects exposed to LMW agents, routine questionnaires coupled with an assessment of bronchial responsiveness could prove useful in detecting the disease at an early stage. There is some evidence that surveillance and early removal of sensitized workers result in a better outcome than no surveillance. However, it is often difficult to determine which component of the surveillance programme is effective. A cost-effectiveness analysis of medical surveillance for diisocianate asthma found a ratio in favour of surveillance.

Drug treatment

Drug therapy of OA or OR does not differ from that indicated in national and international guidelines for other forms of asthma or rhinitis. It is known that taking anti-inflammatory inhaled corticosteroid preparations accelerates clinical, functional, and pathological improvement of OA once removal from exposure has been carried out. The long-term effects of inhaled steroids on OA have seldom been evaluated. There is currently no sufficient evidence that treatment with inhaled corticosteroids and long-acting β_2-agonists is able to prevent the long-term deterioration of asthma in subjects who remain exposed to the agent causing OA. Antiasthma drugs are generally not sufficient to prevent asthma attacks upon re-exposure to the offending agent at work, although they can reduce the severity.

Conclusions regarding the effectiveness of medications in managing OA are difficult to draw, but the effectiveness of the medications studied among workers with sensitizer-induced OA appeared to be similar to that of others with chronic asthma. Treatment with inhaled corticosteroids in addition to removal from exposure may provide slight beneficial effect, but there is insufficient evidence to support a systematic treatment with high-dose inhaled corticosteroids after cessation of exposure.

To date, there is minimal information about pharmacotherapy for OR, whether allergic or non-allergic. Suggested approaches include the daily use of intranasal corticosteroids or the administration of antihistamines and/or intranasal cromolyn immediately before allergen exposure. Specific immunotherapy with HMW occupational agents is currently limited by the unavailability of standardized extracts for most occupational allergens and the lack of information on its effectiveness and adverse effects. The available studies include those on immunotherapy for natural rubber latex in healthcare workers, Hymenoptera venom in beekeepers, wheat in bakers,

pollens in outdoor workers, and cat allergen in animal workers.

Medicolegal aspects: assessment of disability and compensation

Criteria for the clinical diagnosis of OA and medicolegal requirements for the diagnosis of OA have not been uniform among countries. There are several reasons why it is important to confirm the diagnosis of OA both medically and medicolegally. Missing the diagnosis may well result in a worker's continued exposure to the asthma-provoking agent – with all the medical consequences that implies. A diagnosis of OA also has significant social and financial consequences. Unlike pneumoconiosis, OA frequently affects young people. Leaving the job on a physician's advice has a major impact, as it implies retraining for a new occupation. Although it is of the utmost importance to offer retraining programmes to workers, or early retirement with financial compensation, the efficacy and cost of these programmes should also be considered.

OA can lead to permanent asthma, even after removal from exposure. The United States, Canada and most European countries recognize OA as compensable disease. Workers' compensation is generally a no-fault compensation system paid by employers and administered by governmental agencies (in Canada and Europe) or private insurance companies (in the United States). It is clear that the methods for reporting, recognizing, and paying compensation for occupational diseases are far from uniform from one country to the next. The principles of impairment assessment valid for chronic lung diseases (such as pneumoconiosis or chronic obstructive pulmonary disease), which are associated with a stable functional impairment and abnormalities of gas exchange and mechanical parenchymal properties, are inappropriate for subjects with asthma. OA, like other forms of asthma, is characterized by variable air-flow obstruction, amenability to therapy, no radiological abnormalities, no clear relationship with the level of exposure to the offending agent, and triggering by multiple factors in the presence of BHR. A scaling system that includes some of these variables has been proposed by a committee appointed by the American Thoracic Society (Table 15.2). The long-term assessment of impairment should be performed for 2 years after the cessation of exposure, since the maximum rate of improvement occurs within this period of time. However, more prolonged follow-up has been required to demonstrate inprovement in non-specific airway responsiveness.

As with OA, medicolegal requirements for the diagnosis of OR vary by country, with some requiring that objective changes be documented by nasal provocation testing, whereas others consider clinical history with immunological sensitization as supportive of claims for compensation.

Table 15.2 American Thoracic Society guidelines for assessing impairment and disability in asthma and occupational asthma

Score	0	1	2	3	4	5
FEV_1 (% pred.)	>80	79–79	60–69	50–59	<50	
Reversibility of airway obstruction (% change in FEV_1)		<10	10–19	20–29	>30	
Hyperresponsiveness $PC_{20}FEV_1$ (mg/mL)	>8	2–8	0.25–2	<0.25		
Medication needed:						
Bronchodilators	None	Occasional (not daily)	Daily	Daily		
Cromolyn	None	Courses (1–3/year)	Daily			
Inhaled steroid	None	Courses (1–3/year)	Low dose daily	High dose daily	High dose daily	
Systemic steroid	None	None	None	Courses (1–3/year)	Daily	
Summary rating class:						
Class	0	I	II	III	IV	V
Total score	0	1–3	4–6	7–9	10–11	
	Uncontrolled	Uncontrolled				

FEV_1, forced expiratory volume in the first second; $PC_{20}FEV_1$, provocative concentration of histamine or methacholine producing a 20% fall in FEV_1.

In addition, the disability rating for OR may also vary greatly between countries.

Conclusions

Occupational allergy can affect many target organs, including the lungs, nose, eyes, and skin. This chapter focuses on occupational allergy affecting the upper and lower airways – that is, occupational asthma and occupational rhinitis. It has been estimated that >20% of total workforce is exposed to at least one of the numerous asthmogenic products in the workplace. In the general population, the attributable risk fraction for asthma due to occupation represents approximately 15%. Based upon cross-sectional studies, prevalence rates of OR are two to four times more prevalent than OA. Due to its significant medical, social, and (possibly) legal consequences, a definitive diagnosis of occupational allergy, including identification of the causative agent, is imperative. Since all cases of occupational allergy are avoidable, policies related to primary prevention must be encouraged. Elimination of the sensitizing agent(s) is the most effective way of primary prevention, although this is often not practicable. OA and OR can lead to permanent impairment and disability. The early detection of workers with established disease, and their subsequent removal from exposure, is the most effective way to prevent progression to moderate or severe disease with its associated morbidity and disability. An individual diagnosis of OA represents a potential sentinel event for the identification and prevention of other cases of OA. In addition, screening programmes may provide a means to measure the impact of primary prevention measures. Therefore, adequate worker medical surveillance has to be ensured.

Summary of important messages

- Early diagnosis of OA and early removal from exposure to the causative agent in the workplace improve the chance of recovery
- Suspecting work exposure as a cause of asthma in all individuals with new-onset or worsening asthma, and asking key questions about work exposures while history taking, are crucial in the work-up of OA
- Despite the efforts of standardization, the diagnosis of OA and OR still remains complicated and controversial
- OR is frequently present in OA, and may precede development of OA, particularly with HMW sensitizers
- OA and OR can lead to permanent impairment and disability

Further reading

Castano R, Malo JL. Occupational rhinitis and asthma: Where do we stand, Where do we go? Curr Allergy Asthma Rep 2010; 10:135–142.

Dykewicz MS. Occupational asthma: current concepts in pathogenesis, diagnosis and management. J Allergy Clin Immunol 2009; 123:519–528.

Maestrelli P, Boschetto P, Fabbri LM, et al. Mechanisms of occupational asthma. J Allergy Clin Immunol 2009; 123:531–542.

Malo J-L, Chang-Yeung M. Agents causing occupational asthma with key references. In: Bernstein IL, Chang-Yeung M, Malo J-L, et al, eds. Asthma in the workplace, 3rd edn. New York: Taylor & Francis; 2006:825–849.

Mapp CE, Boschetto P, Maestrelli P, et al. Occupational asthma. Am J Respir Crit Care Med 2005; 172:280–305.

Moscato G, Vandenplas O, Gerth Van Wijk R, et al, for the EAACI Task Force on Occupational Rhinitis, Occupational rhinitis. Allergy 2008; 63:969–980.

Quirce S, Lemière C, de Blay F, et al. Noninvasive methods for assessment of airway inflammation in occupational settings. Allergy 2010; 65:445–458.

Siracusa A, Desrosiers M, Marabini A. Epidemiology of occupational rhinitis: prevalence, aetiology and determinants. Clin Exp Allergy 2000; 30:1519–1534.

Tarlo SM, Balmes J, Balkissoon R, et al. Diagnosis and management of work-related asthma: American College Of Chest Physicians Consensus Statement. Chest 2008; 134(3 suppl):S1–41.

16

Drug hypersensitivity

B Kevin Park, Dean J Naisbitt and Pascal Demoly

DEFINITION

Drug hypersensitivity is an immunologically mediated adverse drug reaction. To initiate an immune response, the drug must associate with protein generating an antigen that is presented to T lymphocytes in the context of MHC molecules. Individuals with disease conditions such as HIV and cystic fibrosis are susceptible to a much-increased risk of drug allergy. Furthermore, several strong genetic associations between expression of specific HLA alleles and drug allergy have been discovered.

Introduction

Drug hypersensitivity reactions (DHRs) are the adverse effects of drugs that, when taken at doses generally tolerated by normal subjects, clinically resemble allergy. They are a daily worry for the clinician. Only when a definite immunological mechanism (either drug-specific antibody or T cell) is demonstrated, should these reactions be classified as drug allergy. To simplify classification, DHRs are divided into two types according to the delay of onset of the reaction after the last administration of the drug: (1) immediate reaction – occurring less than 1 hour after the last drug intake – usually in the form of urticaria, angioedema, rhinitis, conjunctivitis, bronchospasm, and anaphylaxis or anaphylactic shock; (2) non-immediate reaction – with variable cutaneous symptoms occurring after more than 1 hour and up to several days after the last drug intake – for example, late-occurring urticaria, maculopapular eruptions, fixed drug eruptions, vasculitis, toxic epidermal necrolysis, Stevens–Johnson syndrome, or drug reaction with eosinophilia and systemic symptoms (DRESS). The first category is mostly mediated through specific IgE, whereas the latter is specifically T cell mediated. To stimulate a reaction the drug might act as a hapten and bind irreversibly to protein. The majority of drugs are not directly protein reactive; in such cases, hapten formation is thought to occur as a consequence of metabolic activation. An alternative hypothesis termed the 'pharmacological interaction' (PI) theory, which evolved from analysis of the response of T-cell clones to drug stimulation, suggests that drugs, although smaller than traditional antigens, might also interact directly with immunological receptors through a reversible interaction with major histocompatibility complex (MHC) molecules and specific T-cell receptors. The tools allowing a definite diagnosis are few in number and include the following procedures: a thorough clinical history, standardized skin tests, reliable biological tests and drug provocation tests. All of these tools, although not always validated or predictive at the individual level – often due to limited availability of relevant drug antigens – and sometimes dangerous have been carefully evaluated by the European Network of Drug Allergy (the European Academy of Allergy and Clinical Immunology drug allergy group of interest). When properly performed in specialized centres, a firm diagnosis is often possible and safe alternative medication can be proposed. Several strong genetic associations between expression of a particular HLA allele and susceptibility to specific forms of drug hypersensitivity have recently been discovered. For the drug abacavir an association between *B*5701* expression and hypersensitivity has prompted the development of predictive testing strategies and labelling changes to drug information sheets.

Disease mechanisms

Drug hypersensitivity can be defined as a serious adverse drug reaction, with an immunological aetiology, to an otherwise safe and effective therapeutic agent. Any drug is assumed to be able to elicit DHRs. However, the frequency differs widely. Antibiotics, non-steroidal anti-inflammatory drugs, antiepileptics and anti-HIV drugs are the most prevalent classes responsible (Table 16.1).

Table 16.1 Drug classes commonly associated with hypersensitivity reactions

Drug class	Drug examples
Antiepileptics	Carbamazepine, phenytoin, lamotrigine
Antibiotics	Penicillins, cephalosporins, sulfonamides, tetracyclines, quinolones
Anti-HIV drugs	Abacavir, nevirapine
NSAIDS	Ibuprofen, diclofenac, piroxicam, celecoxib
General anaesthetics	Neuromuscular blocking agents
Local anaesthetics	Lidocaine (lignocaine), mepivacaine
Contrast media and dyes	Iohexol, iomeprol, patent blue

Fortunately, in most individuals DHRs are rare; however, the incidence rate is increased with certain diseases (e.g. Infectious mononucleosis, HIV, cystic fibrosis). Clinical manifestations of DHRs are numerous and range from maculopapular exanthema to anaphylactic shock (Table 16.2).

Immediate hypersensitivity reactions

Immediate DHRs develop as a result of IgE production by antigen-specific B lymphocytes. The IgE antibody ligates the surface of mast cells and basophils creating a multivalent binding site for the drug antigen (Fig. 16.1). Following subsequent drug exposure the antigen – presumably a hapten protein complex – cross-links bound IgE, stimulating the release of prestored mediators (e.g. histamine) and the production of new mediators (e.g. leukotrienes, cytokines). The prestored mediators stimulate a response within minutes, whereas the inflammatory component develops after several hours – the time required for protein synthesis and the recruitment of immune cells (Fig. 16.2). The most well-defined immediate DHRs are β-lactam-mediated anaphylaxis, angiodema, urticaria, rhinitis, conjunctivitis, and bronchospasm.

Delayed hypersensitivity reactions

Delayed-type DHRs are mediated through the actions of T lymphocytes. Skin is the organ most commonly targeted by drug-responsive T cells. Reactions vary in severity from mild self-limiting rashes to Stevens–Johnson syndrome and toxic epidermal necrolysis, which have fatality rates of 5% and 30% respectively. Skin reactions may occur in isolation or in combination with a variety of systemic symptoms. Diclofenac and several other carboxylic acid non-steroidal anti-inflammatory drugs cause immune-mediated cholestatic liver injury in humans,

Table 16.2 Clinical symptoms and available allergy tests

Clinical symptoms	Potential pathogenesis	Diagnostic tests
Urticaria Angioedema	Type I allergy, non-allergic hypersensitivity, rarely: type III allergy	Prick, intradermal tests, specific IgE, mediator release/cellular tests
Anaphylaxis	Type I allergy, non-allergic hypersensitivity	Prick, intradermal tests, specific IgE, mediator release/cellular tests
Maculopapular exanthem	Type IV allergy	Patch, late-reading intradermal tests, LTT
Vesicular–bullous exanthem	Type IV allergy	Patch tests
Pustular exanthem	Type IV allergy	Patch, late-reading intradermal tests, LTT
Fixed drug eruption	Type IV allergy	Patch tests in affected area

Adapted from Pichler WJ. Delayed drug hypersensitivity reactions. Ann Intern Med 2003; 139:683–693.
LTT, lymphocyte transformation test.

which may be explained by hepatic metabolism and selective covalent modification of hepatocyte protein. It is important to note that the same drug might stimulate different clinical signs in different individuals, despite the drug being administered at the same dose and via the same route.

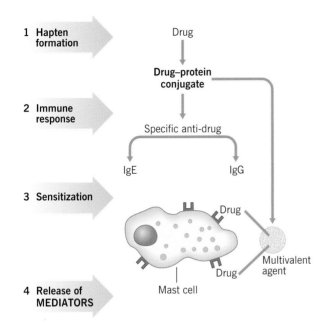

Fig. 16.1 The generation of a multivalent drug antigen and its interaction with mast-cell-associated immunoglobulin E (IgE).

To stimulate naive T cells, dendritic cells 'recognize' the drug antigen. The antigen is then internalized and transported to the regional lymph nodes if the localized microenvironment is rich in maturation signals. Maturation signals, often referred to as 'danger signals' may develop as a result of drug-related stress, disease, or trauma. On arrival at the lymph nodes the antigen is presented to naive T lymphocytes. Drug antigens might also stimulate pathogen-specific T cells, thus avoiding the requirement for T-cell priming. However, this hypothesis is difficult to reconcile with the time between initial drug exposure and the development of clinical signs.

Antigen-specific T cells migrate to target organs and, once re-exposed to the antigen, they are activated to secrete cytokines that regulate the response and cytotoxins (e.g. perforin, granzymes, and granulysins) (Fig. 16.3).

Table 16.3 provides a simple classification system for DHRs.

Chemical basis of drug hypersensitivity

Currently available methods to diagnose drug allergy lack sensitivity, and there are no established methods to predict the immunogenic potential of a drug. It is therefore critical to define the fundamental mechanisms of DHRs and determine whether a drug can act as a hapten, antigen, immunogen, and costimulatory agent (Table 16.4). The development of such mechanistic tools will

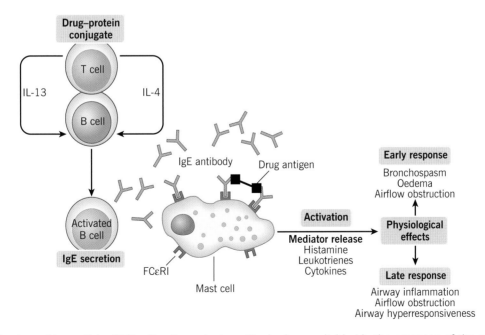

Fig. 16.2 Mechanism of immediate DHRs. B cells undergo antibody class switching in the presence of the cytokines IL-4 and IL-13. Antigen stimulation activates the B cell to secrete high quantities of IgE, which associates with mast cells. Following subsequent drug exposure, cross-linking of IgE stimulates mast cell degranulation. Mediator release stimulates both the early and the late phase of the immediate hypersensitivity reaction. IL, interleukin; FcRI, Fc domain of the high-affinity Ig receptor.

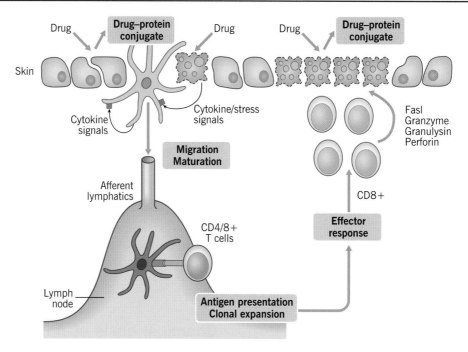

Fig. 16.3 Mechanism of delayed DHRs in skin. Cutaneous dendritic cells take up the drug antigen and in the presence of cutaneous stress signals migrate to draining lymph nodes and present the antigen to naïve T cells. Following subsequent drug exposure, antigen-specific T cells migrate to skin and, when activated through the T-cell receptor, secrete cytokines and cytotoxins. FasL, FS7-associated cell surface antigen.

Table 16.3 Classification of drug hypersensitivity reactions

Type	Type of immune response	Pathophysiology	Clinical symptoms	Chronology of the reaction
I	IgE	Mast cells and basophil degranulation	Anaphylactic shock Angioedema Urticaria Bronchospasm	A few minutes to 1 hour after the last intake of the drug
II	IgG and FcR	FcR-dependent cell death	Cytopenia	5–15 days after the start of treatment
III	IgM or IgG and complement or FcR	Deposition of immune complexes	Serum sickness Urticaria Vasculitis	7–8 days for serum sickness 7–21 days after the start of treatment for vasculitis
IVa	Th1 (IFNγ)	Monocytic inflammation	Eczema	5–21 days after the start of treatment
IVb	Th2 (IL-5 and IL-4)	Eosinophilic inflammation	Maculo-papular exanthema, bullous exanthema	2–6 weeks after the start of treatment for DRESS
IVc	Cytotoxic T cells (perforin, granzyme B, FasL)	Keratinocyte death mediated by CD4 or CD8	Maculo-papular exanthema, bullous exanthema, pustular exanthema	2 days after the start of treatment for fixed drug eruption, 7–21 days after the start of treatment for Stevens–Johnson and TEN
IVd	T cells (IL-8/CXCL8)	Neutrophilic inflammation	Acute generalized exanthematous pustulosis	Less than 2 days

Adapted from Jenkins RE, Meng X, Elliott VL, et al. Characterization of flucloxacillin and 5-hydroxymethyl flucloxacillin haptenated HSA in vitro and in vivo. Proteomics Clin Appl 2009; 3:20–729.

Management

The diagnosis of DHRs is often difficult and requires a stereotypic attitude no matter which drug is involved. It remains largely clinical with the help of certain allergy tests that are available for some of the drug classes. Provocation tests are the gold standard but, because they are cumbersome and possibly harmful, are limited to highly specialized centres. New and validated biological tools for diagnosis that are available to all clinicians are necessary in order to improve care for these patients.

A definite diagnosis of DHRs is required in order to institute proper preventive measures. Whatever the intensity of the clinical reaction, a state of hypersensitivity is shown towards the particular drug with the possibility of a more serious reaction in the future. Diagnosis is important and particularly challenging in vulnerable patients often receiving multiple drugs and/or with a history of multiple DHRs. General preventive measures include a declaration to the Committee on Safety of Medicine Reports. Individual measures include the issue of an 'allergy card' specifying the culprit agent(s), the delivery of a list of drugs to avoid, and the delivery of a list of possible alternatives. The patient is also asked to make his allergies known prior to all prescriptions and surgical operations, and to read the package insert on any drugs to be taken. The lists can never be completely exhaustive, are only indicative, and should be frequently updated. Similarly, questioning (to elicit any history of allergy) of every patient by every clinician prior to issuing a prescription is essential from both a medical and a medicolegal point of view. Preventive measures by premedication (e.g. slow injection and preparations with antihistamines and glucocorticosteroids) mainly concern non-allergic hypersensitivity reactions (for example to vancomycin, certain anaesthetics, and chemotherapy drugs). The possibility of desensitization should always be considered when the offending drug is essential and when either no alternatives exist, or they are unsatisfactory, as in the following cases: sulfonamides in HIV-infected patients, quinolone allergies in some cystic fibrosis patients, serious infections with allergy to penicillins, allergy to tetanus vaccine, haemochromatosis with allergy to desferoxamine, or aspirin and non-steroidal anti-inflammatory drug hypersensitivity in patients for whom there is a clear necessity for these drugs to treat either a cardiac or rheumatoid illness.

Conclusions

Drug hypersensitivity is an adverse drug reaction that is highly variable with respect to frequency and severity. It is of great concern to the physician because the severe forms of the reaction, which include anaphylaxis and toxic epidermal necrolysis, can be life threatening. The development of tests for the prediction of individual susceptibility remains an important goal, for which recent developments in pharmacogenetics provides promise. Both phenotyping and genotyping are particularly important for vulnerable groups of patients on multiple drug therapy; therefore the development of reliable diagnostic tests remains a priority for research in this area.

Summary of important messages

- Drug hypersensitivity reactions are defined as a serious adverse drug reaction with an immunological aetiology to an otherwise safe and effective therapeutic agent
- Drug hypersensitivity reactions are rare; they vary in severity and clinical signs
- Immediate hypersensitivity reactions develop as a result of specific IgE production; delayed reactions are mediated by antigen-specific T cells
- Drug haptens form antigenic determinants by interacting irreversibly with protein
- Diagnosis of drug hypersensitivity reactions should be based on history, clinical manifestations, and if possible skin tests and biological tests
- A patient with a definitive diagnosis of hypersensitivity should be re-exposed to the culprit drug only with extreme caution in an appropriate clinical setting

Further reading

Bircher AJ. Symptoms and danger signs in acute drug hypersensitivity. Toxicology 2005; 209:201–207.

Brander C, Mauri-Hellweg D, Bettens F, et al. Heterogeneous T cell responses to beta-lactam-modified self structures are observed in penicillin-allergic individuals. J Immunol 1995; 155:2670–2678.

Callan HE, Jenkins RE, Maggs JL, et al. Multiple adduction reactions of nitroso sulfamethoxazole with cysteinyl residues of peptides and proteins: Implications for hapten formation. Chem Res Toxicol 2009; 22:937–948.

Castrejon JL, Berry N, El-Ghaiesh S, et al. Stimulation of T-cells with sulfonamides and sulfonamide metabolites. J Allergy Clin Immunol 2010; 125:411–418.

Chessman D, Kostenko L, Lethborg T, et al. Human leukocyte antigen class 1-restricted activation of CD8+ T cells provides the immunogenetic basis of a systemic drug hypersensitivity. Immunity 2008; 28:822–832.

Demoly P, Romano A. Drug hypersensitivity: clinical manifestations and diagnosis. In: Pawankar R, Holgate ST, Rosenwasser LJ, eds. Allergy frontiers: clinical manifestations, vol 3. Tokyo: Springer; 2009:379–392.

Ebo DG, Sainte-Laudy J, Bridts CH, et al. Flow-assisted allergy diagnosis: current applications and future perspectives. Allergy 2006; 61:1028–1039.

Jenkins RE, Meng X, Elliott VL, et al. Characterization of flucloxacillin and 5-hydroxymethyl flucloxacillin haptenated HSA in vitro and in vivo. Proteomics Clin Appl 2009; 3:720–729.

Mallal S, Nolan D, Witt C, et al. Association between presence of HLA-B*5701, HLA-DR7 and HLA-DQ3 and hypersensitivity to HIV-1 reverse-transcriptase inhibitor abacavir. Lancet 2002; 359:727–732.

Pichler WJ. Delayed drug hypersensitivity reactions. Ann Intern Med 2003; 139:683–693.

Anaphylaxis

Phil Lieberman and Pamela W Ewan

DEFINITION

Anaphylaxis is a potentially life-threatening allergic reaction, usually sudden in onset and rapidly progressive, with airway obstruction or hypotension, often with cutaneous features.

Introduction

The definition of 'anaphylaxis' is in flux. It is a potentially life-threatening allergic reaction, usually sudden in onset and rapidly progressive, with airway obstruction or hypotension, and often with cutaneous features. Criteria for the diagnosis of anaphylaxis that mandates adrenaline (US epinephrine) treatment have been established in the United Kingdom (Box 17.1), while in the USA the National Institutes of Health have established criteria for the diagnosis of anaphylaxis.

Classically anaphylaxis was considered to be an immediate hypersensitivity IgE-mediated reaction, but similar events can be mediated without the need for IgE and such events were termed 'anaphylactoid' reactions. More recently it has been suggested that the term 'anaphylactoid' be abandoned, and all events, regardless of the mechanism of production, be called 'anaphylactic episodes'. Table 17.1 summarizes the two terminologies. In this table, anaphylactoid events would be those described as non-IgE-mediated, whether non-immunological or immunological in origin.

Epidemiology

The incidence of anaphylaxis overall remains undetermined and has to be estimated indirectly. However, based on data from real-time prescriptions for adrenaline (US epinephrine), as much as 1% of the population may be at risk for an anaphylactic episode or may have experienced such an episode. Data from attendances at emergency departments show that 1 in 3300 of the population had an anaphylactic reaction in a 1-year period. Data from recorded diagnosis in English primary care databases found the lifetime prevalence to be 1 in 3333 of population. These may be conservative estimates because anaphylactic events are underreported. An American College of Allergy, Asthma and Immunology working group found that the overall frequency of episodes of anaphylaxis using current data lies between 30 and 950 cases per 100 000 persons per year, and the lifetime prevalence is between 50 and 2000 episodes per 100 000 persons, or 0.05–2.0%.

The frequency of anaphylactic events is increasing and hospital admissions in UK increased seven-fold over a decade. The reasons for this are unclear, but are probably related to the increase in allergic disease, including food allergy, that has occurred over the past three decades.

© 2012 Elsevier Ltd
DOI: 10.1016/B978-0-7234-3658-4.00005-6

Box 17.1 Criteria established for the requirement for the diagnosis of anaphylaxis and therefore a mandate for adrenaline* treatment

1. Acute onset of cutaneous symptoms (urticaria, itch, flush, angioedema) and at least one of the following:
   a. respiratory symptoms
   b. reduced blood pressure
2. Two or more of the following that occur rapidly after exposure to a likely antigen:
   a. skin or mucosal involvement
   b. respiratory symptoms
   c. reduced blood pressure
3. Reduced blood pressure, syncope, after exposure to a known allergen

*Adrenaline is called epinephrine in the USA.

Table 17.1 Terminology referring to the classification of anaphylaxis

Traditional	Recently suggested change
IgE-mediated anaphylaxis	Anaphylaxis
'Anaphylactoid'*	Immunological: – IgE-mediated – non-IgE-mediated
'Anaphylactoid'	Anaphylaxis non-immunologically mediated

*The term 'anaphylactoid' refers to a clinically similar event not mediated by IgE.

Several factors affect the incidence of anaphylaxis, as is noted in Table 17.2. Atopy is a risk factor for many causes of anaphylaxis, including food-induced anaphylaxis. Furthermore, it also constitutes a risk factor for other forms of anaphylaxis such as exercise-induced anaphylaxis.

Of interest is the more recently described effect of geography on the incidence of anaphylaxis. In the northern hemisphere, events appear to be more frequent in upper latitudes, and the reverse is true for the southern hemisphere – perhaps implying a role for sunlight exposure and the serum levels of vitamin D. It has been postulated that higher levels of the vitamin are protective based upon this finding.

In children, events are more common in males, but at the time of puberty the reverse becomes true, with females predominating. After menopause, the incidence becomes approximately equal. To date there has been no described racial or ethnic predisposition to anaphylactic events.

Mechanism of anaphylaxis

Mast cell and basophil

The primary event underlying anaphylactic episodes is degranulation of the mast cell and the basophil. The clinical manifestations are the result of the activities of the mediators released from these cells (Fig. 17.1 and see Table 17.3).

These mediators not only exert direct effects on the target organs, but also recruit other inflammatory

Table 17.2 Factors influencing the incidence of anaphylaxis

Factor	Comment
Atopy	Atopy is a risk factor for anaphylaxis in general. Tha incidence of atopy is higher in patients with food-, latex-, and food-dependent exercise-induced anaphylaxis. It is not a risk factor for drug or Hymenoptera allergy
Geographic location	Recently found to be a risk factor in terms of latitude. In the northern hemisphere, episodes are more frequent in higher latitudes. The reverse is true for the southern hemisphere. This implies a role for sunlight exposure and perhaps vitamin D levels
Gender	In children (up to age 15), more common in males. After age 15, more common in females. After menopause, incidence is approximately equal
Socioeconomic status	Some studies suggest that higher socioeconomic status increases the risk of anaphylactic events
Constancy of administration of antigen	Gaps in administration of antigen may predispose to reactions. This has been shown for allergen immunotherapy and insulin therapy. In contrast a short interval between stings increases the risk of a systemic reaction
Chronobiology	No known effect related to time of day
Race/ethnicity	No known effect on the incidence of anaphylaxis

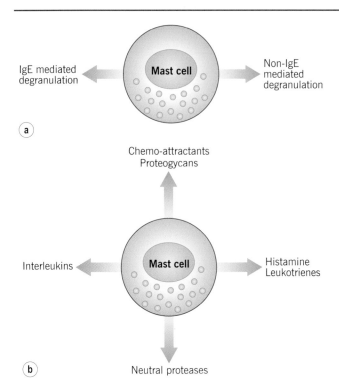

Fig. 17.1 (a) The mast cell can be degranulated by both IgE and non-IgE mechanisms. (b) Upon degranulation, chemical mediators are released that result in the symptoms and signs of anaphylaxis.

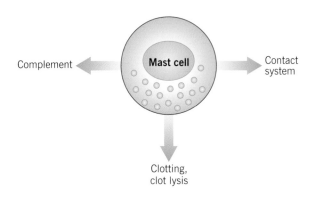

Fig. 17.2 In addition to the activities of mediators directly released from mast cells, there is recruitment of other inflammatory cascades including the complement system, contact system with the formation of bradykinin, and clotting and clot lysis, which can result in intravascular coagulation.

cascades, including complement, the contact system, and the clotting cascade, which can amplify and change the nature of the pathophysiology (Fig. 17.2 and Table 17.3).

Causes of anaphylaxis

The most common causes of anaphylaxis are foods, Hymenoptera stings, and drugs; however, idiopathic anaphylaxis is increasingly common, so that in adults these four causes account for the majority of cases. In children, the picture is different and food allergy accounts for most cases of anaphylaxis. Other causes are physical (e.g. exercise, cold, or pressure induced) or latex allergy. Rarer causes include allergy to seminal plasma. Nut allergy occurs in at least 2% of children and about one-third will suffer anaphylaxis. Peanut is the commonest food to cause fatal or near-fatal episodes. Cow's milk is an important cause of severe anaphylaxis in children, but a wide range of foods cause anaphylactic events. Of drugs, antibiotics – especially β-lactams, non-steroidal anti-inflammatory drugs (NSAIDs), and aspirin – as well as neuromuscular-blocking drugs and other agents used in general anaesthesia, chlorhexidine, diagnostic dyes, and radiocontrast media, can cause them. Fatal anaphylaxis due to penicillin occurs with an incidence of 0.002% and accounts for 500 penicillin-related anaphylactic deaths annually in the USA. Non-fatal reactions occur in 0.7–1.0% of penicillin recipients.

Clinical presentation

Classical clinical presentation

The signs and symptoms of anaphylaxis are noted, in approximate order of frequency, in Box 17.2. Series of anaphylactic events reveal striking similarities, which have allowed us to discern the approximate incidence of each manifestation listed in Box 17.2.

By far, cutaneous and subcutaneous manifestations are the most common. They include urticaria, angioedema, erythema (often referred to as 'flush' in USA), and pruritus. In adults, one (or more) of these manifestations is present in 90% or more of episodes. In children, the incidence of cutaneous manifestations may be slightly lower. Respiratory complaints such as wheeze, dyspnoea, stridor, and rhinitis comprise the next most common group of symptoms. They occur in 40–60% of cases. There is a clear-cut association with severe episodes and mortality when respiratory symptoms are present. This is especially true for asthma. Cardiovascular symptoms are the next most frequent manifestation. Dizziness, syncope, arrhythmia, angina, myocardial infarction, and hypotension occur in about 30–35% of events. Gastrointestinal symptoms have an incidence very close to that of cardiovascular manifestations. Nausea, vomiting, cramping abdominal pain, and diarrhoea are common occurrences, especially if the antigen has been ingested.

The pattern of symptoms varies with the cause. In food-induced anaphylaxis the dominant severe feature is frequently respiratory (laryngeal oedema or asthma), whereas with bee venom or intravenous drugs/agents cardiovascular features (hypotension or loss of consciousness) may predominate. For example, in perioperative

Table 17.3 Anaphylactic mediators and their resultant pathophysiological activities factors directly released from mast cells and basophils

Mediator	Pathophysiological event	Clinical correlate
Histamine and products of arachidonic acid metabolism (leukotrienes, thromboxane, prostaglandins, and platelet-activating factor)	Smooth muscle spasm, mucus secretion, vasodilatation, increased vascular permeability, activation of nociceptive neurons, platelet adherence, eosinophil activation, eosinophil chemotaxis	Wheeze, urticaria, angioedema, flush, itch, diarrhoea and abdominal pain, hypotension, rhinorrhoea, and bronchorrhoea
Neutral proteases: tryptase, chymase, carboxypeptidase, cathepsin G	Cleavage of complement components, chemoattractants for eosinophils and neutrophils, further activation and degranulation of mast cells, cleavage of neuropeptides, conversion of angiotensin I to angiotensin II	May recruit complement by cleaving C3, may ameliorate symptoms by invoking a hypertensive response through the conversion of angiotensin I to angiotensin II and by inactivating neuropeptides. Also, can magnify response owing to further mast cell activation
Proteoglycans: heparin, chondroitin sulphate	Anticoagulation, inhibition of complement, binding phospholipase A2, chemoattractant for eosinophils, inhibition of cytokine function, activation of kinin pathway	Can prevent intravascular coagulation and the recruitment of complement. Also can recruit kinins increasing the severity of the reaction
Chemoattractants: chemokines, eosinophil chemotactic factors	Calls forth cells to the site	May be partly responsible for recrudescence of symptoms in late phase reaction or extension and protraction of reaction
Nitric oxide	Smooth muscle relaxation causing vasodilatation of peripheral vascular bed, bronchodilatation, and coronary artery vasodilatation. In addition, nitric oxide causes increased vascular permeability	Perhaps relief of bronchospasm, but most important effect appears to be the production of hypotension and shock
Tumor necrosis factor α activates NF-κB	Production of platelet-activating factor	Vascular permeability and vasodilatation. Also since it is synthesized and released 'late', has been incriminated in production of late phase reactions
Interleukins 2, 6, 10	These are usually found later in the course of an event than histamine and tryptase, and persist longer. The effects they cause have not been determined. IL-10 may be active in recovery from events	Unknown
Tumor necrosis factor receptor-1	Unknown	Elevated levels have been associated with more profound hypotension
Factors activated by recruitment of other inflammatory cascades		
Activation of the contact system (kinins)	Vasodilatation and vasopermeability	Hypotension and angioedema
Activation of the complement system	C3a/C5a can cause vasopermeability	Possible urticaria/angioedema
Activation of the clotting system (Factor XI, plasmin)	Intravascular coagulation	Disseminated intravascular coagulation

Box 17.2 Signs and symptoms of anaphylaxis

Cutaneous, subcutaneous:

- Urticaria and angioedema
- Erythema*
- Pruritus without rash

Respiratory:

- Wheeze
- Dyspnoea
- Upper respiratory obstruction (angioedema)
- Rhinitis
- Stridor

Cardiovascular:

- Dizziness
- Syncope
- Hypotension
- Collapse
- Loss of consciousness
- Arrhythmia
- Angina
- Myocardial infarction

Gastrointestinal:

- Nausea
- Vomiting
- Diarrhoea
- Cramping abdominal pain

Miscellaneous and rare:

- Incontinence
- Substernal pain
- Seizure
- Visual abnormalities
- Disseminated intravascular coagulation

*Erythema is often referred to as 'flush' in USA.

anaphylaxis, cutaneous symptoms occur less frequently, and cardiovascular collapse is seen more frequently than in events occurring outside the operating theatre.

Symptoms of anaphylaxis usually begin within 5–30 minutes after antigen injection, and within 2 hours after antigen ingestion. However, there can be a delay of several hours after ingestion in some instances. This delay has been noted most commonly related to episodes caused by the ingestion of red meat in which galactose-α-1,3-galactose has been incriminated as the offending allergen. It is felt that the more rapid the onset of symptoms after exposure to allergen, the more severe is the event.

Less-common presentations of anaphylaxis

Hypotension without other manifestations

There are exceptions to these classical manifestations of anaphylaxis. Perhaps the most common of these is cardiovascular collapse with shock, which can occur immediately after exposure to antigen, and which may not be accompanied by any other manifestations. Severely affected patients may experience cardiovascular collapse in the absence of any other manifestation. In 5% of patients who experience cardiovascular collapse other neurological problems are found, including seizures, muscle spasms, and prolonged impairment of consciousness.

Anaphylaxis in children with nausea and palatal itching

It has also been demonstrated that children with food allergies, especially those with asthma, may initially present with misleadingly modest symptoms, such as nausea and palatal itching, and then rapidly progress to severe and potentially fatal episodes with airway involvement.

Prolonged and biphasic anaphylaxis

Anaphylactic events can follow three clinical patterns. The commonest is acute followed by treatment and rapid resolution. Episodes of anaphylaxis can also be prolonged and protracted, lasting hours. This may occur in drug allergy, when after oral administration the drug absorption continues over hours. Secondly, in the case of protracted events there may be remissions followed by exacerbations. Finally, they can be characterized by a resolution in manifestations followed by a recurrence – even in the absence of further antigen exposure (a biphasic reaction).

A biphasic reaction is thus characterized by the recrudescence of symptoms occurring after either a spontaneous remission or a remission due to therapy. It is probably uncommon, most occurring after immunotherapy. The majority of such episodes appear within 8 hours after resolution of the initial symptoms, but they can occur as long as 24 hours later. Factors have been found to be associated with these episodes are seen in Box 17.3.

Anaphylaxis with bradycardia

Classically the cardiovascular manifestations of anaphylaxis are associated with a compensatory tachycardia in response to a decrease in effective vascular volume. This sign is used to distinguish anaphylactic events from vasodepressor (vasovagal) reactions. However, it has been found that anaphylactic events can also present with

Box 17.3 Risk factors for biphasic events

- Inadequate initial treatment
- Delay in adrenaline* administration
- Inadequate adrenaline dosing
- Failure to administer corticosteroids
- Ingested antigen, especially drug or food without vomiting
- Previous biphasic reaction

*Adrenaline is called epinephrine in the USA.

bradycardia. This is not unexpected as bradycardia can be produced by decreased filling of the cardiac ventricles during an anaphylactic event. This activates baroreceptors in ventricular tissue and produces vagal reflex activity.

Anaphylactic events can be associated with depression of the myocardium and a resultant decreased cardiac output. Rarely, coronary artery vasospasm in the absence of coronary artery disease can produce angina. During events, electrocardiographic abnormalities have been recorded.

Anaphylaxis and syncope

Other unusual manifestations of anaphylaxis include syncope. There are a number of cases where there has been delayed recognition of an anaphylactic event when patients have presented only with syncope. This has occurred after Hymenoptera or fire ant stings, exercise-induced anaphylaxis, and in patients with mastocytosis. Such patients lose consciousness without experiencing any other symptom or manifesting any other sign. Unless anaphylaxis is suspected, this presentation often leads to unnecessary neurological and cardiovascular evaluations.

Diagnosis

Anaphylaxis is a 'clinical diagnosis' based on the interpretation of the manifestations. A detailed clinical history should lead to (i) the diagnosis of anaphylaxis and (ii) its cause or type. The history should include assessment of the clinical features, timing and progression, and treatments required. Further, targeted questioning is required to identify triggers, whether allergic or physical or idiopathic. Idiopathic anaphylaxis has a typical picture – often beginning with pruritus of the palms and soles followed by more generalized pruritus and rash, then variable gastrointestinal or cardiovascular features. Progression tends to be slower than with IgE mediated anaphylaxis. The laboratory can be used for confirmation that the event was anaphylactic but, because no acute test is sufficiently sensitive, the failure to obtain confirmation via the laboratory does not rule out the diagnosis. It is important to mention here that many episodes of

anaphylaxis occur without known cause. The incidence of idiopathic anaphylaxis in adults can be as high as 30–40%. The incidence of is far less in children, where most events are food related.

Differential diagnosis

The differential diagnosis of anaphylaxis is summarized in Box 17.4.

Vasovagal syncope

The most common condition confused with anaphylaxis is the vasodepressor reaction (vasovagal syncope). The vasodepressor reaction is characterized by hypotension, pallor, nausea, vomiting, weakness, and sweating. The characteristic bradycardia associated with vasodepressor reactions has been used as a differential diagnostic feature to distinguish them from anaphylaxis. However, for reasons noted above, this single feature does not always occur. Thus, perhaps the most important distinguishing feature between the two types of events is the absence of cutaneous symptoms (erythema, urticaria) in the vasodepressor response. Characteristically, the skin in patients suffering a vasodepressor response is pale and there is a 'cold sweat.'

Flushing syndromes

Since flush occurs relatively frequently in anaphylactic episodes, other flushing syndromes should be considered. These include carcinoid syndrome; postmenopausal flush; alcohol-, nicotine-, drug-, and niacin-induced flush; and vasoactive-polypeptide-secreting tumours.

Direct vasodilatation without stimulation of the sweat glands produces a dry flush, as is seen in the carcinoid syndrome. Other forms of dry flush include those due to niacin, nicotine, catecholamines, and angiotensin-converting enzyme inhibitors. A dry flush can also be seen in vasoactive polypeptide secreting tumours such as occur in the pancreas, other areas of the gastrointestinal tract, and the thyroid (medullary carcinoma). Flushing can also occur due to hereditary angioedema, 'progesterone' anaphylaxis, acquired C1 inhibitor deficiency, neurological causes (seizure), pheochromocytoma, rosacea, capillary leak syndrome, hypoglycaemia and 'red man' syndrome (from vancomycin). Flush is also characteristic of mastocytosis.

Alcohol-induced flush is particularly common. It causes a non-elevated intense erythema more frequently distributed across the trunk, neck, and face, occurring minutes after the ingestion of alcohol. Symptoms usually peak 30–40 minutes after ingestion, and usually subside within 2 hours. There are two forms; one occurs when alcohol is taken simultaneously with certain drugs and in patients with certain illnesses. Such drugs include griseofulvin,

Box 17.4 Differential diagnosis of anaphylaxis

Anaphylaxis

- Anaphylaxis due to exogenously administered agents (e.g., drugs, foods, Hymenoptera stings, latex)
- Anaphylaxis due to physical factors
  - exercise
  - cold
  - heat
  - pressure
  - sunlight
- Idiopathic anaphylaxis
- Food-dependent exercise-induced anaphylaxis
- 'Progesterone' anaphylaxis

Vasodepressor reactions

- Flush syndromes
  - carcinoid
  - postmenopausal
  - alcohol
  - nicotine
  - drugs, e.g.:
    catecholamines
    angiotensin-converting enzyme inhibitors
  - niacin
  - vasointestinal-polypeptide-secreting tumours
    medullary thyroid carcinoma
    gastrointestinal tumours

Other forms of shock

- Cardiogenic
- Haemorrhagic
- Endotoxic

'Restaurant syndromes'

- Scombroidosis
- Monosodium glutamate (MSG)

Non-organic disease

- Panic attacks
- Globus hystericus
- Münchhausen stridor
- Vocal cord dysfunction syndrome
- Undifferentiated somatoform anaphylaxis

Excess endogenous production of histamine syndromes

- Systemic mastocytosis
- Urticaria pigmentosa
- Basophilic leukaemia
- Acute promyelocytic leukaemia (tretinoin treatment)
- Hydatid cyst rupture

Miscellaneous

- Hereditary angioedema
- 'Progesterone' anaphylaxis
- Acquired C1 inhibitor deficiency
- Pheochromocytoma
- Neurological (seizure)
- Capillary leak syndrome
- Hypoglycaemia
- Rosacea
- 'Red man' syndrome (vancomycin)
- Mastocytosis

cephalosporins, and niacin. Conditions predisposing to alcohol-induced flush include lymphoreticular neoplasms, the hypereosinophilic syndrome, and mastocytosis. The second form of alcohol-induced flush is due to a deficiency in acetaldehyde dehydrogenase-2. This enzyme metabolizes acetaldehyde, a metabolite of alcohol. In patients with a deficiency of this enzyme, there is accumulation of acetaldehyde, which results in mast cell degranulation.

Other forms of shock

Other forms of shock including haemorrhagic, cardiogenic, and endotoxic shock are also to be considered. The absence of cutaneous features of course distinguishes these from the majority of episodes of anaphylaxis.

Restaurant syndromes

A group of 'restaurant syndromes' can cause symptoms similar to mastocytosis.

Scombroidosis

Perhaps the most common of these, and the one that resembles anaphylaxis to the greatest degree, is histamine poisoning. This condition, referred to as 'scombroidosis', is produced by the ingestion of histamine contained in spoiled fish. It may be increasing in frequency. Histamine is the major chemical involved in the production of symptoms, but not all the symptoms are caused by histamine alone.

Histamine is produced by histidine-decarboxylating bacteria, which cleave histamine from histidine in spoiled fish. This histamine production occurs shortly after the death of the fish and can therefore occur on the fishing vessel, at the processing plant, in the distribution system, or in the restaurant or home. Such contaminated fish cannot be distinguished by appearance or smell, and cooking does not destroy the histamine.

The onset of symptoms in scombroidosis occurs within a few minutes to several hours after the ingestion of fish. Several members eating at the same table may be affected. The episodes usually last a few hours, but can persist for longer. Symptoms include urticaria, flush, angioedema, nausea, vomiting, diarrhoea, and a fall in blood pressure. Neurological findings can also occur, and rarely wheezing is present. The most common manifestation is face and neck flush accompanied by a sensation of heat and discomfort. The rash can resemble sunburn. Serum tryptase levels are not elevated in histamine poisoning, whereas plasma histamine and 24-hour urinary histamine metabolites are present in increased amounts.

Monosodium glutamate

Although monosodium glutamate (MSG) reactions are not truly similar in manifestations to anaphylactic events, they have been confused with anaphylaxis in the past. They are due to an 'acetylcholinosis' with the production of chest pain, flushing, facial burning, paraesthesias, sweating, dizziness, headaches, palpitations, nausea, and vomiting. Symptoms usually begin no later than 1 hour after ingestion, but they can be delayed for up to half a day. There may be a familial tendency to develop these episodes.

Psychogenic

Non-organic problems that are 'psychologically' based have also been confused with episodes of anaphylaxis. These include panic attacks, globus hystericus, Münchausen stridor, vocal cord dysfunction syndrome, and undifferentiated somatoform anaphylaxis. Panic attacks, except for flushing and sweating, are usually devoid of cutaneous manifestations, but can be characterized by tachycardia, gastrointestinal symptoms, and shortness of breath. There is no pruritus or true airway obstruction, and the absence of urticaria and angioedema is usually a tell-tale sign.

'Undifferentiated somatoform anaphylaxis' is a term used to describe patients who present with manifestations that mimic anaphylaxis, but who lack confirmatory findings and fail to respond to standard therapy. They often have psychological characteristics of other undifferentiated somatoform disorders.

Excess endogenous histamine production

Anaphylaxis can be a result of an underlying disease and not actually due to exposure to an external agent. Such illnesses are systemic mastocytosis, urticaria pigmentosa, basophilic leukaemia, acute promyelocytic leukaemia treated with tretinoin, and a ruptured hydatid cyst.

Miscellaneous

There are a number of miscellaneous conditions that can present with signs that may mimic anaphylactic episodes. These include hereditary angioedema, 'progesterone' anaphylaxis, acquired C1 inhibitor deficiency, pheochromocytoma, neurological disorders such as seizure, the 'red man syndrome' due to vancomycin, and the capillary leak syndrome. For example, rarely patients with hereditary angioedema exhibit an erythematous, serpiginous rash that can resemble urticaria; this rash accompanied by upper airway obstruction can be confused with an anaphylactic episode. The capillary leak syndrome can present with angioedema, gastrointestinal symptoms, shock, and haemoconcentration. Recurrent episodes have mimicked idiopathic anaphylaxis.

Laboratory investigations and tests

Immediate tests; at the time of the reaction

As mentioned, the diagnosis of an anaphylactic event is based upon a clinical interpretation of the manifestations. However, the laboratory may be useful for confirmation. Table 17.4 lists those tests that may confirm the diagnosis

Table 17.4 Tests used to confirm a diagnosis of anaphylaxis

Test	Comment
Serum tryptase	The most useful test. Simple and readily available. Serum tryptase levels usually peak about 60 minutes after the onset of symptoms and may persist for up to 4 hours. However, tryptase levels can occasionally be elevated for as long as 6–24 hours in severe anaphylaxis. Measurement should ideally be obtained between 1 and 2 hours after onset of symptoms
Plasma histamine	Plasma histamine levels rise earlier than tryptase levels, increasing within 5 to 10 minutes after the onset of symptoms. Levels are elevated only evanescently and usually return to normal after 60 minutes. Thus they are of little help if the patient is seen more than an hour after the event began. Not commercially available in UK
24-hour urinary histamine metabolites (*N*-methylhistamine)	Urinary histamine metabolites can be elevated for up to 24 hours after the onset of the event. Not readily available in UK

of anaphylaxis in an event with suggestive clinical manifestations.

Presently, commercially available tests to confirm a diagnosis of anaphylaxis are the serum tryptase, plasma histamine, and 24-hour urinary histamine metabolites (although the latter two are no longer routinely available in the UK). Tests that hold promise, and are being investigated for potential use in diagnosing anaphylactic events include carboxypeptidase A3, platelet activating factor, and platelet activating factor hydrolase. Currently, however, the latter tests have not been validated, or may not be commercially available. The only widely available test is serum tryptase.

Tryptase

By far the most useful and commonly employed biomarker used to confirm a diagnosis of anaphylaxis is the measurement of total serum tryptase. This test lacks sensitivity, but is highly specific. Nevertheless, because of the lack of sensitivity, a normal total tryptase value obtained during an event does not rule out the diagnosis of anaphylaxis. Tryptases are a subgroup of trypsin-family serine peptidases. Almost all human mast cells contain tryptases, and small amounts can be found within the human basophil. Tryptase is specific to these cells and therefore is a useful marker for their degranulation.

Tryptase is secreted constitutively in small amounts. The constitutively secreted tryptase is, for the most part, an immature form of tryptase: β-protryptase. With mast cell degranulation, there is a marked increase in tryptase levels owing to the secretion of mature β-tryptase.

Serum levels peak about 60 minutes after the onset of symptoms and usually persist for up to 4 hours. The optimal time for drawing a serum tryptase is about 1 hour after the onset of symptoms. Ideally two samples should be taken – one immediately after resuscitation then, depending upon the time of presentation, a second sample at 1–2 hours after the start of symptoms. However, in very severe life-threatening episodes elevated serum tryptase levels have been found as long as 24 hours after symptom onset. As noted, anaphylactic episodes have occurred in the absence of detectable elevations of serum tryptase, and, for reasons not clearly understood, elevations are not seen as frequently in food-induced events.

Histamine

Plasma histamine rises much more rapidly than does serum tryptase. Plasma histamine levels can be elevated 5–10 minutes after the onset of symptoms. However, such levels are evanescent, usually returning to normal within 60 minutes after the onset of the event. For this reason, plasma histamine levels are of little help if the patient is seen as long as an hour after the event. In this case, however, a 24-hour urinary collection for histamine metabolites may be useful. Such metabolites can be elevated for as long as a day. However, these assays are not widely available.

Unfortunately, there are disparities between histamine and tryptase levels. If the patient is seen soon enough, plasma histamine levels may be more sensitive and may also correlate better with clinical manifestations. Plasma histamine may be more likely to correlate with cutaneous manifestations as well as wheeze.

Later tests: differential diagnosis

Systemic mastocytosis

Table 17.5 lists tests used to evaluate the presence of other conditions that are considered in the differential diagnosis. Tryptase levels obtained during an asymptomatic phase are a reasonably good screening test to diagnose episodes due to underlying systemic mastocytosis. Patients with mastocytosis may have elevated levels of baseline total serum tryptase (between episodes). However, it should be noted that both mastocytosis and mast-cell-activating syndromes can be present with normal baseline serum tryptase levels.

It was originally thought that a tryptase level of 20 ng/mL was necessary to raise suspicion of mastocytosis, but it has been recently shown that levels far lower, as low perhaps as 11 ng/mL, may reflect an underlying increased burden of mast cells. An elevated tryptase level above 20 ng/mL is highly specific, but again this test lacks sensitivity, and a normal baseline level does not rule out the presence of mastocytosis. Also, the majority of patients suffering from mastocytosis have a point mutation in the *c-kit* receptor (D816V), which can be demonstrated in bone marrow. Other mutations are described. A test for D816V on blood is now available, but this appears to be less sensitive than the same test performed on the bone marrow. It should also be remembered that elevated total serum tryptase can occur in myeloproliferative disorders, the hypereosinophilic syndrome associated with *FIP1L1/PDGFRA* mutations, and end-stage kidney disease.

Carcinoid syndrome

Serum serotonin and urinary 5-hydroxyindoleacetic acid can be measured if the clinician is considering flushing due to the carcinoid syndrome. The measurement of various gastrointestinal vasopeptides is available. These include substance P, neurokinins, vasointestinal polypeptide, pancreastatin, and others. These measurements may be useful to rule out the presence of a vasoactive-peptide-secreting tumour. Octreotide- assisted CT scanning is also useful in this regard.

Pheochromocytoma

Plasma-free metanephrine and urinary vanilmandelic acid are employed if a possibility being considered is a paradoxical response to a pheochromocytoma.

Table 17.5 Tests employed to diagnose other entities considered in the differential diagnosis

Disease	Test	Comment
Mastocytosis	Serum tryptase	Baseline serum tryptase levels (between episodes) are usually elevated in patients with systemic mastocytosis
	Bone marrow	Most definitive test to establish the diagnosis of systemic mastocytosis. Analysis for *c-kit* mutations, mast cell markers, and histology can be done
	Test for mutations in *c-kit* tyrosine-kinase receptor (D816V)	Test for the 816V mutation in *c-kit* is commercially available and can be done on blood. The relative sensitivity of this test has not been documented in large numbers of patients. Test is extremely costly
Carcinoid syndrome	Serum serotonin and urinary 5-hydroxyindoleacetic acid	
Vasopeptide-secreting- tumours	Pancreastatin, vasointestinal polypeptide, substance P, neurokinin, and others	Useful to diagnose a number of tumours that secrete substances that produce events very similar to anaphylaxis. These include medullary carcinoma of the thyroid, pancreatic tumours, and other tumours of the gastrointestinal tract
	Octreotide-enhanced CT of abdomen/bowel	Localizes tumour by octreotide binding
Pheochromocytoma	Plasma-free metanephrine and urinary vanilmandelic acid	Paradoxical responses to pheochromocytoma are rare but can mimic anaphylactic events

Later tests to determine aetiology of anaphylaxis

Allergy testing: skin prick tests

If allergy is suspected from the history, this should be confirmed by skin prick test. This is helpful in food, venom, and latex allergy. For fruits and vegetables prick-prick tests are superior and should be used. Generally skin tests are more helpful than serum-specific IgE; they are more sensitive, and it is important to have the results when the patient is being assessed so that further history can be obtained to distinguish whether a positive test is causal or incidental (e.g. sensitization). In allergy to seminal plasma, specific IgE serology is indicated.

Diagnosis of drug allergy is more complicated as reactions may be IgE-mediated or non-IgE mediated. Drugs such as aspirin and NSAIDs cause anaphylaxis through non-IgE mechanisms. There are no diagnostic tests except challenge, and this would be undertaken only in a monitored setting if there was doubt about the diagnosis from the history and the risk of inducing life-threatening reactions was low. Even in IgE-mediated anaphylaxis, skin prick tests are only sometimes diagnostic and positive results require correlation with the history. Even in suspected β-lactam allergy, intradermal and challenge testing is often required. In patients in whom a penicillin reaction is suspected but skin tests to penicillins are negative, European studies show that up to 30% will have a positive challenge test, whereas in USA this figure is lower at

about 6%. The difference may be due to patient selection. UK and European guidelines suggest that challenge is mandatory in patients with negative skin tests before a diagnosis can be reached.

Other tests

Occasionally other tests such as an ice cube test to confirm a history of cold-induced anaphylaxis, or an exercise test may be required to confirm a diagnosis of exercise anaphylaxis, may be indicated.

Management

Management of anaphylactic events should be divided into two broad categories:

1. prevention of episodes in patients at risk (those who have experienced a previous reaction)
2. treatment of the acute event.

The goals of these two categories of management are the same, but the first category is, of course, prophylactic, and the second is to prevent fatalities during an event.

Prevention of anaphylactic episodes

The key is accurate diagnosis of the aetiology of anaphylaxis. Identification of the trigger (e.g. a food or drug) should allow avoidance and prevent further episodes.

This should be backed up by the provision of an emergency treatment plan with medication for self-treatment should there be a further reaction following inadvertent exposure. A summary of the measures instituted to prevent anaphylactic episodes in the population as a whole, and for those at risk, is given in Box 17.5. It is of course essential to obtain a thorough drug allergy history in all patients. It is also important to record the drug allergy history in a prominent and consistent place in the medical chart. Proper interpretation of the drug allergy history in terms of cross-reacting agents is necessary. Patients should of course be instructed to avoid all agents that might present a risk. When a drug allergy is present, a substitute, non-cross-reactive drug should be administered whenever possible.

Since anaphylactic episodes are usually worse when medications are given by injection rather than orally, oral agents should preferably be administered wherever possible. If an in-office injection of a medication with the potential to cause an anaphylactic reaction is required, the patient should remain under observation for 20–30 minutes after the injection. Theoretically, such an observation period should also be employed when drugs are administered orally.

Patients who are at risk (food-allergic patients, systemic mastocytosis patients, insect-allergic patients, patients with idiopathic anaphylaxis, etc.) should always wear identifying jewellery (e.g. Medic Alert) and carry an identification card in their wallet or purse. All patients at risk should be instructed in the use of an automatic adrenaline injector, and patients should be diligently encouraged to keep their injectors with them at all times. They should also be instructed on the location of expiration dates on their injectors so that they can be refilled at appropriate times. Patients at risk should also, if at all possible, not take drugs that may make an episode of anaphylaxis more severe or interfere with therapy (Table 17.6). These might include β-adrenergic blocking agents, non-cardioselective beta blockers, angiotensin-converting enzyme inhibitors, monoamine oxidase inhibitors, and perhaps some tricyclic antidepressants as well. These drugs can, in some instances, worsen hypotension or complicate therapy by interfering with the activities of adrenaline, accentuating its α-adrenergic while compromising its β-adrenergic activity, and diminish adrenaline catabolism, thus making dosage adjustments difficult.

Patients known to be allergic to drugs who must have them re-administered should be considered for specialized procedures such as pharmacological pretreatment, desensitization, or provocative dosing. For example, pretreatment with antihistamines and corticosteroids may be used to prevent a repeat reaction to radiocontrast media,

---

Box 17.5 Strategies to prevent anaphylaxis and anaphylactic deaths

General measures

1. Obtain thorough history
2. Record drug allergy history in dedicated and prominent portion of chart
3. Administer drugs orally rather than parenterally when possible
4. Check all drugs for proper labelling
5. Patients to remain under observation after injected drugs and vaccines for appropriate intervals of time according to established guidelines. For example, British guidelines state an hour after allergen immunotherapy, whereas US guidelines call for a 30-minute observation period for aeroallergen and a 1-hour period for venom immunotherapy

For patients at risk

A. Ensure allergy referral and accurate diagnosis of aetiology of anaphylaxis
B. Give advice on avoidance of allergen or, if non-immunological, the trigger (e.g. cold, exercise)
C. Be aware of immunological and biochemical cross-reactivity between drugs, and avoid those which may produce events (e.g. all non-steroidal anti-inflammatory drugs in the aspirin-sensitive asthmatic, all β-lactam drugs in the penicillin-sensitive patient)

D. For patients with food allergy, give instructions on how to avoid, including label reading high-risk situations and avoidance of potentially cross-reacting foods (e.g. avoidance of all crustaceans in lobster-sensitive patient)
E. Have patient wear and carry warning identification labels (e.g. Medic Alert)
F. Provide a written emergency treatment plan, which will usually include an adrenaline* autoinjector and an oral antihistamine
G. Teach self-injection of adrenaline
H. Emphasize the need to keep adrenaline autoinjector available at all times
I. In the case of children, provide school staff with training on avoidance and in the recognition and management of anaphylaxis
J. Consider discontinuing, where possible, drugs that may interfere with therapy or potentially worsen an event (e.g. β-adrenergic blocking agents, angiotensin-converting enzyme inhibitors, monoamine oxidase inhibitors, and possibly certain tricyclic antidepressants
K. Employ when indicated special procedures such as desensitization, pharmacological pretreatment, and provocative challenge

*Adrenaline is called epinephrine in USA.

Table 17.6 Drugs that may increase the risk of anaphylaxis, increase the severity of an attack, or complicate therapy

Drug	Potential adverse effect
β-Adrenergic blocking agents	May diminish the effect of adrenaline* used to treat an event. Can potentially make the event worse by preventing the response to endogenously secreted adrenaline and noradrenaline.* While blocking the β-adrenergic effect of adrenaline (bronchodilation), may enhance the α-adrenergic effect inordinately (vasoconstriction) resulting in severe hypertension
Non-cardioselective beta blockers	Anaphylaxis may not respond to adrenaline calling for intravenous salbutamol*
Angiotensin-converting enzyme inhibitors	May prevent the effect of the compensatory secreted angiotensin-converting enzyme, thus worsen hypotension. Also prevents the degradation of bradykinin. Excessive bradykinin activity has been shown to occur during anaphylactic episodes. Has been shown to increase the risk of reactions to venom immunotherapy and perhaps the severity of events due to Hymenoptera stings
Monoamine oxidase inhibitors	May complicate therapy because prevents degradation of adrenaline used to treat an event, thus making the proper dose more difficult to assess. Start with standard dose and titrate dose of adrenaline according to response
Tricyclic antihistamines	Many prevent reuptake of catecholamines and thus can exaggerate effect of adrenaline. Increased risk of arrhythmias. Start with standard dose and titrate dose of adrenaline according to response

*Adrenaline is called epinephrine, noradrenaline is called norepinephrine, and salbutamol is called albuterol in USA.

and desensitization can be used to safely re-administer penicillin. Also, after skin testing has been shown to be negative, a provocative dosing procedure is often employed to administer influenza vaccine.

Assessment of the patient who has experienced an anaphylactic episode and management of an acute event

The allergist deals with anaphylaxis in two settings. The more frequent of these involves the diagnosis and management plan for a patient who has experienced a possible previous anaphylactic event, and who presents to the allergist days to weeks subsequent to this event. The second involves the treatment of an acute event. In most instances, in terms of the allergist, this relates to the treatment of reactions due to allergen immunotherapy or during a diagnostic challenge test (e.g. to drugs or foods).

Approach to the patient who presents for diagnosis and a management plan after having experienced an anaphylactic episode

The approach to the patient presenting after an event for the purpose of establishing the diagnosis, identifying the aetiological agent, and instituting a future management plan is summarized in Figure 17.3.

In the evaluation of a patient who has experienced a previous episode of anaphylaxis, the most important procedure is the history. A detailed history should be obtained that includes elements such as establishing the time of

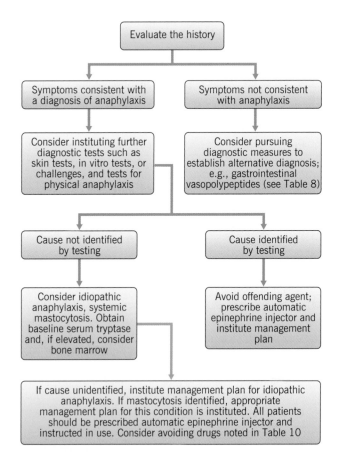

Fig. 17.3 Algorithm for the evaluation of a patient who has experienced an anaphylactic episode.

the occurrence of the attack, the setting in which the attack occurred, the treatment that was required, whether or not an emergency department visit was necessary, and the duration of the episode. The details required to investigate potential causes should include a detailed list of ingestants, including medications, consumed within a few hours of the event, any history of sting or bite, whether or not exercise or sexual activity occurred prior to or during the event, and whether or not there was exposure to heat or cold prior to or during the event. The symptoms should, of course, also be reviewed in detail, and it should be determined as to whether or not the event was biphasic in nature.

If the history is inconsistent with anaphylaxis, and suggests another disorder, appropriate tests should then be ordered (see Table 17.5). If the history is consistent with an anaphylactic event, tests to identify the causative agent should be done if indicated. These would include procedures such as allergy skin tests to foods and/or drugs, or serological tests for specific IgE to food and/or drugs. In addition, in some instances an oral challenge may be considered depending upon the safety of such a challenge and the availability of alternative therapies.

If the allergist is unable to identify the cause, a diagnosis of mastocytosis can be entertained, and a baseline serum tryptase and/or bone marrow biopsy should be undertaken. If no cause can be found despite a diligent search, the patient should be classified as having experienced an episode of 'idiopathic anaphylaxis'.

Of course, if the cause of the attack has been identified, the patient should avoid any further exposure to the responsible agent. A management plan should be provided by the allergist. This will include detailed advice on avoidance. Emergency medication should be carried, together with a written treatment plan. All patients should be taught the self-injection of adrenaline and supplied with an adrenaline autoinjector. Patients need to be trained in recognition of reactions; in the case of a child the parents and school staff should also be trained. There is evidence of efficacy of management plans. In large studies in nut allergy, such a plan produced substantial reduction in reactions, such that further reactions were nearly all mild – requiring only oral antihistamines or no treatment. Where adrenaline was used, it was always effective and only a single dose was required. Similarly clinical experience shows that, with early treatment of reactions, in the majority of situations only a single dose of adrenaline is required. Reactions to intravenous drugs (e.g. during anaesthesia) cause more severe and protracted reactions, some times with asystole-requiring repeated adrenaline, but this is related to a large bolus of allergen (i.e. drug) being given intravenously. Consideration should be given to discontinuation of any drugs that might complicate therapy or increase the severity of a future episode (see Table 17.5).

Treatment of the acute event

The procedure is set out in detail in the UK Resuscitation Guidelines on management of anaphylaxis. An algorithm outlining the management steps for the acute event is seen in Figure 17.4. A list of suggested drugs and equipment for the clinic or office is given in Box 17.6.

The acute management of an anaphylactic event requires immediate recognition and institution of therapy. Initial management is directed to the preservation of the airway and assessment of vital signs. Establishment of the airway should be done immediately, while assessing the vital signs and placing the patient in the recumbent position with legs elevated. If the problem is predominantly respiratory (severe asthma or laryngeal oedema) without features of hypotension, the patient should be kept sitting up. Simultaneously, adrenaline should be administered. Injection in the vastus lateralis muscle (lateral thigh) produces a more rapid rise in blood adrenaline levels and, because of this desirable effect, has been

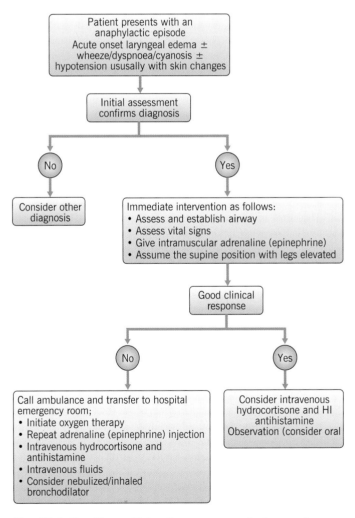

Fig. 17.4 Algorithm outlining the management of an acute anaphylactic event.

Box 17.6 Suggested office/clinic equipment for management of an anaphylactic episode

Oxygen delivery:

- Canister O_2
- Face mask
- Tubing
- Nasal probe

Intravenous supplies:

- Normal saline
- 5% dextrose
- Connection tubing and needles

Medications:

- Adrenaline* for intramuscular use
- Intravenous antihistamine, e.g. chlorphen(ir)amine
- Oral non-sedative antihistamine
- Intravenous hydrocortisone
- Oral prednisolone (prednisone)
- Nebulized β_2-agonist e.g. salbutamol*

Consider other agents (in emergency department or specialist settings):

- Glucagon (can be useful in patients on beta blockers)
- Atropine for injection (useful if severe bradycardia after anaphylaxis)
- Noradrenaline* or metaraminol for intravenous infusion (specialist settings)

*Adrenaline is called epinephrine; noradrenaline is called norepinephrine; salbutamol is called albuterol in the USA.

suggested as the initial route of administration of choice. The dose in an adult is 0.3–0.5 mg [i.e. 0.3–0.5 mL of 1 in 1000 strength (1mg/mL)] intramuscularly. The dose in a young child is dependent on weight (0.01 mg per kg). For children between 1 and 6 years old, 0.15 mL of 1 in 1000 strength should be given.

Once this has been done, further therapy depends on the assessment. It should be emphasized, however, that adrenaline therapy is essential and is the initial drug of choice. There is evidence to suggest that a delay in adrenaline administration can be a risk factor for a fatal event, as well as for a biphasic event. Therefore, this drug should be administered as soon as the diagnosis has been established. The indications for adrenaline therapy are seen in Box 17.1. This is usually followed by intravenous administration of an H_1 antagonist and hydrocortisone.

If the patient responds to the initial treatment, they should be observed for recurrences, and if they remain asymptomatic can be discharged from the clinic. A short course of oral antihistamine and a corticosteroid such as prednisoline (prednisone) may be given on discharge.

The exact time for observation after an attack responding to a single dose of adrenaline has not been established, and remains a matter of clinical judgement. However, as noted above, the majority of recurrent reactions will occur within 8 hours, but these are unlikely after good initial therapy. It would be prudent, however, to observe the patient for a minimum of 2 hours if possible.

If the episode does not respond to a single dose of adrenaline, other therapies should be considered, an emergency call should be placed and the patient taken to hospital. If there is no response within 5–10 minutes, a second dose of adrenaline should be administered, and a third if no response in another 5–10 minutes. Intravenous antihistamine and corticosteroid should be given. At that time, supplemental therapy such as an inhaled bronchodilator, and intravenous fluids should also be considered, depending on the patient's symptoms. For example, an inhaled bronchodilator would be the drug of choice if the persistent symptoms were shortness of breath and wheeze. If hypotension is present, intravenous fluids should be given. If the patient is taking a β-adrenergic blocker and hypotension persists, glucagon may be employed in addition to fluids. Atropine injection may be useful if severe bradycardia is present after the episode. For hypotension not responding to fluid administration, vasopressors such as noradrenaline (norepinephrine) or metaraminol can be employed. For more detail of drugs and doses see Table 17.7.

Traditionally, corticosteroids have been used to treat anaphylactic episodes. It is difficult to conduct studies to assess the efficacy of adding IV hydrocortisone, so data are lacking. Clinical experience shows that steroids are effective in acute tongue angioedema and asthma, and there is some evidence that they may have a role in diminishing the frequency of late phase or recurrent responses.

The use of a tourniquet proximal to the injection site to slow absorption of antigen has been suggested for patients experiencing a reaction due to antigen administered in the limb. Should it be used, the tourniquet should be loosened every few minutes to prevent anoxic injury. It has also been suggested that adrenaline should be injected into the site where allergen was injected, also to slow the absorption of antigen. The suggested dose has ranged from 0.1 to 0.2 mg (in addition to the dose mentioned above administered to treat the acute event). There is no evidence that either of these is an effective measure.

Table 17.7 Drugs used in acute anaphylaxis

Drug	Dose and route of administration	Comment
Adrenaline*	1:1000 0.5 mL IM lateral thigh (adult); 1:1000 0.01 mg/kg or 0.15 mL IM lateral thigh (child aged <6 y): 0.3 mL age 6–12	Initial drug of choice for all episodes; should be given immediately; if no response repeat after 5 min. If no response to IM administration and patient in shock with cardiovascular collapse can consider intravenous administration but *only by experienced specialists* with monitoring and titration of dose using 1 in 10 000 dilution
Antihistamines		
Chlorphen(ir)amine	10 mg slow IV (adult) 5 mg slow IV (child 6–12y) 2.5 mg slow IV (child 6 m–6 y)	Give after adrenaline. Route of administration depends on severity of episode. Also consider oral administration when discharged after response to therapy
Corticosteroids		
Hydrocortisone	200 mg slow IV or IM (adult); 100 mg slow IV (child 6–12 y); 50 mg (6 m–6y); 25 mg (<6 m)	Exact dose not established; other preparations such as methyl-prednisolone can be used; for milder episodes, oral prednisolone 40–60 mg may be given. Also consider oral administration when discharged
β₂ agonists		
Salbutamol* or terbutaline	Nebulized 5 mg (adult); 5–10 mg (adult)	Useful for bronchospasm not responding to adrenaline
Intravenous fluids (normal saline or Ringers lactate)	500–1000 mL rapidly in adults; 20 mL/kg in child; 500 mL rapidly followed by slow infusion in adults	Rate of administration titrated against blood pressure response
Other vasopressors		
Noradrenaline*, metaraminol		Specialist use only. The rate of infusion should be titred against the blood pressure response; continued infusion requires intensive care monitoring
Drugs employed in patients who are beta-blocked		
Glucagon (specialist use only)	Initial dose of 1–5 mg IV followed by infusion of 5–15 µg/min titrated against blood pressure. Child 50–150 µg/kg	Glucagon is probably the drug of choice for shock unresponsive to adrenaline
Atropine sulphate (specialist use only)	0.3–0.5 mg IV; may repeat every 10 minutes to a maximum of 3 mg in adults	Atropine useful for treatment of bradycardia and hypotension
Ipratropium	Nebulized 500 µg (250 µg in child)	Ipratropium may be added to inhaled β-adrenergics for wheezing

*Adrenaline is called epinephrine, noradrenaline is norepinephrine and salbutamol is albuterol in the USA.

Summary of important messages

- The incidence of anaphylactic reactions is increasing
- The commonest causes are foods, drugs, Hymenoptera stings, and idiopathic reactions. In children most anaphylaxis is food induced
- In patients with a history of anaphylaxis, further reactions are common
- Anaphylactic reactions are not easy to study with randomized controlled trials. There are, however, systematic reviews of the available evidence and a wealth of clinical experience to help formulate management
- In the acute episode, early treatment with intramuscular adrenaline is the treatment of choice
- All patients who have had an anaphylactic reaction should be referred to an allergist for identification of the cause or type and institution of a management plan to prevent recurrence or minimize reactions. This includes advice on avoidance, provision of adrenaline for self-administration, training, and control of background asthma. Avoidance of a food or drug can prevent further episodes
- In patients who have experienced anaphylaxis to hymenoptera, desensitization should be considered

Further reading

Bains SN, Hsieh FH. Current approaches to the diagnosis and treatment of systemic mastocytosis. Ann Allergy Asthma Immunol 2010; 104(1):1–10.

Bonadonna P, Perbellini O, Passalacqua G, et al. Clonal mast cell disorders in patients with systemic reactions to Hymenoptera stings and increased serum tryptase levels, 12 January 2009. J Allergy Clin Immunol 2009; 123(3):680–686.

Clark AT, Ewan PW. Good prognosis, clinical features and circumstances of peanut and tree nut reactions in children treated by a specialist allergy center. J Allergy Clin Immunol 2008; 122(2):286–289.

Ellis AK, Day JH. Incidence and characteristics of biphasic anaphylaxis: a prospective evaluation of 103 patients. Ann Allergy Asthma Immunol 2007; 98(1):64–69.

Estelle F, Simons R. Anaphylaxis: recent advances in assessment and treatment. J Allergy Clin Immunol 2009; 124(4):625–636.

Estelle F, Simons R. Anaphylaxis. J Allergy Clin Immunol 2010; 125(2 suppl 2):S161–181.

González-Pérez A, Aponte Z, Vidaurre CF, et al. Anaphylaxis epidemiology in patients with and patients without asthma: a United Kingdom database review, 15 April 2010. J Allergy Clin Immunol 2010; 125(5):1098–1104.

Lieberman P, Kemp SF, Oppenheimer J, et al. The diagnosis and management of anaphylaxis: an updated practice parameter. J Allergy Clin Immunol 2005; 115(3 suppl 2): S483–523.

Mirakian R, Ewan PW, Durham SR, et al, BSACI. BSACI guidelines for the management of drug allergy. Clin Exp Allergy 2009; 39(1):43–61.

Sampson HA, Muñoz-Furlong A, Campbell RL, et al. Second symposium on the definition and management of anaphylaxis: summary report – Second National Institute of Allergy and Infectious Disease/Food Allergy and Anaphylaxis Network symposium. J Allergy Clin Immunol 2006; 117(2):391–397.

Sheehan WJ, Graham D, Ma L, et al. Higher incidence of pediatric anaphylaxis in northern areas of the United States, 25 August 2009. J Allergy Clin Immunol 2009; 124(4):850–852.

Soar J, Pumphrey R, Cant A, et al, Working Group of the Resuscitation Council (UK). Emergency treatment of anaphylactic reactions – guidelines for healthcare providers. Resuscitation 2008; 77(2):157–169.

Stone SF, Cotterell C, Isbister GK, et al, Emergency Department Anaphylaxis Investigators. Elevated serum cytokines during human anaphylaxis: identification of potential mediators of acute allergic reactions, 22 September 2009. J Allergy Clin Immunol 2009; 124(4):786–792.

Paediatric allergy and asthma

John O Warner and Attilio L Boner

This chapter covers the prevalence and natural history of allergic diseases in the paediatric population, as well as the diagnosis and treatment of these diseases in this population. The possibility of primary and secondary prevention of allergic diseases in children is also discussed.

Historical introduction

Allergic diseases in children received relatively scant attention until the 20th century. It was assumed, as stated by Aretaeus the Cappadocian (AD120–180), that 'children recover more readily'. However, Hippocrates (460–375BC) recognized that asthma could occur in children. 'Children are liable to convulsions and asthma which are regarded as divine visitations and the disease itself as sacred.' Periodic references to children can be found in the literature; for example, John Millar in 1769 described a child who had died of asthma with 'an abundance of gelatinous secretions obstructing the bronchi'. He also described another child who had died with asthma, but whose lungs were said to be perfectly normal. In the subsequent 2.5 centuries, little has changed in terms of understanding the reasons for death from asthma. In this respect it is worth noting that the first publication to emphasize that airway inflammation can occur even in mild asthma came from a paediatric study of the ultrastructure of open lung biopsies from two children with asthma who were sampled during a clinical remission. The appearances were similar to those seen in the lung tissue from two children who had died of asthma. All four had cellular infiltrates with eosinophils and loss of airway epithelium. One might even attribute to John Millar the percipient observation that eventually identified inhalant allergy as an important feature of asthma. In discussing potential causes of childhood asthma he wrote 'it is chiefly incident in children especially such as have been lately weaned and that it has been most prevalent in spring and autumn, moist seasons, changeable weather and when the mercury stood low in the barometer'. He suggested that 'disease must depend greatly on the state of the atmosphere'.

It was only in the latter half of the 20th century that attention was focused on the early life origins of allergic disease, as it became clear from epidemiological studies that there have been considerable increases in the prevalence of all allergic diseases in children – initially in the developed world, but more recently in developing countries. Simultaneously with dramatic improvements in the understanding of the immunopathology of allergy, we have witnessed increases in prevalence, morbidity, and in some circumstances mortality. Although this might be viewed as a deficiency in delivery of appropriate services for patients with allergic disease, we must also investigate the

DOI: 10.1016/B978-0-7234-3658-4.00005-6

changes in lifestyle and environment that are affecting the induction and incitement of allergic conditions.

Epidemiology

Increases in all the allergic conditions have been demonstrated in many countries worldwide over a period of 30–40 years. This can be exemplified by studies from south Wales where identical ascertainment was employed in 12 year olds in 1973, 1988, and 2003 showing increases in asthma, eczema, and allergic rhinitis (Fig. 18.1). The international study of asthma and allergies in childhood (ISAAC) has now evolved through three phases. In the first instance, studies comparing prevalence in different countries throughout the world showed higher rates of allergic disease in English-speaking communities, with reducing prevalence going from north to south in Europe and into Africa and from west to east through Asia. More recently, however, the prevalence rates have increased in many developing countries – but, in the first instance, predominantly focused on the more affluent segments of the population.

Migration studies have suggested that early life environment is critical to the expression of disease such that the second-generation immigrants from a low- to a high-prevalence country show far higher prevalence of allergic disease than did their parents who arrived in the country as adults. The adoption of a Western lifestyle appears to be critical and has been associated with adoption of the native language of the country to which families migrate. Retention of the language of the country of origin appears to be associated with also retaining the prevalence rate of allergy of the country of origin. Adopting the native language is therefore clearly a surrogate marker for a whole lifestyle change.

The allergic march

It has been known for well over a century that allergic diseases had a family predisposition. For example, Morrill Wyman in 1872 described his own family's problem with autumnal catarrh. This was clarified by Robert Cooke in 1916 who, with Arthur Coker, coined the term 'atopy' from the Greek 'atopus' or 'no place'. This was a recognition that eczema, asthma, and hay fever often co-existed in individuals and ran in various patterns in families. This evolved into the concept of the 'allergic march' (this was first described by Fouchard in 1973), in which young children presented with atopic eczema, often associated with food allergy, which then improved through early childhood to be replaced by asthma and subsequently allergic rhinitis (Fig. 18.2).

To what extent asthma precedes or follows allergic rhinitis remains to be established. However, evidence from occupational allergic disease would suggest that, following allergic sensitization, rhinitis often develops well before the onset of lower airway manifestations of the allergic reaction. What, however, is very clear is that comorbidity is very common. Thus the UK contribution to ISAAC phase I demonstrated that, amongst the 33% of 12 year olds who had wheezing, 14.4% had in addition rhinoconjunctivitis or eczema, or both (Fig. 18.3).

There is a suggestion that in some countries the rates of increase in asthma prevalence has declined, whereas those for food allergy and anaphylaxis are continuing to increase. Indeed paediatric allergy services are now being flooded with children manifesting a wide array of problems associated with food allergy. This includes not only eczema, but also a range of enteropathies such as eosinophilic oesophagitis and enterocolitis. The subtle variations over time in different environments for each of the allergic disorders suggest that a single factor will not explain the changing global epidemiology of allergic disorders. Rather, there is an interplay of genetics and a host

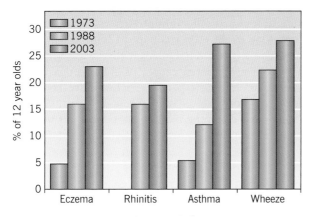

Fig. 18.1 Data from 3 consecutive prevalence studies on 12 year olds in south Wales using identical ascertainment methods. There are large increases in prevalence for the three common allergic conditions. (From Burr ML, Wat D, Evans C. Asthma prevalence in 1973, 1988 and 2003. Thorax 2006; 61(4):296–299.)

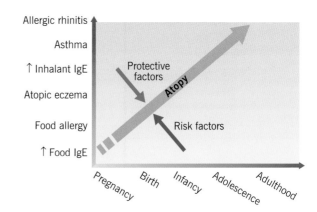

Fig. 18.2 A graphical representation of the atopic or allergic march, suggesting a progression from one manifestation to another but affected by various risk and protective factors.

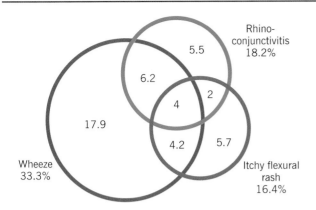

Fig. 18.3 A Venn diagram of the prevalence and comorbidity of the three common allergic conditions in 12-year-old UK children, from the ISAAC 1 survey. (From Austin JB, Kaur B, Anderson HR, et al. Hay fever, eczema, and wheeze: a nationwide UK study (ISAAC, international study of asthma and allergies in childhood). Arch Dis Child 1999; 81(3):225–230.)

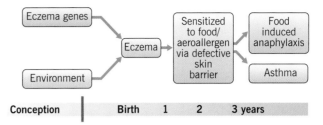

Fig. 18.4 A concept of the allergic march in which eczema as a skin barrier defect is followed by sensitization to food and/or inhalant allergens followed by anaphylaxis and/or asthma.

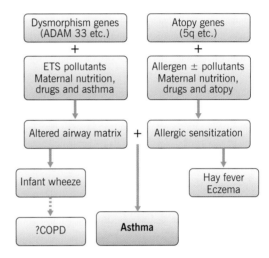

Fig. 18.5 A hypothesis combining the concepts of gene-by-environment interactions independently affecting susceptibility to airway disease, allergy, and allergic asthma.

of environmental factors in which diet, climate, infections, allergen exposures, and pollutants all contribute.

The concept of the allergic march has become even more complex with the identification that there are genetic polymorphisms associated with eczema or asthma, or both, which are apparently independent of the mechanisms associated with an allergic immune response. Thus, it has been shown that, in children not previously sensitized to allergens, eczema (but not asthma or rhinitis) is an independent predictor of allergic sensitization by 5 years of age. The loss of skin integrity associated with polymorphisms in genes such as filaggrin that affect epithelial barrier function is associated with both eczema and susceptibility to allergic sensitization. This suggests that breakdown of the skin barrier, which could be affected by a host of non-allergic triggers, initiates inflammation in the skin through which allergens could gain entry and lead to the induction of sensitization. It is therefore perhaps not surprising that acute severe peanut allergy occurs most commonly in children who had preceding eczema – or, indeed, that asthma and inhalant allergy often follow eczema. Emollients containing *Arachis* oil used to treat eczema have been shown to promote sensitization to peanut. Furthermore, in murine models it is possible to demonstrate that skin application of an allergen will promote sensitization and subsequent systemic allergic responses on further exposure to the allergen (Fig. 18.4).

Asthma has also been associated with genetic polymorphisms that have an effect on airway structure and function rather than inflammatory immune responses. Thus, the gene *ADAM33* (a disintegrin and metalloprotease), polymorphisms which have been associated with asthma, is expressed in airway epithelial cells, fibroblasts, and smooth muscle but not in inflammatory cells.

Interestingly, this gene is first expressed during airway morphogenesis, and polymorphisms may potentially affect airway modelling in the fetus. This suggests that some alteration to airway structure and function is more fundamental to the disease process than is allergic sensitization. However, its combination with allergy confers the highest risk of severe disease and of its persistence through childhood into adulthood (Fig. 18.5).

This is now very clear from very large longitudinal cohort studies evaluating wheezing phenotypes through childhood. Thus, whereas transient wheeze of infancy is common and associated with maternal smoking during pregnancy and premature delivery but not with allergy, early onset and even intermediate and later onset persistent wheezing is commonly associated with allergic sensitization. This and observations of the effects of allergen exposure on eczema suggest that, although both eczema and asthma are a consequence of organ-specific defects, it is allergy that increases the severity and probability of persistence of the diseases (Fig. 18.6). Allergy tests will facilitate prognosis and therefore treatment.

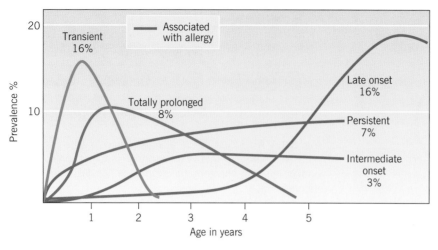

Allergy tests will facilitate prognosis and therefore treatment

Fig. 18.6 Wheeze phenotypes as described in the Avon (UK) longitudinal study. This was based on cluster analysis and showed five phenotypes of which those persisting into later childhood were predominantly associated with allergy. Transient wheeze in infancy was associated with maternal pregnancy smoking and early prolonged wheeze with respiratory syncytial virus bronchiolitis. (From Henderson J, Granell R, Heron J, et al. Associations of wheezing phenotypes in the first 6 years of life with atopy, lung function, and airway responsiveness in mid childhood. Thorax 2008; 63:974–980.)

Eczema

Children with eczema are commonly atopic. Most have positive immediate skin tests and high levels of total serum IgE. Between 20 and 50% go on to develop asthma, and up to 50% have allergic rhinitis. It is, however, unclear to what extent allergy contributes to the immunopathology of eczema in that an allergen will produce a wheal and flare reaction, but not the skin lesions of eczema. It is sometimes possible to replicate lesions by so-called 'atopy patch tests'; in these, either food allergens or aeroallergens are applied to the skin for 48 hours, and then 24 hours later an erythematous vesicular eruption develops with very similar features to eczema. However, the atopy patch test does not increase the sensitivity or specificity of making a specific allergy diagnosis and thus is of little help in identifying clear triggers of the disease.

The distribution of skin lesions varies with age. It is often facial, but sparing the nose, and on the torso in young infants; then in childhood a more flexural distribution develops (Figs 18.7 and 18.8).

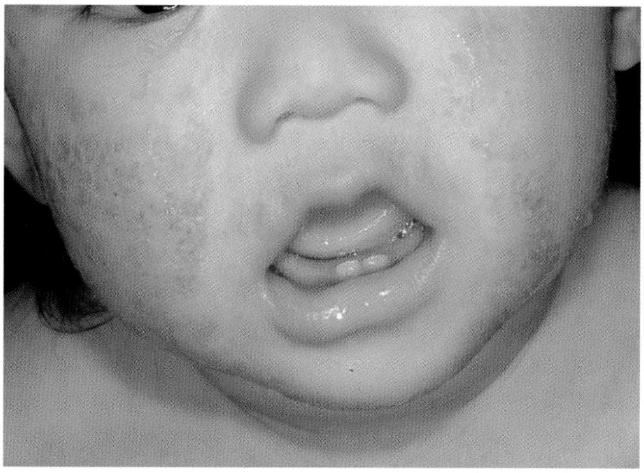

Fig. 18.7 Atopic dermatitis and the headlight sign in early infancy. Note the relative sparing of the midface and immediate perioral area. (From Paller AS, Mancini AJ, Hurwitz clinical pediatric dermatology, 4th edn. Ontario: Elsevier; Ch. 3, Fig. 3.3, July 2011 in press.)

Eczema and allergen avoidance

Some children with eczema do have clear-cut food allergies and exclusion of dietary allergens can achieve some degree of improvement. This is most frequent in children with an onset of eczema below the age of 1 year, and is progressively less likely the older the child. Although the use of dietary modification in children with eczema has been shown in rigorously conducted studies to achieve some benefit, overall the long-term results are often disappointing. Even in highly motivated families with severe eczema associated with food intolerance, up to 20% of children under the age of 3 years and 50% over 3 years will be unable to sustain avoidance diets. This suggests that only simple avoidance diets, such as those excluding dairy products and egg, are likely to achieve long-term benefit. However, in carefully selected cases, more complex diets can be highly effective and are important where there are coexistent gastrointestinal symptoms. It is not infrequent to find degrees of failure to thrive in infants with eczema, and many such children do have multiple food allergies. To what extent avoidance of aeroallergens, which might aggravate eczema via skin contact, will benefit control of eczema is not well established. There are one or two trials of house mite avoidance measures employing bed barrier systems that have demonstrated some degree of improvement in eczema.

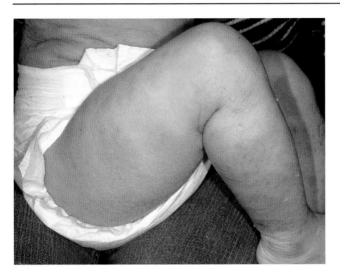

Fig. 18.8 Atopic dermatitis in later infancy. Involvement of the extensor surfaces of the legs and arms are commonly seen during the infantile phase of atopic dermatitis, beginning at about 8 months of age, concomitant with crawling and exposure to irritant and allergenic triggers. (From Paller AS, Mancini AJ, Hurwitz clinical pediatric dermatology, 4th edn. Ontario: Elsevier; Ch. 3, Fig. 3.5, July 2011 in press.)

Management protocol

The primary strategy is focused on effective skin care to reinforce the defective skin barrier function. This must include appropriate use of skin cleansers followed by moisturizers and then application of anti-inflammatory treatment either with topical steroids or with other immunosuppressants such as tacrolimus or pimecrolimus. Many non-specific factors cause a breakdown in barrier function – such as soaps, biological washing powders and fabric softeners, infection, and irritation from synthetic or woollen clothing – and these should be avoided. Inflammation is a consequence and can be controlled with topical immunosuppression. Food allergy is a common aggravator of inflammation in infants with eczema, so avoidance of the relevant allergens, of which hen's eggs and cow's milk are the most common, can be very effective. It is not uncommon for other features of food allergy to coexist in children with eczema including bouts of acute urticaria and angioedema, often triggered by foods. The latter are relatively easy to detect as simple allergy tests (skin prick or IgE antibody tests) usually confirm the diagnosis. Enteropathies associated with failure to thrive, vomiting (with or without gastroesophageal reflux), diarrhoea, or gut motility disorders also occur. These are often not associated with positive allergy tests and require investigation with reflux studies, endoscopy, or biopsy as appropriate. The commonest finding is of eosinophilic inflammation. Under such circumstances, trial dietary avoidance protocols may be the only way of identifying causes. The same may be true of eczema alone – where allergy tests in some circumstance lack sensitivity and specificity.

Skin contact with aeroallergens may also cause exacerbations of eczema and is very notable in pollen-allergic patients. Intensification of topical therapy and regular antihistamine treatment can help reduce acute urticarial reactions. As discussed earlier, avoidance of house mites may be of benefit, but the evidence base is flimsy. It remains to be established whether effective control of eczema will have any impact on the subsequent prevalence of asthma.

Asthma

William Osler is quoted as having failed to appreciate that asthma may end in death: 'the asthmatic pants on into old age'. However, it might equally be assumed that this statement indicates that asthma is a chronic condition that persists well beyond childhood and often into old age. There is a continuing misconception that childhood asthma is a self-limiting disorder with spontaneous improvement during adolescence. However, many longitudinal studies have now shown that a significant percentage persist and, even amongst those who remit in adolescence, large numbers of individuals find their problems recur in later adult life. This has led to the concept that perhaps early intervention in the management of disease will have the best chance of modifying outcomes. Sadly, though, hitherto there is no therapeutic intervention (other than potentially allergen immunotherapy in specific cases) that has been shown to have any impact in modifying its natural history. The Melbourne prospective study of asthma has had the longest follow-up. This study demonstrated that intermittent wheezing in early to mid childhood is a self-limiting condition and is not associated with lung function deficits in mid adult life. The prognosis is less favourable in children with an early onset of frequent severe or prolonged attacks and if there is associated infantile eczema. Other studies have shown that reduced lung function and/or increased bronchial hyperresponsiveness in childhood asthma are associated with a greater lung function deficit in adulthood.

The gender distribution of asthma changes through childhood. In young children, the male to female ratio is progressively higher with increasing severity of disease. Thus severe persistent asthma in children has a 3 : 1 male predominance. In contrast, in adulthood the gender ratio shows a marginal female predominance for severe disease. It is apparent that during adolescence more males are likely to improve, whereas females are more likely to have persistent problems or develop new asthma for the first time. There has been some association particularly in females with new onset asthma and earlier menarche, rapid weight gain, and obesity. Smoking in adolescence decreases the probability of improvement in asthma symptoms amongst patients who have wheezed earlier in childhood, and uptake of smoking in early adulthood increases the risks of a remitted asthmatic having a relapse.

Immunopathology of childhood asthma

Bronchial biopsy studies from children with asthma have shown similar changes to those seen in adult asthmatics, with shedding of the suprabasal epithelial cells and an inflammatory infiltrate dominated by eosinophils with some increases in mast cells and lymphocytes. Remodelling has also been observed consistently in school age asthmatic children who have moderate or severe persistent asthma. This has included thickening of the lamina reticularis, increased collagen within the lamina propria, and sometimes also smooth muscle hypertrophy. These changes do not correlate with duration of disease or, necessarily, with allergic status. There remains some uncertainty about the timing of the appearance of features of remodelling. Some studies suggest that it is already apparent when the disease first manifests, whereas others suggest there is a delay after onset of symptoms before changes occur. Only larger longitudinal studies will elaborate on this. However, what is clear is that the remodelling process is not a consequence of eosinophilic inflammation, but occurs in parallel with the inflammation and could conceivably occur even in advance of inflammation. This latter concept is supported by cohort studies from both Norway and Perth (Australia) that demonstrated an association between diminished lung function with heightened bronchial hyperresponsiveness at around 4 weeks of age and asthma at 6 and 10/11 years. However, the Tucson cohort studies have also shown that diminished lung function in early infancy is associated with virus-induced wheeze, but less so with those who had persistent asthma. These studies suggested that true asthmatics have near-normal lung function in infancy, but progressive deterioration that is detectable by 6 years of age (Fig. 18.9). This evolution of airway function parallels that of symptoms of airway obstruction, which are mostly episodic initially and become progressively more persistent during the preschool years.

Bronchial lavage studies in childhood asthma have shown very similar alterations in inflammatory mediators to those shown in adulthood. Even in infancy those with more severe disease have predominant neutrophil infiltration, and levels of neutrophils correlate with the major neutrophil chemokine interleukin (IL)-8. In addition, there are raised levels of matrix metalloproteinase 9

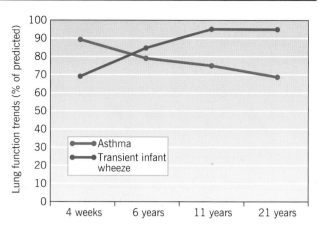

Fig. 18.9 A schematic representation of the evolution of airway function as a percentage of that predicted by age through childhood, in those with transient wheeze in infancy and those with persistent asthma. This is based on a number of longitudinal cohort studies. Transient infant wheeze is a consequence of pre-existing reduced lung function that improves with lung growth and increase in alveolar support to small airways. However, there remains a possibility that such individuals are at increased risk of late adult life lung problems. Those who develop asthma may have early subtle differences in airway structure and function and show a decline over the first few years of life.

(MMP-9), which is predominantly generated by neutrophils. Raised levels of the tissue inhibitor of matrix metalloproteinase 1 (TIMP-1) have been shown to predict persistence of wheezing in infant wheezers, and they also have raised levels of serum soluble intracellular adhesion molecule 1 (ICAM-1). The other pivotal factor, which is also increased in asthma, is transforming growth factor β (TGF-β) as this has a potent effect in stimulating fibroblast activity and the generation of myofibroblasts. This is likely to be important in the remodelling process. The presence of eosinophils in bronchial lavage, and indeed biopsies from young wheezers, has been associated with a much higher probability of persistence – but it is the presence of neutrophils that has been associated with increased severity, both in children and in adults.

Viruses and asthma

It is very clear that virus respiratory infection is the major trigger for exacerbations of wheezing both in infancy and in later childhood. Although respiratory syncytial virus (RSV) is the commonest cause of bronchiolitis and may well be followed by recurrent wheeze through early childhood, for the majority of children this is not associated with ongoing asthma. It is rhinovirus-triggered wheezing in infancy that is most commonly associated with asthma by 6 years of age, as shown in the COAST study (Fig. 18.10). The risk of admission to hospital with an acute exacerbation of asthma is very strongly correlated with rhinovirus infection against a background of

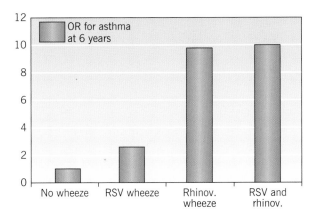

Fig. 18.10 The odds ratio (OR) for asthma at 6 years in relation to the viral triggers of wheeze in infancy. These data from the COAST study show that rhinovirus (rhinov.) rather than respiratory syncytial virus (RSV) is the predominant infecting agent associated with subsequent asthma. OR, odds ratio. (Jackson DJ, Gangnon RE, Evans MD, et al. Wheezing rhinovirus illnesses in early life predict asthma development in high-risk children. Am J Respir Crit Care Med 2008; 178(7):667–672. Reprinted with permission of the American Thoracic Society. Copyright © 2008 American Thoracic Society.)

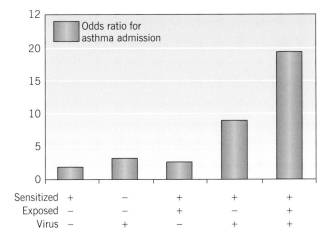

Fig. 18.11 Odds ratios for hospital admission with an acute asthma exacerbation in relation to allergic sensitization, allergen exposure, and viral infection from the Manchester asthma and allergy study. This shows that allergy and allergen exposure enhance the probability that viral infection will induce a significant exacerbation. (From Murray CS, Poletti G, Kebadze T, et al. Study of modifiable risk factors for asthma exacerbations: virus infection and allergen exposure increase the risk of asthma hospital admissions in children. Thorax 2006; 61:376–382.)

allergic sensitization and exposure to the relevant allergen (Fig. 18.11). Rhinovirus gains access to epithelial cells via aggregation with the molecule Intracellular adhesion molecule 1 (ICAM-1). As allergic sensitization and exposure will up-regulate ICAM-1, this perhaps provides an

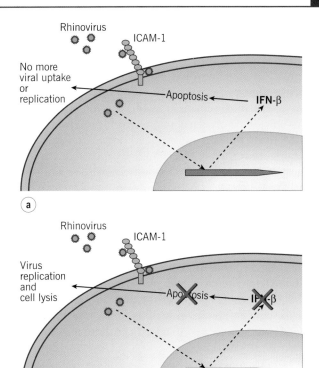

Fig. 18.12 A mechanistic explanation for the effect of rhinovirus-induced asthma exacerbations. (a) A cartoon representation of the route taken by the rhinovirus to translocate into airway epithelial cells via intracellular adhesion molecule 1 (ICAM-1), the expression of which is increased in those with allergic asthma even in infancy. The normal epithelial cell response is to increase expression of interferon-β (IFN-β), which induces cell apoptosis and thereby facilitates clearance of the virus. (b) Failed generation of interferon-β results in further viral replication and disruption of the cell to spread virus through the airway. (Data from Wark PA, Johnston SL, Bucchieri F, et al. Asthmatic bronchial epithelial cells have a deficient innate immune response to infection with rhinovirus. J Exp Med 2005; 201:937–947.)

explanation for the unique susceptibility of the asthmatic to this virus (Fig. 18.12a). Most recently it has been shown that it is one specific subtype of rhinovirus (C) that is uniquely associated with a very high risk of subsequent asthma.

In addition it has been shown, at least in adults with asthma, that when infected with rhinovirus their airway epithelial cells are uniquely deficient in production of type I interferons (IFN), such as IFN-β, and type III IFNs. This results in defective cell apoptosis and consequent cell disruption leading to proliferation of the virus rather than its elimination. These observations provide a clear explanation of the relationship between allergy, viruses, and asthma (Fig. 18.12b).

Allergy, allergen avoidance and asthma

Allergy is an extremely common feature of childhood asthma – with somewhere between 80 and 90% having positive skin prick tests and raised specific IgE levels. House dust mite sensitivity is the commonest allergy in asthmatics in most parts of the world, followed closely by cat, grass and tree pollens, and dogs. Food and mould allergies are relatively less commonly involved. However, in some parts of the world (southern Europe and southern USA) *Alternaria* mould is a significant factor. Given the very common association of allergy and asthma, it would seem self-evident that avoidance of allergen should be a major component of the management strategy. However, two Cochrane reviews of house mite avoidance have suggested that there is not enough evidence to show that current chemical and physical methods aimed at reducing exposure to house dust mite allergens are effective in reducing the severity of asthma. Indeed the most recent review suggested that perhaps there was no reason to consider doing any further trials. However, heterogeneity of outcomes suggested that some forms of physical method of avoidance may be effective in some cases.

This lack of efficacy of single-modality measures to reduce house mite exposure such as employing acaricides, bed barrier system, etc. should be balanced against the observation that being resident in a low-allergen environment can produce dramatic improvements. This has been best demonstrated in studies where children with allergic asthma have been moved to a high-altitude environment that has low humidity and therefore no exposure to house dust mites, or indeed often to other aeroallergens and pollutants. Studies have shown that it is possible to reduce regular prophylaxis dramatically while simultaneously having significant improvements in bronchial hyperresponsiveness and reduction in IgE levels and a host of other inflammation markers (Figs 18.13, 18.14). The critical issue is how to replicate this environment in a normal domestic situation. A recent study of a unique temperature-controlled laminar flow system employed in the bedrooms of patients with house mite, cat- and/or dog-allergic asthma has shown significant improvements in terms of quality of life for asthma and reductions both in exhaled nitric oxide and in IgE levels.

The evidence base from which to recommend any other form of allergen avoidance is non-existent. However, all guidelines suggest that in cat- or dog-allergic patients it would be sensible to remove the pets from the patients' homes. However, it may take many months for the animal allergen to be eliminated from the dust. Furthermore, there is some evidence that a high animal allergen exposure, particularly to cats, will modify the pattern of immune response and confer some degree of protection. Indeed, the relationship between the concentration of exposure and disease outcomes is complex and clearly not linear. It may well be that there is a bell-shaped, with

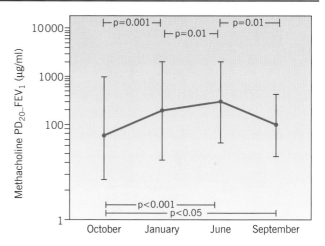

Fig. 18.13 The median and ranges for the dose of metacholine to produce a 20% fall in FEV_1 in a group of house mite sensitive children followed over a 12-month period resident at a high altitude institution (Misurina) from October to June and after a period at home (September). This shows a progressive improvement (increase) in PD20 over 8 months with avoidance of house mites and a deterioration after 3 months at home. (From Peroni DG, Boner AL, Vallone G, et al. Effective allergen avoidance at high altitude reduces allergen-induced bronchial hyperresponsiveness. Am J Respir Crit Care Med 1994; 149(6):1442–1446. Reprinted with permission of the American Thoracic Society. Copyright © 1994 American Thoracic Society.)

both very high and very low exposures conferring some degree of protection.

Allergen immunotherapy

The other allergen-specific approach to the management of asthma is allergen immunotherapy. Cochrane reviews of subcutaneously administered specific immunotherapy (SCIT) for asthma have consistently shown that, compared with placebo, there are significant improvements in asthma symptoms, medication needs, and bronchial hyperresponsiveness for house dust mite, grass and tree pollens, cat, and dog. The data are not quite so clear-cut for other allergens. However, the prevailing concern from regulatory authorities, and therefore expressed in guidelines for the management of asthma, is that there have been no head-to-head comparisons with pharmacotherapy, particularly in relation to risk–benefit profiles. There remain concerns that allergen immunotherapy for asthma is associated with higher risk of serious adverse events compared with its equivalent use for allergic rhinitis alone. While sublingual immunotherapy (SLIT) has an evidence base of efficacy and greater safety than SCIT for allergic rhinitis, it is less secure for asthma.

House mite immunotherapy for house-mite-sensitive childhood asthmatics has been demonstrated to produce significant improvements in control of asthma, with

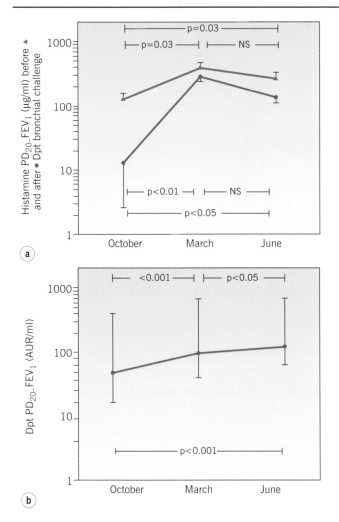

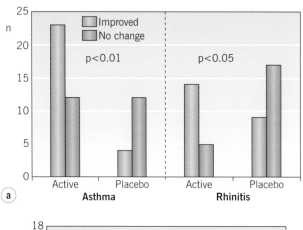

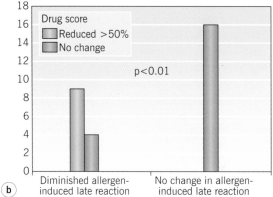

Fig. 18.14 (a) The dose of histamine (PD20) to produce a 20% fall in FEV$_1$ in a group of house-mite-sensitive children before (triangles) and 2 days after (circles) a house mite challenge. In October when the children were first admitted to a high-altitude school (Misurina), the mite exposure enhanced bronchial hyperresponsiveness (BHR) considerably, but after 5 months (March) and 8 months (June) the capacity of a single mite exposure to increase BHR was significantly reduced. (b) The concomitant changes in the dose of house mite allergen to induce a 20% fall in lung function (Dpt PD20 FEV$_1$) in the children resident at high altitude (Misurina) for 8 months. This showed a progressive decrease in sensitivity to the house mite (i.e. increase in PD20). (From Peroni DG, Boner AL, Vallone G, et al. Effective allergen avoidance at high altitude reduces allergen-induced bronchial hyperresponsiveness. Am J Respir Crit Care Med 1994; 149(6):1442–1446. Reprinted with permission of the American Thoracic Society. Copyright © 1994 American Thoracic Society.)

Fig. 18.15 (a) Data from a double-blind placebo-controlled trial of house mite immunotherapy in children with house mite allergy and asthma. A significantly higher number of actively treated children achieved clinical improvements in both asthma and rhinitis symptoms. (b) The most significant clinical improvements in the house mite immunotherapy trial occurred in those children who had a diminished late house-mite-induced late reaction on formal challenge with >50% reductions on pharmacotherapy to control asthma symptoms. (From Warner JO, Price JF, Soothill JF, et al. Controlled trial of hyposensitisation to *Dermatophagoides pteronyssinus* in children with asthma. Lancet 1978; ii(8096):912–915.)

considerable reductions in requirement for asthma medication coincident with a loss of the late allergen-induced asthmatic reaction (Fig. 18.15). There is some evidence that, at least for seasonal allergic rhinoconjunctivitis, 3 years of treatment can be associated with a prolonged carry-over effect after stopping treatment.

One trial has specifically addressed the question of whether allergen-specific immunotherapy will modify the natural history of allergic disease. This focused on administering pollen immunotherapy to children with allergic rhinitis alone but no asthma. The study was unfortunately not placebo controlled, but compared a group of children treated with allergen specific subcutaneous immunotherapy with contemporaneous controls not receiving the treatment. Over a period of 3 years, there was a lower rate of new asthma development in the actively treated patients. Even after a period of stopping therapy, there was a continued carry-over effect, with less new asthma over several years of postimmunotherapy follow-up. Furthermore, studies that have administered allergen-specific immunotherapy to children with a single allergy have shown a very much lower rate of development of new additional allergies, compared with not receiving this treatment. These studies suggest that, in subjects with single-allergen sensitivity, early use of allergen-specific immunotherapy may be more likely to achieve long-term beneficial outcomes than delaying the use of this therapy until disease is well established and multiple allergies are present. It is unknown, however, whether similar effects can be obtained in children with multiple sensitivities or in placebo-controlled studies.

Anti-IgE therapy

The final proof of the concept that allergy and therefore IgE antibodies are important in asthma was established by the use of the anti-IgE agent omalizumab. This modality of treatment has been shown to reduce free circulating IgE, and thereby also the density of high-affinity IgE receptors on mast cells and basophils, therefore reducing mast cell and basophil activation. There is also the potential that this therapy reduces IgE-facilitated antigen presentation so resulting in a slow decline in IgE production. Successive placebo-controlled trials in adults with very severe asthma have shown considerable benefits. This therapy has now been extended to the paediatric age group between 6 and 12 years of age with similar favourable responses.

Management strategies

Although pharmacotherapy forms the mainstay of the management of asthma (Fig. 18.16), it is clear that allergy is an important cofactor in the severity and persistence of the disease. Thus, from the patient's and carers' perspective, identifying triggers and recommending avoidance is a given. It is a tragedy that many health professionals fail to take the needs and expectations of patients into account – even though it is encompassed in the definition of evidence-based medicine. Identification of specific exposures that can trigger asthma symptoms can improve the doctor–patient relationship and thereby improve adherence to pharmacotherapy. However, it must be acknowledged that current single-modality avoidance measures, particularly for house dust mite, have yet to be shown to produce convincing improvements.

Allergic rhinitis and the united airway

Allergic rhinitis (Fig. 18.17) is an extremely common disorder. It occurs in a very high percentage of patients with asthma and this has led to the concept of the 'united airways', which postulates that many of the inflammatory mechanisms present in the lower airways may also be present in the nasal mucosa. In support of this contention, several studies have found that inflammatory markers found in bronchial lavage can also be identified in nasal lavage in patients with allergic rhinitis. Unfortunately, the presence of allergic rhinitis is frequently missed, especially in children with asthma, and its importance as a cause of morbidity is grossly underestimated. Quality of life studies have suggested that impairment in allergic rhinitis is equivalent to that of moderate to severe asthma and worse than that of asthma controlled with low-dose inhaled corticosteroid. Allergic rhinitis has a profound effect on sleep quality and thereby affects

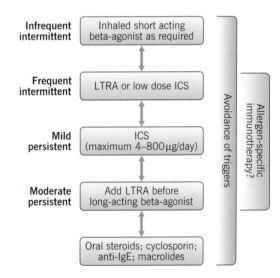

Fig. 18.16 A therapeutic algorithm for the management of childhood asthma indicating the place of allergen avoidance at all levels of severity and a potential place for allergen immunotherapy. Pharmacotherapy remains the mainstay of management. LTRA, leukotriene-receptor antagonist; ICS, inhaled corticosteroid.

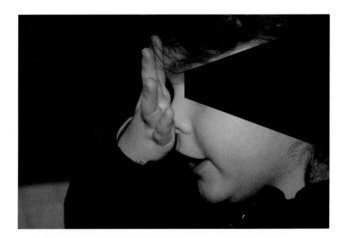

Fig. 18.17 The 'nasal salute' is a typical gesture of patients, especially children, with profuse rhinorrhoea requiring frequent wiping. (From Cauwenberge P, Watelet J-B, Van Zele T, et al. Allergic rhinitis. In: Laurent GJ, Shapiro SD, eds. Encyclopedia of respiratory medicine. New York: Elsevier; 2006:80–91.)

daytime attentiveness, with an increase in somnolence. This has been shown to impair educational attainments. Furthermore, the presence of allergic rhinitis is associated with reduced asthma control in both children and adults. Limited studies suggest that effective treatment of allergic rhinitis improves control of the asthma.

Immunotherapy using SCIT or SLIT has clearly been shown to be of benefit from allergic rhinitis and does have an established place in the treatment algorithm – particularly when focused on tree, grass, or weed pollens – with Cochrane reviews demonstrating considerable improvements in symptom and medication scores. Here the use of 3 years of immunotherapy is associated with a prolonged carry-over benefit. In comparison, the use of pharmacotherapy, although controlling mild to moderate symptoms, has no carry-over effect. However, mostly based on concerns about the risk:benefit ratio associated with immunotherapy, most guidelines reserve it for patients who fail to respond to standard therapy with antihistamines and nasal corticosteroids. Development of safer forms of immunotherapy may modify its current placement in consensus algorithms for the treatment of allergic rhinitis.

In patients with allergic rhinitis and asthma there is concern that the use of topical steroids for the nose and bronchi will have a cumulative effect, and therefore a higher probability of adverse outcomes particularly in relation to growth. There is little doubt that moderate high-dose inhaled corticosteroid can have an impact on growth during childhood. Nevertheless good control of allergic rhinitis can improve asthma control and therefore doses of corticosteroid to nose and lower airways should be carefully titrated to avoid adverse effects. Leukotriene receptor antagonists (LTRAs) such as montelukast can benefit both rhinitis and asthma simultaneously.

Food allergy

Food allergy in childhood has become an increasingly common problem, affecting between 5 and 10% of young children. Up to 2% are affected by allergy to peanut and/or tree nuts, which is associated with the most severe and potentially life-threatening reaction (i.e. anaphylactic shock). Ninety per cent of children with food allergies react to one of eight food groups – that is, eggs, dairy products, peanuts, tree nuts, wheat, soy, fish or shellfish. Allergy to other foods is increasing, as exemplified by reports on sesame and kiwi allergies. Peanut allergy has doubled in prevalence, while peanut sensitization has increased three-fold over the last 5–10 years. There is also an increasing appreciation of oral allergy syndrome in children: patients with birch pollen allergy have cross-reactions to heat-labile proteins in various fruits and vegetables. Allergic reactions to food leading to hospital admissions in the UK have risen by seven-fold in the last 15 years. An association between severe and life-threatening asthma resulting in admission to intensive care or death and the presence of food allergy has also been reported, although a cause–effect relation has not been established. Nevertheless, asthma confers the highest risk of life-threatening anaphylaxis in those with food allergy. Diagnoses of urticaria, angioedema, and anaphylaxis due to food are usually straightforward. A thorough history often shows a very short time interval between exposure and reaction. Furthermore, in the overwhelming majority of patients, skin prick tests and IgE antibody measurement will confirm the diagnosis. However, in some cases timing of exposure and reaction are less clearly temporally associated, and allergy tests provide confusing or equivocal results. This is certainly true in relation to eczema and also to the increasingly common group of enteropathies induced by foods. Often eosinophilic oesophagitis or eosinophilic colitis induced by foods is not associated with positive allergy tests at first presentation in infancy, and the diagnosis can only be established by therapeutic trials of avoidance and rechallenge. Atopy patch tests to foods have not clearly improved diagnostic yield. It is possible that these conditions are not driven through an IgE-mediated mechanism, but are in fact a direct, lymphocyte-induced eosinophil activation through the generation of IL-5. However, recent studies have suggested that local IgE production within the bowel may also be involved.

Food protein-induced enterocolitis syndrome (FPIES) is a relatively recently recognized symptom complex of severe vomiting and diarrhoea caused by non-IgE-mediated allergy to cow's milk, soy, wheat, or other cereals in infants. Symptoms typically begin in the first month of life in association with failure to thrive and may have a catastrophic presentation, with severe dehydration and circulatory collapse due to bowel fluid loss within a few hours of ingestion of the offending food. Symptoms resolve after the causal protein is removed from the diet. Symptoms recur approximately 2 hours after reintroduction of the protein along with a coincident elevation of the peripheral blood polymorphonuclear leukocyte count. The sensitivity is usually outgrown by 3 years of age.

One concept that has arisen out of recent observational studies is that the main route of sensitization to foods may not be via the gastrointestinal tract. Peanut allergy is very uncommon in Israel despite the fact that peanut is used as an early weaning food in infancy. The prevalence has been compared with Jewish children of identical ethnic origin living in London who have very delayed oral exposure to peanuts, but have a much higher prevalence of peanut allergy. This observation would suggest that non-oral exposure to food may be the most important in triggering sensitization and exposures through the skin, particularly among children with eczema, may be the main route of sensitization.

Diagnosis of food allergy

Population surveys have indicated that perceived food allergy/intolerance is very common, with up to 20% of individuals avoiding foods they consider to be causing adverse reactions. However, the true prevalence is around 5% based on double-blind placebo-controlled food challenge (DBPCFC). Thus the remaining subjects with non-reproducible responses are classified as 'food aversion'. There is an imperative in clinical practice to discriminate such cases, which may be possible only by food challenge. It is also important to distinguish intolerance/allergy, which affects only a proportion of the population, from reactions to foods, which occur in the majority if not all and are due to toxins or pharmacologically active components. The latter may sometimes produce symptoms identical to allergic reactions. This is best exemplified by scombroid fish poisoning: tuna and related fish if badly stored will accumulate high levels of histamine, and ingestion will produce a systemic histamine reaction (see Ch. 17). Having distinguished toxic reactions and food aversion, there will also be patients who have reproducible adverse reactions to foods but no evidence of its having an immune mechanism. Such cases may be classified as 'food intolerance' where errors of metabolism may be involved, and these will be reliably diagnosed only by DBPCFC.

Reproducible responses to food, if associated with immunological hypersensitivity, may or may not be IgE mediated. In the former case, diagnostic confirmation can usually be achieved by skin prick tests or IgE antibody measurement. However, careful interpretation of the results is critical. There is a 5% false negative rate, and sensitivity rarely exceeds 85% and varies considerably between different foods. The quality and allergen content of the extract employed for the test are pivotal. Thus patients with oral allergy syndrome reactions to fresh, but not cooked, tree fruit associated with tree pollen allergy will usually not show positive tests to commercial extracts. Skin testing using the fresh fruit is far more sensitive. Therefore an important component of management is the understanding by clinicians of the predictive value of individual food allergy tests. Non-IgE-mediated reactions may be due to immune complex formation or direct activation of eosinophils or lymphocyte. Food-induced eosinophilic oesophagitis is an example of eosinophil activation that is often not associated with detectable circulating IgE or positive skin tests.

A suggested classification of adverse reactions to foods is illustrated in Figure 18.18.

Prevention of food allergy

Hitherto, national advice about weaning practices has suggested that there should be delayed introduction of

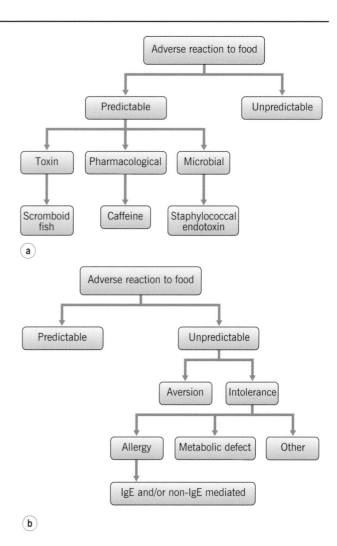

Fig. 18.18 (a) A suggested classification of adverse reactions to food which, though sometimes difficult to distinguish from allergy, is predictable in that it will occur in the majority if not all who are exposed. (b) A classification of adverse reactions to foods that occurs in only a subsection of the population. Food aversion is common, affecting 15% of the population, whereas intolerance and allergy are discriminated by being reproducible on double-blind food challenge. If associated with immunological hypersensitivity, it is allergy that can be IgE or non-IgE mediated.

highly allergenic foods to children born into atopic families. However, this may have paradoxically increased the rate of food allergy. Trials are now in progress to establish whether the exact timing of introduction of allergenic foods may be critical. There is perhaps a greater potential to induce tolerance if there is an overlap between weaning and continued breastfeeding. There is also a precedent from coeliac disease, which suggests that introduction of wheat prior to 4 months of age dramatically increases the prevalence of the condition. There is, however, also an increase in incidence if wheat introduction is delayed beyond 6 months of age. This has led the European Society of Paediatric Gastroenterology, Hepatology and Nutrition to recommend that gluten should be introduced gradually between 4 and 7 months – preferably while the mother is still breastfeeding, as this has the best chance of achieving mucosal immune tolerance.

The degree to which breastfeeding protects against the development of allergy remains unclear. Systematic reviews have suggested that it does reduce early allergic manifestations, and particularly those associated with food allergy, in the first 2 years of life. However, beyond that age there is relatively little evidence of protective effects. It is unlikely that a controlled trial will ever be performed, because many benefits derive from breast-feeding, which extend well beyond those related to allergic disease, and it would thus be unethical to randomize children to a non-breastfeeding arm in a controlled trial. It will be difficult, therefore, to rule out potential confounding factors as an explanation for the results obtained from observational studies. There has been a suggestion, for example, that prolonged breastfeeding may be associated with an increased risk of allergy; however, it is likely that families with the highest risk of allergic disease choose prolonged breastfeeding as an option because they believe it might be protective. There are also now studies demonstrating that variations in the constituents of human breast milk can affect outcomes. Thus it has been shown that lower levels of soluble CD14, which is part of the complex with endotoxin that induces a Th1 and therefore Th2-suppressive immune response, and reduced levels of transforming growth factor β (TGF-β), a regulatory cytokine, are associated with a higher risk of subsequent eczema. In addition, variations in polyunsaturated fatty acid levels in breast milk have been associated with different allergic outcomes. Future studies will need to focus on strategies to improve the allergy-protective qualities of human breast milk.

Systematic reviews of the allergy-preventive effects of hydrolysed milk formulae with or without pre- or probiotics have been hampered by doubts about the accuracy and veracity of some published studies. However, there is evidence that extensively hydrolysed casein formulae and prebiotics do confer some protection.

Treatment of food allergy

The mainstay of management is identification of the cause, and advice and support on avoidance. The latter requires input from a dietitian with expertise in paediatric allergy. Any nutritional inadequacies will need to be covered by appropriate supplements. In this respect, it has become increasingly apparent that vitamin D insufficiency is very common and may increase the likelihood of the development of allergic disease and also enhance its severity. As accidental exposure to food allergens is all too frequent, rescue treatment must also be instantly available. For most this will include antihistamines for a mild reaction, and autoinjector adrenaline (US epinephrine) for more severe reactions. Training in the carriage, storage, and use of the devices is critical. Systemic oral tolerance induction using graded exposures to the offending food allergens is now being employed in research studies and could become part of the therapeutic algorithm, at least for some food allergies. It will not be practical for those with multiple food allergies, however.

Education and allergic disease

The paternalistic approach to doctor–patient relationships is no longer acceptable, and families have every right to expect to participate in management decisions. This requires empowerment of families to handle their child's condition with support and help from health professionals when necessary. Thus the focus is now on concordance rather than compliance. This is a shared responsibility for management between patient, family and clinician.

Provision of appropriate training and education for patients and their families about the causes and management of their allergic disease should be a fundamental component of all consultations. There is a strong evidence base supporting the use of written action plans. It is somewhat less strong for other components of the education package, but has proven benefits in relation to asthma, eczema, and anaphylaxis. Different populations and disease groups will require different approaches, depending on age, ethnicity, and other factors. Modern information technology, which is particularly well used by children, can be of considerable value.

In providing support, education and training, it is important to consider all carers likely to be involved with the child. In the early years this is focused on the family alone, but should include grandparents and sometimes childcare staff. Programmes based on management in schools have been shown to benefit children with asthma and are particularly important for the child with acute food allergy. They must include advice on avoidance of triggers and the provision and use of rescue treatment. Thus training to recognize acute exacerbations and in the use of autoinjectors and inhaler devices will be the primary focus.

Summary of important messages

- Allergic diseases in children have progressively increased in prevalence over the last 50 years – initially involving inhalant allergy associated with asthma and rhinitis, but more recently also food allergy; this has predominantly occurred in affluent environments, but is also now extending to the developing world
- Not only has the prevalence of these diseases increased, but so too has the diversity of allergens involved
- Given that no therapeutic intervention has been conclusively shown to alter the natural history or progression of allergic diseases, much attention now focuses on the early life origins of allergy
- These studies are highlighting potential targets for prevention, but no intervention has yet been shown to affect incidence significantly; allergen avoidance in primary prevention has notably failed in this respect, and there is a suggestion that early allergen exposure may actually be more likely to achieve tolerance – thus management must still concentrate on reducing the severity of disease and improving the quality of life
- Once allergic disease is established, allergen avoidance has an important place in the therapeutic algorithm – mainly when a clear cause–effect relationship can be established between exposure and symptoms
- Pharmacotherapy with anti-inflammatory treatment, mostly in the form of topical corticosteroids, forms the mainstay of therapy
- Much attention should also be devoted to patient and carer education to empower families to handle their allergies effectively

Further reading

Bousquet J, Khaltaev N, Cruz AA, et al. Allergic Rhinitis and its Impact on Asthma (ARIA) 2008 update (in collaboration with the World Health Organization, GA(2) LEN and AllerGen) [Rreview]. Allergy 2008; 63(suppl 86):8–160.

British Thoracic Society, Scottish Intercollegiate Guidelines Network. British Guideline on the Management of Asthma. Thorax 2008; 63(suppl 4):1–121.

Erlewyn-Lajeunesse MDS, Hunt LP, Pohunek P, et al. Bronchoalveolar lavage MMP-9 and TIMP-1 in preschool wheezers and their relationship to persistent wheeze. Pediatr Res 2008; 64:194–199.

Håland G, Carlsen KC, Sandvik L, et al, ORAACLE. Reduced lung function at birth and the risk of asthma at 10 years of age. N Engl J Med 2006; 355(16):1682–1689.

Holt P, Naspitz C, Warner JO. Early immunological influences in prevention of allergy and allergic asthma. In: Johansson SGO, Haahtela T, eds. World Allergy Organization Project report and guidelines. Basel: Karger; 2004:102–127.

Lack G. Epimediologic risks for food allergy. J Allergy Clin Immunol 2008; 121:1331–1336.

Lieberman P, Nicklas RA, Oppenheimer J, et al. The diagnosis and management of anaphylaxis practice parameter 2010 update. J Allergy Clin Immunol 2010; 126(3):477–480.

McCann DC, McWhirter J, Coleman H, et al. A controlled trial of a school based intervention to improve asthma management. Eur Resp J 2006; 27:921–928.

Peroni DG, Boner AL, Vallone G, et al. Effective allergen avoidance at high altitude reduces allergen induced bronchial hyperresponsiveness. Am J Respir Crit Care Med 1994; 149:1442–1446.

Warner JO. Developmental origins of asthma and related allergic disorders. In: Gluckman P, Hanson M, eds. Developmental origins of health and disease. Cambridge: CUP; 2006:349–369.

19

Eosinophilia: clinical manifestations and therapeutic options

Charles W DeBrosse and Marc E Rothenberg

DEFINITION

Eosinophilia is a hallmark of allergic disorders. However, the differential diagnosis for the patient with eosinophilia is broad and patients with eosinophilia require a thoughtful history, physical exam, and laboratory evaluation. This chapter focuses on the diagnosis and management of the most common causes of eosinophilia.

Introduction

Eosinophilic inflammation is one of the hallmarks of allergic disease, and accumulation of eosinophils in affected tissues is a feature of diseases such as allergic rhinitis, asthma, and eosinophilic gastrointestinal disorders (EGIDs). Eosinophils are derived from the bone marrow where they undergo transcriptionally regulated maturation and subsequent expansion, which is primarily driven by interleukin 5 (IL-5). Following maturation and expansion, eosinophils enter the circulation and will accumulate in response to a variety of chemoattractants, including the eotaxin family of chemokines. Eosinophils may accumulate locally or peripherally, and eosinophilia is frequently the product of a Th2-driven response associated with elevated levels of IL-5, IL-4, and IL-13. In addition to atopic diseases, eosinophilia can be associated with autoimmune disorders, parasitic infection, malignancy, drug hypersensitivity, eczema, and a variety of pulmonary disorders (e.g. allergic bronchopulmonary aspergillosis and eosinophilic pneumonia).

Peripheral eosinophilia is defined by the presence of >450 eosinophils/µL of blood (although the exact value depends upon specific laboratories and locations) and can readily be detected by performing a peripheral blood smear. Elevated eosinophil levels in the blood are typically classified as mild (450–1500 cells/mm^3), moderate (1500–5000 cells/mm^3), and severe (>5000 cells/mm^3). Given that the differential diagnosis for eosinophilia is quite broad (Box 19.1), the presence of eosinophilia can present a significant diagnostic challenge to allergists and immunologists. A proposed guide to the evaluation of peripheral eosinophilia is outlined in Figure 19.1. In this chapter, we highlight the clinical features, diagnostic evaluation, and therapeutic approach for the most common causes of eosinophilia.

Hypereosinophilic syndrome

Originally described by Chusid et al, in 1975, hypereosinophilic syndrome (HES) is the best illustration of the important clinical consequences that can arise from eosinophilia. HES is defined as the presence of >1500 eosinophils/µL of blood for a sustained period of time with evidence of eosinophil-mediated end-organ damage. From a clinical standpoint, HES typically affects the dermatological, pulmonary, gastrointestinal, and

© 2012 Elsevier Ltd
DOI: 10.1016/B978-0-7234-3658-4.00005-6

Box 19.1 Differential diagnosis for eosinophilia

Parasitic infection	Eosinophilic gastrointestinal disorders) (EGIDs)	Eosinophilic pneumonia (acute or chronic
Hypereosinophilic syndrome (HES)	Drug hypersensitivity (DRESS syndrome, granulocyte infusions)	Eosinophilia with thrombosis
Asthma	Malignancy (CML, AML, ALL)	Churg–Strauss syndrome
Eczema	Interstitial nephritis	Allergic bronchopulmonary aspergillosis
Systemic mastocytosis	Episodic angioedema	Immunodeficiency (hyper-IgE, Omenn syndrome, immunosuppression)

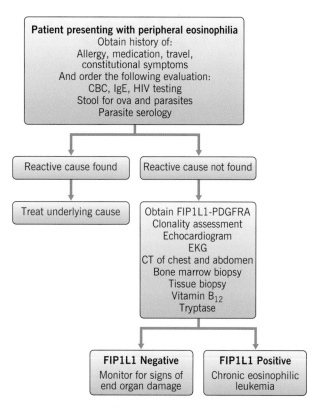

Fig. 19.1 Diagnostic algorithm for eosinophilia. The approach to the evaluation for patients with eosinophilia is outlined. A thorough history and physical exam precede laboratory testing. Laboratory testing is then utilized to identify the most likely diagnosis and to exclude or confirm the presence of malignancy.

of HES demonstrated that the subset of patients possessing this fusion gene is small (11%) and nearly exclusively male. Among HES patients who do not possess the novel fusion gene, aberrant populations of T cells are occasionally identified. It is thought that these T cells may be secreting eosinophil growth factors such as IL-5, which would promote the development of peripheral eosinophilia. For the majority of patients with HES, however, the underlying aetiology remains undefined.

Confirmation of suspected HES includes several evaluations, the first of which are the documentation of persistent peripheral eosinophilia [complete blood count (CBC) with differential] and the identification of suspected end-organ damage. A second critical component of the diagnosis of HES involves excluding common causes of eosinophilia, and in particular parasitic infection. This evaluation typically involves analysing stool for ova and parasites and titres for common parasitic infections. Additionally, the possibility of chronic eosinophilic leukaemia should be excluded through bone marrow biopsy. Serum levels of Vitamin B12 and mast cell tryptase, which are often both elevated in patients with HES, should also be evaluated. There are data to suggest that patients with an elevated Vitamin B12 level tend to have the myeloproliferative form of HES. Bone marrow cells collected at the time of biopsy may also be used to detect the presence of the HES-associated fusion gene, *FIP1L1/PDGFRalpha*. It is reasonable to obtain additional tests [e.g. computed topography (CT) of the chest, abdomen, and pelvis; lactate dehydrogenase (LDH); cardiac troponin, and uric acid] in the initial evaluation of suspected HES in order to rule out the presence of malignancy. T-cell receptor phenotyping can also be helpful to identify whether an aberrant T-cell population is present. IgE and total immunoglobulin analysis can also be helpful, as both substances tend to be elevated in patients with the lymphoproliferative variant of HES. Finally, given the risk of Loeffler's endocarditis, an echocardiogram should be obtained at initial evaluation among patients with persistent peripheral eosinophilia.

Treatment for HES is, in part, dependent upon the results of the diagnostic evaluation. For patients who are positive for the *FIP1L1/PDGFRalpha* fusion gene, imatinib mesylate can be very effective for achieving disease remission. Doses from 100 to 400 mg daily have been

neurological systems. However, it can affect any end organ, and the clinical presentation can be quite variable. In rare circumstances, eosinophils can infiltrate the myocardium, resulting in endocarditis (Loeffler's endocarditis) and/or a pericardial effusion. There are several variants of HES – lymphocytic and myeloproliferative being the two most common subtypes.

The aetiology of HES is not entirely clear. In a subset of HES patients, the disease is the result of a continuously activated tyrosine kinase. This tyrosine kinase results from the fusion of two genes, *FIP1L* and *PDGFRalpha*, and leads to the constant promotion of eosinophil growth and survival. A recent multicentre study suggested in the medical literature. However, a recent, small study suggests that patients receiving at least 400 mg daily are less likely to relapse. The authors suggest that the optimal dose of imatinib should be individualized and that patients should be monitored closely for relapsing disease.

For patients with HES who are negative for the *FIP1L1/PDGFRalpha* fusion gene, corticosteroids are the first-line therapy. There is no consensus on the dose needed for initial therapy or maintenance, though a daily dosing regimen starting at 1 mg corticosteroid per kilogram of body weight and slowly tapering over 3–6 months has been advocated. The majority of patients with HES will relapse once corticosteroid therapy is withdrawn, however. Accordingly, many patients will remain on low doses of corticosteroids indefinitely. Given the many side effects associated with long-term steroid therapy, it is critical for the clinician to identify the minimal effective corticosteroid dose. Monitoring for the development of osteopenia, diabetes, and hypertension among patients on corticosteroids is also an important component of the care of patients with HES. There is a small risk that patients with HES may go one to develop malignancy, or they may go on to have involvement of other organ systems. As such, all patients with HES need to be monitored periodically with physical exams, CBCs and any other clinically indicated testing to monitor for the development of these complications.

An important advance for patients with HES has been the introduction of mepolizumab, a fully humanized anti-IL-5 monoclonal antibody. A multicentre, double-blind, placebo-controlled trial of patients with HES who received mepolizumab demonstrated an excellent therapeutic response: 95% had decreases in their eosinophil counts that yielded levels of less than 600/µL. Additionally, 87% of patients with HES were able to lower their required steroid dose. Among the potential therapies for HES, mepolizumab appears to be the most effective; however, this drug is currently available only through research protocols. A variety of other medications may be attempted including hydroxyurea, vincristine, ciclosporin, and interferon α (IFN-α).

Asthma

Eosinophilic inflammation, mucus hypersecretion, and airway hyperresponsiveness are classic features of allergic asthma. In mouse models of this condition, eosinophils are typically involved in the late phase response. Given their relative abundance in allergen-induced models of asthma, eosinophils have therefore become a target for therapeutic interventions. Anti-IL-5 and anti-IL-13 monoclonal antibodies are currently being tested for the treatment of asthma.

Clinical trials utilizing monoclonal antibodies directed against IL-5, an eosinophil growth factor, have yielded interesting results. The original clinical trials, which did not distinguish patients based on the presence or absence of sputum eosinophilia, did not show improved outcomes in patients who received anti-IL-5 (mepolizumab or reslizumab). When studies tested the effectiveness of mepolizumab among a well-defined group of patients with sputum eosinophilia, however, the data did demonstrate reductions in asthma exacerbations. These data suggest that anti-IL-5 therapy may be efficacious in a well-defined subset of asthmatics with sputum eosinophilia. These findings also emphasize the heterogeneous nature of asthma and nicely illustrate how phenotyping patients based on the presence or absence of sputum eosinophilia may be clinically helpful. There are at least two distinct asthma phenotypes based on sputum eosinophil counts. Attempts to direct asthma therapy based on these phenotypes have been made; Green et al demonstrated that utilizing sputum eosinophils as a marker for asthma control led to decreased asthma exacerbations and hospitalizations compared with conventional management.

Clinical trials testing the efficacy of anti-IL-13 for the treatment of asthma are also underway. IL-13 is a Th2 cytokine with the ability to increase eosinophilic inflammation through up-regulation of eotaxin-3. Anti-IL-13 antibodies hold promise as maintenance medications for the treatment of asthma.

Allergic bronchopulmonary aspergillosis

Peripheral eosinophilia is a common manifestation seen among patients with allergic bronchopulmonary aspergillosis (ABPA). ABPA is the result of hypersensitivity to the ubiquitous fungus *Aspergillus fumigatus*; however, other *Aspergillus* and *Penicillium* species have been implicated in the development of ABPA. Typical presenting clinical symptoms of ABPA include dyspnoea, productive cough, and wheezing. The typical clinical picture of ABPA is that of a patient with poorly controlled asthma despite maximal medical therapy. Chest radiographs will often reveal fleeting pulmonary infiltrates. CT of the chest will display central bronchiectasis – a classic feature of ABPA. The clinical features of ABPA are summarized in Box 19.2.

As with other eosinophilic disorders, treatment with oral corticosteroids is helpful for patients with ABPA. However, when utilized long term, these medications can lead to the development of diabetes, hypertension, decreased bone mineral density, and adrenal insufficiency. Accordingly, patients with ABPA or other conditions requiring frequent oral corticosteroid use should be periodically assessed for the development of these sequelae.

Box 19.2 Clinical features of ABPA

Eosinophilia	Central	Precipitation
Asthma	bronchiectasis	antibodies to
History of	Elevated total	*Aspergillus*
infiltrates on	IgE	Increased serum
chest X-ray	Positive skin	IgE to *Aspergillus*
	prick test to	
	Aspergillus	

To reduce the need for corticosteroids, an empirical trial of itraconzaloe can be utilized as another therapeutic option for patients with ABPA. Ideally, eradication of *Aspergillus* from the airway should lead to airway eosinophilia reduction and symptomatic improvement. In a recent clinical trial, the use of itraconazole for 6 months led to decreased total IgE, decreased eosinophil levels, and decreased need for prednisone in patients with ABPA. However, it was unclear whether this was due to the eradication of *Aspergillus* or whether the administration of itraconazole led to elevated prednisone levels in these patients. Currently, there are no data regarding the effect of anti-IL-5 monoclonal antibodies or anti-IL-5 receptor therapies among patients with ABPA.

Eosinophilic pneumonias

Eosinophilic pneumonias are rare disorders that can manifest as either acute or chronic eosinophilic pneumonia. Little is known about the pathophysiology of either condition. A recently published study demonstrated that galectin-9, an eosinophil chemoattractant, was significantly increased in the bronchoalveolar lavage fluid (BALF) of patients with acute and chronic eosinophilic pneumonia. Although a well-defined mechanism has not been established for acute eosinophilic pneumonia, both antibiotic use and smoking have been associated with its onset.

For patients with acute eosinophilic pneumonia, corticosteroids are the treatment of choice, and patients typically respond quickly when high doses are administered.

Chronic eosinophilic pneumonia is characterized by fever, fatigue, cough, and pulmonary infiltrates on chest X-ray. CT scans may demonstrate non-specific findings such as consolidation, ground-glass-like opacities or band-like subpleural opacities. Clinically, patients with eosinophilic pneumonia are typically middle aged and they are more likely to be female than male. The important clinical finding in the diagnosis of chronic or acute eosinophilic pneumonia is the presence of elevated numbers of eosinophils in the BALF (normally eosinophils are found in low numbers – typically about 1%). Therefore,

higher eosinophil levels suggest an underlying pathology. From a therapeutic standpoint, eosinophilic pneumonia responds readily to treatment with prednisone; however, patients typically require prolonged therapy with this drug as the majority will relapse if it is stopped during the first 12 months. Without therapy, patients experience a chronic disease course marked by recurrent exacerbations. With therapy, the prognosis is generally very favourable.

Drug hypersensitivity

The presence of eosinophilia is common among patients who are experiencing drug hypersensitivity reactions. Drug rash with eosinophilia and systemic symptoms (DRESS) is infrequently encountered, but clinically important, immunological reaction to medications. The mechanism for DRESS is probably a delayed, type IV immune response. This is supported by the observation that symptoms of DRESS typically begin 1–8 weeks after initiation of the offending agent. Antiepileptics and antimicrobials (tetracyclines and sulfonamides) are the most common causes of the condition. Typical symptoms include a prominent exanthema, fever, lymphadenopathy, pharyngitis, and fatigue. Interestingly, only 30% of patients with DRESS develop eosinophilia; thus, the absence of the latter cannot be used to rule out DRESS. Importantly, the inflammatory response leads to the development of hepatitis among 50%, and presence of nephritis in up to 30%, of patients with DRESS. There are also rare reports of fatalities related to severe end organ damage related to DRESS. Accordingly, the treating physician should be aware of its potential severity.

There is some recent evidence to suggest that coinfection with or reactivation of human herpes virus 6 (HHV-6) may be associated with the development of DRESS in a subset of patients. However, the data are limited, and reactivation of HHV-6 does not appear to occur in all patients. Typically, symptoms will resolve with removal of the offending agent. Systemic corticosteroids can also be helpful in the treatment of DRESS.

Eosinophil-associated gastrointestinal disorders

Eosinophil-associated gastrointestinal disorders (EGIDs) are a clinically diverse collection of diseases that share an inappropriate accumulation of eosinophils within the gastrointestinal (GI) tract as a common feature. Approximately 25–50% of patients with EGIDs also have evidence of blood eosinophilia. Eosinophilic oesophagitis (EoE) is the most common of the EGIDs. EoE is an emerging allergic disorder, and the frequency with which it has been diagnosed is clearly on the rise. This increase appears to largely be the result of increasing recognition, primarily manifested by the increased employment of endoscopy and biopsy, which is required for disease diagnosis.

Clinical observations have suggested that the pathogenesis of EoE may be the result of an allergic response to foods or aeroallergens. Children and adults with EoE frequently have positive skin and patch tests to foods, in addition to positive skin prick tests (SPT) to aeroallergens. Patients with EoE often develop other atopic disorders as well. Recent advances suggest that thymic stromal lymphopoietin (TSLP) may play a critical role in the development of EoE as the main genome-wide susceptibility locus maps to the gene encoding TSLP. Although the exact mechanism is unknown, TSLP promotes Th2 responses through increasing antigen presentation by dendritic cells. It is possible that, in patients with EoE, single-nucleotide polymorphisms in TSLP may lead to increased antigen presentation. This would explain, in part, the highly atopic nature of many of these patients and the association of EoE with food and aeroallergens.

A variety of other Th2-related cytokines and allergic chemokines have been implicated in the development of EoE. Specifically, the gene encoding for the chemokine eotaxin-3 is the most highly up-regulated gene in the oesophagus of EoE patients. Eotaxin-3 mRNA transcript levels are higher in the oesophagus of patients with EoE than in those with gastroesophageal reflux disease (GERD) or in normal control individuals. Additionally, the level of eotaxin-3 correlates with eosinophil levels.

The inflammatory process associated with EoE leads to several histological changes that can be observed in the oesophagus. The findings of basal layer hyperplasia, lamina propria fibrosis, surface layering, and eosinophilic microabscesses are common in EoE patients. Importantly, these findings all appear to be reversible with appropriate therapy.

The typical clinical presenting symptoms of EoE vary with age (Box 19.3) and include dysphagia, food impactions, heartburn, chest pain, vomiting, abdominal pain, and failure to thrive. The diagnosis of EoE can be very difficult to distinguish from GERD based on clinical symptoms. In contrast, patients may also have elevated numbers of eosinophils in the oesophagus and be asymptomatic. Because of its wide array of presenting symptoms, it is not uncommon for patients to be symptomatic for several years before the diagnosis of EoE is made. However, patients who present with symptoms consistent with GERD, but fail to respond to therapy with proton pump inhibitors (PPIs), should undergo oesophagogastroduodenoscopy (EGD) with biopsy to rule out the possibility of EoE. This is especially true if the patient is male or has a history of atopic disease: 75% of EoE patients are male, and as many as two-thirds will have allergic rhinitis. It is important to note that among EoE patients the oesophagus may appear grossly normal on endoscopy and that oesophageal biopsy is critical for the accurate diagnosis of EoE. The presence of severe dysphagia and food impaction should also increase the suspicion for EoE. It is not uncommon for patients with EoE, particularly adolescent males, to present with the sudden onset of food impaction. Interestingly, the food impaction can occur in the presence or absence of oesophageal strictures.

To promote the identification and accurate diagnosis of EoE, consensus diagnostic guidelines based upon expert opinion and a review of the available literature were developed in 2007 (Box 19.4). Based upon these guidelines, the diagnosis of EoE requires ≥15 eosinophils/400× high-power field on oesophageal biopsy in association with GI symptoms and in the absence of GERD. Clinically, the contribution of GERD can be excluded if eosinophil levels remain elevated following a 6–8-week trial of PPI therapy or if the patient has a negative pH probe.

There are several effective treatment approaches for patients with EoE. In general, treatment strategies involve swallowed corticosteroids or dietary intervention. Although there are no comparative effectiveness trials available, elimination diets appear to be the most effective treatment. Several uncontrolled clinical trials have demonstrated high rates of success when treating EoE with an elemental diet. However, whereas an elemental diet is frequently tolerated by infants and toddlers, it is often quite difficult for children and adults. Fortunately, there are several other treatment options for patients with EoE. After initiating treatment with dietary elimination or swallowed corticosteroids, patients are followed for 3 months and then rebiopsied to determine whether there has been an improvement in, or resolution of, their oesophageal inflammation.

Box 19.3 Presenting symptoms for patients with EoE

0–3 years old	4–8 years old	>8 years old
Vomiting	Dysphagia	Food impaction
Poor weight gain	Heartburn	Dysphagia
Feeding disorder	Abdominal pain	Heartburn
	Nausea	Abdominal pain
	Vomiting	

Box 19.4 Diagnostic criteria for eosinophilic oesophagitis (EoE)

- Upper GI symptoms are present
- ≥15 eosinophils/400× high-power field on oesophageal biopsy
- Exclusion of gastroesophageal reflux disease (through a negative pH probe or 6–8-week trial of proton pump inhibitor therapy)

For patients in whom dietary therapy is unsuccessful or undesired, treatment with swallowed budesonide and swallowed fluticasone can be successful. Budesonide has been studied at doses of 1 mg once daily for those less than 1.5 m (5 ft) tall and 2 mg once daily for those over this height. Small clinical trials suggest an efficacy of 80–85%. For fluticasone, the 220 μg inhaler is typically prescribed, and patients are advised to take two puffs twice daily. The use of mepolizumab for the treatment of EoE has been investigated. These studies demonstrated a substantial reduction in the number of eosinophils in the oesophagus of mepolizumab-treated patients; however, only a small percentage of patients achieve complete resolution of their EoE. Phase I clinical trials are underway to evaluate the safety and efficacy of anti-IL-13 therapy in the treatment of EoE.

Importantly, eosinophilic disorders of the GI tract are not limited to the oesophagus. Eosinophil levels may become elevated in any segment of the GI tract and may become increased in any layer of the wall of the GI tract. EGIDs may present with abdominal pain, vomiting, diarrhoea, weight loss, or bloating. The original literature regarding EGIDs other than EoE suggests that these disorders begin to manifest during the 3rd or 4th decade of life. However, it is now recognized that EGIDs occur during childhood as well. Diagnosis is dependent upon the identification of elevated numbers of eosinophils on biopsy. Firm diagnostic criteria for EGIDs other than EoE have not been developed. However, the normal number of eosinophils in the GI tract of children without apparent GI disease has been reported and serves as a comparison (Table 19.1).

Similar to EoE, other EGIDs are thought to be associated with atopy. Available data suggest that patients with other EGIDs also respond to treatment with elemental diet and steroids. However, much less is known about the prevalence, natural history, or the most common triggers of other EGIDs in comparison with EoE.

Churg–Strauss syndrome

Churg–Strauss syndrome (CSS) is an autoimmune-mediated vasculitis, often associated with peripheral eosinophilia, which distinguishes CSS from other forms of vasculitis. The diagnostic criteria for CSS are variable; however, it typically manifests in multiple stages. The typical initial symptoms mimic those of allergic rhinoconjunctivitis and asthma. The final stage is characterized by systemic vasculitis.

The respiratory symptoms associated with CSS typically present as refractory asthma. However, CSS patients may also develop transient pulmonary infiltrates and may present with a clinical picture similar to pneumonia. The development of vasculitis is the hallmark of the syndrome. CSS can present with a variety of dermatological manifestations ranging from purpura to urticarial type lesions, or even maculopapular exanthema. There are also case reports of patients with CSS developing vasculitis in the small bowel, as well as eosinophilic inflammation of the GI tract.

Interestingly, the development of CSS following treatment with leukotriene-modifying agents, as well as omalizumab, has been reported. It is postulated that CSS is

Table 19.1 Eosinophil levels in gastrointestinal segments*

Gastrointestinal segment	Lamina propria		Villous lamina propria		Surface epithelium		Crypt/glandular epithelium	
	Mean	Max	Mean	Max	Mean	Max	Mean	Max
Esophagus	N/A	N/A	N/A	N/A	0.03 ± 0.10	1	N/A	N/A
Antrum	1.9 ± 1.3	8	N/A	N/A	0.0 ± 0.0	0	0.02 ± 0.04	1
Fundus	2.1 ± 2.4	11	N/A	N/A	0.0 ± 0.0	0	0.008 ± 0.03	1
Duodenum	9.6 ± 5.3	26	2.1 ± 1.4	9	0.06 ± 0.09	2	0.26 ± 0.36	6
Ileum	12.4 ± 5.4	28	4.8 ± 2.8	15	0.47 ± 0.25	4	0.80 ± 0.51	4
Ascending colon	20.3 ± 8.2	50	N/A	N/A	0.29 ± 0.25	3	1.4 ± 1.2	11
Transverse colon	16.3 ± 5.6	42	N/A	N/A	0.22 ± 0.39	4	0.77 ± 0.61	4
Rectum	8.3 ± 5.9	32	N/A	N/A	0.15 ± 0.13	2	1.2 ± 1.1	9

*Biopsies were obtained from children without apparent gastrointestinal disease. The mean number of eosinophils present in each segment of the GI tract is shown. Under healthy conditions, eosinophils reside in all parts of the GI tract except for the esophagus. Eosinophils are also rarely found in the surface epithelium. The table was adapted with permission of the publisher. (From DeBrosse CW, Case JW, Putnam PE, et al. Quantity and distribution of eosinophils in the gastrointestinal tract of children. Pediatr Dev Pathol 2006; 9:210–218.)
N/A, not applicable.

unmasked in these populations as prednisone doses are frequently decreased after initiation of these medications. However, the possibility that these medications may contribute to the development of CSS in a small subset of patients taking these medications cannot be completely ruled out.

Prednisone, azathioprine, methotrexate, and intravenous immunoglobulin (IVIG) have all been utilized in the treatment of CSS. Interestingly, recently published data support a role for anti-IL-5 in the treatment of CSS. Emerging data also suggests a role for a novel anti-IL-5-receptor-α antibody in the treatment of CSS. Both of these new therapeutic options have been shown to decrease blood eosinophilia significantly in patients with the syndrome.

Eosinophilic renal disease

Interstitial nephritis is an inflammatory response that occurs within the interstitium of the kidney. The common presenting symptoms include fever, arthralgias, rash, and renal failure. Eosinophilia and eosinophiluria are associated with the development of interstitial nephritis –although there is considerable debate over how frequently these findings are present. It has been demonstrated, however, that the presence of eosinophiluria has a specificity of greater than 80%. Eosinophils present on renal biopsy are also suggestive of the condition. The specific role eosinophils play in the pathogenesis of interstitial nephritis is poorly understood.

Medications are the common cause of interstitial nephritis. Those most commonly associated with interstitial nephritis are NSAIDs. A number of penicillin and non-penicillin antibiotics have also been implicated in its development. Removal of the offending agent is helpful in most cases. The role of corticosteroids in the treatment of interstitial nephritis is controversial; however, reports of improvement following treatment with prednisone have been published.

Eosinophilic skin disease

Under healthy conditions, eosinophils typically do not reside in the skin. However, eosinophils are present in a variety of dermatological disorders. These include common conditions such as atopic dermatitis and urticaria, as well as rare conditions such as bullous pemphigoid, episodic angioedema, and eosinophilic cellulitis (Wells syndrome).

Wells syndrome is an uncommon disorder that clinically mimics cellulitis. Diagnosis is made by skin biopsy, which demonstrates the presence of flame figures and a significant eosinophilic infiltrate. Importantly, there is no evidence of vasculitis on biopsy of patients with Wells syndrome. Currently, the aetiology of the syndrome is unclear. Although patients may have several episodes during their lifetime, treatment of acute episodes with low doses of steroids is helpful and the prognosis is generally favourable. However, the physician should be aware that there are reports of Wells syndrome in association with myeloproliferative states.

Immunodeficiency

In rare instances, peripheral eosinophilia can be an ominous harbinger for the presence of immunodeficiency. Omenn syndrome is a rare form of autosomal recessive severe combined immunodeficiency (SCID) that is associated with the presence of profound peripheral eosinophilia and lymphocytosis. Additional presenting symptoms include an eczematous rash, lymphadenopathy, pneumonitis, and chronic diarrhoea. Omenn syndrome stems from mutations in the *RAG1* and *RAG2* genes. These mutations lead to altered VDJ recombination and impaired T- and B-cell maturation. As a result, children with Omenn syndrome have absent to very low levels of circulating T and B cells and subsequently they develop SCID. Due to decreased populations of T and B cells, children with this syndrome also typically have very low levels of immunoglobulin production. A component of immune dysregulation is also present in Omenn syndrome. Thus, these patients may also present with marked peripheral eosinophilia, which is probably due to decreased numbers of T-regulatory cells.

The evaluation of Omenn syndrome typically includes a CBC with differential and T- and B-cell phenotyping. These analyses will reveal the presence of peripheral eosinophilia in addition to reduced numbers of T and B cells. Total immunoglobulin, a CD 45RA/RO ratio, and genetic testing for mutations in *RAG1* and *RAG2* can also be helpful. Recently, genetic mutations in *ARTEMIS*, *IL-7Ralpha*, and *ADA* have been implicated in the development of an Omenn syndrome-like phenotype. Therefore, genetic testing for these mutations may also be useful.

Children with Omenn syndrome typically present with a severe eczema-like rash, failure to thrive, diarrhoea, and recurrent infections. Typically diagnosed in the first 6 months of life, Omenn syndrome can be fatal, and the definitive therapy for involves bone marrow transplantation. Prior to transplantation, the administration of IVIG can be beneficial in the treatment or prevention of infection. Patients should also be monitored vigilantly for signs of infection prior to transplantation.

In addition to Omenn syndrome, other primary immunodeficiencies may also present with eosinophilia. Patients with hyper-IgE syndrome and HIV may also present with elevated peripheral eosinophil levels. Therefore, these immunodeficiencies should be included in the differential diagnosis of patients with eosinophilia.

Parasitic infection

The most common cause of eosinophilia worldwide is parasitic infection. Despite the low occurrence of parasitic infections in developed countries, a thorough history should be gathered from patients with peripheral eosinophilia to uncover any risk factors for the development of parasitic infection.

Parasitic infections that lead to the development of eosinophilia are typically caused by helminthic parasites, but can also be caused by other parasites such as the protozoans *Dientomeba fragilis* and *Isopora belli* and the filarial parasite *Toxicara canis*. To detect these parasitic infections, stool analysis for ova and parasites should be included in the evaluation of patients with peripheral eosinophilia. Importantly, *Strongyloides* infection can become invasive and fatal in patients treated with prednisone. If parasitic infection is a consideration in the patient presenting with eosinophilia, care should be taken to rule out *Strongyloides* infection prior to the initiation of steroid therapy. If this is not possible, an empiric trial of itraconazole can be coadministered. In addition to evaluation of the presence of ova and parasites in stool, titres to many parasitic infections including *Strongyloides* can be measured. If not available locally, titres may be obtained through the Centers for Disease Control (CDC).

Summary of important messages

- A thorough history is required in the evaluation of patients with eosinophilia
- Patients with HES should be monitored closely for signs of end-organ damage or development of malignancy
- Drug reactions associated with eosinophilia typically improve with removal of the offending agent
- Patients with EGIDs can be treated with corticosteroids or dietary modification
- CSS is associated with profound eosinophilia and distinguished from other disorders by the presence of vasulitis
- It is critical to rule out infection with Strongyloides as disseminated infection can be fatal with systemic glucocorticoid therapy

Further reading

Cools J, DeAngelo DJ, Gotlib J, et al. A tyrosine kinase created by fusion of the PDGFRA and FIP1L1 genes as a therapeutic target of imatinib in idiopathic hypereosinophilic syndrome. N Engl J Med 2003; 348:1201–1214.

Eshki M, Allanore L, Musette P, et al. Twelve-year analysis of severe cases of drug reaction with eosinophilia and systemic symptoms: a cause of unpredictable multiorgan failure. Arch Dermatol 2009; 145:67–72.

Fletcher A. Eosinophiluria and acute interstitial nephritis. N Engl J Med 2008; 358:1760–1761.

Furuta GT, Liacouras CA, Collins MH, et al. Eosinophilic oesophagitis in children and adults: a systematic review and consensus recommendations for diagnosis and treatment. Gastroenterology 2007; 133:1342–1363.

Green RH, Brightling CE, McKenna S, et al. Asthma exacerbations and sputum eosinophil counts: a randomised controlled trial. Lancet 2002; 360:1715–1721.

Klion AD, Bochner BS, Gleich GJ, et al. The Hypereosinophilic Syndromes Working Group: Approaches to the treatment of hypereosinophilic syndromes: a workshop summary report. J Allergy Clin Immunol 2006; 117:1292–1302.

Konikoff MR, Noel RJ, Blanchard C, et al. A randomized, double-blind, placebo-controlled trial of fluticasone propionate for pediatric eosinophilic esophagitis. Gastroenterology. 2006; 131:1381–1391.

Ogbogu PU, Bochner BS, Butterfield JH, et al. Hypereosinophilic syndrome: a multicenter, retrospective analysis of clinical characteristics and response to therapy. J Allergy Clin Immunol 2009; 124:1319–1325.

Rosenwasser LJ, Rothenberg ME. IL-5 pathway inhibition in the treatment of asthma and Churg-Strauss syndrome. J Allergy Clin Immunol 2010; 125(6):1245–1246.

Weller PF. Eosinophilia in travelers. Med Clin North Am 1992; 76:1413–1432.

20

Systemic mastocytosis*

Dean D Metcalfe, Sarah Austin and Peter Valent

DEFINITION

Mastocytosis refers to a heterogeneous group of systemic disorders that follows the clonal expansion of mast cells, usually secondary to activating mutations in KIT, the receptor for stem cell factor.

Introduction

Mastocytosis is a disease characterized by the pathological accumulation of mast cells in one or more organ systems. In some cases, mastocytosis presents with episodes of mediator release that are associated with flushing or anaphylaxis. It is a disease that is known to affect all age groups. Its exact prevalence is not known. Mastocytosis is now considered to be a clonal disorder of the haematopoietic system. At the molecular level, recent studies have reinforced the role of activating mutations in *KIT* in the aetiology of mastocytosis. The diagnosis of systemic mastocytosis (SM) is challenging, especially in the absence of cutaneous involvement.

Mastocytosis is variable in respect to the organ systems involved, clinical presentation, symptoms, and association with other haematological diseases. This has dictated the need for a classification scheme to allow assessment of prognosis and therapy. Most patients with mastocytosis have an indolent form of disease (ISM) (Table 20.1; discussed below) and are managed symptomatically using treatments directed toward mast cell mediator-related symptoms. Such patients usually live a normal lifespan without major limitations. Aggressive mastocytosis, in contrast, may lead to disability or even death. Cases of mast cell disease diagnosed in childhood often resolve by adulthood, whereas adult onset mastocytosis usually persists. The diagnosis is now aided by new surrogate markers.

Disease mechanisms

Human mast cells arise from CD34+ pluripotent cells in the bone marrow. Committed mast cell precursors exit the bone marrow into the blood, migrate to the peripheral tissues and mature into mast cells under the influence of stem cell factor (SCF), in addition to cytokines including IL-4, IL-6, IL-9, and nerve growth factor (NGF). SCF is the ligand for KIT. KIT is a tyrosine kinase growth factor receptor (Fig. 20.1) that mediates intracellular signal transduction pathways that promote mast cell growth and maturation.

*This work was in part supported by the National Institute of Allergy and Infectious Diseases Division of Intramural Research, NIH.

DOI: 10.1016/B978-0-7234-3658-4.00005-6

Table 20.1 WHO mastocytosis variants

Variant term	Subvariants
Cutaneous mastocytosis (CM)	Urticaria pigmentosa (UP) = maculopapular CM (MPCM) Diffuse CM (DCM) Mastocytoma of skin
Indolent systemic mastocytosis (ISM)	Smouldering SM Isolated bone marrow mastocytosis
Systemic mastocytosis with an associated clonal haematological non-mast-cell-lineage disease (SM-AHNMD)	SM-AML SM-MDS SM-MPD SM-CMML SM-NHL
Aggressive systemic mastocytosis (ASM)	Lymphadenopathic variant
Mast cell leukaemia (MCL)	Aleukaemic MCL
Mast cell sarcoma	
Extracutaneous mastocytoma	

SM, systemic mastocytosis; AML, acute myeloid leukaemia; MDS, myelodysplastic syndrome; MPD, myeloproliferative disease; CMML, chronic myelomonocytic leukaemia; NHL, non-Hodgkin lymphoma.

Tyrosine kinase domain mutations of *KIT* are detected in mastocytosis, and are believed to contribute to the abnormal growth of mast cells observed in this disease. The D816V *KIT* mutation is the most common mutation found in neoplastic mast cells (Box 20.1). The hypothesis that additional genetic events might be involved in the pathogenesis of mastocytosis is supported by the fact that *KIT* D816V mutations occur in a wide clinical spectrum of mast cell disease.

The increased mast cell burden in patients with mastocytosis is accompanied by an overall increase in the synthesis and release of mast cell mediators, which contributes to the signs and symptoms associated with mastocytosis (Table 20.2). Note, however, that IgE-mediated allergy is not increased in patients with mastocytosis, despite the well-known role for mast cells in allergic disease.

Clinical presentation

General clinical presentation

Two-thirds of all cases of mastocytosis present in childhood with a second peak of onset in the late third to early fourth decade. Although there are more than 50 cases of familial cutaneous mastocytosis reported, most patients report no family history of mastocytosis. The disease occurs in both males and females with roughly equal frequency.

Clinical symptoms follow patterns of organ system involvement, which include the skin, GI tract, lymph nodes, liver, spleen, and bone marrow. The respiratory, reproductive and endocrine systems are not usually involved.

Episodes of flushing and/or life-threatening episodic hypotension may occur. Hypotension can occur spontaneously without an associated trigger, or on a patient-specific basis may be related to ingestion of alcohol, insect stings or bites, certain medications, or contrast materials (Table 20.3). Fatigue, usually mild, is a frequent symptom. Weight loss, fever, and sweats may occur in patients with long-standing mastocytosis, but also may be the presenting symptoms for aggressive disease or mastocytosis with an associated haematological disorder. Headache is a frequent complaint. Chronic symptoms include decreased attention span, forgetfulness, irritability, and depression.

Cytopenias including anaemia, thrombocytopenia, and neutropenia are common in aggressive forms of SM. Neutrophilia, monocytosis, and eosinophilia are also observed in these patients. Central and peripheral lymphadenopathy may occur in aggressive forms, or during long-standing ISM with marked disease burden (smouldering SM, SSM).

Abdominal pain is the most common GI symptom, followed by diarrhoea, nausea, and vomiting. The pathogenesis of abdominal symptoms appears to be multifactorial. Most patients with dyspeptic types of abdominal pain have evidence of gastric acid hypersecretion. Some

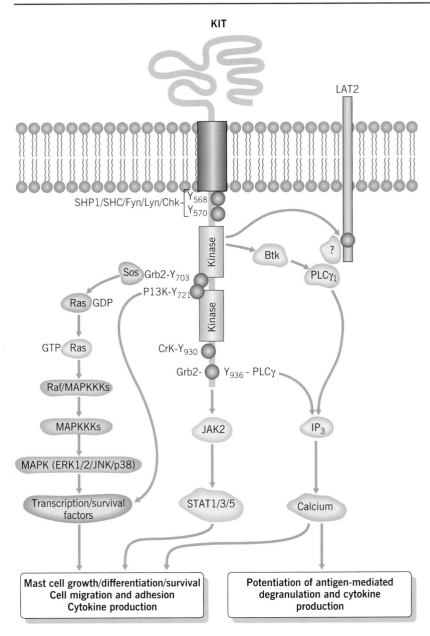

Fig. 20.1 KIT molecule. KIT is a tyrosine kinase growth factor receptor and contains extracellular, transmembrane, and intracellular portions. The intracellular section contains a kinase enzymatic domain. The region between the tyrosine kinase domain and the transmembrane portion is called the juxtamembrane domain and it regulates the enzymatic activity of the tyrosine kinase domain. The extracellular portion of the molecule has five immunoglobulin-like domains. The first two of these domains are involved in binding of KIT to its ligand, SCF. Binding of ligand (homodimer) causes dimerization of two KIT receptors through the immunoglobulin-like domain 4, which in turn activates the intrinsic tyrosine kinase enzymatic activity of the intracellular portion and results in autophosphorylation of the receptor. Phosphorylated receptor then becomes a docking site for downstream signal transduction and regulatory and adaptor proteins.

Box 20.1 Mutations in *KIT* associated with mastocytosis

- *KIT* D816V: all variants; >80% of SM variants
- *KIT* D816Y: SM, SM-AHMD; <5%
- *KIT* F522K: SM; <5%
- FIP1L1/PDGFRA: SM-HES, SM with eosinophilia; <5%
- PRKG2-PDGFRB: SM with basophilia; rare
- GIST* with UP/SM: all variants <1%

*GIST, gastrointestinal stromal tumours.

evidence of malabsorption is found in a minority of patients. Such malabsorption is usually not severe and is manifested primarily as mild steatorrhoea with impaired absorption of *d*-xylose or vitamin B12.

Mild hepatomegaly is often seen in patients with long-standing SM with high mast cell burden, and may be accompanied by normal or mildly elevated levels of liver enzymes. Aggressive forms of mastocytosis are associated with liver fibrosis, cirrhosis, ascites, and portal hypertension. Splenomegaly is reported in systemic disease and is more pronounced in those with high mast cell burden or aggressive mastocytosis.

Musculoskeletal pain is frequently reported. Bone pathology in patients with mastocytosis ranges from

Table 20.2 Major human mast-cell-derived mediators*

Class	Mediators	Physiological effects
Preformed mediators	Histamine, heparin, neutral proteases (tryptase and chymase, carboxypeptidase, cathepsin G), major basic protein, acid hydrolases, peroxidase, phospholipases	Vasodilation; vasoconstriction; angiogenesis; mitogenesis; pain; inflammation; tissue damage and repair; protein processing/degradation; lipid/proteoglycan hydrolysis; arachidonic acid generation
Lipid mediators	LTB_4, LTC_4, PGE_2, PGD_2, PAF	Leukocyte chemotaxis; vasoconstriction; vasodilation; bronchoconstriction; platelet activation
Cytokines	TNF-α, TGF-β, IFN-α, IFN-β, IL-1α, IL-1β, IL-5, IL-6, IL-13, IL-16, IL-18	Inflammation; leukocyte migration/proliferation
Chemokines	IL-8 (CXCL8), I-309 (CCL1), MCP-1 (CCL2), MIP-1αS (CCL3), MIP1β (CCL4), MCP-3 (CCL7), RANTES (CCL5), eotaxin (CCL11), MCAF (MCP-1)	Tissue infiltration by inflammatory cells
Growth factors	SCF, M-CSF, GM-CSF, bFGF, VEGF, NGF, PDGF	Cell proliferation; vasodilatation; angiogenesis

*Examples only. Also, many mediators are identified in human mast cell lines or primary cultures of human mast cells and may not be produced in human tissue mast cells in vivo.

Table 20.3 Examples of triggers of episodes of mediator release*

Triggers	Examples	Comments
Medications	NSAIDS, thiamine, alcohol, narcotics, radiographic dyes, some drugs used in general anaesthesia (induction anaesthetics and muscle relaxants)	NSAIDS may induce mast cell degranulation in some patients and have proved to be effective therapy in others. If radiographic studies are necessary, premedicate patients with H_1 and H_2 antihistamines and glucocorticoids as indicated
Venoms	Insect, snake	Stinging insect venom immunotherapy may be considered with caution
Polymers	Dextran, gelatin	
Physical stimuli	Heat, cold, friction, sunlight	
Emotional factors	Stress, anxiety	
Allergens**	Foods, inhalants	Identifiable allergens should be avoided

*Inciting factors differ from patient to patient. Sensitivities should be listed on a medical alert device or card.
**Applicable to patients with allergies.

osteoporosis to osteosclerosis. Vertebral compression fractures may occasionally be the first presentation of mastocytosis. In patients with aggressive mastocytosis, osteolyses may be observed.

Classification of mastocytosis

The classification of variants of mastocytosis is shown in Table 20.1. Mast cell disease confined to the skin is termed 'cutaneous mastocytosis' (CM). There are three CM subvariants. The most common variant by far is 'maculopapular CM' [MPCM or 'urticaria pigmentosa' (UP)] (Figs 20.2 and 20.3). 'Diffuse cutaneous

mastocytosis' (DCM) is unusual and presents in childhood, as does solitary mastocytoma of skin. 'Telangiectasia macularis eruptiva perstans' (TMEP) is a very rare form of CM and described to occur mainly in adults.

Systemic disease is characterized by variable multiorgan involvement, including the bone marrow, skeletal system, spleen, liver, lymph nodes, and gastrointestinal tract.

The most frequent form of systemic mastocytosis is indolent systemic mastocytosis, which tends to follow a benign course. The term 'smouldering mastocytosis' has been used to define patients with extensive systemic disease, but no evidence of aggressive mastocytosis or

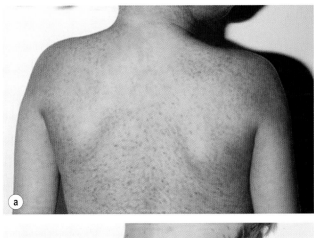

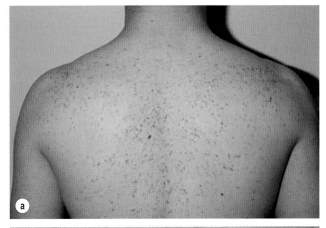

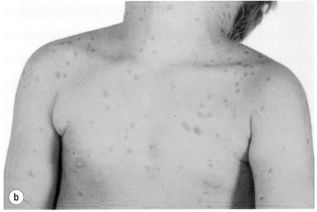

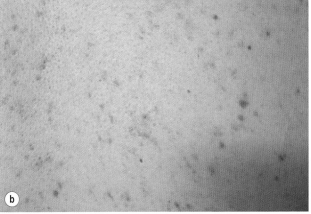

Fig. 20.2 Urticaria pigmentosa lesions in children with cutaneous mastocytosis. (a) Typical urticaria pigmentosa lesions. (b) Urticaria pigmentosa in a child, but somewhat larger and more variable in size.

Fig. 20.3 Urticaria pigmentosa lesions in an adult. (a) Typical urticaria pigmentosa lesions. (b) Close-up of lesions.

associated non-mast cell clonal disease. SM with an associated haematological non-mast-cell-lineage disease (SM-AHNMD), aggressive systemic mastocytosis (ASM), and mast cell leukaemia (MCL) all have a more guarded prognosis.

Diagnosis

The diagnosis of SM is established on the basis of specific criteria determined following a thorough evaluation. The work-up should include a bone marrow biopsy with immunohistochemistry [CD34, tryptase (Fig. 20.4), CD25, CD30], examination of bone marrow smears (percentage and morphology of mast cells) (Fig. 20.5), mutation analysis of *KIT*, flow cytometry of bone marrow cells if the methodology is available, cytogenetics of bone marrow cells, blood count, and serum chemistry including serum tryptase levels. This requires consultation with a haematologist. Extent of disease is determined by an ultrasound of the liver, spleen, and lymph nodes, osteodensitometry, X-ray of bones in cases of suspected focal

osteopathy, and a GI-tract evaluation in consultation with a gastroenterologist when GI-tract involvement is suspected.

Depending on the variant of SM, a number of other diagnoses have to be considered (Table 20.4). This is of particular importance when skin lesions are absent. SM can coexist with other diagnoses, which may complicate disease management. One example is allergy, which may become more severe as the mast cell burden increases. Another example is osteoporosis, which is often difficult to manage when SM is also present. Low-grade SM may also be confused with gastrointestinal, endocrinological, neurological, and even psychiatric disorders, especially when skin lesions are absent. High-grade SM variants, where skin lesions are often absent, may be confused with other bone marrow neoplasms such as myeloproliferative neoplasm, myeloid leukaemia, or myelodysplastic syndrome. Again, SM may coexist with such disorders, in which case the condition is termed 'SM-AHNMD'. Other patients with high-grade SM may be confused with a lymphoma, a solid tumour with metastasis, with multiple myeloma, with a primary liver disease, or with a primary GI tract disease.

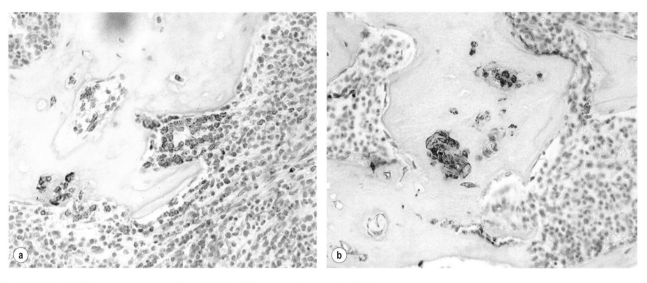

Fig. 20.4 (a, b) Bone marrow sections obtained from a patient with ASM; tryptase immunohistochemistry.

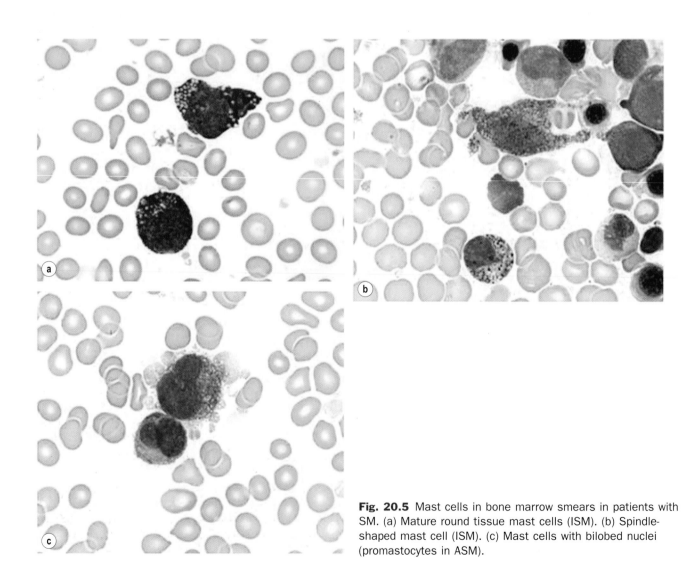

Fig. 20.5 Mast cells in bone marrow smears in patients with SM. (a) Mature round tissue mast cells (ISM). (b) Spindle-shaped mast cell (ISM). (c) Mast cells with bilobed nuclei (promastocytes in ASM).

Table 20.4 Differential diagnoses in low-grade (indolent) SM and high-grade SM

Diagnosis	Major differential diagnosis	Trigger(s) and key findings
Low grade		
Isolated bone marrow mastocytosis (BMM)	Insect venom allergy Idiopathic osteoporosis Mast cell hyperplasia MDS (or SM-MDS)	Specific IgE T score Reactive condition Dysplasia, CFU
Indolent systemic mastocytosis (ISM)	Cutaneous mastocytosis SM-AHNMD	BM infiltrates WHO criteria
Smouldering systemic mastocytosis (SSM)	ISM, SM-AHNMD, MPN Malignant lymphoma*	WHO criteria LN histology
High grade		
Aggressive systemic mastocytosis (ASM)	MCL, SM-AHNMD, SSM Malignant lymphomas* Tumor metastasis, primary liver or GI-tract disease	WHO criteria LN histology Histology Histology
Mast cell leukaemia (MCL)	ASM, SM-AHNMD, AML Tumor metastasis, primary liver or GI-tract disease	WHO criteria Histology Histology
SM with AHNMD (SM-AHNMD)		
SM-MPN, SM-CMML	MPN, CMML, AML	WHO criteria
SM-MDS and SM-AML	MDS, AML, CMML	WHO criteria
SM-CEL and SM-HES	CEL, MPN-eo, HES, NHL, ALL	WHO criteria
SM-NHL, SM-myeloma	NHL, myeloma, MGUS	WHO criteria

*In cases of lymphadenopathic mastocytosis, the differential diagnosis of a (coexisting) malignant lymphoma or Morbus Hodgkin must be considered. Here, it is of importance to be aware of the fact that neoplastic mast cells in these patients frequently express CD30.

SM, systemic mastocytosis; WHO, World Health Organization; AHNMD, associated clonal haematological non-mast-cell-lineage disorder; MPN, myeloproliferative neoplasm; CMML, chronic myelomonocytic leukaemia; AML, acute myeloid leukaemia; CEL, chronic eosinophilic leukaemia; HES, idiopathic hypereosinophilic syndrome; NHL, non-Hodgkin lymphoma; MGUS, monoclonal gammopathy of uncertain clinical significance; CFU, colony-forming units.

A number of investigations and tests are required before a final diagnosis can be established in a patient with suspected SM. Usually these investigations are performed in a stepwise fashion and in concert with a haematologist. The most important preinvasive screening assay is the serum tryptase test. In patients with elevated tryptase or other signs of SM, SM criteria are documented by appropriate investigations of the bone marrow and blood. Then, the subvariant of SM is determined by applying WHO criteria and by asking for the presence of findings indicative of an AHNMD. It is important to note that the diagnosis SM-AHNMD is a prefinal diagnosis. In these patients both the SM component and the AHNMD component of the disease have to be examined in detail to define the exact subvariant (e.g. ISM-CEL) by using WHO criteria. Following this, the patient is examined by defining the organ systems involved. In suspected ASM/MCL, it is important to define whether organ systems are (or are not) involved with mast cell infiltration, and whether mast cell infiltration leads to organ dysfunction or even loss of organ function. Finally, the patient is examined for the presence of relevant comorbidities, such as a coexisting allergy.

The final diagnosis in a patient with mast cell disease should include the subvariant of SM, and the subvariant of AHNMD if present. In addition, the final diagnosis should report on the presence or absence of severe mediator-related symptoms. In patients with ASM it may be preferable to report on the percentage of mast cells in bone marrow smears together with the final diagnosis. This is of importance as those with low mast cell counts (<5%) have a better prognosis compared with patients with a high mast cell count (5–19% – often progressing to MCL within short time). An increase of mast cells in bone marrow smears to greater than 20% is indicative of transformation to MCL.

The final report should also include *KIT* mutation results. Here it is important to say whether or not the *KIT* D816V mutant is detectable and, if not, whether and what other type of mutation in *KIT* was found.

Management

The natural history of disease varies with age and variant of disease. In children, CM tends to resolve with time, whereas systemic disease persists into adulthood. In adults, ISM tends to remain relatively stable or evolve slowly. Transformation from ISM into more aggressive forms of disease is unusual. Aggressive forms of disease such as SM-AHNMD often progress and may require interventional therapy directed at decreasing the mast cell burden and treating the associated haematological disease.

Goals of management

Treatment of those with mastocytosis begins with symptom management with antimediator therapy and avoidance of triggers known to exacerbate symptoms (Table 20.3 and Table 20.5). For those with skin disease, management includes good skin care, with preservation of moisture within the skin. There is no therapy currently available that is effective at selectively reducing the mast cell compartment. Cytoreductive therapies are reserved for the treatment of those with aggressive SM (ASM), MCL, and mastocytosis with an associated haematological disorder.

Patient education

It is crucial that patients with any of the variants of mastocytosis understand the need for a thorough evaluation and that treatment and prognosis depend upon the findings of such an evaluation. Referral to a centre with expertise in managing the more rare forms of disease may also be desirable. Patients must be educated on disease symptoms, complications, and management. Parents of children with cutaneous disease may be reassured by understanding the natural history of CM is for improvement.

Management plan

After having defined the final diagnosis and (sub)variant of SM and all risk factors, a management plan needs to be established. With regard to mediator-related symptoms and anaphylaxis, it is of importance to advise patients and treating physicians that all potential triggering factors and conditions have to be strictly avoided (see Table 20.3). In case a specific IgE and thus allergy is detectable in a symptomatic (or high-risk) patient, specific immunotherapy should be considered. In all non-symptomatic and all symptomatic patients, (prophylactic) histamine receptor antagonists are prescribed (see Table 20.5). In most patients, symptoms can be well controlled using such drugs. If this is not the case, additional antimediator-type drugs such as glucocorticosteroids have to be considered. It is not standard to treat patients with mediator-related symptoms with cytoreductive agents or (KIT) targeted drugs. However, in patients with high-grade SM with a high burden of mast cells and coexisting allergy, it may be preferable to initiate cytoreductive drugs early before progression is seen because of the high risk of life-threatening anaphylactic reactions. Such a decision requires consultation with a haematologist.

In patients with advanced disease (aggressive SM or MCL), cytoreductive drugs, interferon-α, or chemotherapy-agents are usually prescribed. In those with smouldering SM or slowly progressing ASM, 2CdA (cladribine) may produce long-lasting responses. In rapidly progressing ASM and MCL, however, the available cytotoxic drugs are usually without a long-lasting response. The same holds true for various KIT-targeting drugs such as imatinib, midostaurin, or dasatinib. The difficulty with imatinib is that the KIT D816V mutant that is expressed in most patients with SM confers resistance to this drug. Theoretically, resistance can be overcome with midostaurin. However, in advanced disease, KIT-independent oncogenic molecules and related (more malignant) subclones often become predominant (subclone selection).

In rapidly progressing ASM and MCL, polychemotherapy is usually administered and, in those who show a measurable (good) response, stem cell transplantation should be considered if the patient is eligible, young, and fit, and a donor is available. However, stem cell transplantation may not be a curative manoeuvre in all patients, and the mortality rate is substantial. In conclusion, no satisfactory therapy exists for patients with high-grade mastocytosis.

Treatment of emergencies

Mastocytosis can be associated with medical emergencies that represent a challenge for patients, relatives, and the treating physicians. One important emergency is spontaneous hypotension associated with an episode of mediator release (anaphylactic shock), which is managed in the same way as anaphylaxis in allergic patients without mastocytosis. It is sometimes of interest to determine the serum tryptase level during the event and after all symptoms have resolved in these patients in order to verify that mast cell mediator release was the basis of the episode.

Another emergency is gastrointestinal bleeding in a patient with advanced mastocytosis. Especially in patients with ASM and MCL, in whom thrombocytopenia and a coagulopathy develop, life-threatening bleeds may occur. Local mast cell infiltrates in the GI tract may aggravate the situation. In these patients, it is important to stop

Table 20.5 Management of the symptoms associated with mastocytosis

System	Symptom	Management
Skin	Cutaneous mastocytosis	• H_1 and H_2 antihistamines • Consider topical corticosteroids • Consider PUVA for refractory symptoms
Cardiovascular	Hypotension/anaphylaxis	• Intramuscular adrenaline* • For attempted prophylaxis in patients with frequent life-threatening episodes, consider scheduled H_1 and H_2 antihistamines +/− glucocorticoids
Gastrointestinal	Abdominal cramping	• H_2 antihistamines • +/− leukotriene antagonists
	Peptic ulcer disease	• H_2 antihistamines
	GERD	• +/− proton pump inhibitor
	Diarrhoea	• H_2 blocker +/− proton pump inhibitor • +/− leukotriene antagonist • +/− anticholinergics
	Malabsorption	• Cromolyn sodium • Consider glucocorticoids
	Ascites	• Glucocorticoids • Consider protocaval shunt • Consider cladribine or interferon-α
Musculoskeletal	Osteopenia	• Calcium and vitamin D supplementation
	Osteoporosis	• Bisphosphonates (when T score <2) • Consider cladribine or interferon-α in severe osteoporosis
	Bone pain	• NSAIDS or opioids if tolerated • Radiation therapy for severe localized bone pain

*Adrenaline is called epinephrine in the USA. PUVA, psoralen ultraviolet A; GERD, gastroesophageal reflux disease.

bleeding as soon as possible by administering platelet concentrates, coaguloactive medication, heparin antagonists, high doses of histamine receptor antagonists, and proton pump inhibitors, depending on the clinical situation.

A third emergency event to be mentioned is imminent vertebral fracture caused by severe osteoporosis. Here, the most important therapeutic intervention is to introduce early prophylaxis using bisphosphonates based on bone density studies.

Assessment of effectiveness of disease control

It is important to control disease activity in patients with SM. In those with ISM, all disease-relevant parameters, including blood counts, serum tryptase levels, and osteodensitometry, should be followed. It may also be necessary to control disease parameters and clinical symptoms within closer time intervals. In patients with stable SSM, disease parameters are checked every 6–12 months. In patients with ASM and MCL, frequent follow-up visits are required, their frequency depending on the clinical course, therapy, and overall situation. In these patients, the most important follow-up parameter is the serum tryptase level. Similarly, serum tryptase levels are important to document that the disease remains stable (haematologically) in patients with ISM (stable low baseline levels) and SSM (high but still stable tryptase levels). In SSM, high tryptase levels (up to 1000 ng/mL) may remain in a constant stable range over decades without any therapy. Other important follow-up parameters that can be employed as markers of disease control are blood counts, serum chemistry, the T-score, and ultrasound of the spleen.

Conclusions

Mastocytosis is characterized by the abnormal growth and accumulation of mast cells in one or more organ systems and may vary significantly in clinical presentation and severity. The disease affects both males and females in all age groups, and in most cases is not inherited. The heterogeneity of the disease patterns in mastocytosis strongly suggests that more than one biological lesion may occur in the developmental sequence that leads to placement of mast cells in tissues. In most instances, mastocytosis is now considered to be a clonal disorder of the haematopoietic system, and in the majority of cases follows a benign course. The diagnosis of systemic mastocytosis is challenging, especially in the absence of cutaneous involvement and/or the presence of an AHNMD.

Manifestations of the disease are provoked in part by the resultant increase in mast-cell-derived mediators, which lead to a variety of local and systemic effects. Mastocytosis is variable in respect to the organ systems involved, clinical presentation, symptoms, and association with other haematological diseases. Therapy of indolent mastocytosis is mainly symptomatic and palliative. At the molecular level, recent studies have reinforced the role of activating mutations in *KIT* in the aetiology of mastocytosis. These findings provide a conceptual basis for the development of new therapeutic strategies.

Summary of important messages

- Mastocytosis is a clonal disorder of mast cells and thus its diagnosis should follow strict diagnostic criteria. A serum tryptase level alone cannot be used to exclude or make a diagnosis of systemic disease
- Episodes of mast cell mediator release leading to flushing and even anaphylaxis may occur. However, some patients are relatively asymptomatic
- The treatment of mastocytosis is largely symptomatic. Only aggressive forms of disease are treated with cytoreductive agents including tyrosine kinase inhibitors
- Cutaneous mastocytosis in children may resolve with time. In adults, cutaneous disease usually persists and is accompanied by systemic disease
- The management of patients with mastocytosis with documented bone marrow involvement should be performed in concert with a haematologist
- The care of a patient with mastocytosis must include instruction on the consequences of the disease and careful follow-up

Further reading

Bodemer C, Hermine O, Palmérini F, et al. Pediatric mastocytosis is a clonal disease associated with D816V and other activating c-KIT mutations. J Invest Dermatol 2010; 130:804–815.

Brockow K, Jofer C, Behrendt H, et al. Anaphylaxis in patients with mastocytosis: a study on history, clinical features and risk factors in 120 patients. Allergy 2008; 63(2):226–232.

González de Olano D, Alvarez-Twose I, Esteban-López MI, et al. Safety and effectiveness of immunotherapy in patients with indolent systemic mastocytosis presenting with Hymenoptera venom anaphylaxis. J Allergy Clin Immunol 2008; 121:519–526.

Horny HP, Metcalfe DD, Bennett JM, et al, eds. WHO classification of tumours of haematopoietic and lymphoid tissues. London: IARC; 2008:54–63.

Kluin-Nelemans HC, Oldhoff JM, Van Doormaal JJ, et al. Cladribine therapy for systemic mastocytosis. Blood 2003; 102:4270–4276.

Lim KH, Tefferi A, Lasho TL, et al. Systemic mastocytosis in 342 consecutive adults: survival studies and prognostic factors. Blood 2009; 113:5727–5736.

Ma Y, Zeng S, Metcalfe DD, et al. The c-KIT mutation causing human mastocytosis is resistant to STI571 and other KIT kinase inhibitors; kinases with enzymatic site mutations show different inhibitor sensitivity profiles than wild-type kinases and those with regulatory type mutations. Blood 2002; 99:1741–1744.

Metcalfe DD. Mast cells and mastocytosis. Blood 2008; 112:946–956.

Nagata H, Worobec AS, Oh CK, et al. Identification of a point mutation in the catalytic domain of the protooncogene c-kit in peripheral blood mononuclear cells of patients who have mastocytosis with an associated hematological disorder. Proc Natl Acad Sci (USA) 1995; 92:10560–10564.

Niedoszytko M, de Monchy J, van Doormaal JJ, et al. Mastocytosis and insect venom allergy: diagnosis, safety and efficacy of venom immunotherapy. Allergy 2009; 64:1237–1245.

Peavy RD, Metcalfe DD. Understanding the mechanisms of anaphylaxis. Curr Opin Allergy Clin Immunol 2008; 8(4):310–315.

Schwartz LB. Diagnostic value of tryptase in anaphylaxis and mastocytosis. Immunol Allergy Clin North Am 2006; 26(3):451–463.

Ustun C, Corless CL, Savage N, et al. Chemotherapy and dasatinib induce long-term hematologic and molecular remission in systemic mastocytosis with acute myeloid leukemia with KIT D816V. Leuk Res 2009; 33:735–741.

Valent P, Akin C, Escribano L, et al. Standards and standardization in mastocytosis: consensus statements on diagnostics, treatment recommendations and response criteria. Eur J Clin Invest 2007; 37(6):435–453.

Valent P, Sperr WR, Schwartz LB, et al. Classification of systemic mast cell disorders: delineation from immunologic diseases and non mast cell lineage hematopoietic neoplasms. J Allergy Clin Immunol 2004; 114:3–11.

Verstovsek S, Tefferi A, Cortes J, et al. Phase II study of dasatinib in Philadelphia chromosome-negative acute and chronic myeloid diseases, including systemic mastocytosis. Clin Cancer Res 2008; 14:3906–3915.

A

AAM Alternatively activated macrophages that arise from bone marrow precursors under the influence of IL-4 and/or IL-13.

Acute phase proteins Serum proteins whose levels increase during infection or inflammatory reactions.

Adhesion The sticking of migratory leukocytes to endothelial or structural cells by the interaction of complementary adhesion proteins.

Adhesion proteins Complementary cell surface molecules expressed on leukocytes, endothelial, and structural cells that allow leukocyte adherence.

Adjuvant A substance that non-specifically enhances the immune response to an antigen.

Agretope The portion of an antigen or antigen fragment that interacts with a MHC molecule.

AID Activation-induced cytidine deaminase; an enzyme important in immunoglobulin isotype switching in B cells

Airway obstruction reversibility Significant improvement of an airway obstruction detected by spirometry after inhaling a bronchodilator.

AKC (atopic keratoconjunctivitis) A severe scarring conjunctivitis occurring mainly in adults.

A-kinase (cAMP dPK) Cyclic-AMP-dependent protein kinase; a family of enzymes activated by cyclic AMP that catalyse intracellular phosphorylation reactions.

Allele Any one of a series of two or more different DNA sequence variations that occupy the same position (locus) on a chromosome.

Allergen A foreign protein or hapten that induces the formation of IgE antibodies and may precipitate an allergic response.

Allergenic Behaving like an allergen.

Allergy Initially embraced immunology, but now focused on the host tissue-damaging or irritation effects of immunological responses.

Anaphylactoid reaction An allergic-like reaction but one that does not involve IgE.

Anaphylatoxins Complement peptides C3a and C5a, which cause smooth muscle contraction, increased microvascular permeability, leukocyte migration and activation, and degranulation of some types of mast cells.

Anaphylaxis The consequences of a systemic allergic reaction.

Antibody An immunoglobulin molecule produced by the immune system in response to antigen that has the property of combining specifically with the antigen that induced its formation.

Antidromic reflex see Axon reflex.

Antigen A molecule that interacts with immunological receptors.

Antigen presentation The process by which certain cells in the body (antigen-presenting cells) express antigen on their cell surface in a form recognizable by lymphocytes.

Antigen processing The conversion of an antigen into a form in which it can be recognized by lymphocytes.

Antiserum Serum containing antibodies to a specific antigen.

APCs (antigen-presenting cells) A variety of mobile or tissue-fixed cells, usually of the monocyte/macrophage family, which present antigen to lymphocytes through MHC class II molecules.

Apoptosis Programmed cell death in which one cell engulfs another, usually senescent, cell in order to prevent liberation of its potentially toxic constituents.

Arachidonic acid A 20-carbon fatty acid liberated from membrane phospholipid that may be converted into prostaglandins of the 2 series and leukotrienes of the 4 series.

Aspergillus A fungal species found in indoor environments.

Atopic diseases Diseases associated with atopy (atopic dermatitis, allergic asthma, allergic rhinitis, food allergy).

Atopy The ability to produce IgE antibodies to common allergens;

demonstrable by specific IgE in serum or skin prick tests.

Autoallergen Allergenic protein derived specifically from the host per se.

Axon reflex Local propagation of a nerve reflex by retrograde or antidromic stimulation of nerve axons resulting in the release of neuropeptides.

B

B cell A type of lymphocyte that is associated with antibody production. *See also* T cell.

Basophil A member of the granulocytic group of cells found in blood that plays a role in type 1 allergic diseases by releasing a variety of mediators such as histamine. It stains purple with basic dyes and represents less that 0.5% of all white blood cells. *See also* Eosinophil and Neutrophil.

BHR (bronchial hyperresponsiveness) A heightened bronchoconstrictor response to a variety of stimuli.

Bradykinin A vasoactive nonapeptide that is probably the most important mediator generated by the kinin system.

C

C1–C9 The components of the complement classical and lytic pathways that are responsible for mediating inflammatory reactions, opsonization of particles, and lysis of cell membranes.

C domains The constant region domains of antibodies and T-cell receptors. These domains do not contribute to the antigen-binding site and show relatively little variability.

CALT (conjunctiva-associated lymphoid tissue) Lymphoid tissue associated with the conjunctival mucosa.

CD (cluster of differentiation) markers Surface molecules of cells, usually leukocytes and platelets, which are identified with monoclonal antibodies and may be used to distinguish cell populations.

© 2012 Elsevier Ltd
DOI: 10.1016/B978-0-7234-3658-4.00005-6

CD3+ cells T lymphocytes with pan-T-cell marker CD3 on their surface.

CD4+ cells T lymphocytes with CD4 surface marker, usually equitable with helper T cells.

CD8+ cells T lymphocytes with CD8 surface marker, usually equitable with suppressor T cells.

CD14 A cell surface protein that acts as a coreceptor, along with TLR-4 and MD2, for LPS.

CD23 The low-affinity receptor for IgE (FcεRII).

Cell line A collection of cells that divide continuously in culture. May be either monoclonal or polyclonal and may have been transformed naturally or be an artificial hybridization.

CGRP (calcitonin gene-related peptide) A common neuropeptide that is likely to be involved in the neurogenic spread of the skin flare response. CGRP causes vasodilatation and has pro-inflammatory actions, but does not induce histamine release.

Challenge Administration of an implicated allergen to an allergic subject, in order to provoke an allergic response.

Charcot–Leyden crystal Lysolecithin crystals found in sputum of asthmatic subjects.

Chemokine A cytokine/interleukin that is involved in the chemoattraction of cells to sites of inflammation.

Chemokinesis Increased random migratory activity of cells in response to a chemical stimulus.

Chemotaxis Increased directional migration of cells particularly in response to concentration gradients of certain chemotactic factors (chemotaxins).

Chymase A neutral protease of the mast cell granule found only in the MC_{TC} subpopulation of human mast cells.

Ciclosporin (cyclosporin) An immunosuppressive drug with an action primarily on CD4+ lymphocytes.

CLA (cutaneous lymphocyte antigen) Antigen on T-cells that localizes to the skin.

Class I/II/III MHC molecules Three major classes of molecule within the MHC. Class I molecules have one MHC-encoded peptide associated with β2-microglobulin. Class II molecules have two MHC-encoded peptides that are non-covalently associated, and class III molecules are other molecules including complement components.

Class switching The process by which an individual B cell can link new immunoglobulin heavy-chain C genes to its recombined V gene to produce a different class of antibody with the same specificity. This process is also reflected in the overall class switch seen during the maturation of an immune response.

Clone A family of cells or organisms having a genetically identical constitution.

CMI (cell-mediated immunity) A term used to refer to immune reactions that are mediated by cells, usually lymphocytes, rather than by antibody or other humoral factors.

Complement A group of serum proteins involved in the control of inflammation, the activation of phagocytes, and the lytic attack on cell membranes. The system can be activated by interaction with the immune system.

Conjugate A reagent that is formed by covalently coupling two molecules together such as fluorescein coupled to an immunoglobulin molecule.

Contact dermatitis Dermatitis caused by irritants or classical contact allergens. *See also* Hapten.

CPT (conjunctival provocation test) Allergic conjunctival inflammation induced by deliberate application of known dose of allergen to the eye surface.

CR1, CR2, CR3 Receptors for activated complement C3 fragments.

CSFs (colony-stimulating factors) A group of cytokines that control the differentiation of haemopoietic stem cells.

Cytokines A generic term for soluble molecules that mediate interactions between cells.

Cytophilic Having a propensity to bind to cells.

Cytostatic Having the ability to stop cell growth.

Cytotoxic Having the ability to kill cells.

D. Pt. (*Dermatophagoides pteronyssinus*) One of the common species of house dust mites.

DAG (diacylglycerol) A potent protein kinase C activator usually generated from the action of phospholipases on membrane phospholipids.

Degranulation Exocytosis of granular products from inflammatory cells, usually mast cells, basophils, eosinophils, and neutrophils.

Dendritic cells A set of antigen-presenting cells present in epithelial structures and in lymph nodes, spleen, and at low levels in blood, which are particularly active in presenting antigen and stimulating T cells.

Der p 1 The major allergen of dust mite *Dermatophagoides pteronyssinus*.

Desensitization (allergen immunotherapy) A protocol of repeated injections of allergen or modified allergen with the aim of reducing a patient's allergic responsiveness to that allergen.

Desetope The part of an MHC molecule that links to antigen or processed antigen.

Diapedesis The movement of a blood leukocyte through a blood vessel wall into the extravascular compartment.

Domain A region of a protein having a characteristic tertiary structure and/or function. Both immunoglobulins and MHC class I and class II molecules have domains.

DSB (double-strand break) Break in DNA introduced during somatic recombination at immunoglobulin and T-cell receptor loci.

DTH (delayed-type hypersensitivity) The delayed skin reactions associated with type IV hypersensitivity.

ECP (eosinophil chemotactic protein) Protein released following eosinophil degranulation.

Ectoparasites Parasites living outside the body.

EDN (eosinophil-derived neurotoxin) Toxin released following eosinophil degranulation.

Eicosanoids Group name of products derived from 20-carbon fatty acids that includes prostaglandins, leukotrienes, thromboxanes, and lipoxins.

ELAM-1 (endothelial leukocyte adhesion molecule-1; E-selectin) Molecule expressed on vascular endothelial cells, and involved in neutrophil recruitment.

ELISA (enzyme-linked immunosorbent assay) Technique used to quantitate small amounts of material by use of specific antibodies, usually monoclonal antibodies.

Endothelium Cells lining the blood vessels that contract to allow extravasation of plasma proteins and express endothelial adhesion proteins.

Endotoxin A name usually given to components of the outer membrane of Gram-negative bacteria such as LPS and lipooligosaccharides. They are potent immunomodulatory (PAMPs) molecules.

Eosinophil A member of the granulocytic group of cells found in blood that plays a role in type 1 allergic and helminthic diseases by secreting highly toxic granule-associated proteins. They stain red with acidic dyes and represent less that 6% of all white blood cells. *See also* Basophil and Neutrophil.

Epigenetics The study of changes in gene expression that occur without a change in the sequence of the DNA (e.g. DNA methylation and chromatin remodelling).

Epitope A single antigenic determinant. Functionally it is the portion of an antigen that combines with the antibody paratope.

EPO (eosinophil peroxidase) Enzyme released following eosinophil degranulation.

Fab (fragment antigent binding) The part of antibody molecule that contains the antigen-combining site, consisting of a light chain and part of the heavy chain.

Fc (fragment crystallizable) The portion of antibody that is responsible for binding to antibody receptors on cells and the C1q component of complement.

FcεRI A receptor with high affinity for IgE.

Fel d 1 The major allergen of the domestic cat *Felis domesticus*.

Filaggrin A filament-associated protein that binds to keratin fibres in epthelial cells. Mutations in its gene predispose to eczema.

Flare The red area of neurogenic origin, surrounding a skin wheal response to allergen, histamine, or like substance.

FPIES Food protein-induced enterocolitis syndrome.

G-CSF (granulocyte colony-stimulating factor) A cytokine involved in the proliferation and maturation of granulocytes.

Gene A defined DNA sequence that is transcribed to form an RNA product.

Genetic association A term used to describe the condition where particular gene associations are found with particular diseases.

Genome The total genetic material contained within the cell.

Genotype The genetic material inherited from parents; not all of it is necessarily expressed in the individual.

Giant cells Large multinucleated cells sometimes seen in granulomatous type IV hypersensitivity reactions and thought to result from the fusion of macrophages.

GM-CSF (granulocyte-macrophage colony-stimulating factor) A cytokine involved in the proliferation and maturation of granulocytes and macrophages.

GPC (giant papillary conjunctivitis) Distinctive-appearing conjunctivitis caused mainly by contact lens wear.

G-protein A guanosine triphosphate-dependent membrane–protein complex that transduces many receptor-dependent events.

Granulocytopoiesis Production of granulocytes in the bone marrow.

H₁, H₂, and H₃ receptors Subtypes of the histamine receptor family that transduce the action of histamine.

Haplotype A set of genetic determinants located on a single chromosome.

Hapten A small molecule that is incapable of inducing an immune response by itself but can, when bound to a protein carrier, act as an epitope (e.g. penicillin).

Heavy chain Larger molecules of the biheterodimer that comprises an immunoglobulin. Heavy chains are characteristic for each antibody class. Each heavy chain comprises a variable region domain at the N-terminus followed by several constant region domains, usually three or four. *See also* Light chain.

Helminths Parasitic worms living in intestines.

HETE (hydroxyeicosatetraenoic acids) Lipoxygenase products of arachidonic acid, often preceded by a number (e.g. 5- or 15-), which identifies individual chemical structures.

Histamine A major vasoactive amine released from mast cells and basophil granules.

Histocompatibility The ability to accept grafts between individuals.

HLA (human leukocyte antigens) The human major histocompatibility complex.

Humoral Pertaining to the extracellular fluids, including the serum and lymph.

Hybridoma Cell line created in vitro by fusing two different cell types, of which one is a tumour cell. Lymphocyte hybridomas are usually used for making monoclonal antibodies.

5-hydroxytryptamine (5-HT, serotonin) A vasoactive amine present in platelets and some mast cells.

Hyperreactivity A state of increased reactivity to a provoking stimulus (e.g. bronchial hyperreactivity in asthma). Specifically, a greater magnitude of response than normal to a given concentration of stimulus.

Hyperresponsiveness A state of increased responsiveness to a provoking stimulus (e.g. bronchial hyperresponsiveness in asthma). Specifically, the ability to respond, either in magnitude or in sensitivity, to a lower concentration of stimulus.

Hypersensitivity Term synonymous with allergy (by usage).

ICAM-1 intercellular adhesion molecule-1 Molecule expressed on endothelial and other cells that interacts with LFA-1 (CD11b/CD18) expressed on leukocytes.

381

Idiotype A single antigenic determinant on an antibody V region.

IFNs (interferons α, β, γ) Members of the cytokine family originally associated with resistance to viral infections. IFN-γ is now recognized as a pluripotent cytokine, and is particularly associated with cell-mediated immunity.

IgE (immunoglobulin E) Immunoglobulin that binds to Fc$_\epsilon$RI and is associated with allergy.

ILs (interleukins) Members of the cytokine family that were originally conceived as intercellular messengers between leukocytes, but are now perceived as having wider immunological and inflammatory effects.

Immune complex An aggregate of antibody and antigen that may induce a hypersensitivity response, often by stimulating the complement cascade.

Immunity The ability of a host to resist infection.

Immuno CAP A high-capacity solid phase fluorescent technique for measuring IgE.

Immunoblotting A technique of contact transference of proteins from SDS polyacrylamide gel to nitrocellulose so that they may be identified by antibodies.

Immunocytochemistry A technique used to identify cellular constituents by use of specific antibodies.

Immunofluorescence A technique used to identify particular antigens microscopically in tissues or on cells by the binding of a fluorescent antibody conjugate.

Immunogen A molecule that stimulates an immune response.

Immunogenicity The ability of protein/microbe to stimulate an immune response.

Immunotherapy Allergy treatment consisting of allergen administration to modulate the immune system reducing clinical symptoms.

Innate immunity A collection of non-specific and quick-acting defence mechanisms giving rise to protection against invading pathogens.

Integrin A family of cell-adhesion molecules most frequently found on leukocytes, consisting of a common β chain, but different α chains, and involved in leukocyte recruitment.

IPs (inositol phosphates) Intracellular messengers (e.g. inositol 1,4,5-triphosphate) involved in elevation of intracellular calcium from intracellular or extracellular stores.

ISAAC International Study for Asthma and Allergies in Childhood.

ISM (indolent systemic mastocytosis) A common variant of mastocytosis with a favourable prognosis.

Isoelectric focusing Separation of molecules on the basis of charge. Each molecule will migrate to the point in a pH gradient at which it has no net charge.

J chain A monomorphic polypeptide present in, and required for, the polymerization of secretory IgA and IgM.

Kinins A group of vasoactive peptides comprising bradykinin, kallidin (lysyl-bradykinin) and des-arg-bradykinin.

Langerhans' cells Antigen-presenting cells of the skin that emigrate to local lymph nodes to become dendritic cells; they are active in presenting antigen to T cells.

LFAs (leukocyte function antigens) A group of leukocyte adhesion proteins composed of CD11/CD18 heterodimers.

Ligand A linking or binding molecule usually used to define a specific antigenic determinant to which an antibody binds.

Light chains Smaller molecules of the biheterodimer that comprises an immunoglobulin. They may be of κ or λ subtypes, regardless of immunoglobulin class. Present only in the Fab end of the immunoglobulin and composed of both variable and constant regim domains. *See also* Heavy chain.

Lipid transfer proteins (LTP) A group of highly conserved heat-stable proteins of about 9 kDa found in many plants. LTPs may be responsible for cross-reactivity between aeroallergens and foods because they are present in birch pollen and many fruits, including peach, apple, pear, and cherry.

Lipocalins Group of low-molecular-weight lipid transporter proteins.

LPS (lipopolysaccharide) A potent immunomodulatory product of some Gram-negative bacterial outer membrane that can act as a B-cell mitogen.

LTs (leukotrienes) Members of the eicosanoid family, lipoxygenase products, usually of arachidonic acid, with potent myogenic, cardiovascular, and inflammatory effects.

Lymphokines A generic term for molecules other than antibodies that are involved in signalling between cells of the immune system and are produced by lymphocytes (cf. interleukins).

MALT (mucosa-associated lymphoid tissue) Generic term for lymphoid tissue associated with the gastrointestinal tract, bronchial tree, and other mucosae.

MBP (major basic protein) A basic arginine-rich protein making up the electron-dense core of the eosinophil granule, which may be released during eosinophil degranulation.

MC (mast cell) A cell of haematopoietic origin that resides in tissues and is involved in both innate and acquired immune responses.

M-CSF (macrophage colony-stimulating factor) A member of the cytokine family, involved in the proliferation and maturation of macrophages.

MC$_T$ and MC$_{CT}$ Mast cell subtypes defined by their granular content of tryptase (MC$_T$) and tryptase and chymase (MC$_{CT}$).

Mediator A chemical substance released by one cell that stimulates another (e.g. mast cell mediators).

Methacholine A synthetic choline ester that acts as a non-selective muscarinic receptor agonist in the parasympathetic nervous system.

MHC (major histocompatibility complex) A genetic region found in all mammals where products are primarily responsible for the rapid rejection of grafts between individuals, and function in signalling between lymphocytes and cells expressing antigen. *See also* HLA.

MHC class II The histocompatibility antigens expressed on cells of the monocyte/macrophage family that present antigen to the T-cell receptor on T lymphocytes.

MIF (migration inhibition factor) A group of peptides produced by lymphocytes that are capable of inhibiting macrophage migration.

Mitogen A substance that causes cells, particularly lymphocytes, to undergo cell division.

Monoclonal Derived from a single clone, e.g. monoclonal antibodies, which are produced by a single clone and are homogenous.

Muramic acid A component of peptidoglycan from the cell wall of all types of bacteria.

Myeloma A lymphoma produced from cells of the B-cell lineage that produces large qualities of one immunoglobulin.

Neuropeptide Peptides released from nerves following stimulation. The many neuropeptides now recognized include substance P, vasoactive intestinal polypeptide (VIP), neurotensin, and bombesin.

Neutrophil The most common member of the granulocytic group of cells found in blood that plays an important role in innate immunity. They stain blue with neutral stains and account for about 96% of all granulocytes and about 70% of all white blood cells. *See also* Basophil and Eosinophil.

NK (natural killer) cells A group of lymphocytes that have the intrinsic ability to recognize and destroy some virally infected cells and some tumour cells.

Nude mouse A genetically athymic mouse that also carries a closely linked gene producing a defect in hair production.

Oedema Tissue swelling due to extravasation of plasma proteins.

Omalizumab The humanized monoclonal anti-IgE antibody that 'mops up' circulating IgE but does not cause mast cell degranulation. It has been shown to have a number of anti-inflammatory and clinical benefits in patients with asthma, allergic rhinitis, and urticaria.

Opsonization A process by which phagocytosis is facilitated by the deposition of opsonins (e.g. antibody and C3b) on the antigen.

PAC (perennial allergic conjunctivitis) Non-seasonal mild to moderate allergic conjunctival inflammation.

PAF (platelet-activating factor) A lipid-derived product generated by many inflammatory cells that activates platelets and induces bronchial hyperresponsiveness.

PAMPs (pathogen-associated molecular patterns) Characteristic microbial-specific components (e.g. lipopolysaccharide from Gram-negative bacteria and peptidoglycan from Gram-positive bacteria) that stimulate innate and adaptive immune responses via interaction with Toll-like receptors.

Paratope The part of an antibody molecule that makes contact with the antigenic determinant (epitope).

Pathogen An organism that causes disease.

PCA (passive cutaneous anaphylaxis) The technique used to detect antigen-specific IgE, in which the test animal is injected intravenously with the antigen and dye, the skin having previously been sensitized with antibody.

PD 20 FEV₁ The dose of an inhaled substance that produces a 20% fall in lung function – forced expiratory volume in 1 second (FEV_1).

Pectin Cell wall constituents of plants. Complex homo- or heteropolymers of D-galacturonic acid.

PEF (peak expiratory flow) The maximum flow generated during expiration performed with maximal force and started after a full inspiration.

Penicillium A fungal species found in indoor environments.

Peptidoglycan A component from the cell wall of all types of bacteria.

PGs (prostaglandins) Members of the eicosanoid family cyclooxygenase products, usually of arachidonic acid, including PGA_2, PGD_2, PGE_2, and $PGF_{2\alpha}$.

Phagocytosis The process by that cells engulf material and enclose it within a vacuole (phagosome) in the cytoplasm.

Phagolysosome A phagosome containing proteolytic enzymes capable of degrading the ingested particles.

Phagosome An intracellular vacuole containing material ingested by phagocytosis.

Pharmacogenetics The study of genetic determinants of treatment response.

Phenotype The morphological characteristics of a cell or animal resulting from genetic expression.

Pinocytosis The process by which liquids or very small particles are taken into the cell.

PK reaction (Prausnitz–Küstner reaction) The passive transfer of allergic responsiveness to an unresponsive recipient by intradermal injection of serum from an allergic donor.

Plasma cell An antibody-producing B cell that has reached the end of its differentiation pathway.

PNIF (peak nasal inspiratory flow) The maximum nasal flow that can be achieved with a forced inspiratory manoeuvre.

Polyclonal A term that describes the products of a number of different cell types (cf. monoclonal).

Polymorphism A polymorphism is one of two or more alternate forms (alleles) of a chromosomal locus that differ in a nucleotide sequence.

Primary lymphoid tissues Lymphoid organs in which lymphocytes complete their initial maturation steps; they include the fetal liver, adult bone marrow and thymus, and the bursa of Fabricius in birds.

Primary response The immune response (cellular or humoral) following an initial encounter with a particular antigen. Synonymous with sensitization.

Profilins A group of proteins necessary for the structural development of plant and tree cells. All fruits contain profilins, which are frequently allergenic. Thus, fruit profilin allergy sufferers often react to many different fruits.

Promyelocyte A precursor cell of the myelocyte family.

Quality of Life (QoL) An assessment of the effect of a disease and its treatment on the general well-being of a patient.

QoL is assessed either by non-disease-specific questionnaires, such as the SF-36, or by disease-specific questionnaires, such as CUQ2oL for urticaria.

RANTES Regulated on activation, normal T-cell expressed and secreted.

RAST (radioallergosorbent test) A laboratory technique for the detection of circulating IgE with specific allergen determinants.

Receptor A specific protein or group of proteins, usually on the cell surface, capable of recognizing and binding a specific ligand.

Respiratory burst Increase in oxidative metabolism following stimulation of granulocytes, usually by phagocytosis.

RIA (radioimmunoassay) A technique for the laboratory assay of small amounts of materials by competition for antibody binding with known amounts of radioactive substance.

Rhinomanometry Measurement of the air flow and pressure within the nose during respiration.

Rosetting A technique for identifying or isolating cells by mixing them with particles or cells to which they bind (e.g. sheep erythrocytes to human T cells). The rosettes consist of a central cell surrounded by bound cells.

SAC (seasonal allergic conjunctivitis) Allergic conjunctivitis occurring in hay fever.

Safety data sheet A material safety data sheet is a form with data regarding the properties of a particular substance.

SATA-6 Signal transducer and activator of transcription 6.

SCF (stem cell factor) A cytokine released by stromal cells that interacts with the c-kit receptor on mast cells to stimulate cell maturation and activation.

SCIT Subcutaneous immunotherapy.

SDS-PAGE (sodium dodecyl sulphate polyacrylamide gel electrophoresis) A method of separating proteins by gel electrophoresis.

Secondary response The immune response that follows a second or subsequent encounter with a particular antigen.

Sensitization The stimulation of allergic antibody production, usually by an initial encounter with a specific allergenic substance. Synonymous with primary response.

Serotonin (5-hydroxytryptamine, 5-HT) A vasoactive amine present in platelets and some mast cells.

SIT Allergen-specific immunotherapy. *See also* Immunotherapy.

Skin prick test The detection of allergen to specific allergens through the production of a wheal-and-flare response by pricking the skin through droplets of allergen or injecting them intradermally.

SLE (systemic lupus erythematosus) An autoimmune disease of humans usually involving antinuclear antibodies.

SLIT (sublingual immunotherapy) Therapy where drops of allergen are placed under the tongue rather than being injected subcutaneously.

SM (systemic mastocytosis) A clonal disorder of mast cells.

SNP (single nucleotide polymorphism) DNA sequence variations involving substitution, insertion or deletion of a single base pair.

Stratum corneum Outer layer of the skin.

Substance P A common neuropeptide that is likely to be involved in the neurogenic spread of the skin flare response.

Superantigens Microbial products that non-specifically stimulate T-cell activation. They interact with the Vbeta domains of the T-cell receptor and MHC, and may stimulate up to 20% of all T cells.

TCR (T-cell receptor) The T-cell antigen receptor consisting of either a α/β dimer (TCR2) or a γ/δ dimer (TCR1) associated with the CD3 molecular complex.

T-dependent/T-independent antigens T-dependent antigens require immune recognition by both T and B cells to produce an immune response. T-independent antigens can directly stimulate B cells to produce specific antibody.

TGF-β (transforming growth factor β) A cytokine involved in the stimulation of fibroblasts for collagen synthesis.

Th cells (helper T cells) A functional subclass of T cells that can help to generate cytotoxic T cells or cooperate with B cells in production of an antibody response. Helper cells recognize antigen in association with class II MHC molecules.

Th1 cells A subdivision of Th cells involved in cell-mediated immunity and characterized by their production of IFN-γ, TNF-α, and IL-2.

Th2 cells A subdivision of Th cells involved in allergy by their influence on B cells to produce IgE and proinflammatory effects. Characterized by their production of IL-3, IL-4, and IL-5.

TLR (Toll-like receptor) An evolutionarily conserved family of cell surface or cytoplasmic pattern recognition proteins that interact with PAMPs and activate innate immune cell function. There are ten members in humans.

TNF (tumour necrosis factor) A multifunctional cytokine initially identified for its effects on tumour cells.

Tolerance A state of specific immunological unresponsiveness.

Treg T-regulatory cells responsible for controlling the intensity and duration of adaptive immune responses.

Tryptase The major neutral protease of the mast cell granule found in all human mast cells.

TXA₂ (thromboxane A₂) A member of the cyclooxygenase product family of eicosanoids from arachidonic acid. Synthesized by platelets and other cells, its many actions include platelet aggregation and bronchoconstriction.

V domains The variable N-terminal (Fab) domains of antibody heavy and light chains, and the α, β, γ, and δ regions of the T-cell receptor that are responsible for antigen recognition.

VCAM-1 (vascular cell adhesion molecule-1) An adhesion molecule expressed on vascular endothelial cells.

VKC (vernal keratoconjunctivis) A severe allergic conjunctivits in children.

VLA (very late antigen) A series of integrins expressed on the surface of leukocytes involved in cell recruitment, especially T cells and eosinophils.

Wheal An area of oedema produced at the site of intradermal introduction of allergen, histamine, or similar provocant.

Stimulation of axon reflexes in the wheal area gives rise to the larger flare response.

G

H

I